Vascular Malformations

Ajay K. Khanna • Satyendra K. Tiwary
Editors

Vascular Malformations

Springer

Editors
Ajay K. Khanna
Department of Surgery
Institute of Medical Science
Banaras Hindu University
Varanasi
India

Satyendra K. Tiwary
Department of Surgery
Institute of Medical Science
Banaras Hindu University
Varanasi
India

ISBN 978-981-15-9764-0 ISBN 978-981-15-9762-6 (eBook)
https://doi.org/10.1007/978-981-15-9762-6

This Springer imprint is published by the registered company Springer Nature Singapore Pte Ltd.
The registered company address is: 152 Beach Road, #21-01/04 Gateway East, Singapore 189721, Singapore

Preface

Vascular malformations are the abnormalities of blood vessels and lymphatics which have not been well understood. Vascular malformations are one of the classifications of vascular anomalies, the other grouping being vascular tumours. They may cause aesthetic problems as they grow and can continue to grow throughout life.

Vascular anomaly comprises a wide spectrum of lesions as an outcome of disorders in vascular development. They continue to be a challenge in both diagnosis and treatment and need individual and multispecialty treatment programme. The key for proper treatment of these lesions relies on correct diagnosis and classifying the vascular lesion. Vascular anomaly can be described by two abnormal vascular conditions: the congenital vascular malformation (CVM) and vascular tumour that represents neonatal or infantile haemangioma. Both conditions are different in their anatomical, histological and pathophysiological findings and also in their clinical courses, which emphasizes the importance of a precise understanding of these two conditions.

In my clinical practice of more than 40 years, I have seen a large variety of cases of varying type of vascular anomalies and I was really perplexed during their management. Some cases have been really challenging. The patients and their attendants ask for if they will be ever permanently cured of this disease and we doctors are at a loss for words. The majority of the patients will come to us repeatedly and have to be followed for many years. In fact in only less than half of the cases we can promise that this disease can be cured.

The author has vast experience in dealing with the vascular cases and has published his work in international prestigious vascular surgery journals such as *Annals of Vascular Surgery*, *International Angiology*, *Phlebology* and *Acta Phlebologica*. The author has also written books on vascular surgery such as *Manual of Vascular Surgery* by Jaypee, *Ulcers of the Lower Extremity* by Springer and *Varicose Veins Current Trends* by Springer. Hence, the author was approached again by Springer to write a book and they readily agreed to author's vision to compile new thoughts on vascular malformation. With this background we decided to accumulate and compile as much information as possible by inviting a galaxy of medical scientists who deal with these types of patients with the sole aim to provide better treatment and information to my patients regarding what is best for them.

This book has 22 chapters starting from its historical perspective, the epidemiology, the embryology of vascular malformations and the various classifications. Further a chapter is dedicated to how to approach a case of vascular malformation, and then there are individual types of malformations in a full chapter form like arterial malformations, venous malformations, capillary malformations, lymphatic malformations and combined vascular malformations. Further there is a chapter on how to investigate a case of vascular malformation. Then there are chapters on treatment modalities of vascular malformations such as medical treatment, surgical treatment, lasers, endovascular interventions, radiological interventions, sclerotherapy, etc. Then a chapter is dedicated to the complications associated with vascular malformations and also what is the quality of life in patients with vascular malformation.

This book has been designed to answer queries during management of vascular malformation cases by postgraduates, fellows in vascular surgery, general surgeons, paediatric surgeons, vascular surgeons, plastic surgeons, interventional radiologist, phlebologist, orthopaedicians and podiatrists.

I am indebted to my family Dr. Anuradha, Dr. Divya and Dr. Soumya who provided me all the moral support and will forgive me for any negligence which was unavoidable. I am really thankful to my coeditor Dr. Satyendra Tiwary who has been my right hand in bringing out the various publications with me.

We dedicate this book to our patients who have taught us the management of this very complex disease.

It is with our utmost desire that this book becomes a valuable source of understanding of this relatively uncommon and difficult to treat vascular disorder to those students as well as clinical practitioners who may have an interest in vascular anomalies.

Varanasi, India

Satyendra K. Tiwary
Ajay K. Khanna

Contents

About the Editors

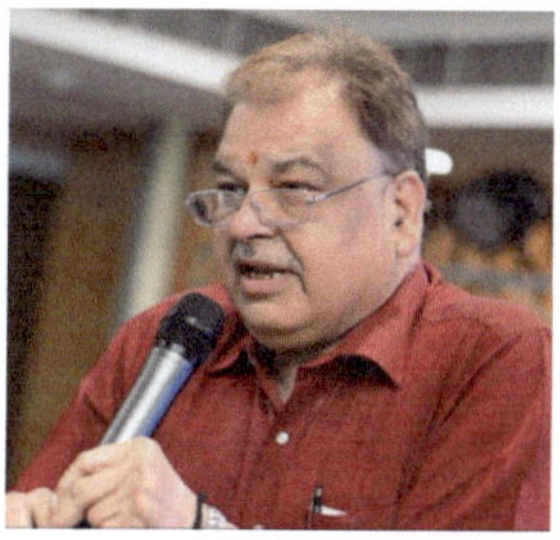

Ajay K. Khanna, MS, FRCS, FAMS, FACS, FICS, FACRSI, MNAMS, MBA, DSc, FRSTMH, FAIS, FUICC, FUWAI, FFIM, FMAS, PDCR, is Professor of Surgery and Ex Head of the Department of General Surgery at the Institute of Medical Sciences, Banaras Hindu University (BHU), Varanasi, India. Prof. Khanna has a teaching experience of more than 40 years and has been awarded with Young Outstanding Teacher and Eminent Surgical Teacher. He is the examiner for MBBS, MS, BDS, DNB and FNB in minimal access surgery and M.Ch in endocrine surgery. He has guided more than 50 theses for MS course. He is fellow/member of 33 societies. He regularly started vascular surgery in the Department of Surgery at BHU.

Prof. Khanna has delivered more than 100 CME lectures, more than 200 guest lectures in various national and international conference in India, UK, USA, Japan, Poland, Egypt, etc., and presented more than 300 presentations in various national and international conferences. He has more than 350 publications in various national and international journals and 60 chapters in various books to his credit. He is the editor of four books.

He served as President of Varanasi Surgical Society, President of Uttar Pradesh chapter of the Association of Surgeons of India (ASI), Governing Council Member of ASI, Vice President of ACRSI and Executive Member of UP chapter of ASI, AMASI, VAI, ATVSI and IASO. He has delivered more than 15 orations. He has received various fellowship awards, viz. Clinical Research Fellowship and Registrar at the Department of Surgery, University of Wales College of Medicine, Cardiff, Wales, UK;

Metrogyl Travelling Fellowship by Gastrointestinal Research Society; Commonwealth Scholarship; and Indo-Czechoslovakian Cultural Exchange Program, among others. Prof. Khanna's name appears in Asia's Who's Who reference book, Marquis Who's Who in the World, Five Hundred Leaders of Influence, International Directory of Distinguished Leadership, Man of the Year and American Biographical Institute, and he received several other awards. He is fellow of the Royal College of Surgeons of England, fellow of United Writers' Association, fellow of the Indian National Science Academy, fellow of the American College of Surgeons, fellow of the International College of Surgeons, fellow of the Association of Colorectal Society of India, fellow of the Royal Society of Tropical Medicine, fellow of the Association of Surgeons of India, fellow of Union Internationale Cancer controlle and fellow of Minimal Access Surgeons of India.

Prof. Khanna was the joint editor of *Indian Journal of Surgery*. He has organized more than 28 conferences and workshops. He was the Chief Inspector for quality assurance review of the Department of Clinical Surgical Sciences, the University of the West Indies, St Augustine Campus, Trinidad and Tobago, and is in the Expert Selection Committee of UPSC, Uttar Pradesh; BPKIMS, Dharan, Nepal; Aligarh Muslim University, Aligarh; KGMU Lucknow; Public Service Commission, J&K; MCI Inspector; DNB Inspector; IGIMS, Patna; PGIMER, Chandigarh; and the Indian Institute of Information Technology, Allahabad.

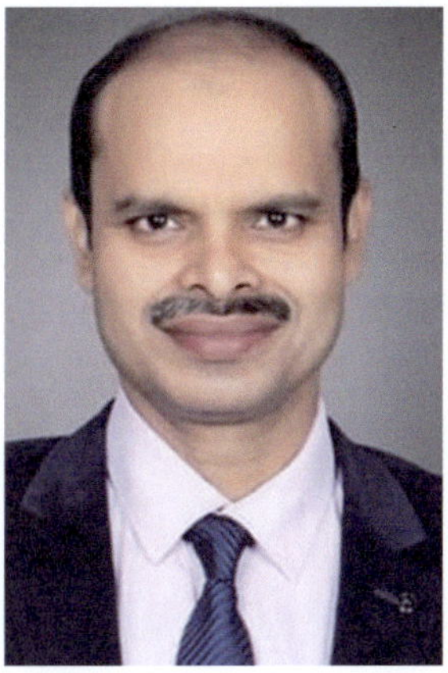

Satyendra K. Tiwary, MBBS (Hons), MS (Surgery), FMAS, FICS, FCLS is Professor of General Surgery at the Institute of Medical Sciences, Banaras Hindu University, Varanasi, India. He graduated and completed his postgraduation from Patna Medical College, Patna, India. Dr. Tiwary has 13 years of teaching experience. He has more than 100 publications in various national and international journals and has delivered numerous oral and poster presentations and invited lectures. He has edited a book *Ulcers of the Lower Extremity* published by Springer in 2016 and another book *COVID-19: Challenges Ahead* published by CBS in 2020 and has published few chapters in international books. He has a keen interest in academics and research with special interest in phlebology, vascular medicine, wound management and lower limb pathology.

Vascular Malformations: Historical Perspective

1

Bhumika Gupta and Arvind Kohli

Vascular anomalies encompass an extremely heterogeneous group of congenital abnormalities of the vascular system. These are a group of common and rare disorders of blood vessel growth leading to identifiable vascular lesions and their associated deformities.

These comprise a wide spectrum of lesions ranging from simple birthmarks to large, disfiguring tumors. Thought to be the result of errors in vessel morphogenesis, these lesions are composed of dysplastic vascular channels.

These vascular anomalies are divided into two groups: vascular tumors and vascular malformations. The vascular tumors are neoplasia of the vasculature. These are characterized by endothelial cell hyperproliferation and can be categorized as benign, locally aggressive/borderline, or malignant based on cellular behavior. These include infantile hemangiomas, rapidly involuting and non-involuting congenital hemangiomas, as well as more aggressive tumors, such as tufted angiomas, Kaposiform hemangioendotheliomas, and angiosarcomas.

The vascular malformations consist of errors in the morphogenesis. In contrast to the rapid growth and involution phases characteristic of vascular tumors, these malformations grow slowly. Usually present at birth and often inconspicuous in appearance, these become more evident with the growth of the child. These malformations can involve arteries, veins, capillaries, lymphatics, or a combination of vessel types. They can occur in any tissue in the body, commonly involving the skin, soft tissues, bones, joint spaces, or viscera. Many of these vascular malformations have been linked with genetic variants.

The nomenclature of vascular anomalies has been challenging and confusing due to the phenotypic variation and complexity. Vascular anomalies are frequently misdiagnosed due to the indiscriminate use of terms such as "angioma," "hemangioma," "hamartoma," and "endothelioma" further complicating classification, and increasing risk of improper management.

The first description of these vascular anomalies has been done by anatomist and obstetrician William Hunter in the mid-eighteenth century in the context of iatrogenic creation of arteriovenous fistulas by phlebotomists [1].

Based on autopsy material, Virchow in 1863 published the first-ever classification of vascular anomalies, defining "*angiomas*" as simple, cavernous, or racemose based on their histologic architecture [2], which he described as neoplasms. He distinguished two large groups: angioma cavernosum, in which there was an absence of parenchyma between the blood vessels; and angioma racemosum (hamartoma), in which vessels were separated by parenchyma.

B. Gupta (✉) · A. Kohli
Department of CTVS, Govt. Medical College, Jammu, India

A. K. Khanna, S. K. Tiwary (eds.), *Vascular Malformations*,
https://doi.org/10.1007/978-981-15-9762-6_1

Virchow Vascular Tumors

1. Angioma cavernosum (absence of parenchyma between the blood vessels).
2. Angioma racemosum (hamartoma—vessels separated by parenchyma)—telangiectasis (thin-walled vessels like capillaries)—angioma racemosum arteriale sive venosum (vascular walls suggest arteries or veins; blood may shortcut artery to vein: arteriovenous aneurysm).

Virchow considered that each one of these types could change into another by cellular proliferation or dilation of blood vessels.

In 1877, Wegener, a student of Virchow, on the basis of these studies, proposed a similar classification for the lymphatic alterations that were used until the end of the twentieth century: lymphangioma simplex, cavernosum, and cysticum.

It attributed the genesis of these lesions to lymphatic inflammation and dilation, and to endothelial malformation or proliferation.

The first clinical observation of a vascular malformation occurred in Germany in 1890 and is described by Berenbruch [3], who operated on a patient with a spinal abnormality. The lesion was not identified as a vascular malformation at surgery, but it was subsequently recognized as a vascular abnormality of the spine at autopsy.

In 1912, Charles Elsberg was the first to attempt to excise a spinal AVM. Elsberg's classification of spinal vascular lesions consisted of three categories: aneurysm, angioma, and dilation of veins. (Elsberg 1916).

Three Categories of Spinal Vascular Abnormalities

1. Aneurysm of spinal vessels.
2. Angioma in which a mass of dilated veins penetrates the spinal cord.
3. Dilation of posterior spinal veins ("hemorrhoids" of the spinal pia mater).

It was not until 1982, when Mulliken and Glowacki introduced a classification system depending upon the pathophysiology of these lesions [4, 5]. This system divided vascular anomalies into two categories: vascular tumors (hemangiomas) and vascular malformations (Table 1.1).

Table 1.1 Mulliken and Glowacki classification of vascular malformations

Simple vascular malformations	
Slow flow	
Capillary	
Lymphatic	
Venous	
Fast flow	
Arterial: Aneurysm, coarctation, ectasy	
Arteriovenous fistulae (with one or more shunts)	
Arteriovenous malformations (with a nidus of multiple shunts)	
Complex vascular malformations	
Regional	Diffuse
Sturge–weber	Mafucci
Klippel–Trenaunay	Solomon
F. P. Weber	Proteus
Syndromes often associated with osseous hypertrophies	

Few years later, in 1988, at the seventh Meeting of the International Workshop on Vascular Malformations in Hamburg, the Hamburg classification system was adopted to classify vascular malformations (Table 1.2). It accounts for the underlying anatomical, histological, and pathophysiological features of congenital vascular malformations (CVM) [6]. It also introduces embryological aspects, further subdividing them into either an extratruncular or truncular form, based on the time of developmental arrest during embryonic life [7].

Lesions are identified first based on the prevailing vascular structure involved- arterial, venous, lymphatic, or capillary, also considering arteriovenous shunting and combined vascular defects [8]. The embryological background of the lesion is then considered for additional delineation [9]. Extratruncular lesions result from developmental arrest in the early reticular embryonic stage, prior to the development of vascular trunks, while the vascular system is still in the reticular stage. They are in fact mesodermal tissue remnants, that retain the potential of angioblasts to grow and proliferate when stimulated. These

Table 1.2 Hamburg classification of vascular malformations

	Lesion form	
Predominant type	Truncular	Extratruncular
Arterial	Aplasia or obstruction Dilatation	Infiltrative Limited
Venous	Aplasia or obstruction Dilatation	Infiltrative Limited
Lymphatic	Aplasia or obstruction Dilatation	Infiltrative Limited
Arteriovenous shunt	Deep Superficial	Infiltrative Limited
Combined/mixed	Arterial and venous without shunt Haemolymphatic with or without shunt	Haemolymphatic Infiltrative or limited

lesions may continue to grow and carry a significant risk of a recurrence even after therapeutic interventions. These may be infiltrating and diffuse or limited and localized.

Truncular lesions result from a defect occurring during the stage of fetal development following the reticular stage, as the vascular trunks are developing. These forms develop from stenosis or obstruction of vascular trunks, with resulting hypoplasia, or dilatation of vascular trunks, which in turn may be localized or diffuse [10]. The presentation includes agenesis or aplasia on the one hand and aneurysms or persistent embryonic channels on the other. These are hence, unable to grow and proliferate and have a minimal risk of recurrence. However, they are often associated with more serious hemodynamic consequences [11, 12].

Truncular lesions are malformations of larger caliber, axial vessels, while extratruncular lesions involve small vessels embedded within the tissue.

The vascular components of Klippel–Trénaunay syndrome (KTS) and F P Weber syndrome (FPWS) have been as "hemolymphatic malformations" using the Hamburg classification system. The CVM in KTS includes venous, lymphatic, and capillary components, while the hallmark of FPWS is arteriovenous shunting, mainly combined with capillary malformations.

The International Society for the study of Vascular anomalies (ISSVA) is the formalization of prior biennial international workshops, which were started in 1976 by Drs. John Mulliken and Anthony Young, of specialists interested in the diagnosis, management, and investigation of these disorders. ISSVA was officially founded in 1992, 2 years after its first International Workshop held in 1990 in Amsterdam.

The International Society for the Study of Vascular Anomalies (ISSVA) adopted the Mulliken and Glowicki classification model for its 1996 classification scheme, to overcome incorrect identification and naming of vascular anomalies occurring across specialties. The ISSVA classification delineated proliferative vascular lesions, or "tumors," from non-proliferative "malformations" [13].

Vascular malformations are thus divided into four groups: simple malformations, combined malformations, malformations of major named vessels, and malformations associated with other anomalies. "Malformations of major named vessels" was the name chosen for those malformations named "truncular" in the Hamburg classification.

The updated ISSVA 2018 classification can be found online at: (http://www.issva.org/classification).

The World Health Organization (WHO) classifications are generally considered as the reference classification for tumors and tumor-like diseases. The WHO classification of skin vascular "tumors" is a nonhierarchical list of a series of different diseases, irrespective of their tumor, malformation, reactive, or infectious nature. The WHO classification of soft tissue tumors uses the word "hemangioma" to describe a tumor or a malformation [14, 15].

These inconsistencies in classification and nomenclature make the WHO classifications misleading and confusing.

1.1 Simple Vascular Malformations

These consist of a single type of vascular channel and are named according to the involved vessel type (e.g., *capillary* malformation, *venous* malformation [VM]). Exceptions include arteriovenous malformations (AVMs) and arteriovenous fistulas (AVFs), which may contain a combination of arterial, venous, and capillary components. Because these lesions are *single* malformations composed of several vessel types, as opposed to a combination of *multiple* malformations, they are more accurately classified as simple vascular malformations.

1.2 Low-Flow Vascular Malformations

Capillary malformations present as non-involuting flat pink or red macules, resulting from abnormal morphogenesis of superficial dermal blood vessels, are the most common group of malformations [16].

These lesions stain positive for fibronectin, von Willebrand factor, and collagenous basement membrane proteins [17].

Particularly, in port wine stains, there is increased expression of vascular endothelial growth factor VEGF-A. Detection occurs at birth, although acquired capillary malformations are rarely identified [18].

Venous Malformations are generally ill-defined, pale-to-dark blue and compressible masses. VMs can affect any tissue, including skin, mucosal surfaces, soft tissue, muscle, and viscera. Distribution may be focal, multifocal, or diffuse. These dysmorphic vascular channels are lined with flattened endothelium [19] and defective smooth muscle, leading to progressive expansion under hydrostatic pressure.

Common VMs, which constitute the vast majority of VMs, are unifocal and sporadic; nearly half of these lesions are associated with somatic mutations in the *TIE2* gene. It is noted that two-thirds of all vascular malformations are venous predominant [20].

1.3 Lymphatic Malformations

Lymphatic malformations arise from abnormal development of the lymphatic system during the early phases of angiogenesis and may be diffuse, often described as lymphedema, or localized, commonly described as a lymphangioma [21].

These malformations are typically large, non-tender masses affecting any area of the body, in the head and neck, they are referred to as cystic hygromas [22]. While most lesions are sporadic, some occur as part of syndromes, such as CLOVES. Lymphatic malformations may be macrocystic, microcystic, or a combination.

1.4 High Flow Vascular Malformations

High flow vascular malformations include macrofistulas, or truncular malformations, consisting of single or multiple arteries directly communicating with outflow veins without an interposed high resistance capillary system. In contrast, arteriovenous malformations, are often extratruncular and consist of a low resistance nidus directing the blood supply from numerous regional inflow arteries to veins. AVM is typically used to describe a nidus or "tangle" of abnormal vessels, while AVF implies a single direct, high flow connection.

Staging of these lesions can be accomplished by scoring according to the Schobinger clinical staging system [23]. Within this system, stage I describes a phase of quiescence where there are a cutaneous blush and skin warmth. In stage II, there is expansion with a darkening blush, lesion pulsation, as well as a bruit or palpable thrill. Stage III is defined by destruction, namely pain, dystrophic skin changes, ulceration, distal ischemia, and steal. Finally, stage IV is marked by decompensation or high output cardiac failure.

1.5 Combined Vascular Malformations

Combined vascular malformations are defined as two or more distinct vascular malformations within a single lesion. The naming convention for combined vascular lesions involves listing the components of the malformation in alphabetical order, with the exception of AVM, which is placed at the end [24].

Combined vascular malformations can contain deep components underlying more clinically apparent surface malformations, and thus these lesions may require radiologic and/or histopathologic evidence to make the correct diagnosis [13].

1.6 Vascular Malformations of Major Named Vessels

Major vessels are subject to the same malformations as smaller caliber vessels. The term "major named vessels" typically refers to large, axial, conducting channels. Arteries, veins, and lymphatics can all be affected. Anomalies include abnormalities of origin, course, number, length, diameter (e.g., hypoplasia, ectasia, or stenosis), and/or valves.

1.7 Vascular Malformations Associated with Other Anomalies

Vascular malformations of all types (simple, combined, involving any type of vessel) can be associated with nonvascular anomalies, most commonly bone, soft tissue, or visceral overgrowth [13].

1.8 Syndromes Associated with Low Flow Vascular Malformations

1.8.1 Klippel–Trenaunay Syndrome

Klippel–Trenaunay syndrome (KTS) is OSCVA syndrome (Overgrowth Syndrome with Complex Vascular Anomalies) with extremity overgrowth, associated with a superficial vascular stain, venous malformations, and usually partial aplasia of the deep venous system and may also involve lymphatic anomalies. The vascular malformations are characterized as truncal malformations, and may be related to the persistence of the embryonic dorsal vein system in the lateral aspect of the extremity (lateral marginal vein in the lower extremity). Large varicosities may result in venous thrombosis and pulmonary embolism. Coagulopathy and Gram-negative sepsis are also complications. Limb gigantism is especially prominent when there is an associated lymphatic malformation.

1.8.2 CLOVES Syndrome

The congenital lipomatous overgrowth, vascular malformations, epidermal nevi, and scoliosis and other skeletal deformities (CLOVES) syndrome consist of truncal lipomatosis, vascular malformations, and acral/musculoskeletal anomalies. Vascular lesions include capillary, lymphatic, venous, and arteriovenous malformation [25].

1.8.3 Blue Rubber Bleb Nevus Syndrome

This syndrome consists of venous malformations of the skin and those within the gastrointestinal tract. Clinical consequences generally result from gastrointestinal venous malformations, which may lead to occult or frank gastrointestinal bleeding.

1.8.4 Maffucci Syndrome

In this syndrome, enchondromas are found coexistent with venous malformations. There is a high frequency of malignant transformation of the enchondromas into chondrosarcomas.

1.8.5 Generalized Lymphatic Anomaly and Gorham–Stout Disease

Generalized Lymphatic Anomaly (GLA) and Gorham–Stout Disease are two different disorders of the lymphatic system with overlapping features. GLA is synonymous with "generalized cystic lymphangiomatosis," "cystic angiomatosis" and "lymphangiomatosis." Features of GLA may include splenic cysts, hepatic cysts, pleural effusions, and macrocytic lymphatic malformations, which may involve several organ systems, including bone [26].

Gorham-Stout disease, which has been called "vanishing bone disease," is also a vascular anomaly of the lymphatics characterized by the proliferation of lymphatic vessels within the bone, resulting in progressive bony destruction.

1.9 Syndromes Associated with High Flow and Mixed Vascular Malformations

Hereditary hemorrhagic telangiectasia (Osler–Weber–Rendu syndrome).

Hereditary hemorrhagic telangiectasia (HHT) is an autosomal dominant disorder involving mutations in the transforming growth factor-beta signaling pathway resulting in irregular cytoskeletal architecture and abnormal vascular tubule formation characterized by telangiectasias and fistulous malformations. Telangiectasias are seen on mucosal surfaces and associated with epistaxis and gastrointestinal bleeding. Arteriovenous fistulas, particularly in the lung, liver, brain, and gastrointestinal tract are a major source of morbidity and mortality [27].

1.9.1 Parkes–Weber Syndrome

Parkes–Weber Syndrome is an OSCVA syndrome, characterized by extremity overgrowth and vascular anomaly. In contrast to the Klippel–Trenaunay syndrome, venous abnormalities are associated with high flow arteriovenous malformations within the hypertrophied extremity. A third component of the syndrome is a cutaneous capillary malformation.

1.9.2 PTEN Hamartoma Syndrome

PTEN mutations promote stimulation of angiogenesis by the Akt/mTOR pathway. PTEN Hamartoma Syndrome (PHTS) usually involves cutaneous lesions, capillary or capillary venous malformations, typically small deep tissue vascular malformations, and multiple high flow AVMs, associated with hamartomatous lesions. Occasionally, lymphatic and venous malformations may be present. High flow AVMs may be present in the limbs, paraspinal region, and dura. They are frequently intramuscular and associated with ectopic fat.

1.10 Unclassified Vascular Anomalies

Several of these vascular anomalies are not yet completely understood. Such lesions therefore remain unclassified in the most recent ISSVA classification scheme.

These entities include.

Intramuscular hemangioma, angiokeratoma, sinusoidal hemangioma, acral arteriovenous "tumor," multifocal lymphangioendotheliomatosis with thrombocytopenia/cutaneovisceral angiomatosis with thrombocytopenia (MLT/CAT) PTEN (type) hamartoma of soft tissue/ "angiomatosis" of soft tissue (PHOST) PTEN Fibro adipose vascular anomaly (FAVA).

1.11 Imaging of Vascular Anomalies

Several noninvasive imaging modalities are useful in characterizing vascular anomalies, contributing information about lesion size, flow characteristics, and relationship to adjacent structures [28].

Ultrasound doppler is indispensable in the evaluation of superficial vascular lesions given its low cost, ease of use, high temporal and spatial resolution, and ability to evaluate flow dynamics [28, 29, 30]. Low flow vascular malformations, including venous and lymphatic malformations, can be differentiated from high flow lesions based on Doppler analysis. Venous malformations appear as hypoechoic or heterogeneous lesions in 80% of cases. Lymphatic malformations are characterized by macrocystic or microcystic spaces with or without debris separated by septae, with no flow, however the septa may contain small arteries and veins US is limited in its ability to evaluate deep lesions and lesions that involve bone.

Contrast-enhanced computed tomography (CT) and CT angiograph are useful in evaluating osseous involvement and phleboliths. It also provides information about enhancement, thrombosis, calcification, vascular anatomy, and involvement of adjacent structures [30]. The use of ionizing radiation and relatively limited ability to provide information about flow dynamics decreases its usefulness. For these reasons ultrasonography (US) and magnetic resonance imaging (MRI) are the primary noninvasive imaging modalities used in the evaluation of vascular anomalies [31].

Magnetic Resonance Imaging (MRI) is the most valuable modality for imaging vascular anomalies due to its superior contrast resolution, ability to characterize flow dynamics, the depiction of deep and adjacent structures, and lack of ionizing radiation [28]. Most information needed to characterize a vascular anomaly can be obtained from T1-weighted, fat-saturated T2-weighted, and gradient-echo MR sequences [30, 32]. Venous malformations are usually hypo- or isointense at T1-weighted MR imaging. In cases of hemorrhage or thrombosis, heterogeneous signal intensity can be observed on T1-weighted images. Abnormal veins can be observed in the area of the malformation. At T2-weighted MR imaging, venous malformations display bright signal intensity. Areas of hypointensity related to thrombosis, septation inside the malformation, or phleboliths can also be observed. Dynamic contrast-enhanced MRI can provide supporting information about flow dynamics [33].

Direct percutaneous phlebography can be performed as a diagnostic procedure in cases of atypical venous malformation. Opacification of abnormal venous cavities allows confirmation of the diagnosis of venous malformation and exclusion of other diagnoses such as benign or malignant soft tissue tumors. It is also performed as the initial step during sclerotherapy [34].

An arteriogram, digital subtraction angiogram (DSA), provide good definition of the central "nidus" of affected vessels and provide access for intravascular treatment when necessary [35].

1.12 Treatment

Low flow malformations can be treated by compression, surgical excision, or sclerosis. Treatment should be reserved for symptomatic or cosmetically disfiguring malformations. Sclerosing agents, which comprise the main form of treatment, include STS, polidocanol, and absolute alcohol [36, 37].

The goal in the treatment of high flow arteriovenous vascular malformations is the eradication of the nidus. This is accomplished with a liquid embolic agent, coils, glue, plugs that will penetrate and occlude the feeding vessels (the nidus) [38, 39].

The surgical management of AVMs requires preoperative supraselective embolization, judicious removal of tissue, and complex reconstructive techniques. In focal lesions, surgical excision has been shown to cure AVM [40, 41, 42, 43].

In essence, AVMs are debilitating vascular malformations that are often misdiagnosed early in life. Despite successful initial therapy, these lesions may recur later making vigilant management necessary.

1.13 Conclusion

Due to different classification systems, inconsistent naming and miscommunication occur among treating physicians and surgeons, which adversely affects the management of these lesions, and so it is required that a single classification system is applied universally. The 2018 ISSVA system adequately serves this purpose, as it represents the most current classification of vascular anomalies and is based on the widely accepted tumor/malformation dichotomy. Also, the accurate diagnosis of vascular malformations and their associated syndromes is important in the formulation of appropriate treatment. The approach thus, requires multidisciplinary team effort, with the important role of imaging in the proper diagnosis and a combined interventional radiologic and surgical treatment methods [44, 45].

References

1. Yaşargil MG. Microneurosurgery: avm of the brain, history, embryology, pathological considerations, hemodynamics, diagnostic studies, microsurgical anatomy. Vol. IIIA: Thieme; 1987.
2. Virchow R. Die Krankhaften Geschwülste. Berlin: A Hirschwald, 1864–1865, pp. 456–463.
3. Berenbruch K. Ein fall von multiplen Angio-Lipomen Kombiniert mit einem angiom des Rückenmarks, Doctoral thesis, Universität Tübingen, 1890.
4. Mulliken JB, Glowacki J. Hemangiomas and vascular malformations in infants and children: a classification based on endothelial characteristics. Plast Reconstr Surg. 1982;69(03):412–22.
5. Mulliken JB, Burrows PE, Fishman SJ. Eds.Mulliken and Young's vascular anomalies: Hemangiomas and malformations. 2nd ed. Oxford, United Kingdom: Oxford University Press; 2013.
6. Belov S. Anatomopathological classification of congenital vascular defects. Semin Vasc Surg. 1993 Dec;6(4):219–24.
7. Lee BB, Laredo J, Lee TS, Huh S, Neville R. Terminology and classification of congenital vascular malformations. Phlebology. 2007;22(6):249–52.
8. Belov S. Classification of congenital vascular defects. Int Angiol. 1990 Jul-Sep;9(3):141–6.
9. Lee BB, Lardeo J, Neville R. Arterio-venous malformation: how much do we know? Phlebology. 2009 Oct;24(5):193–200.
10. Richter GT, Friedman AB. Hemangiomas and vascular malformations: current theory and management. Int J Pediatr. 2012;2012:645678.
11. Mattassi R, Loose DA, Vaghi M. Hemangiomas and vascular malformations, an atlas of diagnosis and treatment. Milan, Italy: Springer Verlag; 2009.
12. Enjolras OJ. Classification and management of the various superficial vascular anomalies: hemangiomas and vascular malformations. Dermatol. 1997 Nov;24(11):701–10.
13. ISSVA Classification of Vascular Anomalies © 2018. International society for the study of vascular anomalies Available at: issva.org/classification.
14. Fletcher CDM, Bridge JA, Hogendoorn PCW, Mertens F. WHO classification of tumors of soft tissue and bone. Lyon, France: IARC Press; 2013.
15. Calonje JE. Hemangiomas. In: CDM F, Bridge JA, PCW H, Mertens F, editors. WHO classification of tumors of soft tissue and bone. Lyon, France: IARC Press; 2013. p. 138–40.
16. Garzon MC, Huang JT, Enjolras O, Frieden IJ. Vascular malformations:- part 1. J Am Acad Dermatol. 2007;56(3):353–70. quiz 371-4
17. Finley JL, Clark RA, Colvin RB, Blackman R, Noe J, Rosen S. Immunofluorescent staining with antibodies to factor VIII, fibronectin, and collagenous basement membrane protein in normal human skin and port wine stains. Arch Dermatol. 1982 Dec;118(12):971–5.
18. Vural E, Ramakrishnan J, Cetin N, Buckmiller L, Suen JY, Fan CY. The expression of vascular endothelial growth factor and its receptors in port-wine stains. Otolaryngol Head Neck Surg. 2008 Oct;139(4):560–4.
19. Eifert S, Villavicencio JL, Kao TC, Taute BM, Rich NM. Prevalence of deep venous anomalies in congenital vascular malformations of venous predominance. J Vasc Surg. 2000 Mar;31(3):462–71.
20. Soblet J, Limaye N, Uebelhoer M, Boon LM, Vikkula M. Variable somatic TIE2 mutations in half of sporadic venous malformations. Mol Syndromol. 2013 Apr;4(4):179–83.
21. Jackson IT, Carreño R, Potparic Z, Hussain K. Hemangiomas, vascular malformations, and lymphovenous malformations: classification and methods of treatment. Plast Reconstr Surg. 1993;91(07):1216–30.
22. Kohout MP, Hansen M, Pribaz JJ, Mulliken JB. Arteriovenous malformations of the head and neck: natural history and management. Plast Reconstr Surg. 1998 Sep;102(3):643–54.
23. Wassef M, Blei F, Adams D, et al. Vascular anomalies classification: recommendations from the International Society for the Study of vascular anomalies. ISSVA board and scientific committee. Pediatrics. 2015 Jul;136(1):e203–14.

24. Jack E, Steiner BS, Beth A, Drolet MD. Classification of vascular anomalies: an update. Semin Intervent Radiol. 2017 Sep;34(3):225–32.
25. Alomari AI. Characterization of a distinct syndrome that associates complex truncal overgrowth, vascular, and acral anomalies: a descriptive study of 18 cases of CLOVES syndrome. Clin Dysmorphol. 2009 Jan;18(1):1–7.
26. Rasalkar DD, Chu WC. Generalized cystic lymphangiomatosis. Pediatr Radiol. 2010 Dec;40(Suppl 1):S47.
27. Dakeishi M, Shioya T, Wada Y, Shindo T, et al. Genetic epidemiology of hereditary hemorrhagic telangiectasia in a local community in the northern part of Japan. Hum Mutat. 2002 Feb;19(2):140–8.
28. Trop I, Dubois J, Guibaud L, et al. Soft-tissue venous malformations in pediatric and young adult patients: diagnosis with Doppler US. Radiology. 1999;212:841–5.
29. Paltiel HJ, Burrows PE, Kozakewich HP, Zurakowski D, Mulliken JB. Soft-tissue vascular anomalies: utility of US for diagnosis. Radiology. 2000 Mar;214(3):747–54.
30. Hyodoh H, Hori M, Akiba H, Tamakawa M, Hyodoh K, Hareyama M. Peripheral vascular malformations: imaging, treatment approaches, and therapeutic issues. Radiographics. 2005 Oct;25(Suppl 1):S159–71.
31. Donnelly LF, Adams DM, Bisset GS. Vascular malformations and hemangiomas: a practical approach in a multidisciplinary clinic. 3rd. AJR Am J Roentgenol. 2000 Mar;174(3):597–608.
32. Rak KM, Yakes WF, Ray RL, et al. MR imaging of symptomatic peripheral vascular malformations. AJR Am J Roentgenol. 1992 Jul;159(1):107–12.
33. Van Rijswijk CS, Van der Linden E, Bloem JL, et al. Value of dynamic contrast-enhanced MR imaging in diagnosing and classifying peripheral vascular malformations. AJR Am J Roentgenol. 2002 May;178(5):1181–7.
34. Dubois JM, Sebag GH, De Prost Y, Teillac D, Chrétien B, Brunelle FO. Soft-tissue venous malformations in children: percutaneous sclerotherapy with Ethibloc. Radiology. 1991;180:195–8.
35. Do YS, Yakes WF, Shin SW, et al. Ethanol embolization of arteriovenous malformations: interim results. Radiology. 2005;235:674–82.
36. Legiehn GM, Heran MK. Venous malformations: classification, development, diagnosis, and interventional radiologic management. Radiol Clin N Am. 2008;46:545–97.
37. Hyodoh H, Hori M, Akiba H, Tamakawa M, et al. Peripheral vascular malformations: imaging, treatment approaches, and therapeutic issues. Radiographics. 2005;25(Suppl 1):S159–71.
38. Rautio R, Saarinen J, Laranne J, et al. Endovascular treatment of venous malformations in extremities: results of sclerotherapy and the quality of life after treatment. Acta Radiol. 2004;45:397–403.
39. Arat A, Cil BE, Vargel I, et al. Embolization of high-flow craniofacial vascular malformations with onyx. Am J Neuroradiol. 2007;28(7):1409–14.
40. Visser TF, Tan ST. Surgical management of arteriovenous malformation. J Plastic, Reconstructive Aesthetic Surg. 2011;64(3):283–91.
41. Lee BB, Baumgartner I, Berlien P, Bianchini G, Burrows P, Gloviczki P, et al. Diagnosis and treatment of venous malformations. Consensus document of the International Union of Phlebology (IUP): updated 2013. Int Angiol. 2015;34:97–149.
42. Coldwell DM, Stokes KR, Yakes WF. Embolotherapy: agents, clinical applications, and techniques. Radiographics. 1994;14:623–43.
43. Wang D, Su L, Han Y, Fan X. Ethanol embolotherapy of high-flow auricular arteriovenous malformations with electrolytically detachable coil-assisted dominant outflow vein occlusion. Eur J Vasc Endovasc Surg. 2014;48:576–84.
44. Lee BB, Do YS, Yakes W, Kim DI, Mattassi R, Hyon WS, et al. Management of arteriovenous malformations: a multidisciplinary approach. J Vasc Surg. 2004;39:590–600.
45. Ponzo LM, Orabona GD, Iaconetta G, Astarita F, Leone G, Cuocolo R, et al. Multidisciplinary approach in the management of head and neck vascular malformations. J Vasc Med Surg. 2017;5:316.

Epidemiology of Vascular Malformations

2

Divya Khanna and Ajay K. Khanna

Vascular anomaly comprises a wide spectrum of lesions as an outcome of disorders in vascular development. They continue to be a challenge in both diagnosis and treatment and need individual and multispecialty treatment program. The key to proper treatment of these lesions relies on correct diagnosis and classifying the vascular lesion [1]. The vascular anomaly can be described by two abnormal vascular conditions: the congenital vascular malformation (CVM) and the vascular tumor that represents neonatal or infantile hemangioma. Both conditions are different in their anatomical, histological, and pathophysiological findings and also in their clinical courses, which emphasizes the importance of a precise understanding of these two conditions [2, 3].

2.1 Classification of Vascular Anomalies

The International Society for the Study of Vascular Anomalies (ISSVA) classification, a widely accepted system, categorizes vascular anomalies into two types: [1] vaso-proliferative or vascular neoplasms such as hemangioma, and [2, 3] vascular malformations. The distinction between the two is histopathological based on the assessment of increased cell turnover. Vascular tumors, earlier termed as hemangiomas, are true neoplasms. They exhibit rapid post-natal pathologic cell proliferation and slow regression and subsequent involution in late childhood in the majority of the cases [1, 4]. Whereas vascular malformations are composed of abnormally formed channels with single endothelial cells lining within a vascular apparatus and they do not undergo abnormal cellular turnover. They are also congenital, but often go unnoticed at birth, never regress, and grow proportionally with the individual [1, 5].

Vascular malformations are thought to result from developmental errors during embryogenesis, such as abnormal signalling processes that control apoptosis, maturation, and growth of vascular cells. These errors cause the persistence of vascular plexus cells with a certain degree of differentiation. There are four major categories of vascular malformations based on their flow characteristics: slow flow (1) capillary malformation, (2) venous malformation, (3) lymphatic malformation, and fast-flow (4) arteriovenous malformation. However, these lesions often have components of multiple malformations, such as a mixed lymphatic-venous malformation which further adds to the confusion in nomenclature [1, 6].

D. Khanna (✉)
Department of Preventive Oncology, Homi Bhabha Cancer Hospital (HBCH) and Mahamana Pandit Madan Mohan Malviya Cancer, Centre (MPMMCC), TATA Memorial Centers, Varanasi, India

A. K. Khanna
Department of Surgery, Institute of Medical Science, Banaras Hindu University, Varanasi, India

A. K. Khanna, S. K. Tiwary (eds.), *Vascular Malformations*,
https://doi.org/10.1007/978-981-15-9762-6_2

2.2 Epidemiology of Vascular Malformations

Infantile hemangiomas represent the most common tumors of infancy. The true incidence of infantile hemangiomas is unknown but estimated to occur in 5–10% of all neonates and in 30% of prematurely born children. They are found 3–9 times more often in girls than in boys [7]. Complicated hemangiomas are even more likely to occur among female infants, for reasons that are unknown [8]. Infantile hemangiomas are often noticed in the first few days to months of life [9]. Most hemangiomas occur sporadically but familial transmission in an autosomal-dominant fashion has also been reported [10]. The frequency of hemangioma occurrence is higher among white non-Hispanic infants than other racial groups. The incidence of hemangiomas is higher in preterm infants and the most significant risk factor appears to be low birth weight [11]. Multiple hemangiomas more common in products of multiple gestations. Maternal associations include older maternal age, placenta-previa, pre-eclampsia, and other placental anomalies [11, 12].

On the other hand, vascular malformations appear definitely less often with no gender-wise frequency difference. Vascular malformations are often observed at the time of birth or they may appear in early childhood. They enlarge proportionally to the child's growth and a sudden expansion can be triggered by an infection, hormonal changes (puberty or pregnancy), or trauma [7, 13].Contrary to hemangiomas, vascular malformations do not regress spontaneously. Moreover, their abrupt increase may result in the impairment or deformation of integral anatomical structures, osseous deformities (slow flow malformations), osteolysis (rapid flow malformations), respiratory tract obstruction (neck or head malformations), pain, thrombosis (venous malformations), infection, or ulceration [7, 14]. This chapter will focus primarily on the epidemiology of vascular malformations. The prevalence of congenital vascular malformations (CVM) is 1.2–1.5%, which is higher than other inborn errors Nearly two-third of CVM are predominantly venous, and a quarter of these lesions are completely or partly of lymphatic origin and are called as low-flow malformations, the remaining are high-flow malformations. The lesions range in size from small to extensive [15].

It is difficult to extract accurate epidemiologic data (incidence and prevalence) of CVM due to confusing nomenclatures and definitions used in the available epidemiologic literature. To describe the epidemiology of CVMs, we have to rely on the data of symptomatic patients with clinically apparent CVM. Some CVM may remain quiescent throughout the remaining life. However, most of the CVM lesions grow with age and some of them may show sudden expansion cause of reasons stated earlier. It is still not known what is the exact mechanism that stimulates the dormant CVM lesion. Hence, an exact incidence of CVM cannot be estimated at the time of birth. European Surveillance of Congenital Anomalies (EUROCAT) is a network of population-based registries (http://www.eurocat-network.eu/aboutus/whocollaboratingcentre) for the epidemiologic surveillance of congenital anomalies which covers about 30% of all births in the European Union. Still with the EUROCAT data, it is difficult to estimate an exact incidence of CVM because vascular malformations are not listed separately as a congenital anomaly and included in the skin anomaly, limb defect, or aortic coarctation as well [16].

In 1988, at the seventh Meeting of the International Workshop on Vascular Malformations in Hamburg, a modern classification system, the "Hamburg Classification," was proposed, which was based on the work of Degni and Malan (Table 2.1). This classification differentiates between truncular and extratruncular malformations. The Hamburg Classification System classifies CVMs taking into account the underlying anatomical, histological, pathophysiological, and hemodynamic status of the defects. Modern technology and improved diagnostic studies have aided in accurate diagnosis of these lesions. This classification has its clinical applicability and has been well accepted as the modern classification system. CVMs are classified into one of five types based on its predominant

Table 2.1 Hamburg classification of congenital vascular malformation

A:
Predominant arterial defects
Predominant venous defects
Predominant arteriovenous shunting defects
Predominantly lymphatic defects
Combined vascular defects
B:
Extratruncular Forms
Infiltrative, diffuse, limited, localized
Truncular Forms
Aplasia or obstruction
Hypoplasia, aplasia, hyperplasia, stenosis, membrane, congenital spur
Dilatation
Localized (aneurysm), diffuse (ectasia)

vascular component: arterial malformation, venous malformations, arteriovenous malformations, lymphatic malformations, and combined vascular malformation. The most common combined or mixed malformation is the hemolymphatic malformations [2, 3].

As per the Bogota Congenital Malformations Surveillance Program (BCMSP) between January 2005 and April 2012, congenital anomalies at birth were detected in 1.66% (4682 out of 282,523 births). Vascular anomalies (0.03%) were the most frequent reported congenital anomaly, followed by hypospadias (0.028%), and anorectal malformations (0.022%). Majority (84%) of the vascular anomalies was blood vessel origin and the rest (15%) was the lymphatic origin. Craniofacial lesions were the most common anatomical site followed by vascular anomalies at the extremities, thorax, and abdomen. However, they did not differentiate CVM from the infantile hemangioma [16, 17].

Similarly, Kennedy et al. reported the incidence of CVM as 1.08% (0.83–4.5%) based on a systematic review of 238 studies reporting more than 20 million births. The information was obtained from hospital records, birth certificates, and retrospective questionnaires from examinations of children. However, this study highlighted the variability in reporting methods due to differences in terminology and inconsistent diagnostic criteria [18]. A study by Tasnadi et al. reported an overall incidence of the CVM is 1.2% based on a study conducted on 3573 three-year-old children. According to them, infiltrating/localized vascular malformation and/or AVM is 0.45%, the capillary malformation is 0.42%, lymphatic malformation or primary lymphedema is 0.14%, and mixed from CVM representing phlebectasias, nevi, and limb length discrepancies is 0.34% [19]. Among venous predominant vascular malformations, *Eifert* et al. also reported the prevalence of deep venous anomalies (truncular VM) among the VMs using duplex ultrasonography, venography, CT, MRI, and arteriography. Among 392 patients with CVMs, 65.5% were confirmed as truncular VM with deep venous anomalies including phlebectasia, aplasia, or hypoplasia of venous trunks, aneurysms, and avalvulia of the deep vein system [20]. Malformations are reported as the most common type of CVMs, which has been reported to occur in one of 5000–10,000 childbirths [21].

2.3 Capillary Malformation

The capillary malformation is a macular pink or purple blanchable cutaneous vascular anomaly present since birth which tends to darken with time and leads to the overgrowth of tissues beneath the stain. Capillary malformations (CMs) are low-flow vascular malformation affecting the capillaries in the papillary dermis that persists throughout life. CMs are found in 0.5% of the population with similar prevalence frequency in both genders [1]. In a prospective study and literature review, capillary malformations occurred in 0.1 to 2% of newborns without sex predilection [22]. They are generally sporadic, but familial cases have been reported.. RASA1 mutations have been attributed with hereditary capillary malformations without arteriovenous malformations [23, 24]. They were initially referred to as "port-wine stain," which is inaccurate, but has persisted due to its widespread use in literature. The majority of CMs appear in the face and mostly in the trigeminal nerve distribution, especially ophthalmic (V1) and maxillary (V2) divisions. They should not be confused with infantile hemangiomas. In contrast with infantile hemangiomas, capillary malformations do not regress with time but grow in proportion to the child's growth and become thicker and darker in color during adulthood [1].

2.4 Venous Malformation

Venous malformations (VMs) are the most frequent slow flow vascular malformations observed amongst the vascular anomalies affecting 1% to 4% of individuals. Although epidemiologic data are lacking, their incidence has been estimated at 1 in 2000 to 5000 births. There is no sex predilection. Clinically they appear as a bluish, soft, compressible lesion typically found on the face, limbs, or trunk. Venous malformations are dependent lesions thus they expand and contract based on patient positioning. They also tend to grow proportionally with the child and often increase in size with puberty, hormonal changes, or infection. They result from inborn errors in the development of the venous network, leading to deficient smooth muscle cells which cause dilated and dysfunctional veins. However, more than 90% of VMs occur sporadically and are unifocal lesions. Multifocal lesions are seen in patients with rare inherited forms with the autosomal-dominant transmission, such as cutaneo-mucosal venous malformation and glomuvenous malformation (1 and 5% of all VMs, respectively), and in two very are sporadic forms namely multifocal venous malformation and blue rubber bleb nevus syndrome (Bean syndrome) [1, 25, 26].

2.5 Lymphatic Malformation

Lymphatic malformations (LMs) are vascular channels, pouches, or vesicles with a single endothelial lining filled with lymphatic fluid. Majority (75%) occur in the cervico-facial region. They were earlier referred to as "lymphangioma," which is a misnomer because LMs lack cellular hyperplasia. Lymphatic malformations are categorized based on their size of the lymphatic chamber as macrocystic (>2 cm), microcystic (<2 cm), or mixed. LMs never regress in size but expand and contract based on the amount of lymphatic fluid present and the presence of bleeding or inflammation. These lesions are mostly evident at birth and appear as small, crimson dome-shaped nodules as a result of intra-lesional bleeding. The majority of LM is present at birth, with the remainder presenting by 2 years of age. Often macrocystic LMs enlarge significantly leading causing anatomical distortion of underlying soft tissues and bones of the face. Distortion, frequent bouts of bleeding, and cellulitis will call for intervention [1].

The common clinical types of pure lymphatic malformation (LM) are namely lymphedema (diffuse LM) and lymphangioma (localized, macrocystic LM). Primary lymphedema is divided into three types based on the age of presentation: congenital familial lymphedema (Milroy's disease), lymphedema praecox (present during adolescence), and lymphedema tarda (presents after 35 years of age). Macrocystic LMs (cystic hygroma) are usually visible at birth and can also be detected by prenatal ultrasound assessments. They are frequently located on the neck, axilla, retroperitoneum, or mesentery. According to a study of 305 patients with lymphangioma, their anatomic distribution was head and neck (46.2%) followed by trunk surface and extremity (44.6%) and intraabdominal or mediastinal (9.2%) and showed male predilection by 1.4: 1. More often, LM is seen in combination with other forms of CVM such as VM, CM, or AVM. Lee et al. conducted a review on the subtypes of the LM separately among 1203 CVM patients. Predominant LM lesion accounted for 32.6% of all patients with CVM which included 271 (69%) patients with truncular LM and 122 (31%) patients with extratruncular LM lesions. Of 122 patients with extratruncular LM, 89 (73%) had the macrocystic type with a predilection for the head, neck, and thorax. Of the 271 patients with truncular LM, 247 (91%) patients showed lymphatic channel aplasia or hypoplasia and a predilection to occur in the lower extremity [16].

2.6 Arteriovenous Malformation

Arteriovenous malformations (AVM) represent vascular malformations that develop from an identifiable source vessel called as "nidus," which allows an abnormal connection of arterial and venous systems. This type of shunt is usually present at birth but is not apparent till first or second decade of life. Arteriovenous malformations can be slightly compressible and pulsatile with a palpable thrill. This kind of lesion is most commonly found intracranially and can expand on stimulus such as trauma or puberty. Clinically, AVMs appearing in soft tissues or bone are typically not accompanied by pain, but rather frequent episodes of bleeding. They have a reliable natural history consisting of four distinct stages namely: quiescent, growing, symptomatic, and decompensating [1].

AVMs can present as an isolated feature or as part of a syndrome; the most common is hereditary hemorrhagic telangiectasia (HHT) and capillary malformation (CM)-AVM. HHT or Osler–Weber–Rendu syndrome (MIM187300) is a known autosomal-dominant, genetically heterogeneous disorder characterized by AVMs, typically in the liver and lung and associated with cutaneous and mucosal telangiectasias. CM-AVM (MIM608354) is an autosomal-dominant disorder with high penetrance and variable expressivity presenting as small multifocal cutaneous CMs.

In a study done on 2971 CVM registered patients at Samsung Medical Center (SMC), VM or venous predominant CVM was the most common type of CVM (53%). Among the VM patients, the lower extremity was the most frequently affected site (42%), followed by head and neck (26%), upper extremity (16%), trunk (9%), and multiple site involvement (6%). Among extremity VM patients, 93% was extratruncular and 13% was truncular form VM. LM and lymphatic dominant CVM comprised of 29% of all CVM patients. It was also most prevalent in the extremities (51%) followed by head and neck (29%) and trunk (14%). AVM accounted for 17% of CVM patients and most frequently found in the extremities (55%) followed by head and neck (34%) and trunk (11%). AVM is known as the least common type of CVMs representing approximately 10–15% of all clinically significant CVM lesions [27]. Among them, "extratruncular" form comprises the vast majority of AVM lesions. Most of the current data regarding the incidence and prevalence of AVMs include AVM lesion affecting CNS [28].

Regarding the age of an initial presentation, the investigators found that patients with AVM or LM presented at a later age than patients with VM or CM. AVMs are also known to occur with equal frequency in males and females. About half of the AVM lesions are recognizable at birth, and 30% become clinically apparent during childhood. They have a predilection to the head and neck area than in other locations. Currently, there is no racial, demographic, or environmental risk factors for CVMs have been identified to date [16, 29].

2.7 Genetic Syndromes Associated with Vascular Malformations

A substantial number of angiogenesis-related genes (i.e., TIE2, VEGFR-3, RASA1, KRIT1, MGC4607, PDCD10, glomulin, FOXC2, NEMO, SOX18, ENG, ACVRLK1, MADH4, NDP, TIMP3, Notch3, COL3A1, and PTEN) have been identified in the pathogenesis of vascular malformations to provide a new base for further scientific epidemiological evaluation. Still, further studies are needed to explore involved molecular mechanisms which may lead to the development of therapeutic strategies for treating Klippel–Trenaunay syndrome (KTS). Several syndromes are associated with slow flow malformations namely Klippel–Trenaunay syndrome (KTS) or Klippel–Trenaunay–Weber syndrome, Parkes–Weber syndrome, Sturge–Weber syndrome, Gorham–Stout syndrome, Proteus syndrome, and Maffucci's syndrome [16, 30].

2.7.1 Sturge–Weber Syndrome

Sturge-Weber syndrome (SWS) is a rare congenital disorder characterized by the classic triad of facial port-wine stain, leptomeningeal angiomatosis, and ocular involvement. The discovery of the somatic mutation in *GNAQ* associated with SWS has raised the hypothesis of somatic mosaicism in SWS [31, 32].

Klippel–Trenaunay Syndrome
Capillary malformations, venous and lymphatic malformations, and soft tissue and bone hypertrophy involving a limb are prominent features of Klippel–Trenaunay syndrome (KTS) [26, 33].

Parkes–Weber Syndrome
Parkes–Weber syndrome is characterized by a large capillary malformation on an extremity, soft tissue and bone hypertrophy of the affected limb, and multiple, microscopic, fast-flow arteriovenous shunts [34].

Servelle-Martorell Syndrome
Servelle–Martorell syndrome is a rare congenital angiodysplastic disease. It manifests with capillary malformations and varicosities similar to KTS, but is associated with progressive limb hypotrophy rather than overgrowth [35].

Proteus Syndrome
Proteus syndrome is an extremely rare disorder characterized by asymmetric and disproportionate overgrowth of body parts. Mosaicism for a somatic activating mutation in the *AKT1* oncogene is thought to be the cause of Proteus syndrome. Cutaneous findings are present in approximately 40% of neonates and include capillary, lymphatic, or venous malformations, epidermal nevi, connective tissue nevi, lipomas, and café au lait macules. The vascular malformations are usually extensive, covering a large portion of the body, and may be associated with visceral vascular malformations [36].

CLOVES Syndrome
Congenital lipomatous overgrowth, vascular malformations, epidermal nevi, spinal/skeletal anomalies/scoliosis (CLOVES) syndrome is a very rare congenital disorder caused by somatic mosaic activating mutations in the *PIK3CA* gene [37–39].

Bannayan–Riley–Ruvalcaba Syndrome
Bannayan-Riley-Ruvalcaba syndrome, which is incorporated into Cowden syndrome-1 (MIM #158350), is an autosomal-dominant disorder caused by mutations in the tumor suppressor gene *PTEN*. Cutaneous features include capillary, venous, and lymphatic malformations as well as lipomas and pigmented macules on the genitalia. Associated findings include macrocephaly, pseudopapilledema, mental retardation, and juvenile intestinal polyposis [40].

Capillary Malformation-Arteriovenous Malformation Syndrome
Capillary malformation-arteriovenous malformation (CM-AVM) syndrome is an autosomal-dominant disorder caused by mutations in the *RASA1* gene. CM-AVM syndrome is characterized by atypical cutaneous capillary malformations in conjunction with an AVM. The AVM can be localized or diffuse and can be located in the soft tissues, muscles, bones, brain, or spine [41, 42].

2.8 Conclusion

Vascular anomaly comprises a wide spectrum of lesions as an outcome of disorders in vascular development. They continue to be a challenge in both diagnosis and treatment and need individual and multispecialty treatment program. The vascular anomaly can be described by two abnormal vascular conditions: the congenital vascular malformation (CVM) and vascular tumor that represents neonatal or infantile hemangioma. As such hemangiomas are much more common than vascular malformation.

References

1. Cox JA, Bartlett E, Lee EI. Vascular malformations: a review. In Seminars in plastic surgery. Thieme Medical Publishers. 2014 May;28(02):058–63.
2. Lee BB, Laredo J, Lee TS, Huh S, Neville R. Terminology and classification of congeni-

tal vascular malformations. Phlebology. 2007 Jan;22(6):249–52.
3. Mulliken JB, Young AE. Vascular Birthmarks: Hemangiomas and Malformations. Philadelphia, PA: WB Saunders; 1988.
4. Van Aalst JA, Bhuller A, Sadove AM. Pediatric vascular lesions. J Craniofac Surg. 2003;14(4):566–83.
5. Mulliken JB, Glowacki J. Hemangiomas and vascular malformations in infants and children: a classification based on endothelial characteristics. Plast Reconstr Surg. 1982;69(3):412–22.
6. Cohen MM Jr. Vascular update: morphogenesis, tumors, malformations, and molecular dimensions. Am J Med Genet A. 2006;140(19):2013–38.
7. Wojcicki P, Wojcicka K. Epidemiology, diagnostics and treatment of vascular tumours and malformations. Adv Clin Exp Med. 2014 May 1;23(3):475–84.
8. Enjolras O, Gelbert F. Superficial hemangiomas: associations and management. Pediatr Dermatol. 1997 May;14(3):173–9.
9. Ricci KW. Advances in the medical management of vascular anomalies. In Seminars in interventional radiology 2017 Sep (Vol. 34, No. 03, pp. 239–249). Thieme Medical Publishers.
10. Blei F, Walter J, Orlow SJ, Marchuk DA. Familial segregation of hemangiomas and vascular malformations as an autosomal dominant trait. Arch Dermatol. 1998 Jun 1;134(6):718–22.
11. Group TH, Haggstrom AN, Drolet BA, Baselga E, Chamlin SL, Garzon MC, Horii KA, Lucky AW, Mancini AJ, Metry DW, Newell B. Prospective study of infantile hemangiomas: demographic, prenatal, and perinatal characteristics. J Pediatr. 2007 Mar 1;150(3):291–4.
12. Munden A, Butschek R, Tom WL, Marshall JS, Poeltler DM, Krohne SE, Alió AB, Ritter M, Friedlander DF, Catanzarite V, Mendoza A. Prospective study of infantile haemangiomas: incidence, clinical characteristics and association with placental anomalies. Br J Dermatol. 2014 Apr;170(4):907–13.
13. Fishman SJ, Mulliken JB. Hemangiomas and vascular malformations of infancy and childhood. Pediatr Surg. 1993;40:1177–200.
14. Boyd JB, Mulliken JB, Kaban LB. Sceletal changes associated with vascular malformations. Plast Reconstr Surg. 1984;74:789–97.
15. Puig S, Casati B, Staudenherz A, Paya K. Vascular low-flow malformations in children: current concepts for classification, diagnosis and therapy. Eur J Radiol. 2005 Jan 1;53(1):35–45.1,2.
16. Kim YW, Lee BB. Epidemiologic Aspect of Congenital Vascular Malformation. In: Congenital Vascular Malformations. Berlin, Heidelberg: Springer; 2017. p. 31–4.
17. Correa C, Mallarino C, Pena R, Rincon LC, Gracia G, Zarante I. Congenital malformations of pediatric surgical interest: prevalence, risk factors, and prenatal diagnosis between 2005 and 2012 in the capital city of a developing country. Bogota, Colombia. J Pediatr Surg. 2014;49(7):1099–103.
18. Kennedy WP. Epidemiologic aspects of the problem of congenital malformations. In: Persaud TNV, editor. Problems of birth defects. Baltimore: Publisher University Park Press; 1977. p. 35–52.
19. Tasnadi G. Epidemiology and etiology of congenital vascular malformations. SeminVasc Surg. 1993;6(4):200–3.
20. Eifert S, Villavicencio JL, Kao TC, Taute BM, Rich NM. Prevalence of deep venous anomalies in congenital vascular malformations of venous predominance. J Vasc Surg. 2000;31(3):462.
21. Vikkula M, Boon LM, Mulliken JB. Molecular genetics of vascular malformations. Matrix Biol J Int Soc Matrix Biol. 2001;20(5–6):327–35.
22. Kanada KN, Merin MR, Munden A, Friedlander SF. A prospective study of cutaneous findings in newborns in the United States: correlation with race, ethnicity, and gestational status using updated classification and nomenclature. J Pediatr. 2012 Aug 1;161(2):240–5.
23. Hershkovitz D, Bercovich D, Sprecher E, Lapidot M. RASA1 mutations may cause hereditary capillary malformations without arteriovenous malformations. Br J Dermatol. 2008 May;158(5):1035–40.
24. Eerola I, Boon LM, Watanabe S, Grynberg H, Mulliken JB, Vikkula M. Locus for susceptibility for familial capillary malformation ('port-wine stain') maps to 5q. Eur J Hum Genet. 2002 Jun;10(6):375.
25. Nguyen HL, Bonadurer GF, Tollefson MM. Vascular malformations and health-related quality of life: a systematic review and meta-analysis. JAMA Dermatol. 2018 Jun 1;154(6):661–9.
26. Wassef M, Blei F, Adams D, Alomari A, Baselga E, Berenstein A, Burrows P, Frieden IJ, Garzon MC, Lopez-Gutierrez JC, Lord DJ. Vascular anomalies classification: recommendations from the International Society for the Study of Vascular Anomalies. Pediatrics. 2015 Jul 1;136(1):e203–14.
27. Lee BB, Baumgartner I, Berlien HP, Bianchini G, Burrows P, Do YS, et al. Consensus document of the International Union of Angiology (IUA)-2013. Current concept on the management of arteriovenous management. Int Angiol J Int Union Angiol. 2013;32(1):9–36.
28. Al-Shahi R, Warlow C. A systematic review of the frequency and prognosis of arteriovenous malformations of the brain in adults. Brain J Neurol. 2001;124. (Pt 10:1900–26.
29. Kohout MP, Hansen M, Pribaz JJ, Mulliken JB. Arteriovenous malformations of the head and neck: natural history and management. Plast Reconstr Surg. 1998;102(3):643–54.
30. Delis KT, Gloviczki P, Wennberg PW, Rooke TW. Driscoll DJ (2007) Hemodynamic impairment, venous segmental disease, and clinical severity scoring in limbs with Klippel-Trenaunay syndrome. J Vasc Surg. 2006;45(3):561–7.
31. Tallman B, Tan OT, Morelli JG, Piepenbrink J, Stafford TJ, Trainor S, et al. Location of port-wine stains and the likelihood of ophthalmic and/or central nervous system complications. Pediatrics. 1991;87(3):323.

32. Shirley MD, Tang H, Gallione CJ, Baugher JD, Frelin LP, Cohen B, et al. Sturge-Weber syndrome and port-wine stains caused by somatic mutation in GNAQ. N Engl J Med. 2013;368(21):1971. Epub 2013 May 8
33. Garzon MC, Huang JT, Enjolras O, Frieden IJ. Vascular malformations. Part II: associated syndromes J Am Acad Dermatol. 2007 Apr;56(4):541–64.
34. Boon LM, Mulliken JB, Vikkula M. RASA1: variable phenotype with capillary and arteriovenous malformations. Curr Opin Genet Dev. 2005 Jun 1;15(3):265–9.
35. Marsden N, Shokrollahi K, Maw K, Sierakowski A, Bhat FA, Mathur B. Congenital vascular malformation associated with multiple cranial, vertebral and upper limb skeletal abnormalities. Ann R Coll Surg Engl. 2010;92(5):W18–20. Epub 2010 Jun 7
36. Turner JT, Cohen MM Jr, Biesecker LG. Reassessment of the Proteus syndrome literature: application of diagnostic criteria to published cases. Am J Med Genet A. 2004;130A(2):111.
37. Sapp JC, Turner JT, van de Kamp JM, van Dijk FS, Lowry RB, Biesecker LG. Newly delineated syndrome of congenital lipomatous overgrowth, vascular malformations, and epidermal nevi (CLOVE syndrome) in seven patients. Am J Med Genet A. 2007;143A(24):2944.
38. Alomari AI. Characterization of a distinct syndrome that associates complex truncal overgrowth, vascular, and acral anomalies: a descriptive study of 18 cases of CLOVES syndrome. Clin Dysmorphol. 2009 Jan;18(1):1–7.
39. Kurek KC, Luks VL, Ayturk UM, Alomari AI, Fishman SJ, Spencer SA, et al. Somatic mosaic activating mutations in PIK3CA cause CLOVES syndrome. Am J Hum Genet. 2012;90(6):1108–15. Epub 2012 May 31
40. Marsh DJ, Dahia PL, Zheng Z, Liaw D, Parsons R, Gorlin RJ, et al. Germline mutations in PTEN are present in Bannayan-Zonana syndrome. Nat Genet. 1997;16(4):333.
41. Eerola I, Boon LM, Mulliken JB, Burrows PE, Dompmartin A, Watanabe S, et al. RASA1 mutations. Am J Hum Genet. 2003;73(6):1240. Epub 2003 Nov 24
42. Thiex R, Mulliken JB, Revencu N, Boon LM, Burrows PE, Cordisco M, et al. A novel association between RASA1 mutations and spinal arteriovenous anomalies. AJNR Am J Neuroradiol. 2010;31(4):775.

3 Embryology of Vascular Malformation

Soumya Khanna and Ajay K. Khanna

3.1 Introduction

The era of the study of embryological development of circulatory system began in the nineteenth century. At that time various dyes like India ink, silver nitrate and Prussian blue were used for the demonstration of minute vessels [1, 2]. The samples were then fixed and histological investigations was conducted. The development of vascular system was mapped meticulously by the careful and extensive observations of the researchers.

It is a prerequisite for all the vascular specialists to have a thorough understanding of vascular system. But the field of venous embryology is often ignored despite the fact that all mature and named vessels originate from their precursor, embryonic vessels and vascular anamolies are closely correlated with them. The reason behind the ignorance of venous embryology might lie in the rarity of occurrence of vascular anomalies and moreover the difficulty in understanding and interpreting them. Thus it still remains to be one of the most neglected fields of basic science in medicine despite its immense value in explaining many obscure conditions related to vascular anatomy (e.g., Budd–Chiari syndrome is caused by membranous occlusion of suprahepatic inferior vena cava [3, 4] and Chronic cerebrospinal venous insufficiency can occur due to defective development causing narrowing of jugular azygous vein system [5, 6]).

To recognize and interpret various vascular anomalies it is essential to have a basic knowledge of vascular embryology especially the evolutional and involutional development of the vessels involved in maturation of truncal vessels [7, 8]. The prevalence of defective development in the vascular structure of the newborn is in the range of 1% to 3%.

3.2 Development of the Blood Vascular System

Third week of intrauterine development marks the establishment of uteroplacental circulation where the lacunar spaces in syncytiotrophoblast facilitate diffusion and blood vascular system starts to develop as a seperate entity. The first blood cells are formed by induction of mesodermal cells to *hemangioblasts* (common precursor for blood cells and vessels). Later *definitive hemopoetic stem cells* develop in the bone marrow. The blood vessels develop by two processes, i.e., *vasculogenesis and angiogenesis* [9].

S. Khanna (✉)
Department of Anatomy, Institute of Medical Sciences, Banaras Hindu University, Varanasi, India

A. K. Khanna
Department of Surgery, Institute of Medical Science, Banaras Hindu University, Varanasi, India

A. K. Khanna, S. K. Tiwary (eds.), *Vascular Malformations*,
https://doi.org/10.1007/978-981-15-9762-6_3

Vasculogenesis begins in the yolk sac and it is the process of differentiation of hemangioblasts into endothelial cells, leading to formation of primitive vascular network. The mesenchymal cells differentiate into angioblast cells. The angioblast cells then clutter up to form blood islands. Later clefts appear in the blood islands and these clefts communicate with each other to form capillary plexus. Reorganization of cells in the islands lead to formation of blood cells and blood vessels. The capillary plexus of the yolk sac is connected to the heart via the dorsal aorta which is formed inside embryo, thus leading to completion of circulation loop.

Angiogenesis is the process of sprouting of new vessels from existing ones. It begins at day 21 of embryogenesis, when the heart begins to beat and blood starts circulating in the capillary plexus. Angiogenesis begins first in yolk sac wall during third week. The erythrocytes produced in yolk sac have nuclei. On the other hand angiogenesis inside the embryo begins in the fifth week and the erythrocytes produced hereby lack nuclei.

Vascular remodeling occurs due to biomechanical and hemodynamic factors. The capillary plexus is remodeled into a functional structure that includes *large caliber vessels* for low resistance rapid flow and *small caliber capillaries* for diffusional flow. This remodeling happens due to various processes happening simultaneously like regression, sprouting, splitting, or fusion of preexisting vessels leading to formation vessels with arterial and venous identities.

Thoma, a pioneer angiogenesis researcher, emphasized the importance of biomechanical factors and fluid dynamics in angiogenesis by showing that increase in blood flow led to the increase in vessel diameter and decrease in blood flow caused shrinkage of the diameter of the vessel [10]. Murray proposed that vessel caliber is proportional to the amount of shear stress at the vessel wall [11].

3.3 Development of the Arterial System

After the heart starts circulating blood through the primitive vascular network, right and left *primitive aortae is* formed. They are continuous with the two endocardial heart tubes. Each primitive aorta consists of three parts: ventral aorta, arched part lying in the first pharyngeal arch and dorsal aorta.

The fusion of the two endocardial tubes is followed by partial fusion of the two ventral aortae to form *aortic sac*. The unfused parts of the right and left ventral aortae forms the *right and left horns* of the sac respectively.

Fusion of two *dorsal aortae* starts in the middle section and then extends cranially and caudally; thus the single dorsal aorta develops. The dorsal aorta communicates with the vitelline arteries in the mid portion and to the umbilical arteries in the caudal portion. In the cranial portion of the embryo, five pairs of *aortic arches* form sequentially at both sides. They originate from the aortic sac and connect to the ipsilateral dorsal aorta (Fig. 3.1).

These arches give rise to major arteries of the head and neck and of thorax in following manner

- The greater part of the first and second arch arteries regresses. The remaining portion of the first and second arch artery forms maxillary and stapedial artery respectively.
- The fifth arch artery also regresses.
- The aortic sac after disappearance of first, second, and fifth arch arteries remains connected to arteries of third, fourth, and sixth arches.
- The third and fourth arch arteries open into ventral part and the sixth arch artery into dorsal part of aortic sac.
- The spiral septum which is formed in the truncus arteriosus extends into the aortic sac and fuses with its posterior wall. The orientation of spiral septum is in such manner that blood from pulmonary trunk passes only into the sixth arch artery, while that from ascending aorta passes into the third and fourth arch arteries.

The arterial arches follow a series of changes to attain the adult pattern (Fig. 3.2). They are as follows:

- The two dorsal aortae extend cranially, beyond the point of attachment of first artery.

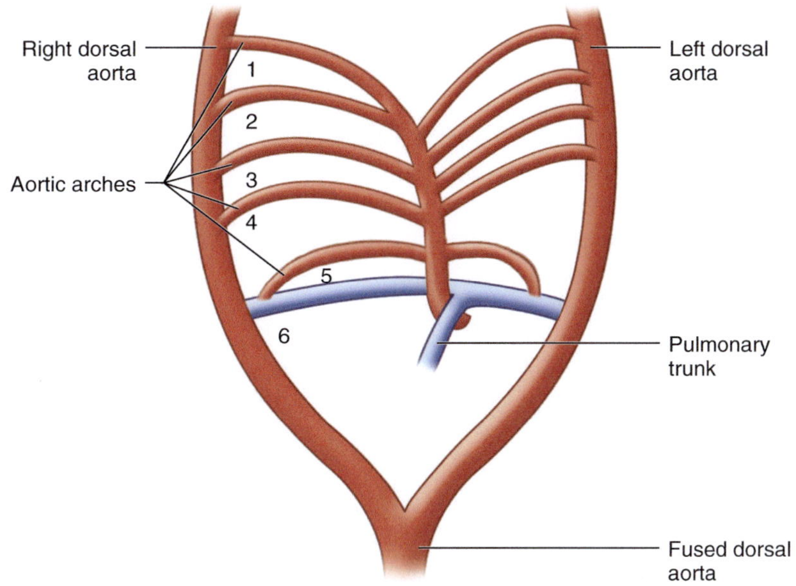

Fig. 3.1 Shows the relation of aortic arches with dorsal aorta. Each arch connects aortic sac to dorsal aorta. It is to be noted that all arches are never present at the same time. The sixth arch appears when first and second arches have regressed

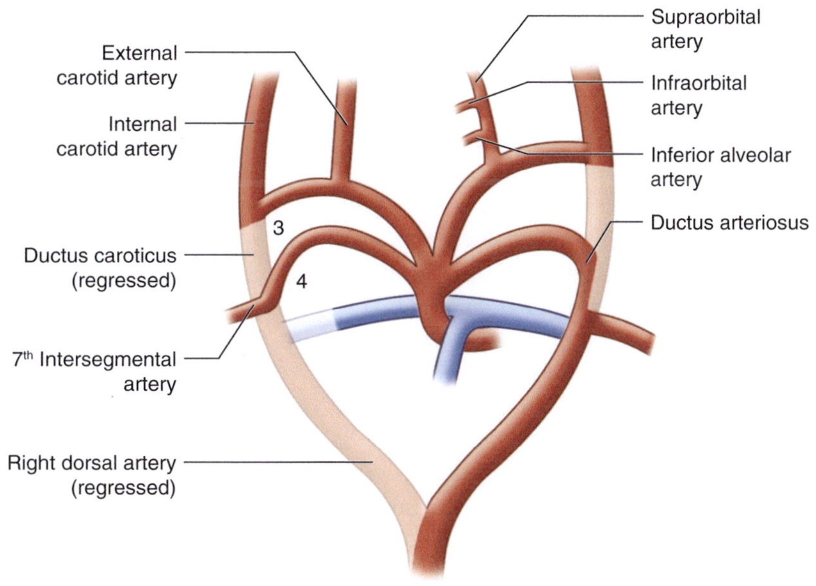

Fig. 3.2 Shows final fate of aortic arches

- The region of dorsal aorta between attachment of the third and fourth arteries (*ductus caroticus*), disappears on both sides.
- A bud arises from each third arch artery that grows cranially to form the external carotid artery.
- The segment of the right dorsal aorta located between the fourth arch artery and the fused dorsal aorta, disappears.
- Both the sixth arch artery gives off an artery to the developing lung bud.
- On the right side, the portion of the sixth arch artery lying between the lung bud and dorsal aorta disappears. On the left side this part remains patent to form *ductus arteriosus*. The ductus arteriosus is responsible for transport of blood from right ventricle to the dorsal aorta. It is obliterated

after birth and is then called *ligamentum arteriosum*.
- The dorsal aorta gives off numerous lateral intersegmental branches to the body wall. Out of these, the seventh cervical intersegmental artery supplies the upper limb bud.

The embryogenesis of the main arteries can be summarized as follows

- The *ascending aorta* and the *pulmonary trunk* arise from truncus arteriosus.
- The ventral part of the aortic sac, its left horn and left fourth arch artery forms the *arch of aorta.*
- The left dorsal aorta, below the attachment of fourth arch artery, along with fused median vessel forms the *descending aorta.*
- The right horn of aortic sac forms the *brachiocephalic artery.*
- Right fourth arch artery gives rise to proximal part of *right subclavian artery* whereas rest part of it is derived from the seventh cervical intersegmental artery.
- Unlike right subclavian artery, *left subclavian artery* is entirely derived from seventh cervical intersegmental artery.
- The *right and left common carotid artery* is derived from the respective part of third arch artery, proximal to external carotid bud.
- The *external carotid artery* arises as a bud from the third arch artery.
- The *internal carotid artery* is formed by the portion of the third arch artery distal to the bud, along with the original dorsal aorta cranial to the attachment of the third arch artery.
- The portion of sixth arch arteries lying between pulmonary trunk and branches to the lung bud will give rise to *pulmonary arteries.*

3.4 Anomalous Development of Pharyngeal Arch Arteries

Owing to the complex nature of the evolution and involution that occurs during the development of the major arteries and the fact that multiple processes must occur in a correct sequence, anomalous conditions of the aortic arch can occur. Some of these anomalies are as follows:

- *Double aortic arch* occurs when all parts of the right dorsal artery persist and this results in an arterial ring which may compress trachea and esophagus.
- *Right aortic arch.*
- *Interrupted aortic arch* occurs when both fourth aortic arches involute and then and the right dorsal artery caudal to the seventh intersegmental artery persists.
- The ductus arteriosus which normally should obliterate soon after birth may continue to remain patent *(patent ductus arteriosus*). It is one of the most common abnormalities occurring in around 8 out of 10,000 births [12].
- *Coarctation of aorta* is another commonly found anamoly with occurrence of 3.2 out of 10,000 births [12]. The aorta may show a localized narrowing of its lumen leading to complete or even partial obstruction to blood flow. The most common location is near the attachment of the ductus arteriosus to the aorta. This abnormality is classified into two types:
  - Preductal: proximal to the attachment.
  - Postductal: distal to the attachment.
- *Abnormal origin of the right subclavian artery* occurs when the right fourth aortic arch and a part of the right dorsal artery cranial to the seventh intersegmental artery involute and the right dorsal artery caudal to the seventh intersegmental artery persists.
- The ductus caroticus may persist. As a result, the left internal carotid arises directly from the aortic arch and the right internal carotid arises from subclavian artery.

3.5 Development of the Venous System

In the fourth week of gestation clusters of angiogenic cells aggregate together to form an extensive network of blood vessels throughout the embryonic body and then they establish a communication with extra embryonic vessels to create a primitive vascular system: the Vitelline–Umbilical–Cardinal vein system [13, 14].

The primitive vascular structure arranged in capillary and reticular plexuses is soon replaced by the newly developed paired *cardinal veins* as an axial, truncal venous system. The *vitelline* vessels arising from yolk sac develop into hepatic portal system. While the paired *umbilical* vessels present in the chorion and body stalk form the ductus venosus. All the three veins namely cardinal, vitelline, and umbilical drain into sinus venosus.

Vitelline veins are also known as omphalomesenteric veins.With the appearance of hepatic bud in septum transversum, the vitelline veins are divided into infrahepatic, intrahepatic, and suprahepatic parts (Fig. 3.3). As the liver develops in the septum transversum, proximal parts of the vitelline and umbilical veins are broken up to form numerous small channels that later on form sinusoids of liver. These sinusoids drain into the sinus venosus via terminal part of the vitelline veins that are now named as *right and left hepatocardiac channels*. The proximal portion of the umbilical veins lose their communication with the sinus venosus. Later on the left horn of the sinus venosus undergoes regression resulting in disappearance of left hepatocardiac channel. As a result the blood from vitelline and umbilical veins now enter the sinus venosus through right hepatocardiac channel (also known as common hepatic vein). This vein later on forms the cranial most portion of inferior vena cava.

With the regression of right umblical vein , all blood from the placenta reaches the developing liver via left umblical vein. A direct passage called ductus venosus is created by enlargement of some of the sinusoids and this passage connects the left umbilical vein to the right hepatocardiac channel. (Fig. 3.4).

The infrahepatic parts of the vitelline veins lie on left and right sides of developing duodenum. The two veins soon get connected with each other by means of three transverse Anastomosis. The cephalic and caudal Anastomosis lie ventral to duodenum and middle Anastomosis lie dorsal to duodenum. Thus forming a figure of eight around the U shaped duodenum. The superior mesenteric and splenic veins (which develop independently) join the left vitelline vein at a short distance caudal to dorsal anastomosis. Most of the parts of the vitelline vein involutes and what remains forms the left and right branch of portal vein along with the main trunk.

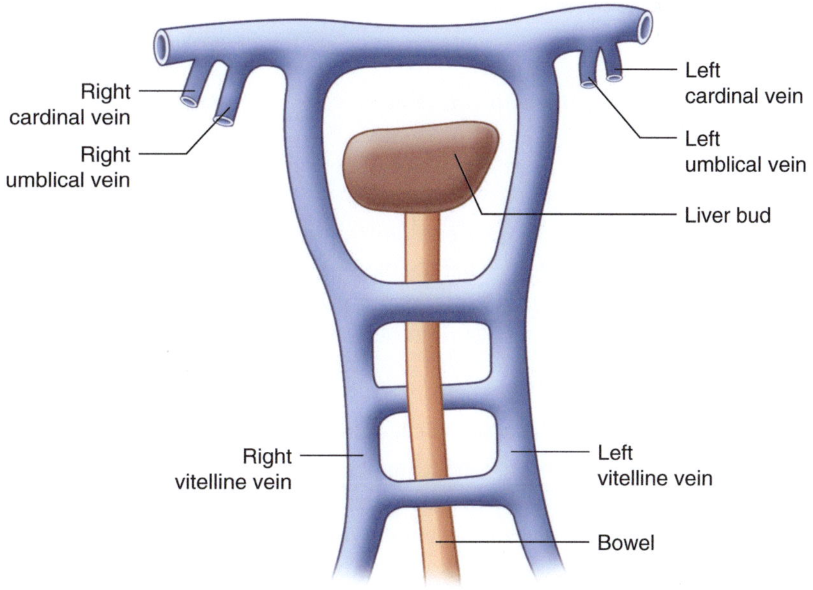

Fig. 3.3 Depicts the initial phase of development of portal vein. Right and left vitelline are joined by 3 transverse anastomosis upper ventral, middle dorsal and lower ventral

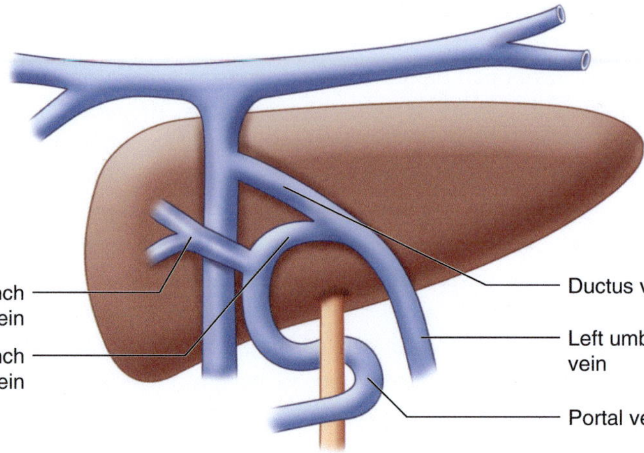

Fig. 3.4 Shows the final fate of portal vein which is formed by part of left vitelline vein, dorsal anastomosis and part of right vitelline vein. The upper ventral anastomosis becomes left branch of portal vein. Right vitelline vein cranial to upper ventral anastomosis forms right branchs of portal vein

The trunk of the portal vein is formed by

- Left vitelline vein between the entry of the superior mesenteric vein and splenic vein and the dorsal anastomosis.
- Dorsal anastomosis itself.
- The right vitelline vein located between dorsal anastomosis and the cranial ventral anastomosis.

Left branch of portal vein is formed by

- The cranial ventral anastomosis.
- A part of left vitelline vein cranial to cranial ventral anastomosis.

Right branch of portal vein is formed by

- Right vitelline vein cranial to cranial ventral anastomosis.

  The left umbilical vein now ends in the left branch of the portal vein whereas the ductus venosus connects the left branch of the portal vein to the inferior vena cava right hepatocardiac channel)

Cardinal veins are responsible for draining the blood to the embryo. The head, neck, upper torso and upper limbs are drained by bilateral *anterior cardinal veins* also known as *precardinal vein* whereas the caudal portion of the body (body and lower limbs) drains through bilateral *posterior cardinal veins* also known as *postcardinal veins* [15, 16].

The precardinal and postcardinal veins of each side unite to form the corresponding common cardinal vein (or duct of Cuvier), which opens into corresponding horns of the sinus venosus. The anterior cardinal veins join with the subclavian vein of respective sides to drain into the upper limbs. Later the anterior cardinal veins become interconnected by a transverse anastomosis proximal to their junction with subclavian veins. The part of left cardinal vein caudal to anastomosis along with left common cardinal disappears.

Superior vena cava is formed from right anterior cardinal vein, distal to the transverse anastomosis with the left anterior cardinal and right common cardinal vein.

Right brachiocephalic vein is formed from the right anterior cardinal vein, between the points of its joining with the subclavian vein and the point of joining with the transverse anastomosis.

Left brachiocephalic vein is derived from the part of left anterior cardinal vein located between point of junction with the subclavian vein and point of junction with the transverse anastomosis; and the transverse intercardinal anastomosis.

Internal jugular veins are derived from the portion of anterior cardinal veins cranial to their junction with the subclavian veins.

Similar to the intersegmental branches of dorsal aorta, the anterior and posterior cardinal veins receive a series of intersegmental veins from the body wall. The subclavian veins are formed by considerable enlargement of one of these veins in the region of the forelimb.

Near the caudal ends of posterior cardinal vein, the veins of the lower limb bud (external iliac) and of the pelvis (internal iliac) drains into it.. A transverse anastomosis is formed between the caudal ends of two posterior cardinal veins.

Subcardinal veins are formed in relation to mesonephros and receive the veins from developing kidneys. They communicate with posterior cardinal vein cranially and caudally. The two subcardinal are interconnected at the level of the renal veins by a transverse intersubcardinal anastomosis.

The cranial part of the right subcardinal vein also establishes an anastomosis with the right hepatocardiac channel.

Supracardinal veins (also known as thoracolumbar veins) like subcardinal vein communicate with posterior cardinal veins. They also form anastomosis with the subcardinal vein.

Many parts of these longitudinal venous channel involutes and what remains form inferior vena cava, renal veins, veins of gonads and suprarenal vein.

Inferior vena cava is derived from the following in caudal to cranial sequence (Fig. 3.5)

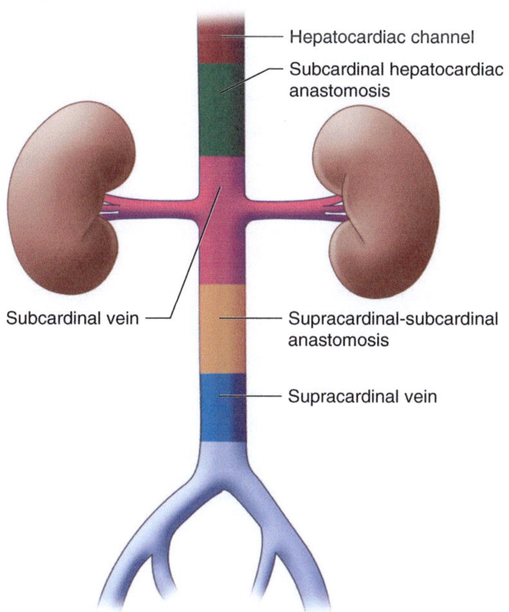

Fig. 3.5 Depicts the contribution of various structure with different colors in formation of inferior vena cava. Red: hepatocardiac channel. Green: subcardinal–hepatocardiac anastomosis. Purple: subcardinal vein. Orange: supracardinal–subcardinal anastomosis. Blue: supracardinal vein

- Inferiormost part of the right posterior cardinal vein (between its junction with the supracardinal, and the anastomosis between the two posterior cardinals).
- Inferior part of the right supracardinal vein (between its junction with the posterior cardinal, and the supracardinal–subcardinal anastomosis).
- Right supracardinal–subcardinal anastomosis.
- Right subcardinal vein (located between the supracardinal–subcardinal anastomosis and the anastomosis between the subcardinal vein and the right hepatocardiac channel). This forms the renal segment of the vena cava.
- Subcardinal–hepatocardiac anastomosis.
- Right hepatocardiac channel–forms the hepatic segment of inferior vena cava.

Common iliac Veins

- Left common iliac vein is formed froms the anastomosis between the two posterior cardinal veins.
- Right common iliac vein is formed from the most caudal part of the right posterior cardinal vein.

The azygous venous system is initially derived as veins of the azygous line which drain cranially into the posterior cardinal veins. The azygous vein is derived from the right supracardinal vein together with the distal portion of the right posterior cardinal vein to form the arch of azygous vein. The left supracardinal vein converts to hemiazygous vein and accessory azygous vein. The accessory hemiazygous vein drains into hemizygous vein and then the blood from hemiazygous vein is drained to azygous vein on right side and subsequently to superior vena cava.

The development of venous system in the lower extremities occur in three phases; [17, 18].

1. First phase: a lateral/posterior fibular (peroneal) vein detains the blood from lower limb to posterior cardinal vein; it is the first embryonic vein of the limb.
2. Second phase: the primitive peroneal vein develops two branches: the anterior tibial vein and the connecting branch. The anterior tibial

vein later on becomes the main deep vein of the calf. The anterior tibial vein along with primitive fibular veins together form sciatic vein which is the second embryonic vein. A small portion of primitive peroneal vein which lies distal to anterior tibial vein develops into short/lesser saphenous vein.

3. Third phase: a connecting branch arise from the middle of the sciatic vein and it connects with a new proximal medial vessel that will become the femoral vein (third embryonic vein) and forms the definitive deep venous system. The sciatic vein regresses. The femoral vein continues in leg as posterior tibial vein and is also the precursor of long/greater saphenous vein.

3.6 Anamolies of the Venous System

The complex involutional process of formation of superior vena cava from the three different cardinal veins makes it prone to defective development. *Double superior vena cava* occurs due to persistence of the left caudal anterior cardinal vein proximal to brachiocephalic anastomosis [19]. *Left superior vena cava* is the outcome that results from failure of retrogression of anterior and common cardinal veins. As a result the left superior vena cava opens into right atrium via a large coronary sinus. Due to the absence of the right proximal superior vena cava, the blood from right upper body drains into left superior vena cava via right brachiocephalic vein.

There are different congenital anamolies of the Inferior Vena Cava involving its length, location, duplication, abnormal connection and draining, etc. *Double inferior vena cava* occurs as a result of bilateral persistence of supracardinal and subcardinal veins [20, 21]. *Left inferior vena cava* occurs when there is caudal regression of the right supracardinal vein and left supracardinal vein persists to form inferior vena cava [22, 23]. In azygous continuation of inferior vena cava there is absence of hepatic segment of the inferior vena cava. It occurs due to nondevelopment of the anastomosis between the right subcardinal vein and the right hepatocardiac channel. In this condition the upper part of the inferior vena cava follows the course of the azygous vein and opens into the superior vena cava. The hepatic veins open into the right atrium at the usual site of the inferior vena cava.

Regarding the variations in lower limb veins; if defect occurs in second phase the primitive fibular vein will persist and become the marginal vein. This marginal vein is always valve less and can cause severe reflux leading to chronic venous hypertension/stasis as well as an increased risk of venous thrombosis and subsequent pulmonary embolism among Kilippel–Trenaunay syndrome patients [24, 25]. A defect in the third phase can lead to persistence of sciatic vein as the main vein draining the lower limb.

3.7 Development of the Lymphatic System

After the development of primitive vascular system, lymphatic system development begin in the sixth or seventh week of embryogenesis. The first sign of the lymphatic system are seen in the form of a number of endothelium lined lymph sacs which are derived from mesenchyme. There are six major lymph sacs that can be identified. The right and left jugular sacs lie near the junction of the anterior cardinal vein and subclavian veins (i.e., at the future junction between the internal jugular vein and subclavian vein. The right and left posterior (or iliac) sacs lie around the corresponding common iliac veins. The retroperitoneal sac is an unpaired sac and is located in relation to root of mesentery. Another unpaired sac is the *cisterna chyli* which lies in the midline at a distance caudal to the retroperitoneal sac. Lymphatic vessels are derived either by extension from the sacs or may form de novo and penetrate into various tissues. Later on all the sacs are converted to lymph nodes by the infiltration of connective tissue and lymphocytes except cisterna chyli. The *thoracic duct* develops from right and left channels that join the cisterna chyli to the corresponding jugular sac. The two channels anastomose across the midline. The thoracic duct is derived from the caudal part of the right channel, the anastomosis between the right and left channels and the cranial part of left channel. The cranial part of the right channel becomes the *right lymphatic duct*.

3.8 Anomalous Development of the Lymphatic System

The malformations in lymphatic system often manifest clinically as congenital or heredity lymphedema. Truncal lymphatic malformations do not always result in an evident morphological defect of the lymphatic system. In *Milroy–Meige syndrome* lymphedema occurs right after birth but there is no anatomical defect of the lymphatic system rather it is the functional impairment at the capillary lymphatic or initial lymphatic level [26]. In *lymphedema distichiasis syndrome* the endoluminal valves are defective leading to lymphatic reflux. Other clinical features associated with this syndrome are cleft palate, cardiac malformations, ptosis, double eyelashes and yellow nails.

References

1. Gladstone RJ. Development of the inferior vena cava in the light of recent research, with especial reference to certain abnormalities, and current description of the ascending lumber.
2. Barry A. The aortic arch derivatives in the human adult. Anat Rec. 1951;111:221–38.
3. Lee BB, Villavicencio L, Kim YW, et al. Primary Budd-Chiari syndrome: outcome of endovascular management for suprahepatic venous obstruction. J Vasc Surg. 2006;43:101–8.
4. Romagnoli R, Bertolani M, Saviano M, Pantusa M, Modena MG, Benassi A. Developmental interruption of the intra-hepatic segment of the inferior vena cava with azygos-hemiazygos continuation. Eur J Radiol. 1984;4:244–7.
5. Zamboni P, Galeotti R, Menegatti E, et al. Chronic cerebrospinal venous insufficiency in patients with multiple sclerosis. J NeurolNeurosurg Psychiatry. 2009;80:392–9.
6. Lee BB, Laredo J, Neville R. Embryological background of truncular venous malformation in the extracranial venous pathways as the cause of chronic cerebrospinal venous insufficiency. Int Angiol. 2010;29:95–108.
7. Leu HJ. Pathoanatomy of congenital vascular malformations. In: Belov S, Loose DA, Weber J, editors. Vascular Malformations, vol. 16. Reinbek, Germany: Einhorn-Presse Verlag; 1989. p. 37–46.
8. Woolard HH. The development of the principal arterial stems in the forelimb of the pig. ContribEmbryol. 1922;14:139–54.
9. Flamme I, Frolich T, Risau W. Molecular mechanisms of vasculogenesis and embryonic angiogenesis. J Cell Physiol. 1997;173:206–10.
10. Thoma R. Untersuchungenuber die histogenese und histomechnikdesgefasssystems. Stuttgart: Ferdinand Enke; 1893.
11. Murray PDF. The development in vivo of the blood of the early chick embryo. R Soc Med (London Ser B). 1932;3:497–521.
12. Sadler TW. Langman's medical embryology. 12th ed. Philadelphia: Lippincott Williams & Wilkins, a Wolters Kluwer business; 2012.
13. Langman J. Medical embryology. 5th ed. Baltimore, MD: Williams andWilkins; 1985. p. 212–7.
14. Warwick R, Williams P. Gray's Anatomy. 37th ed. Edinburgh, London,Melbourne, New York: Churchill Livingstone; 1989. p. 326–7.
15. Collins P. Embryology and development. In: Williams PL, Bannister LH, Berry MM, et al., editors. Gray's anatomy: the anatomical basis of medicine and surgery. 38th ed. Edinburgh: Churchill Livingston; 1995. p. 327.
16. Padget DH. The development of the cranial venous system in man, from the viewpoint of comparative anatomy. ContribEmbryolCarneg Inst Washington. 1957;36:79–140.
17. Lewis FT. The development of the veins in the limbs of rabbit embryo. Am J Anat. 1905;5:1–120.
18. Wyman J. On symmetry and homology in. Limbs. Proc Boston Soc Nat Hist. 1867;11:246–78.
19. Beattie J. The importance of anomalies of the superior vena cava in man. Canad Med AssocJ. 1931;25:281.
20. Hashmi ZA, Smaroff GG. Dual inferior vena cava: two inferior vena cava filters. Ann Thorac Surg. 2007;84:661663.
21. Esposito S, Mansueto G, Amodio F, et al. Duplication of the vena cava inferior with a continuation into the vena azygos. A report of a rare case. Minerva Chir. 1999;54:261–5.
22. Munechika H, Cohan RH, Baker ME, Cooper CJ, Dunnick NR. Hemiazygos continuation of a left inferior vena cava: CT appearance. J Comput Assist Tomogr. 1988;12:328–30.
23. Honma S, Tokiyoshi A, Kawai K, Koizumi M, Kodama K. Left inferior vena cava with regressed right inferior vena cava. AnatSci Int. 2008;83:173178.
24. Gloviczki P, Stanson AW, Stickler GB, et al. Trenaunay syndrome: the risks and benefits of vascular interventions. Surgery. 1991;110:469–79.
25. Noel AA, Gloviczki P, Cherry KJ Jr, Rooke TW, Stanson AW, Driscoll DJ, et al. Surgical treatment of venous malformations in Klippel-Trenaunay syndrome. J Vasc Surg. 2000;32:840847.
26. BB L. Lymphatic malformations. In: LL T, CL N, BB L, et al., editors. Lymphedema: diagnosis and treatment. London: Springer-Verlag; 2008. p. 31–42.

4 Classification: General Overview

BB Lee and James Laredo

Congenital vascular malformation (CVM) is a unique clinical condition as the result of defective development during various stages of embryogenesis of the circulation system. Hence, CVM represents a group of "birth defects" involving any part of the entire circulation system: arterial, venous, lymphatic, and capillary [1, 2]. It may therefore, present either as an independent lesion affecting only one of three circulation systems (e.g., venous malformation) or as a mixed lesion of two or three different types of CVMs affecting more than one circulation system (e.g., hemolymphatic malformation) [1–4].

CVM presents as an abnormal vascular structure anywhere throughout the body in different conditions, shapes, extents, and severities, with different characteristics and behaviors depending upon the circulation system involved and its location [1–4]. Due to such a wide range of clinical presentations with extreme variety and degree of severity and location, the CVM remains with a notorious reputation as a most difficult and confusing diagnostic and therapeutic clinical entity among the vascular disorders. Indeed, the CVM has been known as an enigma in modern medicine due to unpredictable clinical courses by its embryonic characteristics with the erratic response to treatment with high recurrence adding endless confusion.

Since the turn of the last Century, many clinicians challenged this enigma based on their limited knowledge and described most CVMs based on the clinical findings alone and named after the clinicians who described them (e.g., Klippel and Trenaunay syndrome). However, these name-based eponyms (e.g., Servelle and Martorell syndrome; Sturge–Weber–Krabbe syndrome) failed to provide proper anatomical and pathophysiological information to define the critical characteristics among the CVMs [5–8].

Such name-based eponyms as the base of old classification did not take into account the etiology, anatomy, and pathophysiology so that it added more confusion to resulting in often mistaken terminology (e.g., cavernous/capillary hemangioma versus infantile/neonatal hemangioma) [9, 10]. Hence, a new classification system based on accurate anatomic, embryologic, and pathophysiologic information of the CVMs was mandated for appropriate diagnosis and treatment with modern concepts [11–14].

A consensus workshop was held in Hamburg in 1988 to seek a new, more logical classification

B. Lee (✉)
Department Surgery, George Washington University, Washington, DC, USA

Center for the Lymphedema and Vascular Malformation, George Washington University, Washington, DC, USA

Uniformed Services University of the Health Sciences, Bethesda, MD, USA

J. Laredo
Department Surgery, George Washington University, Washington, DC, USA

A. K. Khanna, S. K. Tiwary (eds.), *Vascular Malformations*, https://doi.org/10.1007/978-981-15-9762-6_4

system and a new effort to replace the old name-based eponyms bore two new classifications to meet the needs for contemporary management of the CVMs [2–4, 15, 16].

A new era for modern classification of the CVMs began with two new classifications following the Hamburg Consensus to seek for precise evaluation, diagnosis, and therapeutic implementation: Hamburg Classification [17–20] and ISSVA* Classification [21–24].

* ISSVA: International Society for the Study of Vascular Anomalies.

4.1 Hamburg Classification [17–20] (Table 4.1)

In 1988, St. Belov initiated a consensus conference in Hamburg, Germany to create a classification of congenital vascular malformations, which should be simple, clearly arranged, comprehensible, and implementable in clinical practice.

Malan and Puglionisi proposed a new classification to distinguish the difference among venous, arterial, and other associated malformations [11–14] stating that "vascular malformations were differentiated into a number of anatomo-clinical pictures, each with a precise definition of the vascular abnormality, of its evolution and of the therapeutic possibilities," which served as the basis of the Hamburg Classification and ISSVA Classification.

Malan further introduced the concept of the "predominant type of the involved vessel" since he noticed that very rarely only one type of vessel is affected alone in vascular malformations and in most cases multiple vessels/vascular systems get involved.

Based on the involvement of the main vessel trunks, they identified two different types of lesions: lesions with a direct communication with the main vessel trunks, named as "truncular" forms, and lesions occurring peripherally as separate defects with no direct involvement of main trunk of the vessels, named as "extratruncular" forms.

Belov et al. borrowed an old embryologic term: "extratruncular," from the old embryology school (Sabin F.R. 1917) [25] and introduced back to describe the lesions remaining as vascular tissue clusters derived from the "early stage" of embryogenesis [17–20], which stopped the confusion by *misleading* old term of "angioma" (c.f. hemangioma).

For the lesions derived from the "later stage" of embryogenesis for the vascular trunk formation [1–4], they also borrowed the embryologic term: "truncular" (Woolard H.H.1922), since the lesions are directly involved to the main trunk of often "named" vessels (e.g., iliac-femoral) [26].

Accordingly, the Hamburg Classification was formulated based on the consensus through the Hamburg workshop as a new classification to replace old concept and adopted this new interpretation of the CVM lesions based on embryological characteristics as an outcome of the developmental arrest of the vascular system during two different stages of angiogenesis. Its initial definition was further modified later to add the capillary/microvascular form known as the

Table 4.1 Hamburg classification of congenital vascular malformations (CVMs)

Primary classification[a]
• Arterial malformation
• Venous malformation
• Arteriovenous malformation
• Lymphatic malformation
• Capillary/microvascular malformation
• Combined vascular malformation: Hemolymphatic malformation
Embryological subclassification[b]
Extratruncular forms (former "angioma")
• Diffuse, infiltrating
• Limited, localized
Truncular forms
• Obstruction and/or stenosis
– Aplasia; hypoplasia; hyperplasia
– Membrane; congenital spur
• Dilatation
– Localized (aneurysm)
– Diffuse (ectasia)

[a]Modified based on the consensus on CVM through the international workshop in Hamburg, Germany 1988 and Seoul, Korea 1995

[b]Developmental arrest at the different stages of embryonal life: earlier stage—extratruncular form; latter stage—truncular form

[b]Both forms may exist together; may be combined with other various malformations (e.g., capillary, arterial, AV shunting, venous, hemolymphatic, and/or lymphatic); and/or may exist with hemangioma

"modified" Hamburg Classification. (Table 4.1) and now accepted worldwide and recommended for contemporary management of the CVMs [2–4, 24–27].

One of the most notable contributions of Hamburg Classification is it removed the decade long confusions caused by the term of "angioma" (e.g., cavernous/capillary hemangioma) once and for all; this new classification distinguished two morphologically different lesions; one remaining peripherally with no direct involvement of the vessel trunk, previously called "angioma," and another involving the main vessel trunks per se, based on the embryologically different characteristics as the "extratruncular" and "truncular" lesions [28–31].

Extratuncular lesions, regardless of the type of the CVM, present clinically as a cluster of amorphous vascular tissue as an embryonic tissue remnant of an "undifferentiated capillary network," arising from the "*earlier*" stages of embryogenesis where the primitive vascular structures are still in the reticular plexiform stage. Hence, all the extratruncular lesions will possess mesenchymal cell characteristics with the unique evolutional potential to grow when stimulated. [8, 9, 32–35] On contrary, *Truncular* lesions are the result of defective development that occurs during the "*later*" stages of embryogenesis so that they no longer possess this evolutional potential (e.g., popliteal aneurysm) [30, 31, 36, 37].

Indeed, Malan and Belov convinced the concept that the truncular and the extratruncular forms are the results of a defect in the embryonic phase of development of the vessels, based on the morphological observation. However, the relationship between vessel embryology and genetic mutations affecting vessel development would need to be further clarified based on the recent data on genetic mutations involving vascular malformation pathogenesis obtained through molecular- and genetic research [2–4]. Nevertheless, the relationship/linkage between the process of vasculogenesis and the classification of vascular malformation based on anatomical and pathological characteristics will remain the same regardless of the genetic mutation involved [2, 3].

4.2 ISSVA Classification [21–24] (Tables 4.2 and 4.3)

Following the Hamburg Consensus workshop, Mulliken et al. also established another new concept to lead a new classification system for "vascular anomaly" as a whole. On the contrary to the Hamburg Classification limited its scope only to the vascular malformations, this new classification accommodated both vascular tumors and vascular malformations together under the one umbrella/classification [21–24].

Another word, despite vascular malformation and vascular tumors representing the group of hemangiomas is two entirely different vascular disorders with distinctly different anatomical, histological, and pathophysiological characteristics and clinical behavior, both were classified as "Vascular Anomalies." Subsequently, this new classification accommodating both vascular tumors that proliferate and vascular malformations that are developmental aberrations was adopted by ISSVA (International Society for the Study of Vascular Anomalies) officially as the ISSVA Classification (1996) [2–4, 34, 35, 38, 39].

For the first time, through ISSVA Classification, the term "hemangioma" was correctly designated only for the "vascular tumor" of benign nature that originates from endothelial cells. And its use is limited only to the group of "infantile/neonatal" hemangioma and "con-

Table 4.2 ISSVA Classification of CVM—Original

Vascular Malformations:
• Fast-flow lesions:
• Arterial malformation (AM)
• Arteriovenous malformation (AVM)
• Arteriovenous fistula (AVF)
• Slow-flow lesions:
• Capillary malformation CM (port-wine stain, telangiectasia, angiokeratoma).
– Venous malformation (VM)
– Lymphatic malformation (LM)
• Combined vascular malformation (CVM, CLM, CLVM, CAVM, CLAVM)
Vascular Tumors:
• Infantile hemangioma
• Congenital hemangioma
• Others

Table 4.3 ISSVA Classification of Vascular Anomalies, 2014 Updated

Vascular Anomalies				
Vascular tumors	Vascular malformations			
	Simple	Combined	Of major named vessels	Associated with other anomalies
Benign Locally aggressive or borderline Malignant	Capillary malformations Lymphatic malformations Venous malformations Arteriovenous malformations Arteriovenous fistula	Capillary-venous, Capillary-lymphatic, Lymphatic venous, Capillary-lymphatic-venous, Capillary-arteriovenous, capillary-lymphatic-arteriovenous	(aka "channel-type" or "truncal" vascular malformations) Further characterized by involvement of artery, lymphatic, or vein, And by anomaly of origin, course, number, length, diameter, etc.	For example, Klippel Trenaunay Sturge–Weber Mafucci CLOVES Proteus Bannayan-Riley-Rubacalva Others

Benign vascular tumors
Infantile hemangioma/hemangioma of infancy Congenital hemangioma Rapidly involuting (RICH) [a] Non-involuting (NICH) Partially involuting (PICH) Tufted angioma [a] [°] Spindle-cell hemangioma Epithelioid hemangioma Pyogenic granuloma (aka lobular capillary hemangioma) Others
Locally aggressive or borderline vascular tumors Kaposiform hemangioendothelioma [a] [°] Retiform hemangioendothelioma Papillary intralymphatic angioendothelioma (PILA), Dabska tumor Composite hemangioendothelioma Kaposi sarcoma Others
Malignant vascular tumors Angiosarcoma Epithelioid hemangioendothelioma Others

issva.org/classification for the interactive comprehensive classification
°Many experts believe that these are part of a spectrum rather than distinct entities
N.B. Reactive proliferative vascular lesions are listed with benign tumors
[a]Some lesions may be associated with thrombocytopenia and/or consumptive coagulopathy see details

genital" hemangioma. Indeed, the term "hemangioma" had been misused over many decades to describe the CVMs (e.g., "cavernous/capillary" hemangioma) erroneously adding the confusion [9, 10].

"Hemangioma" is a vascular tumor that originates from the endothelial cells and it is not the result of defective development like vascular malformation; it is therefore appears in the early neonatal period in its majority as a de novo lesion which did not exist on birth like an inborn error. Hemangioma has also a distinctive growth cycle characterized by a proliferation phase of early rapid growth followed by an involutional phase of slow regression [34, 35, 38, 39]. A majority of hemangioma has "self-limited" growth and subsequent involution occurs usually before the age of 5–10 years (cf. CVMs).

On contrary, the vascular malformation is an inborn vascular defect as the result of defective embryologic development so that it is generally recognizable on birth. As embryologic tissue remnants, it possesses the unique characteristic of "self-perpetuating" growth so that it tends to grow continuously at a proportional rate to the growth rate of the body regardless of its type and will never regress (cf. hemangioma).

ISSVA Classification classified the vascular malformation based on the flow status; Fast and Slow flow. The arteriovenous (AV) malformation was further subclassified to "AV Fistula and AV malformation," despite both of which represent [21] same AV malformation but derived from two different stages of embryogenesis, which is appropriately classified by the Hamburg Classification.

Such classification of the AV malformation into "AV fistula (AVF) and AV malformation (AVM)" allows a misunderstanding to recognize them as two different AVMs, one as *fistulous* and another as *non-fistulous*, and mistakenly identify the AVM group of ISSVA Classification as a "non-fistulous" lesion [4, 16, 40]. Indeed, all the AVMs regardless of its type, truncular or extratruncular, are "fistulous" condition to allow the arteriovenous shunting due to the lack of normal physiological capillary system development.

The "AVF" lesion defined by ISSVA Classification is equivalent to the "truncular" form of AV malformation lesion, defined by the Hamburg Classification, to allow direct communication between the artery and vein with no nidus in between (e.g., Ductus Botalli, pulmonary AVM). And the "AVM" defined by ISSVA Classification is equivalent to the "extratruncular" AVM lesion with various conditions of the nidus, correctly defined by the Hamburg Classification [16, 40].

Lately, ISSVA Classification recognized the value of original concept of "extratruncular and truncular" lesions belatedly, adopting/quoting the term "truncular" for the lesions involved to the major vessels. Indeed, "truncular" lesion was defined by Woolard (1922) based on the embryological concept with the two stages of embryogenesis [26]. But, disappointingly, the updating of ISSVA Classification done lately [23] failed to adopt the second embryologic term: "extratruncular" as well to properly name/define two morphologically and functionally different groups of CVMs as truncular and extratruncular forms as done by Hamburg Classification, ignoring the critical difference on its clinical implication.

In addition, many name-based eponyms (e.g., Klippel Trenaunay Syndrome) through the last century were remained/adopted by the ISSVA classification as a part of "syndromic" form of vascular malformations mainly for the role of the coexisting non-vascular anomaly. So, naturally it also inherited much liability of century-old confusion at the same time. Indeed, such name-based classifications and syndromes have been strongly advocated to be abandoned by many experts in order to reduce ongoing confusion through many decades (e.g., Hamburg Consensus Workshop of 1988).

Although the major advantage of ISSVA Classification remains in differentiating vascular tumors/hemangiomas from the vascular malformations, this complexity of continued use of numerous name-based syndromes as a part of a new vascular malformation classification undoubtedly becomes a major liability to this excellent classification system, limiting its capability of clinical implementation in the management of vascular malformations [2, 16].

Hence, further improvement of the current classification system which is far from perfect is mandated as our knowledge of the etiology, anatomy, embryology, histo-pathophysiology, hemodynamics, and genetics in the field of vascular anomaly continues to advance [2].

References

1. Lee BB, Laredo J, Lee TS, Huh S, Neville R. Terminology and classification of congenital vascular malformations. Phlebology. 2007;22(6):249–52.
2. Lee BB, Baumgartner I, Berlien P, Bianchini G, Burrows P, Gloviczki P, Huang Y, Laredo J, Loose DA, Markovic J, Mattassi R, Parsi K, Rabe E, Rosenblatt M, Shortell C, Stillo F, Vaghi M, Villavicencio L, Zamboni P. Diagnosis and treatment of venous malformations consensus document of the International Union of Phlebology (IUP): updated 2013. Int Angiol. 2015;34(2):97–149.
3. Lee BB, Antignani PL, Baraldini V, Baumgartner I, Berlien P, Blei F, Carrafiello GP, Grantzow R, Ianniello A, Laredo J, Loose D, Lopez Gutierrez JC, Markovic J, Mattassi R, Parsi K, Rabe E, Roztocil K,

Shortell C, Vaghi M. ISVI-IUA consensus document - diagnostic guidelines on vascular anomalies: vascular malformations and hemangiomas. Int Angiol. 2015;34(4):333–74.
4. Lee BB, Baumgartner I, Berlien HP, Bianchini G, Burrows P, Do YS, Ivancev K, Kool LS, Laredo J, Loose DA, Lopez-Gutierrez JC, Mattassi R, Parsi K, Rimon U, Rosenblatt M, Shortell C, Simkin R, Stillo F, Villavicencio L, Yakes W. Consensus document of the International Union of Angiology (IUA)-2013. Current concept on the management of arterio-venous management. Int Angiol. 2013 Feb;32(1):9–36.
5. Lee BB, Laredo J, Lee SJ, Huh SH, Joe JH, Neville R. Congenital vascular malformations: general diagnostic principles. Phlebology. 2007;22(6):253–7.
6. Lee BB. Changing concept on vascular malformation: no longer enigma. Ann Vasc Dis. 2008;1(1):11–9.
7. Lee BB, Kim HH, Mattassi R, Yakes W, Loose D, Tasnadi G. A new approach to the congenital vascular malformation with a new concept: how the pioneer prof. Stefan Belov enlightened us through the Seoul consensus. Int J Angiol. 2003;12:248–51.
8. Lee BB. Critical issues on the management of congenital vascular malformation. Annals Vasc Surg. 2004;18(3):380–92.
9. Lee BB. Venous malformation and haemangioma: differential diagnosis, diagnosis, natural history and consequences. Phlebology. 2013;28(Suppl 1):176–87.
10. Lee BB, Laredo J. Hemangioma and venous/vascular malformation are different as an apple and orange! Editorial. ACTA PHLEBOL. 2012;13:1–3.
11. Malan E, Puglionisi A. Congenital angiodysplasias of the extremities, note II: arterial, arterial and venous, and hemolymphatic dysplasias. J Cardiovasc Surg. 1965;6:255–345.
12. Malan E. History and nosography. In: Malan E, editor. Vascular malformations (Angiodysplasias). Milan, Italy: Carlo Erba Foundation; 1974. p. 15–9.
13. Villavicencio JL. Congenital vascular malformations: historical background. Special Issue: Phlebology. 2007;22:247–8.
14. Malan E, Puglionisi A. Congenital angiodysplasia of the extremities. Note I: generalities and classification; venous dysplasias. J Card Surg. 1964;5:87–130.
15. Lee BB, Laredo J. Classification of congenital vascular malformations: the last challenge for congenital vascular malformations. Phlebology. 2012;27(6):267–9.
16. Lee BB. New classification of congenital vascular malformations (CVMs). Rev Vasc Med. 2015;3(3):1–5.
17. Belov S. Classification of congenital vascular defects. Int Angiol. 1990;9:141–6.
18. Belov S. Classification, terminology, and nosology of congenital vascular defects. In: Belov S, Loose DA, Weber J, editors. Vascular Malformations. Reinbek, Germany: Einhorn-Presse; 1989. p. 25–30.
19. St B. Anatomopathological classification of congenital vascular defects. Semin Vasc Surg. 1993;6:219–24.
20. Van Der Stricht J. Classification of vascular malformations. In: St B, Loose DA, Weber J, editors. Vascular Malformations. Reinbek: Einhorn-Presse Verlag GmbH; 1989. p. 23.
21. Enjolras O, Wassef M, Chapot R. Introduction: ISSVA classification. In: Color atlas of vascular tumors and vascular malformations. New York: Cambridge University Press; 2007. p. 1–11.
22. Mulliken JB, Glowacki J. Hemangiomas and vascular malformations in infants and children: a classification based on endothelial characteristics. Plast Reconstr Surg. 1982;69:412–22.
23. Wassef M, Blei F, Adams D, Alomari A, Baselga E, Berenstein A, et al. Vascular anomalies classification: recommendations from the International Society for the Study of vascular anomalies. Pediatrics. 2015;136(1):e203–14.
24. Mulliken JB. Classification of vascular birthmarks. In: Mulliken JB, Young AE, editors. Vascular birthmarks: Hemangiomas and malformations. Philadelphia: WB Saunders; 1988. p. 24–37.
25. Sabin FR. Origin and development of the primitive vessels of the chick and of the pig. Cont Embriol Carnegie Inst. 1917;6-7:61–7.
26. Woolard HH. The development of the principal arterial stems in the forelimb of the pig. Contrib Embryol. 1922;14:139–54.
27. Bastide G, Lefebvre D. Anatomy and organogenesis and vascular malformations. In: Belov S, Loose DA, Weber J, editors. Vascular malformations. Reinbek: Einhorn-Presse Verlag GmbH; 1989. p. 20–2.
28. Lee BB, Laredo J. Venous malformation: treatment needs a bird's eye view. Phlebology. 2013;28:62–3.
29. Lee BB, Bergan J, Gloviczki P, Laredo J, Loose DA, Mattassi R, Parsi K, Villavicencio JL, Zamboni P. Diagnosis and treatment of venous malformations - consensus document of the International Union of Phlebology (IUP)-2009. Int Angiol. 2009 December;28(6):434–51.
30. Leu HJ. Pathoanatomy of congenital vascular malformations. In: Belov S, Loose DA, Weber J, editors. Vascular malformations, vol. 16. Reinbek, Germany: Einhorn-Presse Verlag; 1989. p. 37–46.
31. Lewis FT. Development of the veins in the limbs of rabbit embryos. Am J Anat. 1906;5:113–20.
32. Lee BB, Laredo J, Kim YW, Neville R. Congenital vascular malformations: general treatment principles. Phlebology. 2007;22(6):258–63.
33. Lee BB. Advanced management of congenital vascular malformation (CVM). Int Angiol. September 2002;21(3):209–13.
34. Mulliken JB. Cutaneous vascular anomalies. Semin Vasc Surg. 1993;6:204–18.
35. Boon LM, Enjolras O, Mulliken JB. Congenital hemangioma: evidence of accelerated involution. J Pediatr. 1996;128:329–35.
36. Lee BB. Venous embryology: the key to understanding anomalous venous conditions. Phlebolymphology. 2012;19(4):170–81.

37. Lee BB, Laredo J, Neville R. Embryological background of truncular venous malformation in the extracranial venous pathways as the cause of chronic cerebrospinal venous insufficiency. Int Angiol. 2010 April;29(2):95–108.
38. Enjolras O, Riche MC, Merland JJ, Escandej P. Management of alarming hemangiomas in infancy: a review of 25 cases. Pediatrics. 1990;85:491–8.
39. Mulliken JB. Treatment of hemangiomas. In: Mulliken JB, Young AE, editors. Vascular birthmarks, Hemangiomas and malformations. Philadelphia, Pa: WB Saunders; 1988. p. 88–90.
40. Lee BB, Lardeo J, Neville R. Arterio-venous malformation: how much do we know? Phlebology. 2009;24:193–200.

5 Approach to a Case of Vascular Malformation

Mohd Zeeshan Hakim and Ajay K. Khanna

5.1 Introduction

Vascular Malformations are often misdiagnosed, misinterpreted, and neglected in general practice; their nomenclature has often been after the names of their discoverers, like Klippel–Trenaunay, Maffucci, Parkes–Weber, while few have origins after Latin or Greek terms, eponyms such as "port-wine stains," "strawberry hemangioma" have rapidly gained popularity in the past.

A practical approach encompasses a thorough evaluation and examination. Identifying the origin of the malformation in lymphatic, arterial, and venous system is as important as understanding the nature of the lesion (proliferative versus non-proliferative, involuting or causing hemodynamic effects) and predicting the response to therapy. The biological classification first introduced by Mulliken and Glowackzi [1], later adopted and amended by the International Society for the Study of Vascular Anomalies (ISSVA) (Table 5.1) has been used frequently to classify the lesions on the basis of their biological behavior, i.e., proliferative lesions or tumors and non-proliferative lesions or malformations [2]. Various other classifications have been discussed in this book, which have served to further stratify the anomalies. Of note, the flow rate is an important perspective and terms such as low flow and high flow lesions more frequently encountered both in practice and in the classifications. The classification by Hamburg detailed the subdivisions into Truncal and Extra-Truncal Malformations to signify the clinical difference in their presentation and outcomes.

Our current approach discusses the various types of vascular anomalies and their diagnosis in view of providing a general outline, Hemangiomas have also been described as part of the anomalies, as they need to be differentiated from vascular malformations (Table 5.2).

Table 5.1 ISSVA classification of Vascular Malformations and Vascular Tumors

Vascular Malformations
Fast flow lesions
• Arterial malformations
• Arteriovenous malformations
• Arteriovenous fistula
Slow flow lesions
• Capillary malformations (port-wine stains, telangiectasia)
• Venous malformation
• Lymphatic malformation
Combined vascular malformations
Vascular Tumors
Infantile hemangiomas
Congenital hemangiomas
Others

M. Z. Hakim (✉)
General Surgery, Trauma Center, Institute of Medical Sciences, Banaras Hindu University, Varanasi, India

A. K. Khanna
Department of Surgery, Institute of Medical Science, Banaras Hindu University, Varanasi, India

A. K. Khanna, S. K. Tiwary (eds.), *Vascular Malformations*,
https://doi.org/10.1007/978-981-15-9762-6_5

Table 5.2 Modified Hamburg classification of vascular malformations

Primary Classification	Embryological Classification
1. Arterial malformations	*Extra-Truncal*
2. Venous malformations	– diffuse
3. Arterio-venous malformations	– limited
4. Capillary malformations	*Truncal*
5. Lymphatic malformations	– obstructing/narrowing
6. Combined vascular malformations	– stenosis by hypoplasia/ Coarctation/spurs
	– dilation (aneurysm/ Ectasia)

5.1.1 Molecular Basis of Vascular Anomalies

Much is to be understood behind the genetic and molecular basis of vascular anomalies; *germline mutations* in genes for tyrosine kinase receptor TIE2, angiopoietins1,2 platelet-derived growth factor-2 and have also been found in venous malformations themselves; in arteriovenous malformations such as ENDOGLN, ACTIVIN RECEPTOR-LIKE KINASE 1[ALK1], RASA1, SMAD4 (in patients with HHT), PTEN hamartoma syndromes (including Cowden's syndrome, Bannayan–Riley–Ruvalcaba Syndrome) and many more mutations are frequently noted.

The development of AVMs following trauma or venous thrombosis is another aspect of the study that is being researched. Histochemical evidence of increased activity of endothelial receptors for growth factors, upregulation of VEGF, MMP-9, and inflammatory markers have also been noted [3].

Brouillard Pet al [4]. noted that several patients with familial lymphedema have been noted to have mutations in VEGFR3/FLT4, VEGFD, FOXC2, CCBE1, SOX18, and others.

Somatic mutations occur in the zygote rather than being transmitted by the parental genes, these mutations have also been implicated in several vascular anomalies. In particular, the presence of mosaic expression of somatic GNAQ mutation as deduced by Shirley et al. [5] in cutaneous capillary malformations associated with Sturge–Weber Syndrome and Port-wine stains serves as an example.

Similarly, Patients with Parkes–Weber Syndrome (capillary malformation, arteriovenous malformation, soft tissue overgrowth), Sturge–Weber syndrome (facial capillary malformation in trigeminal distribution, leptomeningeal angiomatosis, glaucoma, and seizures) and Proteus Syndrome (asymmetric progressive, disproportionate overgrowth syndrome, hyperostosis, cerebriform connective tissue nevus, vascular malformation, cystic lung disease) have been found to have somatic mutations associated with RASA1, GNAQ, and AKT1 mutations. [LINDHURST MJ et al., 2011]. Sapp et al. in 2017 described the syndrome of Congenital Lipomatous Overgrowth, Vascular Malformation, Epidermal nevus, scoliosis (CLOVES), which has PIK3CA somatic mutation (termed PROS-"PIK3CA-related overgrowth spectrum," includes both vascular and non-vascular anomalies), common with Klippel– Trenaunay Syndrome and the gene pathway has been utilized in studies using sirolimus for therapeutic purposes in these mutations as a prospect for future use.

These findings will nonetheless favor towards a genetic model, which may be utilized to identify particular gene mutations at the germ line level and correct it beforehand or by modify its expression, reduce their deleterious effects (Fig. 5.1).

5.1.2 Clinical Presentation

A thorough history and clinical examination should always precede any investigation. Detail of to the time of onset, whether since birth or in the first year of life helps in identifying whether the lesion is congenital or infantile, the rate of growth is also important. The presentation in newborn, infants, children, and adults differ remarkably in their symptoms and signs. The rapidly involuting and non-involuting congenital hemangioma is an exceptional case, since they demonstrate high proliferation in-utero occasion-

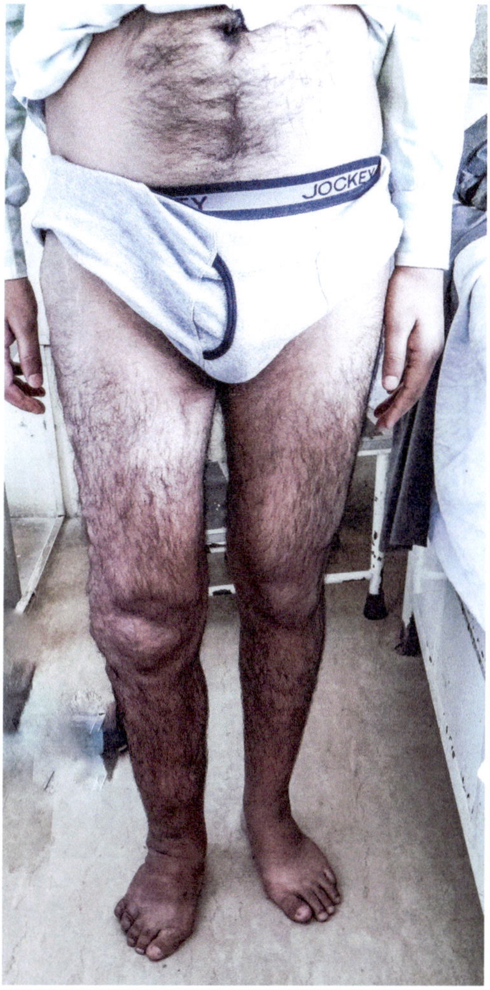

Fig. 5.1 A patient with Klippel–Trenaunay Syndrome

ally leading to high output states and thrombocytopenia.

In a Mayo Clinic Study by Schwartz et al., of the 185 cases with vascular malformations enrolled, the most common sign was found to be skin discoloration (43%) and the most common symptom was pain (37%), while 34% had limb hypertrophy, 35% had a palpable mass. 20% had a skin ulceration or necrosis and 26% had an audible bruit. The presence of additional signs such as increased skin temperature, decreased distal pulsations, and edema with pulsatile veins were also noted.

The physical examination should include a thorough systematic inspection, palpation, and auscultation of the lesion, be it arterial, venous, lymphatic, or mixed. Palpation of pulses, systolic blood pressure assessment in all four limbs, noting visible varicosities in the affected extremity, and complete assessment up to the trunk, it is imperative that the patient should be fully informed and completely exposed to track all the visible abnormal vessels, often pulsatile vessels can be noted in large malformations, apart from this, the skin must also be examined for the presence of superficial thrombophlebitis, edema, skin color and pigmentation, temperature, presence of ulcers, digit loss (often seen with large malformations), atrophic and hypertrophic changes to the entire limb, which may hint towards multiple system anomalies than an isolated vascular anomaly. Clinical progress of lesions should always be documented with photographs that help keep track of the size and changes. Patients with pelvic involvement often present with hematuria or rectal bleeds.

"Growth spurts" are often the time when the limb length discrepancies can become highlighted, Puberty is a triggering factor that may cause progression in a previously quiescent vascular anomaly, Kulungowski et al. [6] found an increased expression of hormone receptors on various arterial, venous, and lymphatic malformations, suggesting that puberty related development of these malformations as a result of hormonal changes.

Two important clinical implications that can result from large malformations and high flow lesions are the development of heart failure due to significantly large AV malformation that results in large preload to the right heart as a consequence of reduced systemic vascular resistance; this is often compensated initially by an increase in circulating volume and heart rate, but is later followed by a gradual enlargement of the heart and ultimately, without intervention cardiac failure becomes inevitable. Another phenomenon (steal) is the short circuiting of blood in a more proximal lesion causing distal limb vascularity to be compromised, may vary from mild ischemic changes to frank ulceration and gangrene of the extremity distal to the malformation. Often described as a classical sign of AV fistula with

Table 5.3 Differentiating between a Hemangioma (Vascular Tumor) and a Vascular Malformation

	Hemangioma	Vascular Malformation
Biological nature	Vascular tumors (proliferative)	Non-proliferative
Age at presentation	Birth/infancy	Variable, may present at birth or early adulthood
Categories	Focal/segmental, superficial/deep	Arterial/venous/capillary, Truncal/extra-truncal
Clinical appearance	Discolored/pinkish nodules, plaques, patches	Superficial lesions as cluster of vessels, pulsations may be visible with AVM, bluish discolored veins soft compressible in venous malformations, deep-seated lesion present as audible bruits or as venous edema of extremity
Natural history	Proliferative and involution phases	Tend to grow proportionately with age, disproportionate growth at pregnancy/adolescence, rarely involute
Duplex findings	Proliferative: High flow Involution: Low flow	High/low flow depending on arteriovenous/ venous/ lymphatic
MR angiography	Proliferative: Low signal intensity lobulated mass on T1 and high intensity on T2 weighted images, flow voids with T1 SE Involution: High signal intensity masses on T1	AVM: Demarcated feeding vessels and abnormal venous return venous malformation: Low signal intensity in T1 weighted images, high intensity on T2 weighted images and flow voids in T2 weighted fat-saturated images

significant output, the *Nicoladoni-Branham sign* can be elicited by proximal compression over the fistula or proximal truncal vessel resulting in a reduction in heart rate by more than 4beats/minute [7].

Pregnancy has been associated with its own challenges in patients with lower extremity malformations, although the presence of hereditary hemorrhagic telangiectasia has not been associated with miscarriages more than the general population [8], it is known that the presence of large malformations can make the patient susceptible to intravascular thrombosis, so can the use of estrogen-containing OCPs, the risk of intracerebral thrombosis has been minimal, however, the use of prophylactic anti-coagulation is often recommended by many for patients with Klippel–Trenaunay and May–Thurner syndrome (an anatomical variation).

A history of trauma has also been implicated as a cause for aggravating vascular malformations, especially lymphatic malformation. Boccara et al. [9] found in their retrospective review of 26 pediatric cases that following surgical intervention in these patients, there was often a delayed wound healing, lymphatic oozing would be present and functional impairment was frequently seen. Large vascular anomalies are known to be associated with thrombocytopenia, known as *Kasabach-Meritt syndrome*, as such these subgroups should be addressed carefully during any medical intervention (Table 5.3).

5.1.3 An Overview of Major Vascular Anomalies

5.1.3.1 Vascular Tumors (Hemangiomas)

As previously mentioned, the term Hemangioma is strictly limited to the anomalies that exhibit a proliferative phase (Growth) followed by resolution and even complete involution. Vascular Malformations, on the other hand, are localized errors in development, they do not exhibit a growth phase nor do they resolve spontaneously.

The *Infantile Hemangiomas* typically arise in the first few weeks after birth and are not present since birth, they may be focal, segmental (plaque-like) or intermediate with superficial, deep, or mixed variety of involvement of skin and subcutaneous tissues. They have a period of rapid growth during the infancy (up to 12 months) followed by quiescence and spontaneous regression beginning at 2-3 yrs. and by 9 yrs., 90% have said to be resolved. Remnants of the lesion in form of telangiectasias or fibrofatty protuberance is noted in the rest of the cases. Problem areas such as eyes, nose, lips, and genitals can often be affected by these hemangiomas, causing the risk of amblyopia or astigmatism in the eyes, nasal deformities, ulcers, and deformities over lips and genitals. PHACES (Posterior Fossa Anomalies, Hemangioma, Arterial Anomalies, Cardiac, Eye, and Sternal defects) affects usually girls, with large facial hemangiomas. Hemangiomas in the lumbar region may be associated with spinal dysgraphia and urogenital defects. Such Infantile Hemangiomas located at critical locations must be treated early to prevent functional defects later on in life.

Congenital Hemangiomas present at birth itself. These are rare vascular tumors and have been sub-classified into rapidly involuting (undergo involution n first few months of life) and non-involuting varieties (transitional variety, with partial regression with age). They typically appear as a bluish nodule with superficial telangiectasias and an anemic halo. These congenital hemangiomas are initially managed with routine follow-up, a pictographic record is often maintained to allow comparison. Rarely, large RICH lesions may be a source of high output fistula and need surgical intervention [10].

Other Vascular tumors are rare, including Kaposiform Hemangioendothelioma, Spindle cell Hemangioendothelioma, Tufted Angiomas, Pyogenic Granulomas, and Hemangioendotheliomas Not Otherwise Specified. Many are large and may also be associated with thrombocytopenia as discussed before.

5.1.3.2 Congenital Vascular Malformations

Vascular malformations have been categorized based upon their flow rate as deduced from a duplex scan. The ISSVA classification involves the following categories of vascular malformations:

5.1.3.3 Arteriovenous Malformations and Arteriovenous Fistulas

Simple AVMs derive from a developmental anomaly leading to abnormal connection between arteries and veins without a well-formed intermediary capillary framework. These lesions can be small, presenting in the extremities, leading to a swelling with the surrounding vascular bunch, a palpable thrill and an audible bruit are common, deep-seated malformations are difficult to identify clinically and will always require radiological confirmation. It is well known that large arteriovenous shunting may result in a steal phenomenon leading to pallor over the skin, even stunting of growth or claudication in an extremity. Ulceration is common at fingers and in the foot. The development of high output cardiac failure is another complication associated with these lesions.

Hemorrhage can be a presenting sign in occult arteriovenous malformations. Truncal malformations may present with hemoptysis, as in hereditary hemorrhagic telangiectasia where pulmonary arteriovenous malformation can produce small bleeding episodes leading to hemoptysis. The manifestation of intracranial bleeding in these patients is mostly in the form of sub-arachnoid hemorrhage. As such patients of HHT have AVMs located in the lungs (50%), Liver (30–70%), Brain (10%), and rarely in the spinal cord (<1%) [11]. Pelvic hemorrhage manifesting as hematuria or per rectal bleed is another example of how truncal AVM may present.

The association of soft tissue and bony hypertrophy causing limb enlargement with limb length discrepancy on the affected side may produce complex syndromes which will be discussed in consequent chapters (Fig. 5.2).

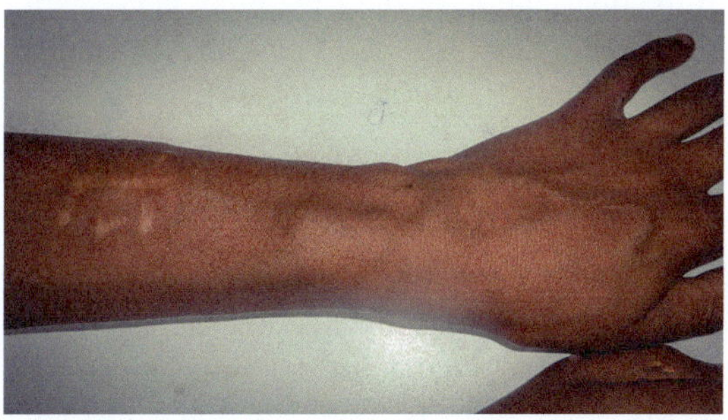

Fig. 5.2 Arteriovenous Malformation on the dorsal forearm. Dilated veins are visible at the wrist

5.1.3.4 Venous Malformations

On an overall, venous malformations are one of the most commonly encountered variety of congenital vascular malformations with an incidence of 1 to 2 per 10,000 population and a prevalence of 1%, they constitute roughly two thirds of all congenital vascular malformations. They are inherently slow-flow lesions and may be subcategorized as Microcystic, Macrocystic, or mixed pattern based on their morphology. These malformations are essentially veins, with abnormal and sparsely distributed smooth muscles in their walls, insufficient valves, and with a haphazard branching pattern. Superficial lesions appear bluish, soft, compressible and may have palpable phleboliths (intralesional calcifications forming as a result of stasis and inflammation, considered pathognomonic of venous malformations) [12], swelling and pain (phlebitis is common in these malformations) in the extremity are accompanying features; the swelling may increase in size on dependent limb placement or with Valsalva maneuver or in pregnancy. There is no hyperemia or pulsation or thrill. These lesions present in childhood or early adult life, being distributed equally in the head–neck region and extremities (40% in each) and roughly 20% occur in the trunk. They represent enlarged post-capillary structures and are susceptible to thrombosis or may induce coagulopathy by stasis in large lesions [13].

5.1.3.5 Capillary Malformations

The frequently encountered birthmarks or the "port-wine" stains or "nevus flammeus," seen mostly in the head and neck regions, especially in the distribution of the trigeminal nerve especially the ophthalmic (V1) and maxillary divisions (V2). At birth, these lesions are flat with pinkish discoloration, however, it may evolve into a reddish or purple raised lesion. These vascular malformations grow with the child and have no chance of spontaneous involution. The clinical progression depends on the site of the lesion and there is often an association with AVMs, VMs, or LMs. With age, the stains tend to darken and thicken producing a "cobblestone" appearance that can distort the facial features, sometimes even the facial bones may become deformed as a result. Location in the Ophthalmic division territory or midline facial lesions have a propensity for associated intracranial or meningeal arteriovenous/capillary malformations and may be associated with seizure disorder as well. A thorough physical examination of the newborn with this congenital anomaly must be done to ascertain its extent and to rule out a syndromic association with Sturge–Weber syndrome, Klippel– Trenaunay and Parkes–Weber syndromes and other congenital anomalies. The evaluation must be done keeping in mind the possible therapeutic measure to be planned [14, 15].

5.1.3.6 Lymphatic Malformations

Lymphatic malformations are essentially dilated lymphatic channels in the form of pouches and vesicles with single endothelial lining and lymphatic fluid as content. More than three fourth of these lesions present in the head and neck region at birth. The previous term "lymphangioma" was a misnomer because the malformation does nott have any proliferative or hyperplastic component. These malformations never regress spontaneously and have been classified according to their lymphatic chamber size into "Macrocystic" (>2 cm), "Microcystic" (<2 cm), or mixed varieties. There is an increase or reduction in size corresponding to the amount of lymphatic flow and presence of hemorrhage into the malformation. Macrocystic lesions are known to enlarge greatly causing significant anatomical distortion of the face, sometimes even the bones are deformed. Most cases are clinically obvious, requiring investigations only in cases that are no clear. There have been various advancements in therapeutics which will be discussed in subsequent chapters as these lesions are often not amenable to complete surgical resection [15].

5.1.4 Imaging in Vascular Malformations

Imaging modalities form the cornerstone for diagnosing vascular malformations. The various methodologies each have their own advantages and disadvantages, however, with the continued development in technology, not only is the diagnosis based on imaging, treatment institution by interventional radiology and planning surgical interventions.

5.1.4.1 Conventional Radiology

Conventional radiology involves multiple views of the lesion taken without contrast administration. It gives a highlight of the bony erosions, periosteal reaction and pathological fractures, phleboliths can be seen on plain skiagrams. Although not routinely performed, the conventional radiograph serves to provide essential bone involvement as described.

5.1.4.2 Duplex Ultrasonography

Ultrasonography combined with doppler ultrasound (the duplex scan) is the main investigation in vascular anomalies. It is a cost-effective, albeit operator-dependent modality with specific protocols, no exposure to ionizing radiation, and is widely available. Use of duplex scans in a dedicated vascular laboratory provides a better diagnostic yield and reveals all aspects and complexities in the lesion, including the extent, depth (may be underestimated with duplex scan), presence of intraluminal phleboliths, air in case of lungs; flow rate and hemodynamics are best assessed with this modality categorizing lesions into low flow and high flow. The extremities must be examined in both supine and standing posture to ascertain any filling with gravity; the high-frequency linear transducer probe is usually suitable for extremity/superficial lesions.

Hemangiomas can be categorized on their sonographic findings to be proliferating, demonstrating high flow in a highly vascular soft tissue mass and involuting, demonstrating low flow characteristics in a residual tissue that is hyperechoic due to fatty degeneration with lesser vessels. Hemangiomas in deep-seated locations may mimic venous and capillary malformations and flow characteristics along with tissue architecture will help in differentiating them.

The arteriovenous malformation typically present with a non-compressible with *active spontaneous flow*, axial arterial trunks providing feeder vessels, pseudoaneurysms, and aneurysmal dilations can be mapped out and outflow veins with morphological changes such as aneurysmal dilation, hypoplasia, or valvular incompetence may be identified; persistent embryonic vessels like the sciatic artery which may lead to Sciatic nerve compression, distal embolization and acute ischemia secondary to thrombosis of an aneurysmal sac in the remnant can also be identified and looked for in truncal lesions [16].

The venous malformation can be characterized based on the size of their venous channels, presence, and absence of valves, and communication with deep venous system. The presence of heterogenous and hypo- or anechoic vascular spaces typically represents *compressible* subcutaneous or intra-muscular vascular spaces which are the hallmarks of venous malformation on B-mode ultrasound. Flow can be assessed on compression, change of posture and Valsalva, induced flow is a hallmark of slow-flowing venous malformation that is typically noted after complete emptying by the change of posture or simple probe pressure followed by gentle release, flow augmentation by postural changes is also appreciable by duplex sonography [13, 17].

Lymphatic Malformations appear as dilated lymphatic channels with anechoic/hypoechoic cysts, with no spontaneous flow, augmentation and distal compression may show some movement of the cyst, however, the directional flow as classically seen with venous malformations is absent. Cyst size characterization is also possible, Microcystic lymphatic malformations tend to present with a diffuse hyperechoic appearance [18].

Besides diagnosis, the duplex scan is also useful in mapping out complete malformation for ultrasound-guided interventions and post-procedural screening of patients undergoing procedures. It can be safely said that the use of Duplex Sonography is the *investigation of choice* for vascular anomalies and fulfills to serve both purposes of diagnostic and therapeutic interventions.

5.1.4.3 Computed Tomography and CT Angiography

Computed Tomography combined with angiography protocols providing three-dimensional images of the vascular anomalies have been used more frequently to provide excellent spatial images that can describe the entire lesion and help in planning out therapeutic interventions. The use of CT provides useful information regarding bony involvement in high flow lesions, bone hypertrophy, and erosions. Arterial and arteriovenous malformations can be identified quickly. Venous malformations appear as hypodense to heterogenous lesions with slow enhancement beginning at the peripheral areas after contrast injection. It may identify obstructed, atretic, or even absent veins and large vein truncal anomalies. It can also delineate variations in normal anatomy that may be crucial to the diagnosis; the presence of intravascular thrombosis and phleboliths can also be seen. Lymphatic malformations on the other hand are seen as low attenuation masses with fluid-filled cavities, fluid-fluid levels, and peripheral contrast enhancement at the walls [19].

5.1.4.4 Magnetic Resonance Imaging (MRI) and MR Angiography (MRA)

Magnetic resonance imaging has several advantages, it can differentiate the soft tissue to a resolution far greater than the conventional CT scan, muscles, bones, fat, and vasculature are clearly demarcated without the use of harmful ionizing radiation. Axial, coronal, and sagittal images are generated to recreate the tissue architecture, gadolinium enhancement provides high-quality angiographic details in MR angiography, high flow, and low flow anomalies can be differentiated. The disadvantages of using MR angiography is the prolonged, noisy, and potentially frightening examination, especially in children, who struggle often needing sedation for the procedure.

The appearance of Hemangioma in an MRI is a characteristic low signal intensity lobulated mass on T1 and high intensity on T2 weighted images, early homogenous enhancement can be seen with flow voids in T1 SE (spin echo) sequence. The involuting hemangiomas appear as high signal intensity masses on T1 weighted images due to fat replacement and decreased enhancement.

Venous malformations on the other hand appear as septated lobulated mass with low signal intensity in T1 weighted images, high intensity on T2 weighted images, and flow voids in T2 weighted fat-saturated images, with slow gradual enhancement on delayed contrast images. The presence of signal voids in T2 weighted images is suggestive of hemosiderin, dystrophic calcification, and phleboliths, which are characteristic of venous malformations.

Lymphatic malformations are very similar to venous malformation, however, the lack of phleboliths is evident, also, the septal and rim enhancement is seen only with the macrocystic variety, enlarged lymph nodes are easily appreciated. Arteriovenous malformations show characteristic large feeding arteries and draining veins, with early enhancement on T1W SE sequence [20]. (Figs. 5.3 and 5.4).

5.1.4.5 Invasive Imaging

Three principle techniques have been employed for assessing vascular anomalies, ascending/descending and segmental phlebography, standard/selective angiography and percutaneous direct puncture lymphography/varicography/phlebography/angiography.

Invasive investigations are reserved for those candidates who are planned for embolization or venous interventions and are generally considered only if the non-invasive testing is unable to confirm the diagnosis or delineate important anatomical detail of the malformation.

Contrast phlebography (venography) is performed by multiple injections in the affected limb or vein territory, use of tourniquet or Esmarch bandage helps visualize the deep system as well. It can determine flow characteristics and differentiate the anatomical variations that may need consideration. A simple angiographic classification by Puig et al. [21] describes the venous malformations on venography as Type I: Isolated without peripheral drainage, Type II:

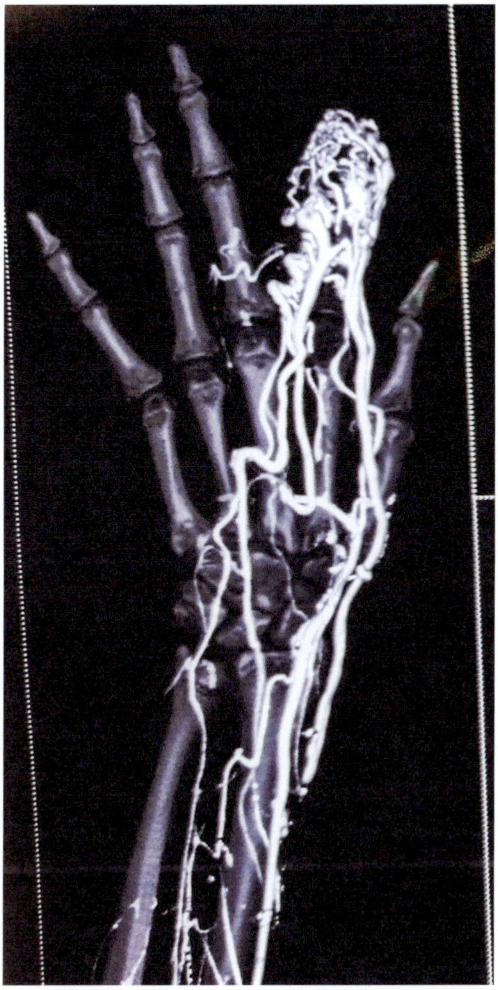

Fig. 5.3 CT Angiogram demonstrating arteriovenous malformation of the forearm and hand

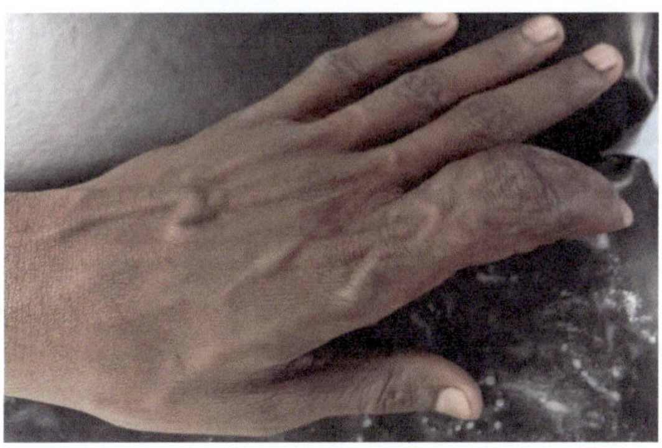

Fig. 5.4 Clinical photograph of arteriovenous malformation at the forearm and hand of the same patient. (note the skin discoloration and thin skin at dorsal aspect of finger)

Malformation draining into normal veins, Type III: Malformation drains into dysplastic veins, and Type IV: Dysplastic malformation. This simple classification can serve as a guidance tool to determine the extent of intervention needed in the treatment. The procedure can also be done in standing position and the absence of valves in an embryological sciatic vein can be assessed by descending phlebography. Ascending phlebography is more useful for truncal and obstructive venous pathologies associated with truncal venous malformations [22].

The use of arteriography is now reserved for candidates planned for embolization. The size of feeding vessels, arteriovenous shunting, flow volume can all be assessed and arteriographic classification can be done to guide further therapy.

Lymphography has been used rarely to confirm the differential diagnosis; coupled with CT, conventional oil contrast based lymphography has been used in selected cases of chylous dysplasia and chylous reflux to ascertain the site and pattern of lymphatic and chylous leakage and extent of the pathology (as for cases of chylothorax, chylous ascites, and protein-losing enteropathy). (Boccardo F et al. [23], Campisi C et al. [24]).

Lymphoscintigraphy has mostly replaced lymphography for evaluation of most cases of lymphedema, there has been some revival of lymphography for use of lymphocele and chylous reflux assessment and as therapeutic USG guided lipoidal infiltration into lymph nodes that produce some degree of inflammation, which may be potentially curative. (Nadolski GJet al [25]) (Fig. 5.5).

5.1.5 Conclusion

A general framework should be kept in mind while addressing a patient with vascular anomalies; Table 5.4 provides one such example, however, the surgeons' own preference may guide the investigational pathways.

The first step for the clinician is to differentiate the malformation from the vascular tumors. It

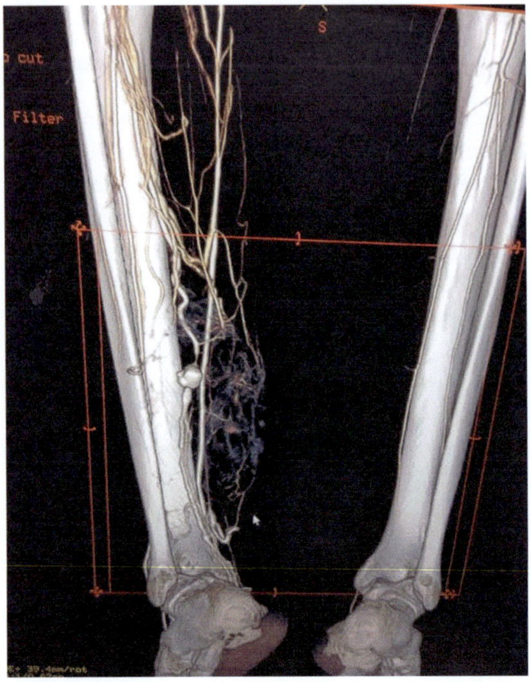

Fig. 5.5 CT angiogram demonstrating arterial malformation in the calf with Posterior Tibial artery Pseudoaneurysm in patient following trauma

is obvious in the pediatric age groups and hemangioma is the only differential diagnosis for vascular tumors in almost all instances. The various clinical features described before will point towards the same.

The next step is to identify the type of malformation, high flow versus low flow, the predominance of veins in the malformation or presence of lymph filled cysts will determine the type of lesion and the surgeon should then proceed to clinically delineate the entire lesion. Many a times only a small part is visible on the surface or the clinical symptoms of a truncal malformation without any external manifestations so that a more extensive imaging will be needed to define the extent of the lesion before its flow characteristics may be ascertained.

Investigating a case of vascular malformation establishes a diagnosis and creates a road map for the vascular surgeon/interventionist to work on. Planning a proper sequence of investigation is most essential. The first investigation is almost always an ultrasonography with color doppler

Table 5.4 Diagnostic algorithm for vascular malformations

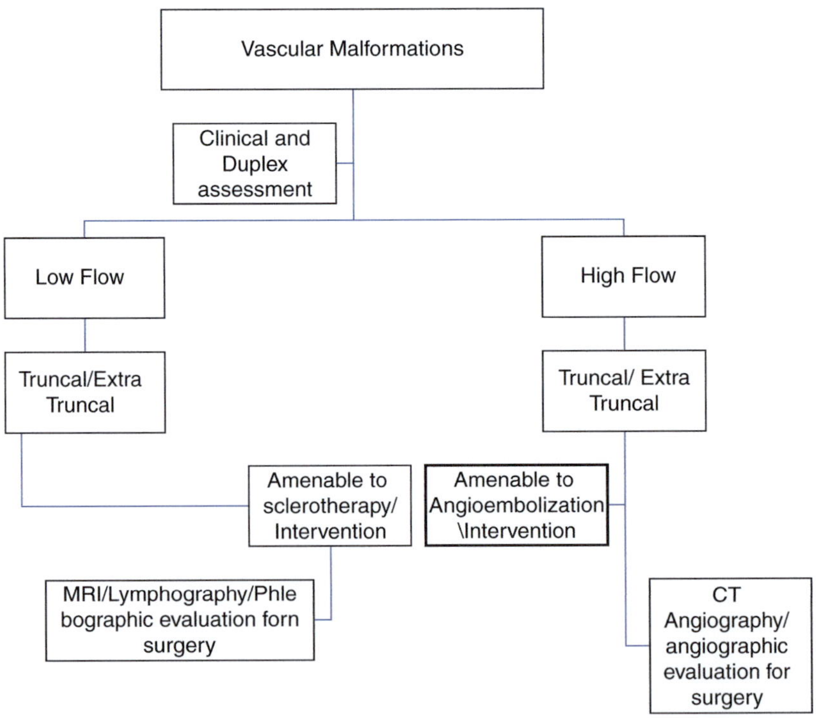

assessment (duplex scan). With the characterization of the lesion type, the proper modality of treatment can be planned with only a meticulously performed duplex scan. The use of CT angiographic evaluation has often served to identify and plan surgical intervention, ultrasound-guided angio-embolization for arteriovenous malformations, and sclerotherapy in cases of venous malformations. MR angiogram and CT angiogram have often been used interchangeably for proper assessment and often both the investigations are done in doubtful cases, however, each carries its own risks and merits and is largely a matter of protocol for the operating vascular surgeon. Detailed assessment and management are provided in forthcoming chapters with regard to the specific malformation.

References

1. Mulliken JB, Glowacki J. Haemangioma and vascular malformations in infants and children: a classification based bon endothelial characteristics. Plast Reconstr Surg. 1982;69:412–22.
2. Rutherford RB. Classification of peripheral congenital vascular malformations. In: Ernst C, Stanley J, editors. Current therapy in vascular surgery. 3rd ed. St. Louis, Mo: Mobsy; 1995. p. 834–8.
3. Burrows PE. Angiogenesis and vascular malformations. In: Kim Y-W, et al., editors. Congenital vascular malformations. Germany: Springer; 2017.
4. Brouillard P, et al. Genetics of lymphatic anomalies. J Clin Invest. 2014;124(3):898–904.
5. Shirley MD, et al. Sturge-weber syndrome and port-wine stains caused by somatic mutation in GNAQ. N Engl J Med. 2013;368(21):1971–9.
6. Kulungowski AM, et al. Expression of androgen, oestrogen, progesterone, and growth hormone receptors in vascular malformations. Plast Reconstr Surg. 2012;129(6):919e–24e.
7. Pandey KK. Arteriovenous fistulas and Malformations. In: Khanna AK, Puneet, editors. Manual of Vascular Surgery. India: Jaypee; 2010.
8. Wain K, et al. Hereditary haemorrhagic telangiectasia and risks for adverse pregnancy outcomes. Am J Med Genet A. 2012;158A(8):2009–14.
9. Boccara O, et al. (April 26–29, 2016) is surgery a triggering factor for clinical worsening of lymphatic malformations? 21st workshop, International Society for the Study of vascular anomalies (ISSVA). Buenos Aires: Argentina; 2016.
10. Theiler M, et al. Vascular Anomalies-A Practical Approach. J Ger Soc Dermat. 2013;11(5):397–405.
11. Govani FS, Shovlin CL. "Hereditary Haemorrhagic telangiectasia": a clinical and scientific review. Eur J Human Genetics. June 2009;17(7):860–71.
12. Hochman M, et al. Current knowledge and management of vascular anomalies, II: malformations. Arch Facial Plast Surg. 2011;13(6):425–33.
13. Behravesh S, et al. Venous malformations: clinical diagnosis and treatment. Cardiovasc Diag Ther. 2016;6(6):557–69.
14. Berwald C, et al. Port wine stains or capillary malformation: surgical treatment. Ann Chir Plast Esthet. 2006;51(4–5):369–72.
15. Cox JA, et al. Vascular malformations: a review. Semin Plast Surg. 2014;28:58–63.
16. Laroche JP, et al. Quality standards for ultrasonographic assessment of peripheral vascular malformations and vascular tumours. Reports of the French society for vascular medicine. J Mal Vasc. 2013;38(1):29–45.
17. Lee BB, Laredo J. Editorial: venous malformation: treatment needs a bird's eye-view. Phlebology. 2013;28:62–3.
18. Lee BB. Lymphedema-Angiodysplasia syndrome: a prodigal form of lymphatic malformation. Phlebolymphology. 2005;47:324–32.
19. Dubois J, et al. Soft tissue venous malformations in adult patients: imaging and therapeutic issues. Radio Graphics. 2001;21(6):1519–31.
20. Konez O, et al. Paediatric techniques and vascular anomalies. In: Rofosky NM, editor. Rubin GD. Lipincott: CT and MR angiography; 2009. p. 1118–87.
21. Puig S, et al. Vascular low-flow malformations in children: current concepts for classification, diagnosis and therapy. Eur J Radiol. 2005;53(1):35–45.
22. Rutherford RB. Congenital Vascular Malformations: Diagnostic evaluation. Semin Vasc Surg. 1993;6:225–32.
23. Boccardo F, et al. The Lymphatics in the pathophysiology of thoracic and abdominal surgical pathology: immunological consequences and the unexpected role of microsurgery. Microsurgery. 2007;27(4):339–45.
24. Campisi C, et al. Diagnosis and management of primary chylous ascites. J Vasc Surg. 2006;43(6):1244–8.
25. Nadolski GJ, et al. Feasibility of ultrasound-guided intranodal lymphangiogram for thoracic duct embolization. J Vasc Int Radiol. 2012;22(9):1300–5.

Arterial Malformations

6

Ravul Jindal, Manpal Loona, Taranvir Kaur, Shabjot Dhillon, and Piyush Chaudhary

6.1 Introduction

Vascular malformations are classified into various entities including arterial, venous, arteriovenous malformations [AVM], and vascular tumors. Since the initial attempt made by Rudolf Virchow in 1863, several classifications have been given over time to classify vascular malformations [1]. Hamburg [Germany] classification (1988) was most widely accepted with its practical approach which was later accepted by the International society for the study of vascular anomalies [ISSVA]. Hamburg classification was modified with time by several authors and used extensively [2]. In 1982 Mulliken and Glowacki also classified vascular anomalies based on hemodynamics termed as "biological classification" [3–6]. ISSVA classification accepted in April 2014 (Melbourne) has been recently revised and updated in May 2018 which imposes pure arterial lesions as separate entity [7].

Congenital Pure arterial malformations are rare entities, which can be further subdivided into three subdivisions: arterial course anomalies, aneurysms, stenosis and hypoplasia.

R. Jindal (✉) · M. Loona · T. Kaur · S. Dhillon
P. Chaudhary
Department of Vascular and Endovascular surgery, Fortis Hospital, Mohali, Punjab, India

6.2 Congenital Course and Origin Anomalies

Variations in course and origin of arteries have been seen throughout the body. Most of these variations have been documented as case reports, which had been either autopsy findings or incidental findings during imaging studies. Most of these variations remain asymptomatic for complete life or may present later in ages with some abnormalities confined to localized sites. These variations require no surgical intervention till they impose any local problems or any symptoms, interrupting day to day activities.

6.2.1 Cranial Vessels

6.2.1.1 Intracranial Vessels

Intracranial variations of course and origin anomalies include maxillary artery branches, ophthalmic artery, basilar artery, and circle of Willis with their variations related to course.

- *Persistent stapedial artery* is a rare anomaly. It originates from the extracranial part of the internal carotid artery, enters the skull medial to the styloid process and runs into the middle ear through the osseous canal, is surrounded by the stapes and reaches the middle cerebral fossa, and ends as a middle meningeal artery [8–10].

A. K. Khanna, S. K. Tiwary (eds.), *Vascular Malformations*,
https://doi.org/10.1007/978-981-15-9762-6_6

6.2.1.2 Extracranial Vessels

The variations of common carotid origin are seen rarely, with its origin being seen near patent ductus arteriosus [11]. Another reported anomaly is common carotid originating from the main pulmonary trunk [12, 13]. These lesions are most commonly seen involving the left common carotid artery. Variations of course of the common carotid artery and its division have also been seen, just above thyroid cartilage in 12.5%, at the upper border of cartilage in 60% cases, and below thyroid cartilage in 27.5% cases [14]. In the usual manner, the left common carotid artery divides into left internal and external carotid branches; a case has been reported with left-sided separate origin of external and internal carotid directly arising from the aortic arch [15].

- *External carotid artery [ECA]* with its branches has also been documented with variations; most common being superior thyroid artery originating from common carotid artery [16] and origin of the lingual artery as a common trunk with facial artery [17].
- *Internal carotid artery [ICA]* also shows many variations. Origin of ascending pharyngeal artery arising directly from ICA [18]. Other anomalies have been seen with occipital arteries and posterior auricular arteries arising directly from the internal carotid artery [19]. Most of these documented cases were either incidental findings or remained asymptomatic, thus not requiring any treatment or surgical interventions.
- *Vertebral artery [VA]* origin anomalies usually involve the left side [20] (Fig. 6.1). Various vertebral artery anomalies have been reported in past with its origin directly between the left subclavian and left common carotid, or distal to left Subclavian, or from left external carotid arteries. Rare cases have also been reported with the right vertebral artery arising from the right common carotid artery [20–23].
- *Vertebral arteria lusoria* is a rare entity, in which the right vertebral artery arising distal

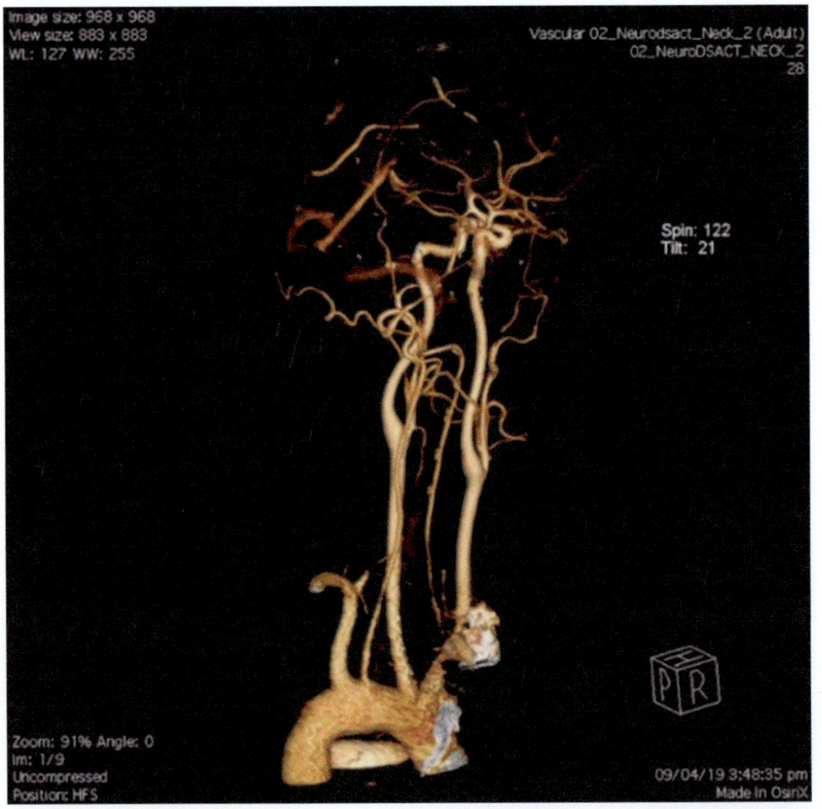

Fig. 6.1 Abnormal origin of left vertebral artery directly from Aortic arch

to the left subclavian artery imposes a life-threatening condition similar to subclavian arteria lusoria [24].
- *Dual origins of VA* has also been reported that imposes significant neurological symptoms which should be managed in preoperative evaluation of patients with extracranial vascular disease [25].

6.2.2 Aorta and its Branches

6.2.2.1 Aortic Arch Anomalies

They can present as double aortic arch, right aortic arch, the cervical aortic arch which forms vascular ring and sling which can lead to obstructive lesions with local symptoms. These anomalies are most commonly managed surgically using hypothermic arrest [26–29].

- *Aberrant right subclavian artery, or arteria lusoria, or dysphagia lusoria* is an aberrant right Subclavian artery that originates distal to left subclavian and courses between the esophagus and thoracic spine [30] (Fig. 6.2). Patients complain of dysphagia due to compression of the esophagus. Symptomatic patients need surgical treatment as transposition of the subclavian artery into the ipsilateral common carotid artery, or reimplantation on the aortic arch [31, 32]. Endovascular hybrid techniques have also been introduced, in which carotid-subclavian bypass is done along with catheter plugging of the anomalous artery to remove decompression symptoms [33].

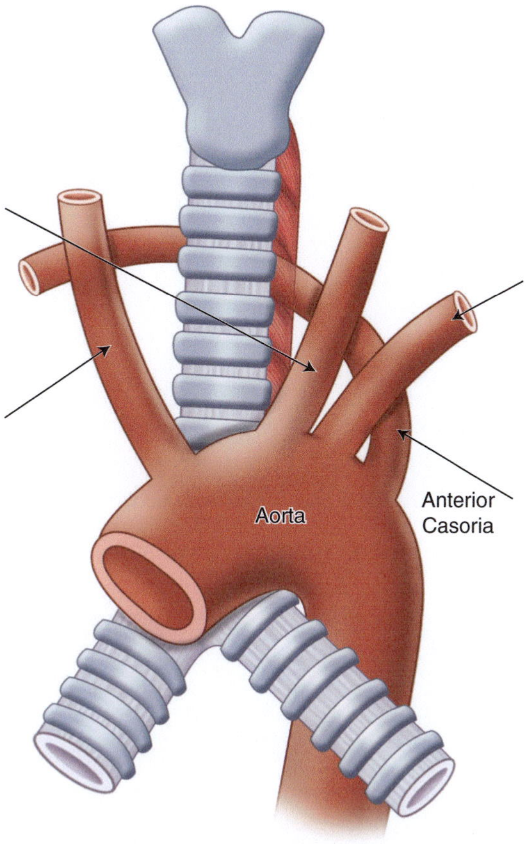

Fig. 6.2 Anterior Casoria: abnormal origin of right subclavian artery distal to left subclavian from Aorta

6.2.2.2 Visceral Arteries

Anomalous origin and branching patterns of various arteries have also been seen from descending aorta. The inferior phrenic arteries can arise directly from the coeliac trunk [34]. Celiac Trunk in its normal course is seen with its trifurcation pattern, but its variations include absent trunk, bifurcation, or quadrification [35]. Variations among the origin of the common hepatic, splenic, hepatic arteries have also been observed from the mesenteric arteries [36] (Fig. 6.3). The right renal artery usually originates at lower level in comparison to the left, but certain variations have been seen with bilateral renal arteries originating at the same level [37] (Fig. 6.4). Variations of origin of gonadal arteries have also been documented from renal, lumbar, or suprarenal artery [38].

6.2.3 Peripheral Arteries

6.2.3.1 Variations in Lower Limb

Anomalies of the lower limb may involve branching pattern of the common femoral artery (which normally divides into superficial femoral artery [SFA] &Profunda femoral artery [PFA]), PFA (which normally give large perforator vessels, medial & lateral circumflex arteries), popliteal,

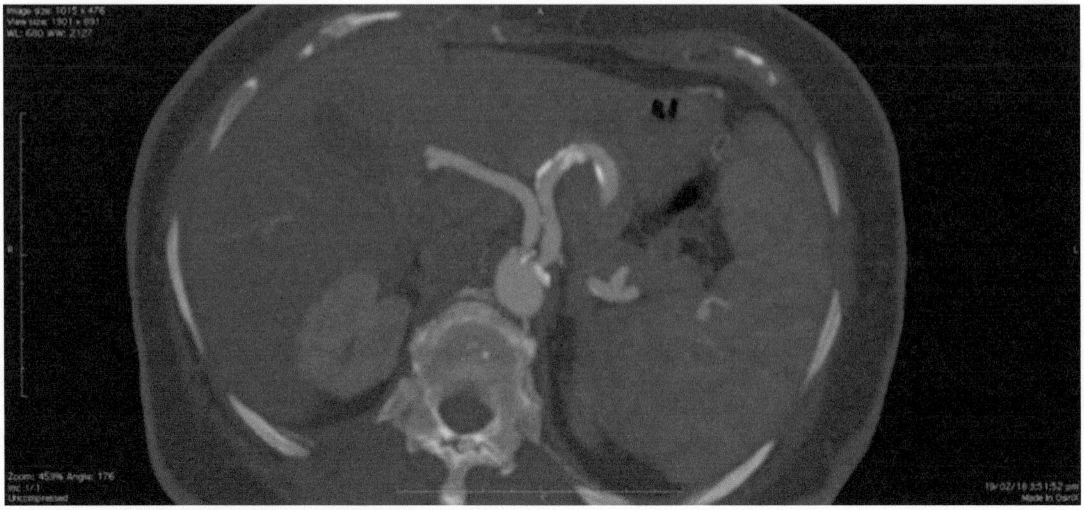

Fig. 6.3 Abnormal origin of the splenic artery directly from Aorta

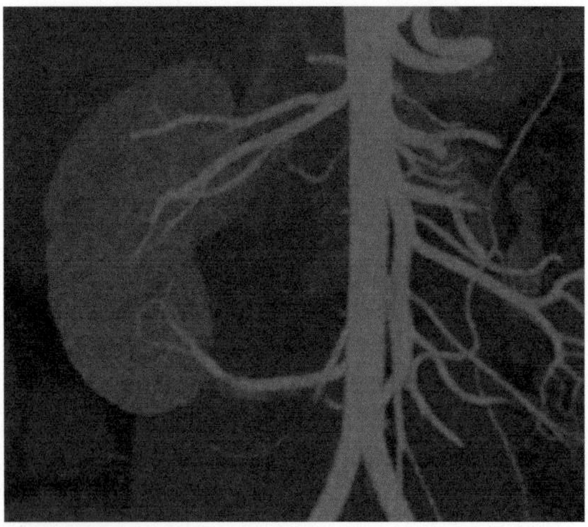

Fig. 6.4 Dual renal arterial supply to the right kidney

peroneal and tibial arteries. These are seen as bifurcation, trifurcation anomalies, or different origin patterns of medial and lateral circumflex arteries from PFA or SFA [39].

- *Popliteal artery* usually divides below the knee into the anterior Tibial artery and the common trunk further dividing into the posterior Tibial artery and the peroneal artery.

  Variations have been seen in the branching of these arteries at different levels above and below the knee [40]. In other sorts of variations seen are, posterior Tibial artery is absent and being replaced by communicating branches of peroneal artery entering tarsal tunnel above the medial malleolus to perfuse the foot. With other less common variants, where the anterior Tibial artery was absent, thick branches of the peroneal artery were seen replacing the anterior Tibial artery to give rise to dorsalis pedis artery [41].
- *Persistent sciatic artery* [PSA] is a rare congenital anomaly. Normally, the sciatic artery regresses during embryonic development. PSA is usually an incidental finding which can be present bilateral with presenting complaints of pain in the thigh, ischemia, claudication, poor capillary refill, cool extremities; black toes; and neurologic symptoms with motor or sensory deficits. It can also present as aneurysms with pulsatile mass, or thromboembolism. "Cowie sign" helps to delineate the diagnosis clinically, with the absence of femoral pulse and the presence of distal pulses. These anomalies can present as complete or incomplete variation, as in complete it is the main artery to supply lower limb, and in incomplete variation, it supplies lower limb with femoral artery and collaterals.

Treatment is confined to surgical repair in symptomatic patients with aneurysms with the restoration of blood supply to the distal limb [42].

6.2.3.2 Variations in Upper Limb Arteries

They are not uncommon, with its branching pattern and level of division. Several reports have been documented in past with early branching of brachial artery, superficial accessory branches, duplication of radial, or ulnar artery. Most of these arterial variations are asymptomatic and may be associated with other congenital anomalies. These are usually incidental findings and may present unilateral or bilateral. Most of these anomalies require no interventional until any symptoms appear. But this carries important significance for vascular surgeons to identify these variations especially during interventions [43, 44].

- *Persistent median artery* occurs with the median nerve. The median artery frames the arterial axis of the forearm during the early embryonic life. After the second embryonic month, it regresses to become a small slender artery "comitans nervi median." It is found accompanying the median nerve in the forearm, but it may sometimes even perforate the median nerve. This anomaly usually presents with complaints of compression similar to carpal tunnel syndrome. When symptomatic this needs to be decompressed surgically for better outcomes [45, 46].

6.3 Congenital Arterial Aneurysms

Congenital arterial aneurysms have been reported with variable incidences involving various arteries over the complete body. These aneurysms have been documented involving intracranial, extracranial, aorta including ascending, thoracic, abdominal, peripheral arteries including renal artery, iliac vessels, visceral arteries, upper limb, and lower limb arteries.

6.3.1 Aneurysms of Cranial Vessels

6.3.1.1 Congenital Intracranial Aneurysms

Congenital Intracranial aneurysms remain to be with low incidence which can present in neonates or young age as ruptured aneurysms in less than 1% which further can lead to subarachnoid hemorrhage in 1% of the patients [47, 48]. The most common site for such aneurysms are located at bifurcation between anterior, middle, and posterior cerebral artery [49]. Male dominance is seen as compared to females [50].

Types of intracranial aneurysms: (a) saccular, (b) micro-aneurysm, (c) Giant, and (d) fusiform.

Aneurysms are the result of undue congenital factors as changes in the vessel wall and hemodynamic stress. Large congenital medial defect could be the initiating cause of aneurysms that appears early in life [51, 52]. Congenital aneurysms usually develop from remnants of small vascular trunks originating from arterial bifurcation [53]. Congenital Cerebral aneurysms have been associated with head trauma (including birth trauma), fibromuscular dysplasia, collagen vascular disease, Ehlers–Danlos syndrome, Marfan syndrome, and tuberous sclerosis [54].

Infants usually present with irritability, lethargy, vomiting, and seizures. Children can present with aneurysmal rupture as subarachnoid hemorrhage with compression effects on the brain from the aneurysm [54].

Management—There are currently three imaging modalities widely used in the diagnosis of intracranial aneurysms: intra-arterial digital subtraction angiography (IADSA) as gold standard imaging modality and others include computed tomography angiography (CTA) and magnetic resonance angiography (MRA) [55].

Obliteration of the aneurysmal sac with a metal clip is considered as a gold standard method for the treatment of cerebral aneurysms at any age. However, congenital aneurysms at a young age have fragile vessels. Other techniques can also be considered like micro anastomosis, bypass and hypothermic arrest for giant aneurysms, endovascular approach, and basilar artery occlusion [55–57].

Morbidity and mortality are lower in children presumably due to less vasospasm and underlying atherosclerotic disease [55].

6.3.1.2 Congenital Extracranial Aneurysms

In comparison to intracranial aneurysms, extracranial aneurysms are less commonly found. Among extracranial vessels, ICA and CCA aneurysms are more frequently involved in comparison to ECA [58–60].

Congenital aneurysms are usually associated with structural defects of the arterial wall as in connective tissue disorder like Marfan syndrome and Ehlers–Danlos syndrome type IV [59].

Most of the time aneurysms are asymptomatic, but these can present in variable forms like the pulsatile mass of the neck, ruptured or leaking aneurysms leading to hematemesis, young age parapharyngeal abscess, or upper airway obstruction [61–65].

Management of such aneurysms is managed with various treatment modalities such as ligation of carotid vessel, surgical resection, and end-to-end anastomosis, clip ligation, using PTFE / saphenous vein patch graft, coil embolization, and endovascular obliteration [59].

6.3.2 Aortic Aneurysms

Congenital aortic aneurysms are rare, but well-documented entities with high mortality in the pediatric population [66]. These aneurysms may involve ascending, thoracic, and abdominal aorta with most commonly involving abdominal aorta as separate congenital defects [66]. Ascending and thoracic aorta are usually dilated in association with congenital heart defects such as congenital aortic stenosis, truncus arteriosus, etc.

The abdominal aorta is defined as dilated when its size is more than 30 mm or more than 50% greater than normal size aorta [66]. These aneurysms can also be seen in association with other multiple sites such as iliac vessels, renal vessels, and superior mesenteric artery [67]. Congenital abdominal aortic aneurysms are usually found at infrarenal sites [66]. Males are found more affected as compared to females.

Congenital Ascending aortic aneurysm [AAA] has been documented at birth with benign nodular fibromyoblastic lesions. Congenital AAA is associated with various predisposing factors, including congenital connective tissue disease (Loeys–Dietz syndrome, Marfan syndrome, Ehlers–Danlos syndrome, collagen disorder, and tuberous sclerosis), trauma (umbilical artery catheterization), and vasculitis (Takayasu arteritis, polyarteritis nodosa, giant cell arteritis, and Kawasaki's syndrome). The etiology of congenital AAA still remains unclear, but it has been shown that it is associated with a genetic defect of transforming growth factor-β (TGF-β) signaling pathway, which controls cellular proliferation, growth, and differentiation of the connective tissue. Marfan syndrome and Loeys–Dietz syndrome rare congenital connective tissue disorders caused by mutations in the genes encoding for TGF-β2 or TGF-β receptor (TGFBR) I or II and fibrillin-1 gene defect leading to thoracic and abdominal aortic aneurysms [66–69].

Clinical presentation varies from asymptomatic, pulsatile abdominal mass, respiratory distress, failure to pass meconium, shock, vomiting, and irritability, rupture with hemodynamic instability [66–69].

Management involves evaluation of the patient with ultrasound abdomen and thorax as a screening modality, thin-cut computed tomographic Aortogram, which helps to delineate anatomy and extent of lesions with associated anomalies. Magnetic resonance angiography (MRA) is considered safe in impending renal failure patients.

There are no definite criteria for the surgical intervention and no standard operative approach for when to intervene. Ascending aortic aneurysm in children and young pediatric patients are treated surgically with associated congenital heart lesions. Abdominal aortic aneurysms are treated using the open repair or endovascular aneurysm repair. Surgical modalities include Aneurysmoraphy, an artificial graft, a new generation decellularized cryopreserved allograft. Endovascular techniques for congenital aneurysms are under evaluation. Recently an endovascular treatment of congenital thoracic aortic aneurysm in a premature newborn has been done with successful results using stent-assisted coil deployment [70]. This provides us better hopes of endovascular repair of congenital aortic aneurysms in near future. Patients on conservative management pose high risk of death due to pulmonary hypertension, cardiac dysfunction, cardiac failure, renal failure, rupture, and thrombosis of the aneurysm [66].

6.3.3 Aneurysms of Major Branch Vessels and Peripheral Arteries [Non-Aortic Aneurysms]

Non-aortic aneurysms have been found involving various peripheral arteries including renal, femoral, iliac, superior mesenteric, brachial, popliteal, axillary, celiac, ulnar, common hepatic, and temporal. It is more commonly found in male children as compared to females.

Factor considered responsible for aneurysms are birth trauma, infection umbilical catheterization, inflammatory disorder, connective tissue diseases(such as Ehlers–Danlos type IV), Kawasaki disease, NF-1, and Klippel–Trenaunay syndrome inherited disorders with genetic mutations involving: ACTA2, CBS, COL3A1, FBN1, FBN2, FLNA, MYH11, MYLK, SKI, SLC2A10, SMAD3, TGFB2, TGFBR1, and TGFBR2 [71, 81].

Such patients present most commonly as asymptomatic, or can present as pulsatile mass, localized pain, or as an incidental finding being evaluated for another problems. Splanchnic artery and iliac artery aneurysms involving intestinal arteries were associated with pain abdomen, jaundice, localized pulsatile mass, or compression problems to other organs [78]. Renal artery aneurysms present as refractory hypertension, pulsatile mass, or incidental findings [81–83]. Upper limb arterial aneurysms present as localized mass, distal hand paresthesias, local compression syndromes, pulsatile mass, deformity with associated anomalies, or incidental with variable sizes [71, 76]. Lower limb arterial aneurysms present as localized mass, distal hand paresthesias, local compression syndromes, pulsatile mass, deformity with associated anomalies, or incidental with variable sizes [74, 81].

Various cases have been reported with multiple arterial aneurysms involving multiple sites in an individual [73, 75, 85]. Delayed presentation had high morbidity and mortality chances [76].

Management involves evaluation of the patient with ultrasonography, catheter-based digital subtraction arteriography, magnetic resonance angiography; thin-cut computed tomography arteriography which helps to delineate anatomy and multiple complex lesions. Indications for intervention include increase in size, impending rupture, localized pressure symptoms, potential thrombosis or embolization of aneurysmal thrombus, nerve compression, and secondary hypertension in the case of renal artery aneurysms.

Treatment option includes aneurysm resection with re-anastomosis, reimplantation, or angioplasty closure, interposition grafts or bypass conduit grafts, ligation, plication, endovascular treatment, and nephrectomy involving severely renal aneurysmal disease, secondary interventions causing restenosis at original aneurysm repair sites and adjacent new aneurysmal development [86–92].

Postoperative patients had low morbidity, mortality, and complications, as compared to those remained untreated or presented late in age. This imposes that non-aortic aneurysms have better outcomes, when diagnosed and managed within time, with good life expectancy rates.

6.4 Congenital Stenosis, Hypoplasia, and Aplasia

6.4.1 Intracranial and Extracranial Vessels

Vertebral arteries followed by carotids are the most commonly involved vessels getting affected with stenosis, hypoplasia, and aplasia in the head and neck but overall still very rare [93, 94].

6.4.1.1 Intracranial Vessels

- *Aberrant ICA in the middle ear* is present in 1% of the population. Patients are usually without symptoms but may present with symptoms like loss of hearing, pulsatile tinnitus, earache, and aural fullness. The treatment of this condition depends on the patient's symptoms and investigation results [95].
- *Hypoplasia of multiple cerebral arteries* involves the circle of Willis. The posterior part of the circle of Willis (Posterior cerebral Arteries and the posterior communicating arteries) is the most variable structure [96].

  Hypoplasia can be mild (average diameter 1.6 mm) or extreme (average diameter 0.9 mm). Both types are usually associated with 81.8% of cases affecting the circle of Willis [97].

  Hemodynamic causes these anatomic variations in these vessels. If a selected part of the brain does not develop, the change in the hemodynamic demand will affect the development of some cerebral arteries [98].
- *Atresia of the right vertebral artery* plays an important role in migraine pathogenesis. It is an additional factor leading to hypoperfusion of the posterior circulation [99].

6.4.1.2 Extracranial Vessels

The major congenital abnormalities of the internal carotid artery (ICA) can be classified as agenesis, aplasia, and hypoplasia. They can be unilateral or bilateral. Agenesis, aplasia, and hypoplasia of the internal (ICA) are rare congenital anomalies, occurring in less than 0.01% of the population [100, 101].

- *Ectopic ICA* is a very rare variation. The ectopic ICA poses a risk during both major oral tumor resection and less extensive procedures, such as tonsillectomy or adenoidectomy. It usually occurs in the temporal bone. Ectopic ICAs should be differentiated from other vascular lesions like angiosarcoma. Diagnosis is done with CT, MRI, or Doppler scan [102].
- *Absent Internal carotid artery* (ICA) is a rare congenital anomaly. Patients remain asymptomatic but some patients may present with transient ischemic attacks. Recognition of this anomaly during planned carotid or trans sphenoidal surgery, in thromboembolic disease and in the surveillance and detection of associated cerebral aneurysms can be very important clinically [103].
- *Congenital absence of bilateral ICA is a rare phenomenon.* ICA supplies two thirds of the brain volume. Bilateral internal carotid artery (ICA) agenesis is an extremely rare congenital anomaly. Most patients with a congenital absence of ICA are detected incidentally by cerebral angiography performed for other reasons. Usually, they have no neurological deficit because of a good collateral blood supply to the affected side but when present, signs and symptoms attributable to acute ischemia are most common [104].

6.4.2 Aorta

6.4.2.1 Interruption of Aortic Arch (IAA)

The absence of lumen between ascending and descending aorta is termed as interruption of the aortic arch. There may be sometimes a fibrous cord. The source of blood flow to the descending thoracic aorta is mostly via the patent ductus arteriosus (PDA). Three types on the basis of the level of interruption are reported. The treatment involves surgical repair using a bypass graft, stent, or end-to-end anastomosis [105].

6.4.2.2 Hypoplastic Aortic Arch

Hypoplasia of arch is described relative to the external diameter of ascending aorta, assuming ascending aorta is of the normal caliber. For the proximal arch hypoplasia, the external diameter is <60%, for distal arch <50% and for the isthmic segment, it is <40% of the external diameter of the ascending aorta [106].

6.4.2.3 Aortic Coarctation

The coarctation of the aorta is a tight narrowing just distal to the left subclavian artery (juxta ductal). This coarctation is hemodynamically significant if the blood pressure gradient is more than

20 mmHg between the upper and lower extremity. It leads to the development of the intercostal collateral vessels that serve to bypass the site of coarctation in order to maintain blood flow to the distal descending thoracic aorta. CTA is the investigation of choice. For postoperative evaluation following stent placement, CT is the better choice as compared to MRA. Similarly, for functional evaluation, MRA is a better choice compared to CT as phase-contrast MRA can assess the collateral flow by comparing the flow in the proximal abdominal aorta with the flow just proximal to the narrowed aortic segment. Coarctation of the aorta is commonly associated with the bicuspid aortic valve, arch hypoplasia, ventricular and atrial septal defects, and mitral valve abnormalities [107].

6.4.3 Non-Aortic

6.4.3.1 Pulmonary Artery Anomalies

Congenital pulmonary artery anomalies are infrequent but are not uncommonly encountered by cardiothoracic imagers. These anomalies have a variable presentation which is often dependent on the underlying nature of the vascular abnormality [108].

- *Pulmonary artery stenosis* causes obstruction of flow from the right ventricle to the pulmonary arteries. Congenital pulmonary stenosis is often asymptomatic when diagnosed. The most common finding on radiograph is the enlargement of the pulmonary trunk and left Pulmonary artery (LPA), which is due to post stenotic dilatation. It is often associated with cardiac abnormalities [109].
- *Unilateral Pulmonary artery agenesis* (UPAA) may be isolated or seen in association with congenital heart disease cases in <1% of cases, which include right-sided aortic arch, septal defects, truncus arteriosus, and tetralogy of Fallot. UPAA is often asymptomatic during early childhood. When symptomatic, they present as recurrent pneumonia, hemoptysis, exercise intolerance, and pulmonary hypertension of the contralateral lung. Early surgical repair of UPAA is desirable as the patent ductus arteriosus often regresses by 6–12 months of age and the intrapulmonary arteries then become hypoplastic, limiting surgical options and long-term outcomes [110, 111].

Idiopathic dilatation of the pulmonary artery (IDPA) is a rare congenital abnormality. It is abnormal enlargement of the pulmonary trunk, with or without enlargement of the right and left pulmonary arteries. Patients are usually asymptomatic. It is a diagnosis of exclusion. As most of these patients are asymptomatic, conservative medical management is often required. However, when the PA reaches a diameter of 60 mm or more, surgical repair is considered [112].

6.4.3.2 Visceral Artery Anomalies

- *Hepato-splenomesenteric trunk* is the common origin of the common hepatic artery, splenic artery, and superior mesenteric artery. The incidence of HSMT is 0.5%. The Left gastric artery may arise directly from the abdominal aorta (6.7%) [113].
- *Agenesis of Celiac Axis (AGCA)* is a rare anomaly of the abdominal aorta with an estimated incidence of 0.1 to 2.5%. One study shows that 31 cases of AGCA have been reported till now of which one-third were detected on angiography and two-third on anatomical dissection. The knowledge about this anomaly is helpful while performing various transplantation, laparoscopy, interventional, and arterial graft procedures [114].
- *Iliac artery anomalies* involve congenital anomalies of the iliac and femoral arteries are rare and usually discovered incidentally at autopsy or suggested by chronic ischemia of the lower limbs [115]. Most reported cases have been iliofemoral aplasia associated with a persistent sciatic artery or atresia with residual cord. Congenital malformation of the external iliac artery has been classified into three groups by Tamisier et al. [116].

		Symptoms
Group 1	Anomalies in origin or course of the artery	Disorders are unlikely to cause chronic ischemia of the leg and are most often discovered at autopsy.
Group 2	Hypoplasia or atresia compensated for by persistent sciatic artery	High incidence of aneurysm formation and arteriosclerosis of the sciatic artery associated with acute occlusion and embolization has been documented for group
Group 3	Isolated hypoplasia or atresia	Disorders are most likely to be suspected because of chronic ischemia of the leg.

6.4.3.3 Lower Limb

- *Femoral Artery hypoplasia or aplasia* is rare. Congenital femoral artery hypoplasia or atresia may appear alone or with an anomaly of the iliac arteries. A persistent sciatic artery with superficial femoral artery (SFA) hypoplasia or aplasia, atresia of the common femoral artery (CFA) and SFA, duplication of the CFA just above the femoral bifurcation, SFA hypoplasia, bilateral SFA hypoplasia combined with the deep femoral artery (DFA) hypoplasia, congenital fibrous ringing of the SFA, SFA duplication, DFA aplasia, bilateral or unilateral DFA duplication, abnormal origin of the DFA and bilateral DFA aplasia have been reported [117].
- *Tibial artery anomalies* are very rare. The knowledge of the popliteal artery and its branches is important for the surgeons. Popliteal and peroneal arteries arise from the axial artery whereas the ATA and PTA arise from the femoral system [118].

The PTA is often the main arterial supply to the foot in patients with clubfoot. Cases with the absence of the PTA associated with idiopathic clubfoot in children have been described in the literature as well [119].

The physical examination alone is not sufficient for the detection of the anatomic variations in the lower extremity arteries. Palpable arterial pulses at the level of the ankle do not exclude congenital absence of even the whole artery. This concurs with studies showing that clinical examination is not independently sufficient to include or exclude a diagnosis of peripheral artery disease. Moreover, normal ABPIs and toe pressures and no symptoms of the peripheral arterial disease do not exclude the Posterior Tibial Artery (PTA) absence. Arterial duplex study and magnetic resonance angiography remain as the studies of choice to exclude hypoplastic vessels, total aplasia, or variations in arterial anatomy. In conclusion, absent tibial arteries may present totally asymptomatic. In addition, normal arterial pulses and normal ankle-brachial pressure index (ABIs) do not exclude PTA absence. Therefore, there is a need for a detailed preoperative investigation of arterial patency and its normal anatomy before specific types of reconstructive procedures or when endovascular techniques are indicated [120, 121].

References

1. Virchof R. Angiome. In: Die Krankhaften Geschwülste. Berlin: Hischwald; 1863.
2. Lee BB, Laredo J, Lee TS, et al. Terminology and classification of congenital vascular malformations. Phlebology. 2007;22:249–52.
3. Mulliken JB, Glowacki J. Hemangiomas and vascular malformations in infants and children: a classification based on endothelial characteristics. Plast Reconstr Surg. 1982;69:412–20.
4. Mulliken J. Cutaneous vascular anomalies. Semin Vasc Surg. 1993;6(4):204–18.
5. Mulliken JB. Classification of vascular birthmarks. In: Grainger RG, Allison DJ, editors. Vascular birthmarks, haemangiomas, and malformations. Philadelphia: WB Saunders; 1988. p. 24–37.
6. Mulliken JB, Burrows PE, Fishman SJ. Vascular anomalies. Hemangiomas and malformations. New York: Oxford University Press; 2013.
7. ISSVA Classification of Vascular Anomalies. International Society for the Study of Vascular Anomalies Available at "issva.org/classification" © 2018.
8. Hitier M, Zhang M, Labrousse M, Barbier C, Patron V, Moreau S. Persistent stapedial arteries in human: from phylogeny to surgical consequences. Surg Radiol Anat. 2013;35(10):883–91.
9. Thiers FA, Sakai O, Poe DS, Curtin HD. Persistent stapedial artery: CT findings. AJNR Am J Neuroradiol. 2000;21(8):1551–4.
10. Guinto FC Jr, Garrabrant EC, Radcliffe WB. Radiology of the persistent stapedial artery. Radiology. 1972;105(2):365–9.

11. Joshi AR, Joshi S, Kale K, Jain R, Bava JS. Isolation of left common carotid artery with its origin proximal to patent Ductus Arteriosus presenting in adult age. Case Reports in Radiology. 2016;2016:4149365–4.
12. Manner J. Isolated left common carotid artery arising from the main pulmonary artery: where is the ductus arteriosus: an embryologist's view. World J Pediatric and Congenital Hearth Surg. 2013;4(4):460–1.
13. Kaushik N, Saba Z, Rosenfeld H, et al. An isolated left common carotid artery from the main pulmonary artery: possible malseptation of the truncoaortic sac. Pediatr Cardiol. 2005;26(5):707–9.
14. Rohita S, Krishnakumari KS. Anatomical variations in the origin of common carotid artery and the branching pattern of the external carotid artery. Indian J Appl Res. 2017;7(9):2249–555X.
15. Cakirer S, Karaarslan E, Kayabali M, Rozanes I. Separate origins of the left internal and external carotid arteries from the aortic arch: MR angiographic findings. AJNR Am J Neuroradiol. 2002;23:1600–2.
16. Smith SD, Benton RS. A rare origin of the superior thyroid artery. Acta Anat (Basel). 1978;101(1):91–3.
17. Gupta V, Agarwal R. Anomalous branching pattern of the external carotid artery in cadavers. Int J Sci Stud. 2014;2(1):28–31.
18. Sirasapalli CN, Mandapal T, Parida S, Belman M. Anatomical variant. Ascending pharyngeal artery arising from the Extracranial internal carotid artery. Indian J Vasc Endovasc Surg. 2017;4:127–8.
19. Özgür Ö, Sindel M, Hizay A, Öztürk S, Aytaç G, Sindel T. Occipital artery arising from the internal carotid artery: a case report. Surg Radiol Anat. 2017 Feb 20;39(2):219–22.
20. Yuan S-M. Aberrant origin of vertebral artery and its clinical implications. Braz J Cardiovasc Surg. 2016;31(1):52–9.
21. Palmer FJ. Origin of the right vertebral artery from the right common carotid artery: angiographic demonstration of three cases. Br J Radiol. 1977;50(591):185–7.
22. K N, Chitravanshi N, Duffis EJ, Prestigiacomo CJ, Gandhi CD. Anomalous origin of the right vertebral artery from the right common carotid artery associated with an aberrant right subclavian artery. J Neurointerv Surg. 2013 Sep 1;5(5):e34.
23. Sartor K, Freckmann N, Böker DK. Related anomalies of origin of left vertebral and left inferior thyroid arteries: report of three cases. Neuroradiology. 1980;19(1):27–30.
24. Lacout A, Khalil A, Figl A, Liloku R, Marcy PY. Vertebral arteria lusoria: a life-threatening condition for oesophageal surgery. Surg Radiol Anat. 2012;34(4):3813.
25. Komiyama M, Nakajima H, Yamanaka K, Iwai Y. Dual origin of the vertebral artery: case report. Neurol Med Chir (Tokyo). 1999;39(13):932–7.
26. Türkvatan A, Büyükbayraktar FG, Olçer T, Cumhur T. Congenital anomalies of the aortic arch: evaluation with the use of multidetector computed tomography. Korean J Radiol. 2009;10:176–84.
27. Arazińska A, Polguj M, Szymczyk K, Kaczmarska M, Trębiński Ł, Arazińska LS, et al. Right aortic arch analysis – anatomical variant or serious vascular defect. BMC Cardiovasc Disord. 2017;17:102. https://doi.org/10.1186/s12872-017-0536-z.
28. Alsenaidi K, Gurofsky R, Karamlou T, Williams WG, McCrindle BW. Management and outcomes of double aortic arch in 81 patients. Pediatrics. 2006 Nov;118(5):e1336–41.
29. Guha S, Grover V, Aiyer P, Dhull J. A unique case of right cervical aortic arch with anomalous left common carotid artery and absent right common carotid artery. Ann Med Surg. 2016;9:58–60.
30. De Luca L, Bergman JJ, Tytgat GN, Fockens P. EUS imaging of the arteria lusoria: case series and re view. Gastrointest Endosc. 2000 Nov;52:670–3.
31. Kieffer E, Bahnini A, Koskas F. Aberrant subclavian artery: surgical treatment in thirty three adult patients. J Vasc Surg. 1994;19:100–9.
32. van Son JA, Vincent JG, van Oort A, Lacquet LK. Reimplantation of an aberrant right subclavian artery into the ascending aorta in dysphagia lusoria in childhood, vol. 56. Tijdschr Kindergenees kd; 1998. p. 126–9.
33. Shennib H, Diethrich EB. Novel approaches for the treatment of the aberrant right subclavian artery and its aneurysms. J Vasc Surg. 2008;47:1066–7.
34. Di G, Ko G, Hk Y, Kb S, Jm L, Sj R, Seo M, Jc S, Gj L, Hk K. Inferior phrenic artery: anatomy, variations, pathologic conditions, and interventional management. Radiographics. 2007;27(3):687–705.
35. Chen H, Yano R, Emura S. Shoumura., anatomic variation of the celiac trunk with special reference to hepatic artery patterns. Ann Anat. 2009;191(4):399–407.
36. Oran I, Yesildag A, Memis A. Aortic origin of right hepatic artery and superior mesenteric origin of splenic artery: two rare variations demonstrated angiographically. Surg Radiol Anat. 2001;23:349–52.
37. Raikos A, Paraskevas GK, Natsis K, Tzikas A, Njau SN. Multiple variations in the branching pattern of the abdominal aorta. Romanian J Morphol Embryol. 2010;51:585–7.
38. Çiçekcibaşi AE, Salbacak A, Seker M, Ziylan T, Büyükmumcu M, Ii U. The origin of gonadal arteries in human fetuses: anatomical variations. Ann Anat. 2002;184(3):275–9.
39. Prakash KJ, Kumar BA, Jose BA, Kumar YS, Singh G. Variations in the origins of the profunda femoris and the medial and the lateral circumflex femoral arteries. A cadaver study in Indian population. Romanian J Morphol Embryol. 2010;51:167–70.
40. Tomaszewski KA, Popieluszko P, et al. The evidence-based surgical anatomy of the popliteal artery and the variations in its branching patterns. J Vasc Surg. 2017;65:521–9.

41. Zheng M, Chen C, Qiu Q, Wu C. Ultrasound in the diagnosis of anatomical variation of anterior and posterior tibial arteries. Med Ultrason. 2016;18(1):64–9.
42. Shaffer W, Maher M, Maristany M, Ustunsoz B, Spieler B. Persistent sciatic artery: a favorable anatomic variant in a setting of trauma. Ochsner J. 2017;17:189–94.
43. Rodriguez-niedenfu M, Vazquez t, Nearn L, Ferreira B, Parkin I, Sanudo JR. Variations of the arterial pattern in the upper limb revisited: a morphological and statistical study, with a review of the literature. J Anat. 2001;199:547±566.
44. Shivanal U, et al. A study of variations in brachial artery and its branching pattern. Int J Res Med Sci. 2015 Jun;3(6):1392–6.
45. Shree B, Khullar M, Kumar A, Singh Z. Study of palmar type of median artery and its fate: Int. J Anat Res. 2015;3(3):1267–72. ISSN 2321- 4287
46. Singla RK. Neelamjit Kaur, Gurvinder Singh Dhiraj. Prevalence of the persistent median artery. J Clin Diagn Res. 2012 November;6(9):1454–7.
47. Norris JC, Wallace MC. Paediatric intracranial aneurysms. Neurosurg Clin North Am. 1998;9:557–63.
48. Weir B, Macdonald RL. Intracranial aneurysms and subarachnoid haemorrhage: an overview. Neurosurgery, Vol II. New York: McGraw-Hill; 1996. p. 2191–213.
49. Gerosa M, Licata C, Fiore DL. Intracranial aneurysms of childhood. Child Brain. 1980;6:295–302.
50. Locksley HB. Natural history of subarachnoid hemorrhage, intracranial aneurysms and arteriovenous malformations. Based on 6368 cases in the co-operative study. J Neurosurg. 1966;25:219–39.
51. Sekhar L, Heros R. Origin, growth and ru p t u re of saccular aneurysms: a review. Neurosurgery. 1981;8:248–60.
52. Lipper S, Morgan D, Krigman MR. Congenital saccular aneurysm in a 19-day-old neonate: case report and review of the literature. Surg Neuro. 1978;10:161–5.
53. Bremer JL. Congenital aneurysms of the cerebral arteries. An embryologic study. Arch Pathol. 1943;35:819–31.
54. Wani AA, Behari S, Sahu RN, Jaiswal AK, Jain VK. Paediatric intracranial aneurysms. J Pediatr Neurosci. 2006;1:11–5.
55. Pinto FCG, Valiengo L, Santos PPML, Matushita H, et al. Intracranial arterial aneurysms in childhood. Arq Neuropsiquiatr. 2006;64(3-A):676–80.
56. ter Brugge KG. Neurointerventional procedures in the pediatric age group. Childs Nerv Syst. 1994;15:751–4.
57. Zhao J, et al. Current treatment strategies for intracranial aneurysms: an overview. Angiology. 2018;69(1):17–30.
58. Jarvis SJ, Parker AJ. External carotid artery aneurysm in an infant presenting with oropharyngeal haemorrhage. J Laryngol Otol. 2001;115:500–1.
59. Pourhassana S. Extracranial carotid arteries aneurysms in children,Single-center experiences in 4 patients and review of the literature. J Pediatr Surg. 2007;42:1961–8.
60. John W, Hammon JR, Donald Silver W, Glenn Young JR. Congenital aneurysm of the Extracranial carotid arteries. Ann Surg. 1972 Dec;176(6):777–81.
61. Misra BK, Shaw JF. Haematemesis from distal extracranial carotid aneurysms. Case report and literature review. Childs Nerv Syst. 1986;2:329–32.
62. Unal OF, Hepgul KT, Turantan MI, et al. Extracranial carotid artery aneurysm in a child misdiagnosed as a parapharyngeal abscess: a case report. J Otolaryngol. 1992;21:108–11.
63. Hazarika P, Sahota JS, Nayak DR, et al. Congenital internal carotid artery aneurysm. Int J Pediatr Otorhinolaryngol. 1993;28:63–8.
64. Meulenbroeks AAWM, Vos GD, Van der Beek JMH, et al. An unexpected cause of upper airway obstruction. J Laryngol Otol. 1995;109:252–4.
65. James AL, O'Malley S, Milford CA. Extracranial internal carotid artery aneurysm in a child: a diagnostic and surgical challenge. J Laryngol Otol. 1999;113:373–5.
66. Wang Y, Tao Y. Diagnosis and treatment of congenital abdominal aortic aneurysm: a systematic review of reported cases. Orphanet J Rare Dis. 2015;10:4.
67. Sirisabya A, et al. Congenital abdominal aortic aneurysm in a term neonate: a case report. Asian Biomed. 2017 April;11(2):163–7.
68. Ono M, Goerler H, Boethig D, Westhoff-Bleck M. Current surgical Management of Ascending Aortic Aneurysm in children and Young adult. Ann Thorac Surg. 2009;88:1527–33.
69. Bell P, Mantor C, Jacocks MA. Congenital abdominal aortic aneurysm: a case report. J Vasc Surg. 2003;38:190–3.
70. Ferrara SL, et al. Endovascular treatment of a congenital thoracic aortic aneurysm in a premature newborn. J Vasc Interv Radiol. 2012;23(10):1330–4.
71. Bahcivan M, Yuksel A. Idiopathic true brachial artery aneurysm in a nine-month infant. Interact Cardiovasc Thorac Surg. 2009;8:162–3.
72. Callicutt CS, Rush B, Eubanks T, Abul-Khoudoud. Idiopathic renal artery and infrarenal aortic aneurysms in a 6-year-old child: case report and literature review. J Vasc Surg. 2005;41:893–6.
73. Checinski P, Henschke J, Pawlak B, Karwowski A, Samolewska E. Multiple aneurysms in childhood - case report and review of the literature. J Vasc Endovasc Surg. 2000;20:108–10.
74. Chithra R, Sundar RA, Velladuraichi B, Sritharan N, Amalorpavanathan J, Vidyasagaran T. Pediatric isolated bilateral iliac aneurysm. J Vasc Surg. 2013;58:215–6.
75. English WP, Edwards MS, Pearce JD, Mondi MM, Hundley JC, Hansen KJ. Multiple aneurysms in childhood. J Vasc Surg. 2004;39:254–9.
76. Got C, Tan TW, Thakur N, Marcaccio EJ Jr, Eberson C, Madom I. Delayed presentation of a brachial artery pseudoaneurysm after a supracondylar humerus fracture in a 6-year-old boy: a case report. J Pediatr Orthop. 2010;30:57–9.

77. Kaye AJ, Slemp AE, Chang B, Mattei P, Fairman R, Velazquez OC. Complex vascular reconstruction of abdominal aorta and its branches in the pediatric population. J Pediatr Surg. 2008;43:1082–8.
78. Ruddy JM, Dodson TF, Duwayri Y. Open repair of superior mesenteric artery mycotic aneurysm in an adolescent girl. Ann Vasc Surg. 2014;28:1032.e21–4.
79. Sarkar R, Coran AG, Cilley RE, Lindenauer SM, Stanley JC. Arterial aneurysms in children: clinicopathologic classification. J Vasc Surg. 1991;13:47–56.
80. Sheppard DG, Wilkinson AG. Syndrome of idiopathic childhood aneurysms: a case report and review of the literature. J Vasc Interv Radiol. 2000;11:997–1004.
81. Akagi D, Ishii S, Kitagawa T, Nagawa H, Miyata T. Popliteal arterial aneurysm associated with Klippel-Trenaunay syndrome: case report and literature review. J Vasc Surg. 2006;43:1287–9.
82. Stanley JC, Criado E, Upchurch GR Jr, Brophy PD, Cho KJ, Rectenwald JE. Pediatric renovascular hypertension: 132 primary and secondary operations in 97 children. J Vasc Surg. 2006;44:1219–29.
83. Milas ZL, Dodson TF, Ricketts RR. Pediatric blunt trauma resulting in major arterial injuries. Am Surg. 2004;70:443–7.
84. Hobbs DJ, Barletta GM, Mowry JA, Bunchman TE. Renovascular hypertension and intrarenal artery aneurysms in a preschool child. Pediatr Radiol. 2009;39:988–90.
85. Short DW. Multiple congenital aneurysms in childhood: report of a case. Br J Surg. 1978;65:509–12.
86. Gumustas S, Ciftci E, Bircan Z. Renal artery aneurysm in a hypertensive child treated by percutaneous coil embolization. Pediatr Radiol. 2010;40:1285–7.
87. de Leeuw K, Goorhuis JF, Tielliu IF, Symoens S, Malfait F, de Paepe A, et al. Superior mesenteric artery aneurysm in a 9-year-old boy with classical Ehlers-Danlos syndrome. Am J Med Genet A. 2012;158A:626–9.
88. Oderich GS, Panneton JM, Bower TC, Lindor NM, Cherry KJ, Noel AA, et al. The spectrum, management and clinical outcome of Ehlers-Danlos syndrome type IV: a 30-year experience. J Vasc Surg. 2005;42:98–106.
89. Gray RJ, Stone WM, Fowl RJ, Cherry KJ, Bower TC. Management of true aneurysms distal to the axillary artery. J Vasc Surg. 1998;28:606–10.
90. Godwin SC, Shawker T, Chang B, Kaler SG. Brachial artery aneurysms in Menkes disease. J Pediatr. 2006;149:412–5.
91. Zimmermann A, Kuehnl A, Seidl S, Eckstein HH. Idiopathic aneurysm of the common iliac artery in an 11-year-old child. J Vasc Surg. 2009;50: 663–6.
92. Taketani S, Imagawa H, Kadoba K, Sawa Y, Sirakura R, Matsuda H. Idiopathic iliac arterial aneurysms in a child. J Pediatr Surg. 1997;32:1519–21.
93. Mattassi R, Loose DA, Vaghi M. Hemangiomas and vascular malformations.An atlas of diagnosis and treatment. Italia: Springer Verlag; 2003. p. 209–14.
94. Paskoy Y, Vatansev H, Seker M, et al. Congenital morphological abnormalities of the distal vertebral arteries (CMADVA) and their relationship with vertigo and dizziness. Med Sci Monit. 2004;10:316 323.
95. Alharethy S. Aberrant internal carotid artery in the middle ear. Ann Saudi Med. 2013;33(2):194–6. https://doi.org/10.5144/0256-4947.2013.194.
96. Sakellaropoulos A, Mourgela S, Kyrlesi A, Warnke J-P. Hypoplasia of multiple cerebral arteries: report of an unusual case. J Stroke Cerebrovasc Dis. 2008;17:161–3. https://doi.org/10.1016/j.jstrokecerebrovasdis.2008.01.011.
97. Marinkovic´ S, Kovacevic´ M, Milisavljevic´ M. Hypoplasia of the proximal segment of the anterior cerebral artery. Anat Anz. 1989;168:145–54.
98. Abbie AA. The morphology of the forebrain arteries with reference to the evolution of the basal ganglia. J Anat. 1934;68:433–70.
99. Lovrencić-Huzjan A. Role of vertebral artery hypoplasia in migraine. Cephalalgia. 1998;18:684–6.
100. Afifi AK, Godersky JC, Menezes A, Smoker WR, Bell WE, Jacoby CG. Cerebral hemiatrophy, hypoplasia of internal carotid artery, and intracranial aneurysm: a rare association occurring in an infant. Arch Neurol. 1987;44:232–5.
101. Chen CJ, Chen ST, Hsieh FY, Wang LJ, Wong YC. Hypoplasia of the internal carotid artery with intercavernous anastomosis. Neuroradiology. 1998;40:252–4.
102. Prokopakis EP, Bourolias CA, Bizaki AJ, Karampekios SK, Velegrakis GA, Bizakis JG. Ectopic internal carotid artery presenting as an oropharyngeal mass. Head Face Med. 2008;4:20. https://doi.org/10.1186/1746-160X-4-20.
103. Given CA, Huang-Hellinger F, Baker MD, Chepuri NB, Pearse Morris P. Congenital absence of the internal carotid artery: case reports and review of the collateral circulation. AJNR Am J Neuroradiol. 2001 Nov/Dec;22:1953–9.
104. Gonzales Cuyar LF, Lam Himlin D, Tavora F, et al. Bilateral internal carotid absence: a case report of a rare congenital anomaly. Cardiovasc Pathol. 2008;17:113 116.
105. Dillman JR, Yarram SG, D'Amico AR, et al. Interrupted aortic arch: spectrum of MRI findings. AJR Am J Roentgenol. 2008;190:1467–74.
106. Hanneman K, Newman B, Chan F. Congenital variants and anomalies of the aortic arch. Radio Graphics. 2017;37:32–51.
107. Singh S, Hakim FA, Sharma A, et al. Hypoplasia, Pseudocoarctation and Coarctation of the aorta – a systematic review. Heart Lung Circ. 2015;24:110–8.
108. Hirsig LE, Sharma PG, Verma N, Rajderkar DA. Congenital pulmonary artery anomalies: a review and approach to classification. J Clin Imaging Sci. 2018;8:29. https://doi.org/10.4103/jcis.JCIS_9_18.
109. Castaneda-Zuniga WR, Formanek A, Amplatz K. Radiologic diagnosis of different types of pulmonary stenoses. Cardiovasc Radiol. 1977;1:45–57.

110. Apostolopoulou SC, Kelekis NL, Brountzos EN, Rammos S, Kelekis DA. "Absent" pulmonary artery in one adult and five pediatric patients: imaging, embryology, and therapeutic implications. AJR Am J Roentgenol. 2002;179:1253–60.
111. Turner D, Vincent J, Epstein M. Isolated right pulmonary artery discontinuity. Images Paediatr Cardiol. 2000;2:24–30.
112. Desmukh M, Guvenc S, Bentivoglio L, Goldberg H. Idiopathic dilatation of the pulmonary artery. Circulation. 1960;21:710–6.
113. Sridhar Varma K1, Pamidi N, Vollala VR, Bolla SR. Hepato-spleno-mesenteric trunk: a case report. Romanian J Morphol Embryol. 2010;51(2):401–2.
114. Rastogi R, Meena GL, Gupta Y, Majid A, Joon P. Agenesis of celiac Axis – a rare clinical entity. Clin Gastroenterol J. 2016;1:103.
115. Koyama T, et al. Congenital anomaly of the external iliac artery. J Vasc Surg. 37(3):683–5.
116. Tamisier D, Melki JP, Cormier JM. Congenital anomalies of the external iliac artery: case report and review of the literature. Ann Vasc Surg. 1990;4:510–4.
117. Narverud G, Myhre HO. Congenital hypoplasia of the lower limb arteries. A report of two cases. Scand J Thorac Cardiovasc Surg. 1974;8(1):70–2.
118. Senior HD. The development of the arteries of the human lower extremity. Am J Anat. 1919;25(1):54–95.
119. Dobbs MB, Gordon JE, Schoenecker PL. Absent posterior tibial artery associated with idiopathic clubfoot. A report of two cases. J Bone Joint Surg: Series A. 2004;86(3):599–602.
120. Khan NA, Rahim SA, Anand SS, Simel DL, Panju A. Does the clinical examination predict lower extremity peripheral arterial disease? J Am Med Assoc. 2006;295(5):536–46.
121. Karaolanis G, Galyfos G, Karanikola E, Palla VV, Filis K. Absence of clinical and hemodynamic consequences due to posterior Tibial artery congenital aplasia. Case Reports in Vasc Med. 2015;2015:821094–3. https://doi.org/10.1155/2015/821094.

7 Venous Malformations

Sandeep Raj Pandey

7.1 Introduction

The subtype of vascular malformation affecting the venous vasculature is called Venous malformation [1]. They are low-flow vascular malformations due to abnormalities in the development of veins. They vary in size and location within the body (Figs. 7.1,7.2, and 7.3). They are usually congenital and found at birth and may manifest clinically in infancy, childhood, or adulthood. Depending on their location, they may remain asymptomatic throughout life. They are treated by open excision, sclerotherapy, or laser therapy.

7.2 History

The history of vascular birthmarks and anomalies is marked by misconceptions, confusing nomenclature, and folklore extending centuries into the past [2]. Birthmarks were believed to be secondary to "maternal impressions." The unborn child could be imprinted with the mother's past experiences, fears, emotions, or objects of desire. Mothers were therefore to blame for the "nevus maternus," or mother's mark. These beliefs continue to exist in many cultures around the world.

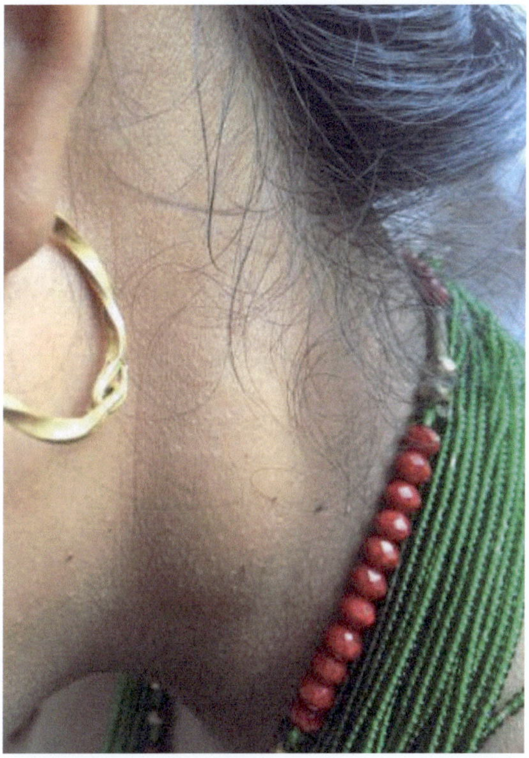

Fig. 7.1 Neck venous malformation

The past two decades have seen great advances in the understanding of the pathophysiology, classification, nomenclature, and treatment of all vascular lesions [3, 4]. In that vein, avoid using synonyms, as they have confused the diagnosis, classification, and management of these vascular

S. R. Pandey (✉)
Vascular & Endovascular Specialist, Annapurna Hospital, Kathmandu, Nepal

A. K. Khanna, S. K. Tiwary (eds.), *Vascular Malformations*,
https://doi.org/10.1007/978-981-15-9762-6_7

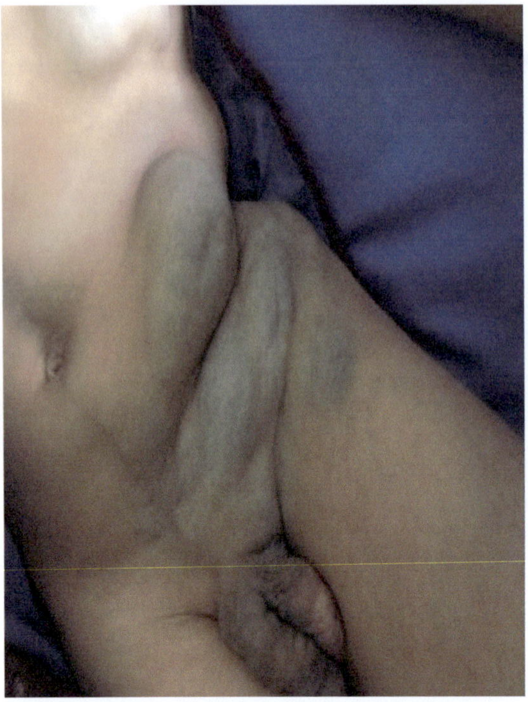

Fig. 7.2 Abdomen and genital venous malformation

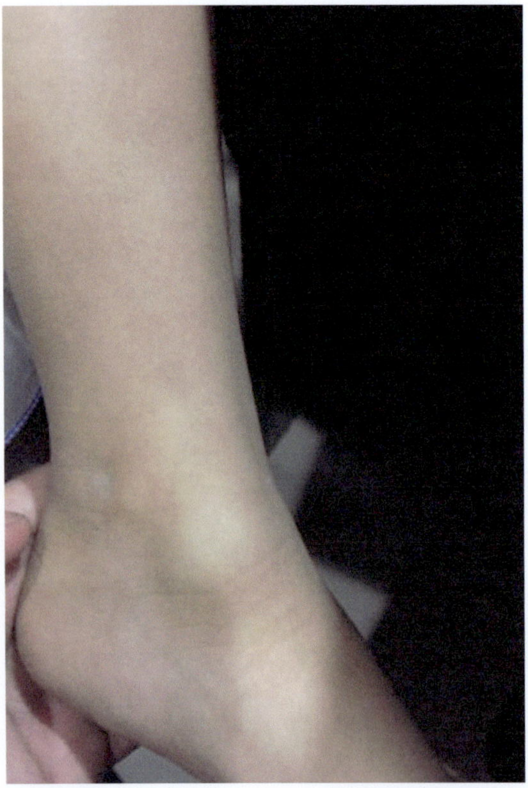

Fig. 7.3 Ankle venous malformation

tumors. Use the appropriate terminology instead, as advocated with passion by Dr.Mulliken [5].

7.3 Etiology

Hundred percent of venous malformations are present at birth, although not all are clinically apparent. Venous malformations are developmental errors composed of dysmorphic channels lined by flattened endothelium exhibiting slow turnover. They are usually singular and solitary isolated events but may occur in multiple areas. If they are present in multiple areas, take a family history, because the autosomal dominant transmission has been described for a subtype of venous malformation termed multiple glomangiomas. In addition, at least one mutation for venous malformations has been identified in a gene that codes for an endothelial receptor on chromosome 9p [6].

Patients with Turner syndrome may have venous malformations of the intestine and feet. Another rare dominant form is represented by the familial cutaneous-mucosal venous malformation. Cerebral cavernous venous malformations could also be familial.

A better understanding of the molecular mishaps that lead to vascular malformations, such as deficient tyrosine kinase receptors, may lead to new therapeutic interventions [7]. Breugem and colleagues have written a thorough overview of the molecular basis of the development of vascular malformations with a discussion of the clinical implications of this new knowledge [3].

7.4 Pathophysiology

Venous malformations usually manifest by childhood or early adulthood. They grow commensurately with the developing child. Unlike hemangiomas, they do not regress [8, 9]. They are by definition "slow-flow" lesions and sometimes are not obvious at birth. They can expand in response to trauma, following incomplete surgical resection [10], or in altered hormonal states (pregnancy, puberty, steroid use). They also may expand following thrombosis or in sepsis.

The following cellular characteristics are important to remember:

- Flat endothelium, slow turnover
- Normal mast cell count
- Dysplastic walls
- Thin basement membranes
- No expression of vascular endothelial growth factor (VEGF) or basic fibroblast growth factor (bFGF)
- Low urinary bFGF

A retrospective study by Koo et al. indicated that the likelihood of localized intravascular coagulopathy occurring in venous malformations is greater in patients in whom such lesions, as seen on magnetic resonance imaging (MRI), are larger, have visualized phleboliths, are located on the trunk rather than the extremities and have a spongiform morphology. Such characteristics suggest that coagulopathy is related to larger capacitance, slower flow, and reduced physiologic compression in these malformations. The study involved 70 patients, including 37 with localized intravascular coagulopathy (Fig. 7.4) [12].

7.5 Clinical Presentations

Venous malformations present in various ways, from a vague blue patch to a soft blue mass. They are easily compressible and usually swell in the dependent position or when venous pressure increases (i.e., when a child cries). They may be relatively localized or quite extensive within an anatomic region. Venous malformations typically involve the skin of the face, limbs, or trunk but also are found in the internal viscera and bones. They have also been identified in skeletal muscle (Fig. 7.5) [13, 14].

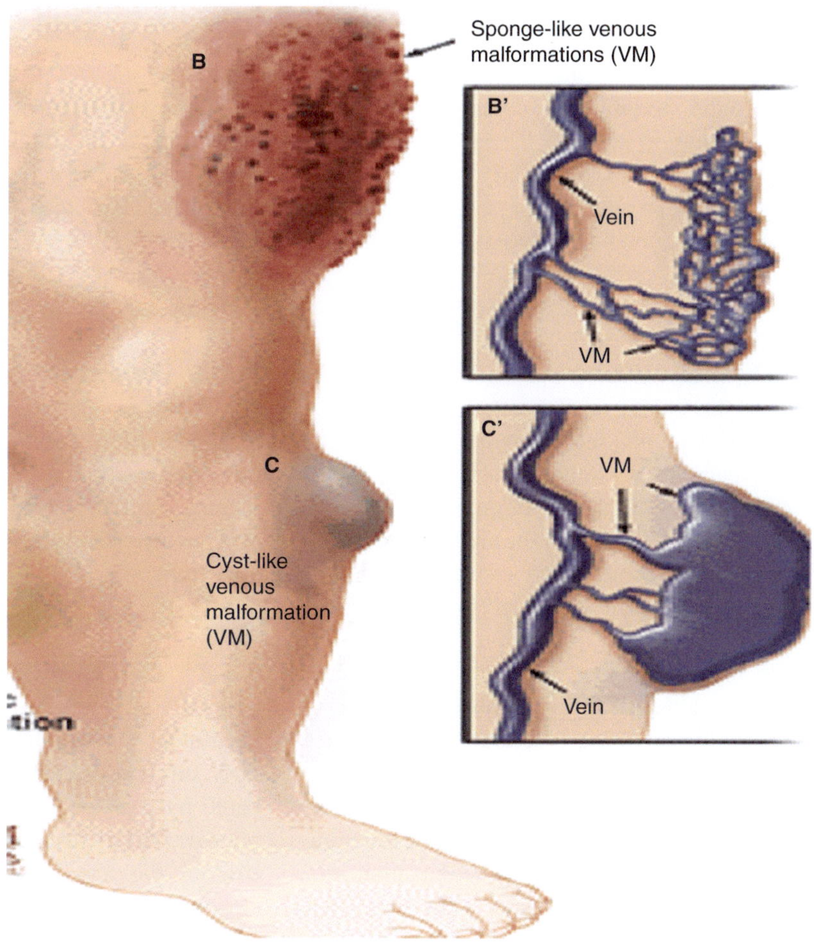

Fig. 7.4 Pathophysiology of venous malformation [11]

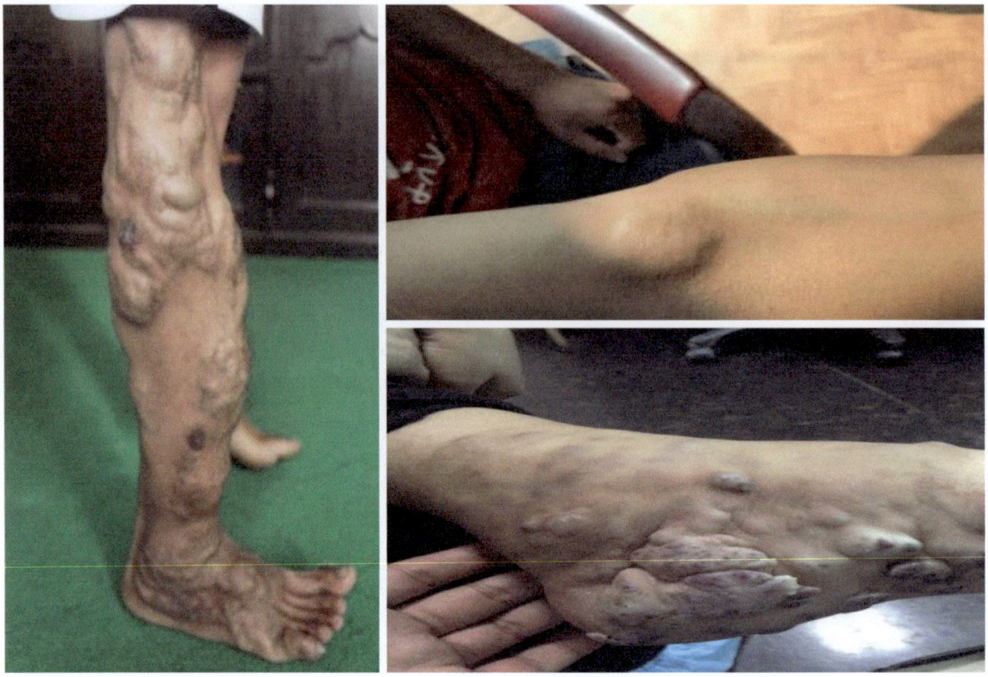

Fig. 7.5 Clinical presentations of VM in form of engorged and dilated superficial veins in lower and upper limbs

Episodic thromboses commonly occur in venous malformations. These are low-flow lesions. Phleboliths, secondary to phlebothrombosis, have been observed in patients as young as 2 years. They might be recognizable with plain radiography.

7.5.1 Indications

The most common indication for medical or surgical treatment of a venous malformation is pain. Pain is likely secondary to thrombosis of the malformation but depends on the size and location of the lesion. Discomfort and stiffness, particularly in the morning, are associated with many larger and deep cutaneous or intramuscular malformations. Intraoral venous malformations can bleed, distort speech or dentition, or obstruct the airway. Venous malformation involving the GI tract or internal viscera can bleed, requiring intervention. Finally, treatment of venous malformations may be indicated to improve appearance or function.

Symptoms associated with venous malformations and indications for intervention vary with the organ system involved. A 3-cm venous malformation of the thigh may be asymptomatic, while the same size intracranial lesion may thrombose and lead to swelling and a life-threatening mass effect requiring emergency intervention.

7.5.2 Relevant Anatomy

Venous malformations represent vascular developmental errors and can occur anywhere. Their management becomes increasingly complex as they involve structures with significant neurovascular function.

7.5.3 Contraindications

Treatment of venous malformations, particularly surgical resection, is often greatly complicated by their deeper involvement with critical neurovascular structures. This is particularly true in the head and neck, intracranial, and extremity malformations. Surgery is often con-

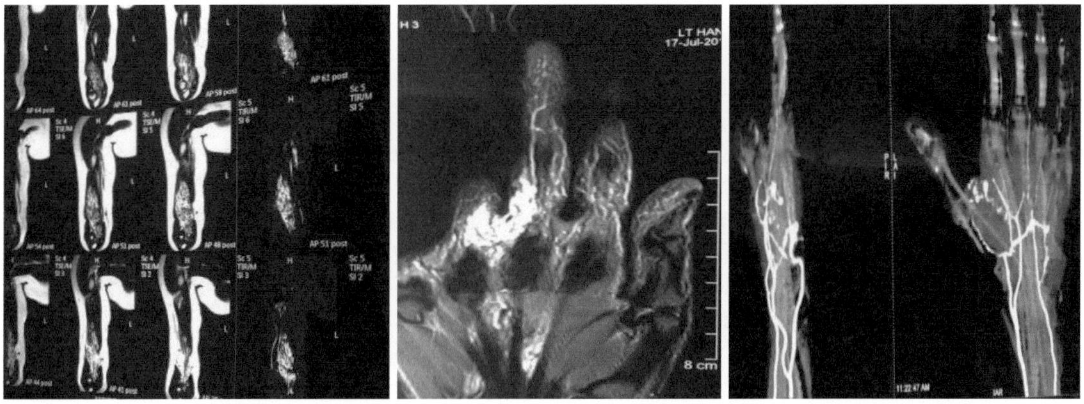

Fig. 7.6 Imaging of VM with contrast are hypoattenuating or heterogenous lesions in lower and upper limbs

traindicated if risks associated with the resection outweigh the presumed improvement in appearance or function that may be derived from surgery.

7.5.4 Laboratory Studies

- Typically, no laboratory tests are indicated for cutaneous venous malformations. Clotting studies and CBC may be indicated in an occasional visceral lesion that is bleeding. If a particular anomaly is a diagnostic dilemma, urinary bFGF rarely may be indicated as part of the work-up.
- A 2005 study was able to differentiate between proliferating hemangiomas and vascular malformations based on serum vascular endothelial growth factor (VEGF) levels [2].
- Perform a coagulation profile on children with extensive disease, as there is a risk for low-grade, localized intravascular coagulopathy (LIC). Disseminated intravascular coagulopathy (DIC) is rare.

7.5.5 Imaging Studies

- Plain radiographs—Phleboliths pathognomonic
- MRI
  - Most informative modality
  - Hyperintense on T2-weighted images [14, 15]
  - No flow voids
  - Inhomogeneous contrast enhancement (like CT)
- CT scan
  - Inhomogeneous contrast enhancement (like MRI)
  - Phleboliths easily seen
- Ultrasound—Hypoechogenic, septated mass (Fig. 7.6)

7.5.6 Diagnostic Procedures

- Arteriography has little or no role in venous malformation unless the diagnosis is unclear.

7.5.7 Histologic Findings

- If the diagnosis is in doubt, biopsy the lesion!
- Most venous malformations are diagnosed based on a good history and physical examination; all of the above studies are ancillary.

7.6 Management

7.6.1 Medical Therapy

Sclerotherapy is the primary form of nonsurgical intervention for venous malformations. [15, 16] Larger lesions usually are treated with 95% ethanol, while cutaneous and smaller lesions are treated with sodium tetradecyl sulfate (1%). Sclerotherapy is often performed by an interventional radiologist under general anesthesia. Multiple sclerotherapeutic sessions often are needed. Venous malformations have a propensity for recanalization and recurrence.

An alternative to standard sclerotherapy using sclerosant foam has recently been described [16]. For example, a retrospective study by Park et al. found sclerotherapy with sodium tetradecyl sulfate foam to be effective against venous malformations, reducing both pain and malformation size. According to the study, which involved 86 patients (91 venous malformations), positive responses with regard to pain and mass reduction were 49.5% and 52.7%, respectively [17].

In a retrospective analysis of facial paralysis caused by ethanol sclerotherapy, Hu et al. concluded that the zygomatic and temporal branches of the facial nerve were the most vulnerable to injury after ethanol sclerotherapy and suggested surgeons to pay close attention when performing ethanol sclerotherapy in those areas [18].

Compression garments are a mainstay of treatment for extremity venous malformations, particularly the lower extremity. Venous malformations of the GI tract also have been managed by sclerotherapy or endoscopic banding.

Laser therapy has shown promise in selected situations. Argon and yttrium-aluminum-garnet (YAG) lasers have been used to treat intraoral lesions [19]. This approach seems more appropriate for smaller lesions (Figs. 7.7 and 7.8) [20].

7.6.2 Surgical Therapy

Surgery is indicated in isolated, symptomatic venous malformations or the following sclerotherapy to improve form or function. Surgical results are a function of the size and location of the malformation. Recurrence following surgery is more common with diffuse malformations and when excision is incomplete [10, 21]. In general, surgery or sclerotherapy is more successful when dealing with pure venous malformations than when dealing with combined malformations [20].

A study by Kang et al. involving 109 patients with slow-flow vascular malformations determined that total excision could generally be carried out in venous malformations but that only partial excision was typically possible for lymphatic and combined vascular malformations, with lymphatic malformations in many cases not being operable at all (Fig. 7.9) [22].

7.6.3 Follow-Up

Complicated or large venous malformations are best treated at a referral center staffed by a multidisciplinary team of diagnostic and interventional

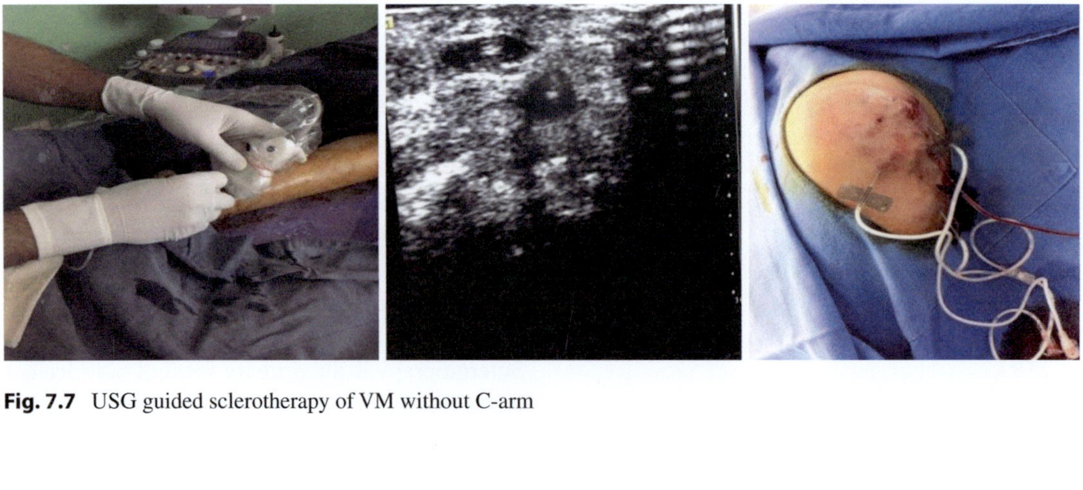

Fig. 7.7 USG guided sclerotherapy of VM without C-arm

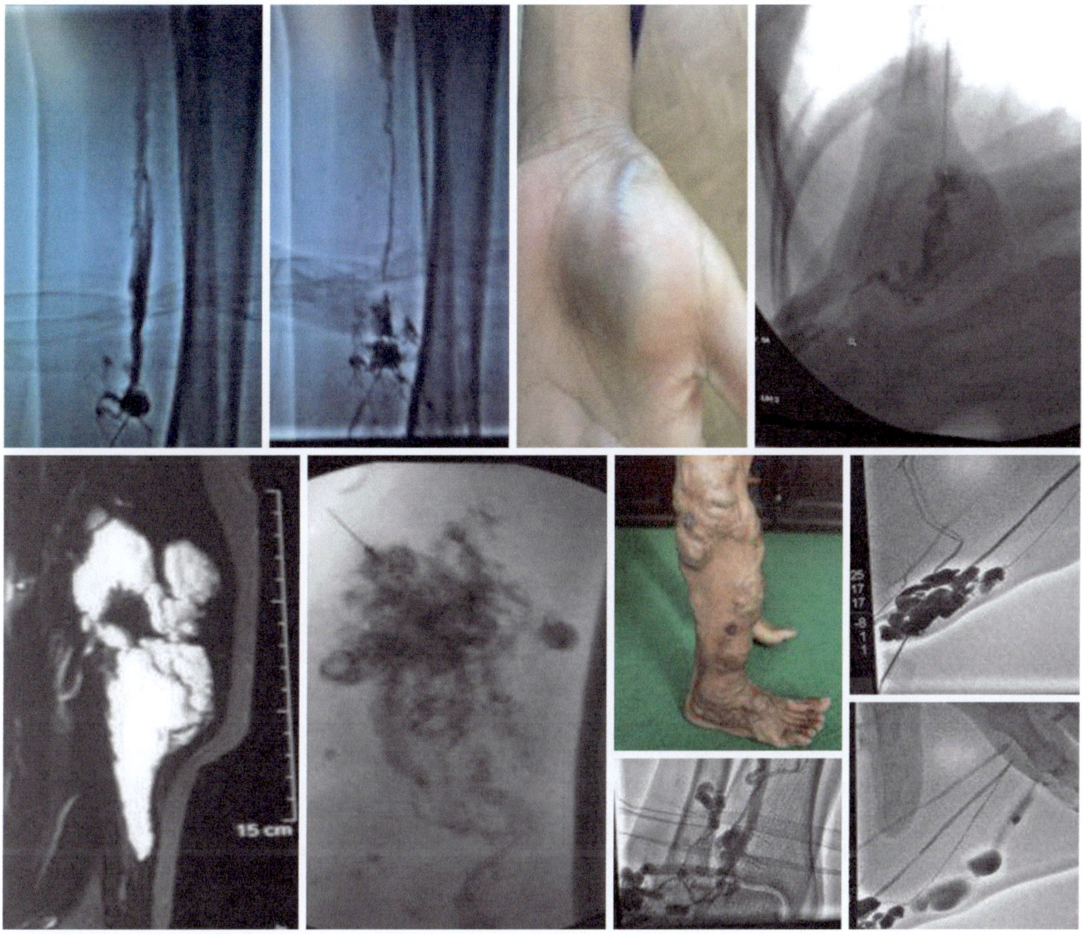

Fig. 7.8 Fluoro guided sclerotherapy of VM with C-arm

radiologists, plastic surgeons, and interested ablative surgeons (e.g., neurosurgery).

7.6.4 Complications

The type and severity of complications depend on the size and location of the malformation and type of intervention chosen. Greater complications are seen with more difficult resections that involve vital structures. Recurrence is a common complication of therapy.

7.6.5 Outcome and Prognosis

The outcome and prognosis are most closely related to the size and location of the venous malformation. The likelihood of significant perioperative morbidity and recurrence increases with more diffuse malformations and with malformations intimately involving vital neurovascular structures.

7.6.6 Future and Controversies

The future holds great promise for the diagnosis and treatment of all vascular malformations, including venous malformations. Advances in molecular genetics are adding to the understanding of vascular malformations and hopefully will elucidate the mechanism of origin of the developmental abnormalities associated with these anomalies [23]. Several inherited disorders have been identified and defective

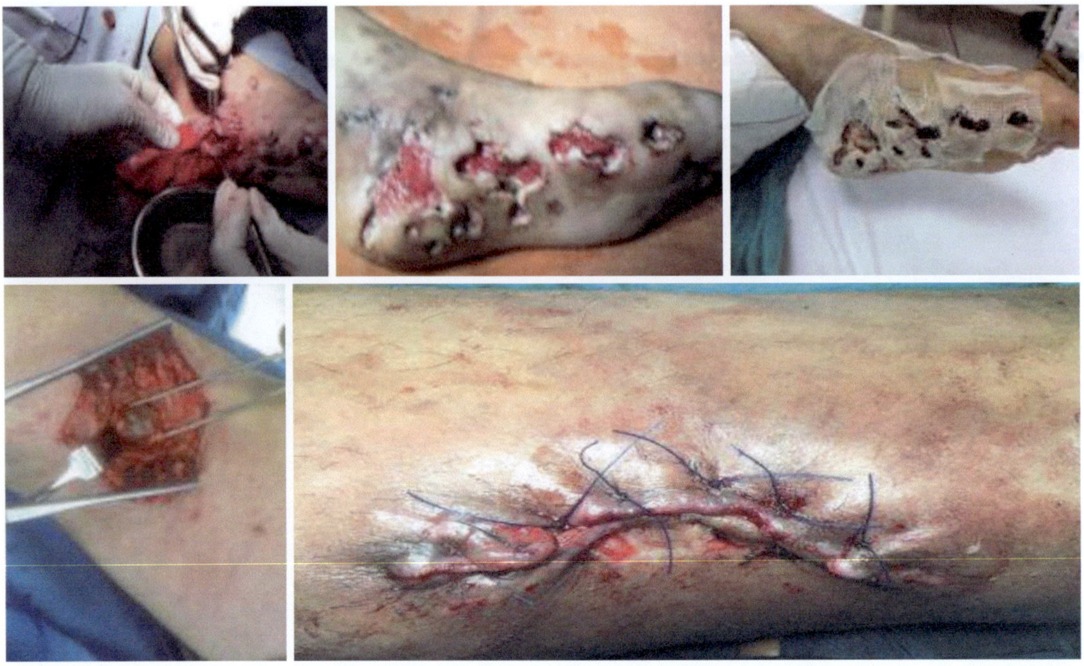

Fig. 7.9 Open surgical excision of VM

genes have been located [6]. Additional information is expected as work on the human genome continues. This new knowledge hopefully will elucidate the pathogenesis of vascular malformations and lead to fresh approaches to therapy [23].

The field of angiogenesis continues to mature, and new antiangiogenesis drugs are in clinical trials that may lead to fresh treatment modalities for these vascular anomalies [23].

7.7 Conclusion

Congenital venous malformations must be diagnosed and treated during childhood. Conservative and resective treatments are useful in different cases. Accurate diagnosis and treatment improve long term results. Vascular malformations are a source of great concern and anxiety not only for patients and their families, but also for treating physicians. Proper identification as well as multidisciplinary approach is paramount for proper treatment. Understanding the clinical aspects, tools available for diagnosis, and options for interventions of each subtype of the lesion will enable appropriate care to be provided and results to be maximized.

References

1. Wassef M, Blei F, Adams D, Alomari A, Baselga E, Berenstein A, Burrows P, Frieden IJ, Garzon MC, Lopez-Gutierrez JC, Lord DJ, Mitchel S, Powell J, Prendiville J, Vikkula M, ISSVA Board and Scientific, Committee. Vascular anomalies classification: recommendations from the International Society for the Study of vascular anomalies. Pediatrics. 2015 July;136(1):e203–14. https://doi.org/10.1542/peds.2014-3673.
2. Breugem CC, van Der Horst CM, Hennekam RC. Progress toward understanding vascular malformations. Plast Reconstr Surg. 2001 May;107(6):1509–23.
3. Mulliken JB, Glowacki J. Hemangiomas and vascular malformations in infants and children: a classification based on endothelial characteristics. Plast Reconstr Surg. 1982 Mar;69(3):412–22.
4. Dubois J, Garel L. Imaging and therapeutic approach of hemangiomas and vascular malformations in the pediatric age group. Pediatr Radiol. 1999 Dec;29(12):879–93.
5. Boon LM, Mulliken JB, Vikkula M, et al. Assignment of a locus for dominantly inherited venous malformations to chromosome 9p. Hum Mol Genet. 1994 Sep;3(9):1583–7.

6. Vikkula M, Boon LM, Carraway KL, et al. Vascular dysmorphogenesis caused by an activating mutation in the receptor tyrosine kinase TIE2. Cell. 1996 Dec 27;87(7):1181–90.
7. Hassanein AH, Mulliken JB, Fishman SJ, Alomari AI, Zurakowski D, Greene AK. Venous malformation: risk of progression during childhood and adolescence. Ann Plast Surg. 2011 May 27;
8. Greene AK, Liu AS, Mulliken JB, Chalache K, Fishman SJ. Vascular anomalies in 5,621 patients: guidelines for referral. J Pediatr Surg. 2011 Sep;46(9):1784–9.
9. Hill RA, Pho RW, Kumar VP. Resection of vascular malformations. J Hand Surg (Br). 1993 Feb;18(1):17–21.
10. Koo KS, Dowd CF, Mathes EF, et al. MRI phenotypes of localized intravascular coagulopathy in venous malformations. Pediatr Radiol. 2015 Jul 5;
11. https://www.hopkinsmedicine.org/interventionalradiology/conditions/malformations/index.html
12. Hein KD, Mulliken JB, Kozakewich HP, et al. Venous malformations of skeletal muscle. Plast Reconstr Surg. 2002 Dec;110(7):1625–35.
13. Fraulin FO, Flannigan RK, Sharma VK, McPhalen DF, Harrop RA. The epidemiological profile of the vascular birthmark Clinic at the Alberta Children's hospital. Can J Plast Surg. 2012 Summer;20(2):67–70.
14. Frischer JM, Göd S, Gruber A, Saringer W, Grabner G, Gatterbauer B, et al. Susceptibility-weighted imaging at 7 T: improved diagnosis of cerebral cavernous malformations and associated developmental venous anomalies. Neuroimage Clin. 2012 Sep 14;1(1):116–20.
15. Pappas DC Jr, Persky MS, Berenstein A. Evaluation and treatment of head and neck venous vascular malformations. Ear Nose Throat J. 1998 Nov;77(11):914–6, 918-22.
16. Park HS, Do YS, Park KB, et al. Clinical outcome and predictors of treatment response in foam sodium tetradecyl sulfate sclerotherapy of venous malformations. Eur Radiol. 2015 Aug;26
17. Hu X, Chen D, Jiang C, Jin Y, Chen H, Ma G, et al. Retrospective analysis of facial paralysis caused by ethanol sclerotherapy for facial venous malformation. Head Neck. 2011 Nov;33(11):1616–21.
18. Rebeiz E, April MM, Bohigian RK, Shapshay SM. Nd-YAG laser treatment of venous malformations of the head and neck: an update. Otolaryngol Head Neck Surg. 1991 Nov;105(5):655–61.
19. van derVleuten CJ, Kater A, Wijnen MH, SchultzeKool LJ, Rovers MM. Effectiveness of Sclerotherapy, surgery, and laser therapy in patients with venous malformations: a systematic review. Cardiovasc Intervent Radiol. 2013 Nov 7;
20. Waner M, O TM. The role of surgery in the management of congenital vascular anomalies.Tech Vasc Interv Radiol. 2013 Mar. 16(1):45–50.
21. Kang GB, Bae YC, Nam SB, Bae SH, Sung JY. The usefulness of surgical treatment in slow-flow vascular malformation patients. Arch Plast Surg. 2017 Jul;44(4):301–7.
22. Fishman SJ, Mulliken JB. Vascular anomalies. A primer for pediatricians. Pediatr Clin North Am. 1998 Dec;45(6):1455–77.
23. Blei F. Medical and genetic aspects of vascular anomalies. Tech Vasc Interv Radiol. 2013 Mar;16(1):2–11.

8 Capillary Malformation

Ajay Narayan Gangopadhyay and Preeti Tiwari

8.1 Introduction

The diagnosis and management of vascular anomalies have been plagued by confusing classification and terminologies. The standard treatment guidelines were very much lacking before the classical work of Mulliken and Glowacki which paved the way for the International Society for the Study of Vascular Anomalies (ISSVA) classification in 1996 [1, 2]. Updated in 2014, this classification divides vascular anomalies into vascular tumors and vascular malformation on the basis of histopathological and blood flow characteristics, in addition to the clinical appearance and disease course.

The vascular malformations have limited postnatal endothelial mitotic activity. The current ISSVA classification stratifies vascular malformations as "simple" or "combined." So, as per ISSVA term, *capillary malformation* (CM) is a simple low flow vascular malformation. The most common and well characterized by the capillary malformations is the port-wine stain (PWS). PWS is clinically and histologically distinctive cutaneous capillary malformation and is caused by GNAQ somatic mutation. Port-wine stain, when combined with ipsilateral leptomeningeal and/or choroidal involvement, comprises Sturge–Weber syndrome. Various other mutations and syndromes have been described in association with capillary malformations.

8.2 Classification

Capillary malformations have been divided into subtypes in ISSVA-2018 classification (Table 8.1) [2].

8.3 Pathophysiology

Capillary malformations result from aberrant morphogenesis and are composed of dilated vessels of mature capillary type [3]. These vessels progressively dilate, fill with blood, and become round. The vessels are lined by thin endothelium and pericytes. Well-developed smooth muscle cells are also present in between the endothelial cells with no evidence of increased mitotic activity. The immunohistochemical evaluation of capillary malformation for endothelial and pericytic markers shown no differences when compared to normal skin. Further, there is no difference between skin and

A. N. Gangopadhyay (✉)
Department of Paediatric surgery, Institute of Medical Sciences, Banaras Hindu University, Varanasi, U.P, India

P. Tiwari
Department of Oral and Maxillofacial surgery, Faculty of Dental sciences, Institute of Medical Sciences, Banaras Hindu University, Varanasi, U.P, India

A. K. Khanna, S. K. Tiwary (eds.), *Vascular Malformations*,
https://doi.org/10.1007/978-981-15-9762-6_8

Table 8.1 Capillary malformation classification (ISSVA-2018)

Subtype	Mutation
Nevus simplex/salmon patch, “angel kiss,” “stork bite”	
Cutaneous and/or mucosal CM (“port-wine” stain)	
Non-syndromic CM	GNAQ
CM with CNS and/or ocular anomalies (Sturge–Weber syndrome)	GNAQ
CM with bone and/or soft tissues overgrowth	GNA11
Diffuse CM with overgrowth (DCMO)	GNA11
Reticulate CM	
CM of MIC-CAP (microcephaly-capillary malformation)	STAMBP
CM of MCAP (megalocephaly-capillary malformation-polymicrogyria	PIK3CA
CM of CM-AVM	RASA1 / EPHB4
Cutis marmorata telangiectatica congenita (CMTC)	
Others	
Telangiectasia[a]	
Hereditary hemorrhagic telangiectasia (HHT)	*HHT1*ENG, *HHT2*ACVRL1, *HHT3*, *JPHT*SMAD4
Others	

[a]The CM nature of some subtypes of telangiectasia is debated. Some telangiectasia may be reclassified in other sections in the future

vascular malformation with respect to the basement membrane proteins and fibronectin [4]. Typically there is a progressive thickening of the vascular wall with dense fibrosis with very little or no proliferation of vessels. With time the vessel wall develops a thick coat of smooth muscle fibers, usually associated with soft tissue hypertrophy along with the development of complex epithelial, mesenchymal, and neural hamartomatous changes [3].

Multiple genetic mutations have been implicated in the development of these malformations and hence their association with various syndromes. A somatic activating mutation encoding a p.Arg183Gln amino acid substitution in GNAQ has been shown to be the etiology of capillary malformations [5]. This specific mutation is found in the lesion of non-syndromic capillary malformations. This is also found in the lesion and affected brain tissue of patients with Sturge-Weber syndrome (SWS). GNAQ is a q class of G-protein alpha subunits that mediates signals between G-protein-coupled receptors and their downstream effectors. Apart from the mutation, there is also a higher density of the *GNAQ* mutation in the malformation tissue when compared to the other affected tissue. Other mutations in this G-protein have been identified in blue nevi, nevus of Ota, and in uveal melanoma. This G-protein is in the MAP/MEK cell proliferation pathway. The mutations affect the expression of different growth factors, their receptors, and enzymes. Vascular endothelial growth factor (VEGF-A) expression has been found to be significantly up-regulated in patients with capillary malformation. Further, the expression of the most active receptor of VEGF-A is also increased [6]. The higher expression of these growth factors and their receptors indicate their role in the pathogenesis of these malformations and their role as a potential therapeutic target. Few reports have questioned the higher expression of these factors as there is a very minimal or no proliferation of the endothelial cell in these disorders. Tyrosine kinase receptor (Tie2) and its ligand angiopoietin-1 are extremely important regulators of vascular remodeling during angiogenesis [7]. Their mutation has also been implicated in different vascular malformation. The decreased vascular tone and the progressive dilatation of these vessels have been postulated due to the abnormal sympathetic innervations. The sympathetic nervous system influences the composition and functional properties of the vessel wall during the development of vessels. Studies have proven the role of the neural system in the development and progression of capillary malformations. There is a significant decrease in the density of perivascular nervous tissue in these lesions on immunohistochemical studies of capillary malformations.

8.4 Genetic Mutations and Syndromes

Multiple mutations have been described in relation to capillary malformations in syndromic and non-syndromic patients. The timing of these mutations explains the extent of tissue involvement and the severity of the condition. In the cases where the mutation occurs at an early period of development, it is associated with syndromes and in non-syndromic patients, the mutations take place at a later stage of development. The most common and well-recognized mutation is *GNAQ* somatic mutation. It is found in both syndromic and non-syndromic port-wine stains. This specific cutaneous vascular malformation, when combined with ipsilateral leptomeningeal and/or choroidal involvement, comprises Sturge–Weber syndrome. Other syndromes with capillary/venulocapillary components but known genetic associations are Cowden's and Bannayan–Riley–Ruvalcaba syndromes (germline PTEN mutations) [8], Capillary malformation-arteriovenous malformation and Parkes–Weber syndrome (germline RASA1 mutations) [9], and Klippel–Trenaunay syndrome (somatic PIK3CA mutations) [10].

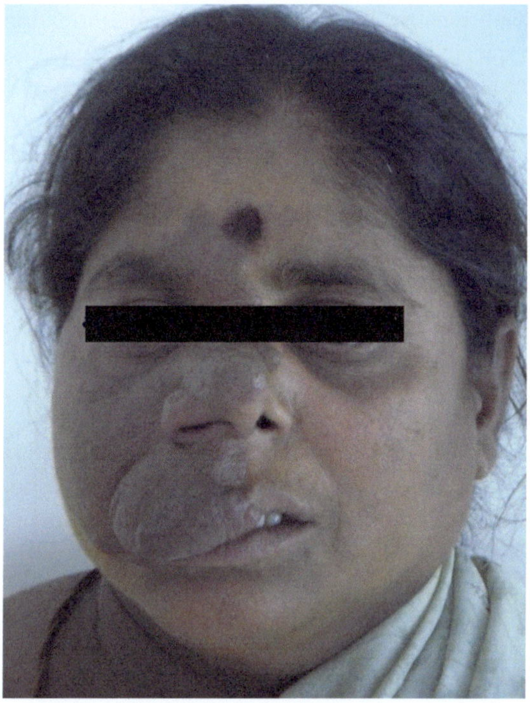

Fig. 8.1 35 year female with Sturge–Weber syndrome with hypertrophied lesion with classical distribution

8.5 Sturge–Weber Syndrome (SWS)

SWS is a neurocutaneous syndrome with the classical triad of a facial capillary malformation with characteristic distribution over the ophthalmic branch of the trigeminal nerve, ipsilateral leptomeningeal vascular malformation, and choroidal vascular malformation of the eye (Fig. 8.1). This is associated with somatic mutation of GNAQ gene. Approximately 6% to 10% of patients with a CM in the ophthalmic distribution have SWS. SWS is associated with a high incidence of congenital glaucoma of the ipsilateral eye, phthisis bulbi, intracranial vascular malformation of the brain with calcification, and atrophy of the underlying cerebrum with associated seizure disorders in 75% of patients (Fig. 8.2). In severe cases, there may be associated with mental retardation and hemiparesis [11, 12].

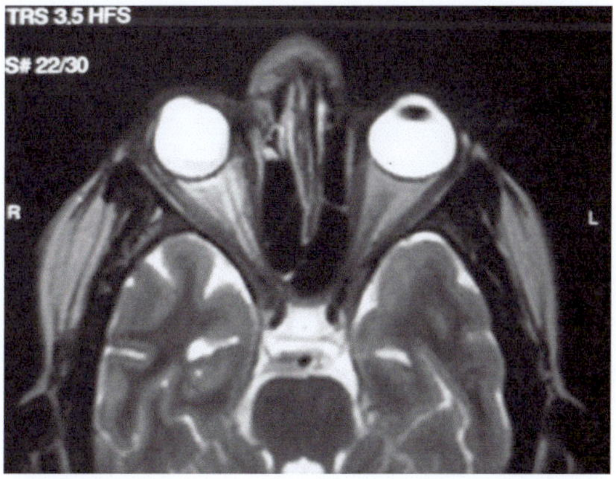

Fig. 8.2 MRI showing hyperintense lesion on the face with phthisis bulbi

8.6 Macrocephaly Capillary Malformation (M-CM)

M-CM is a rare, sporadic syndrome characterized by macrocephaly, hypotonia, developmental delay, and capillary malformation [13]. There can be persistent nevus simplex in place of capillary malformation in few cases. The malformation typically involves the face; philtrum and glabella. Other associated features include hydrocephalus, seizures, developmental delay, connective tissue defects (soft skin and joint hypermobility), toe syndactyly, frontal bossing, and, rarely, hemihypertrophy [14, 15].

8.7 Capillary Malformation-Arteriovenous Malformation (CM-AVM)

CM-AVM is an autosomal dominant condition due to an inactivating mutation of *RASA1* on 5q. RASA1 encodes a GTPase-activating protein, which negatively regulates Ras activity [16, 17]. The syndrome is characterized by multifocal, small CMs which are randomly distributed. The lesions are characteristically pink to dull red in color with annular plaques and a surrounding halo of vasoconstriction. These are associated with underlying arteriovenous fistulas and occasionally Parkes–Weber syndrome [18]. A Doppler examination is extremely helpful to pick these underlying AVM. Genetic counseling may be indicated in these patients [19].

8.8 Klippel–Trenaunay Syndrome (KTS)

Maurice Klippel and Paul Trenaunay described this entity as a classic triad of port-wine stains, lower extremity soft tissue and, bone hypertrophy, and lower extremity varicose veins [20]. KTS effects sporadically with unknown etiology and there is no known genetic or chromosomal linkage. It equally affects male and female with infrequent familial occurrence. Most cases present with a well-defined violaceous plaque with nodularity over the lesion (lymphatic bleb). The lesion thickens and darkens over time (Fig. 8.3, a-b).

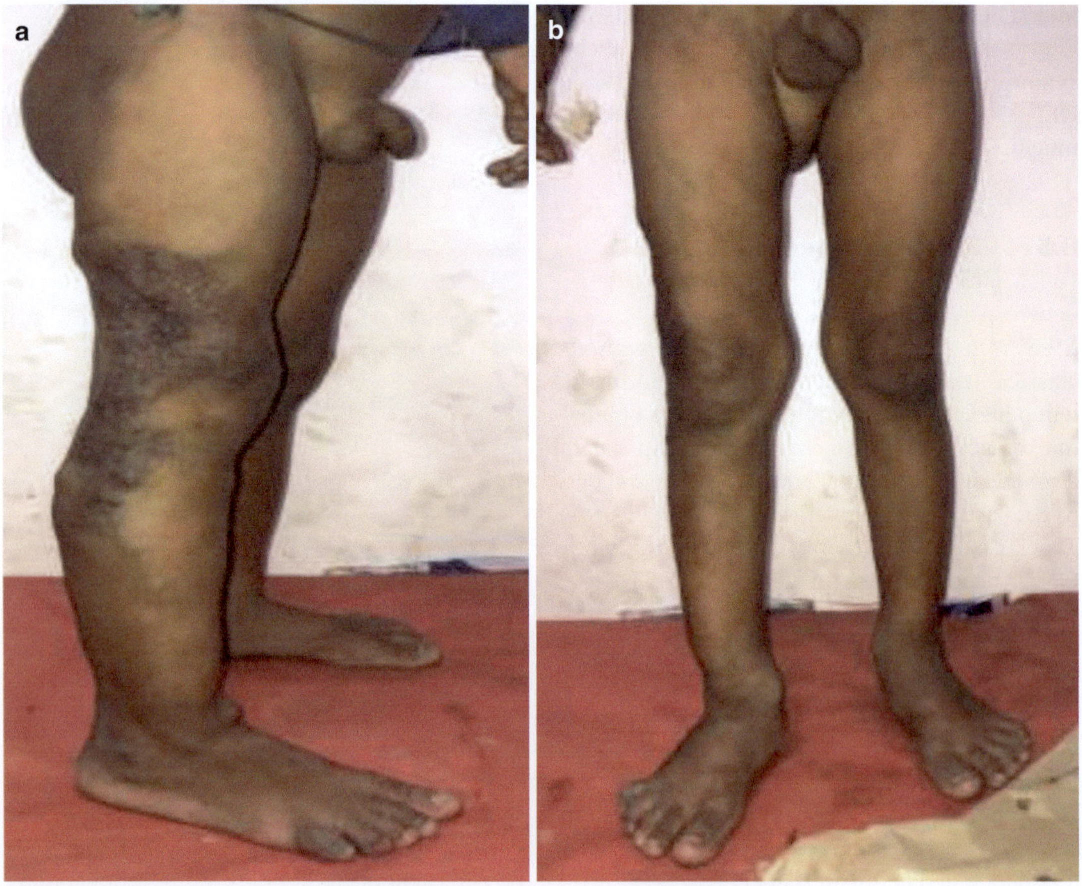

Fig. 8.3 (**a-b**) 5 year male with Klippel–Trenaunay Syndrome (Lateral view and AP)

There is a progressive worsening of the venous stasis ulceration, coagulopathy, and thrombosis resulting in pulmonary emboli, and pulmonary artery hypertension [21]. The diagnosis is made based on history and physical examination alone. Imaging helps in confirming the diagnosis and monitoring of disease progression. Doppler examination of the limb helps to define and determine the patency of the deep and superficial venous systems and characterize any aberrant anatomy such as hypoplasia, atresia, aneurysms, and persistent embryonic veins. The disease has a progressive nature and requires a multidisciplinary approach. The treatment is largely conservative with compression therapy, in the form of elastic, graduated compression garments. Different sclerosants like OK-432, absolute alcohol, sodium tetradecyl sulfate, and polidocanol have been used with good efficacy [22, 23].

8.9 Cutis Marmorata Elangiectatica Congenital (CMTC)

CMTC is a rare vascular disorder of unknown etiology and genetic basis. It is a hypoplasia form of the CVM in contrast to the Klippel– Trenaunay which is the hyperplasia form [24]. It is characterized by a distinctive deep purple color lesion which is depressed in a serpiginous reticulated pattern. These malformations have a regional distribution and usually involve the extremities. There is atrophy of involved skin and with persistent deep vascular staining and diffuse ectasia of the veins in the involved extremities [25]. Limb asymmetry is the most common complaint due to hyperplasia or hyperplasia of the affected limb. Other less frequent associated anomalies are syndactyly, arterial stenosis, and ophthalmologic anomalies. There is a tendency of stain to spontaneously improve with time but limb discrepancy requires orthopedic intervention [26].

8.10 Clinical Features

Port-wine stains affect 0.3% of all newborns at birth [27]. Male and females are equally affected. They present as flat lesions, mostly in the head and neck region, and frequently involve single segment, but can be multi-segmental also. The lesions do not involute with time [12]. They gradually thicken over time and become irregular and nodular and extend to deeper vessels. Most commonly associated syndrome, SWS is present in approximately 6% of children with port-wine stain. The chances of SWS rise up to 26% when there is PWS involving the ophthalmic branch of the trigeminal nerve [28]. The symptoms of associated symptoms like seizures and ocular complications (glaucoma) in SWS should be looked for in children with CM asymptomatic at the time of presentation. Long-standing lesions are associated with soft tissue hypertrophy or limb hypertrophy.

8.11 Natural Course

The capillary malformations are congenital and are always present at birth. The lesions are flat (macular) pink patch which blanch on pressure. They most commonly involve the head and neck region followed by the trunk. Around 45% of these head and neck lesions affect one of the three divisions of the mandibular nerve. Usually, capillary malformations are unilateral with fairly sharp midline cutoffs. Sometimes they may cross the midline or present bilaterally depending on the involvement of one or more than one division of the nerve. The lesions are pink at birth and may be missed due to anemia or plethora in the neonatal period. The lesions vary in color, consistency and undergo changes with age, but never involute with time and persist throughout life. As the child reaches adulthood, the color gets darker and attains a red color [29]. The surface of the lesions also becomes nodular, irregular, and attains cobblestone appearance. The nodular lesion develops as the vasculature dilates and may develop underlying soft tissue or bony hypertrophy [30]. The tissue hypertrophy may result from the development of arteriovenous malformations with time. Long-standing arteriovenous malformations also show hypertrophic nodules. This may also explain the resistant of the long-standing lesions to the pulsed-dye laser treatment, in contrast to infants, which showed a more favorable response [31].

8.12 Imaging Studies

In cases with isolated capillary malformation, diagnosis is clinical and there is no need for imaging. Patients with low-risk lesions, i.e., isolated capillary malformation, either no imaging or color Doppler is reasonable for follow-up. Association of lumbosacral cutaneous anomaly requires imaging studies as there is a much higher risk of associated anomalies. Imaging is indicated in patients with Sturge–Weber syndrome or other syndromes to evaluate the extent of involvement, associated anomalies, and soft tissue hypertrophy. Further, imaging is indicated in lesions with suspected associated AV malformations, complex malformations to plan different treatment modalities [28]. Ultrasound, CT scan, and MRI are used (alone or combined) to evaluate vascular malformations. Ultrasound is usually the first line of investigation as it is easily available and avoids radiation in children. CT scan with or without contrast provides variable degrees of diagnostic accuracy. MRI is the imaging modality of choice for the confirmation, characterization, and differentiation between vascular malformations and their subtypes. As capillary malformations are low flow, they enhance with contrast and normally do not contain flow voids. Capillary malformations have characteristically augmented intraluminal signal on T2-weighted images. This helps to delineate the extent of the malformation throughout the involved tissues and also helps in planning for treatment. MRI with gadolinium enhancement is the optimal diagnostic imaging technique for the screening of Sturge–Weber syndrome. Positive findings include accelerated myelination, gyral enhancement with or without calcification, enlargement, and enhancement of the ipsilateral choroid plexus, and progressive cortical atrophy. These findings may be missed in the early course and so scan should be repeated in suspicious cases [32].

8.13 Medical Management

8.13.1 Imiquimod

Imiquimod is an immunomodulatory agent that is known to inhibit revascularization. It inhibits angiogenesis through various pathways including activation of the innate immune system through Toll-like receptor-7 (TLR-7) to induce interferon alpha (IFN-α), tumor necrosis factor alpha (TNFα), interferon gamma, and tissue inhibitor of matrix metalloproteinase. Further, it induces apoptosis. It is used in the treatment of cutaneous malignancies and many skin conditions from viral HPV infection. Topical imiquimod has been reported to result in improvement in infantile hemangiomas in several case reports and small uncontrolled case series. Its anti-angiogenic potential can be used in patients with CM. One study reported a better result when pulse dye laser and Imiquimod were used concomitantly [33, 34].

8.13.2 Rapamycin

Rapamycin is an inhibitor of angiogenesis. It acts via the mammalian target of rapamycin pathway that downregulates hypoxia-inducible factor and vascular endothelial growth factor. It was originally developed as an antifungal agent, but his target changed when it was demonstrated an immunosuppressive and anti-proliferative effect [35]. The drug to prevent rejection following renal transplant and improves coronary stenting by developing sirolimus-eluting stents. It has been successfully used in children with complicated vascular malformation. Its potential adverse reaction includes immunosuppression, interstitial pneumonitis, and glucose intolerance. It may prove effective as a topical agent in conjunction with PDL in the future. More studies are needed to demonstrate safety and efficacy [36].

8.14 Surgical Management

The decision to treat a patient of CM surgically depends on multiple factors. Both the treatment modality and the extent of treatment depend on the site of involvement, associated syndromes, and complication. The modality and timing of treatment are highly dependent upon the size and location of the lesion. As these lesions do not involute with time, their differentiation from other lesions is must and parents should be counseled about their prognosis. CMs that are not on visually prominent areas may never become an esthetic concern to the patient and thus treatment may not be necessary [37].

The parents of the patients who need treatment because of the involvement of face or esthetically sensitive area should be counseled regarding the natural history of CM. They should be made aware of the potential risks and benefits of any treatment and should be given realistic expectations regarding specific therapies. The timing of treatment is also very important. Though early intervention does not reduce complications, such as overgrowth of the underlying bone or soft tissue or darkening/thickening of the CM, studies have pointed out the development of psychosocial problems in these children with time. The teasing by fellow children can cause stress in these children leading to lowered self-esteem abnormal psychosocial development. The treatment in a pre-school age avoids any such problems and children can involve with their peers normally [38].

8.15 Flashlamp-Pumped Pulsed-Dye Laser (PDL)

Flashlamp-pumped pulsed-dye laser (PDL) is the treatment modality of choice for patients with capillary malformations [31]. Different studies have reported complete response in about 20–25% cases and so it is important to disclose these facts to parents before embarking on treatment. However, there is a considerable lightening of stain in about another 50% of patients, so response rates with PDL alone go up to the tune of 70% (Fig. 8.4, a-b). The response also varies depending on the size and site of the lesion. Thicker lesions with nodularity and deeper extent have a poor response to PDL, which only penetrates to approximately 1 mm in depth. A small lesion with large vessel size along with underlying tissue hypertrophy responds better. The lesion involving the maxillary division of the trigeminal nerve has a better response to PDL for unknown reasons. Further, the response on the torso, hand, and arm is poorer than neck and face [39].

Most PDL units have a wavelength of 595 nm. They function at a setting of 0.45- to 1.5-ms pulse duration, 6- to 10-J/cm2 fluences, and 7- to 10-mm spot size. When this monochromatic yellow light falls on the abnormally dilated superficial dermal blood vessels, oxyhemoglobin in the vessels absorbs it. This causes intravascular coagulation and rupture of some smaller vessels, resulting in the selective destruction of these superficial target blood vessels. Later these are absorbed and replaced by collagen. The surrounding dermis and epidermis are preserved as the thermal relaxation time of the vessels s higher than that of the ultrashort laser pulses but ideally, a coolant system (dynamic cooling device) should be used [39, 40].

The treatment should be started before the pre-school age group because of the psychosocial perspective. Few studies have reported the results to better if treatment was started less than 1 year, but few studies do not support this fact. The other advantage of initiation of treatment before age of 6 months is that the child can undergo this procedure without general anesthesia. So few cycles can be given without general anesthesia and thus overall reduce the number of times a child has to undergo general anesthesia. Treatment can be started as early as 7–14 days of life without any complications [41].

Most children recover nicely without any adverse reaction. But there is edema and purpura of overlying skin immediately after the procedure. This takes around 1–2 weeks to subside and the treatment can be repeated after this gap. Few studies have advocated that a 3-month interval between two sessions has superior efficacy. Thus, PDL can be repeated between 2 weeks and 3 months. Again a shorter gap will mean increased number of sessions without general anesthesia prior to age 6 months, thereby reducing the number of subsequent treatments needed under general anesthesia. Immediately after treatment, the child can complain of pain (a hot snapping sensation) which characteristically increase with repeated pulses. There can also be burning of hair-bearing areas in the presence of increased ambient oxygen. Few children can develop adverse reactions like pigmentation alterations,

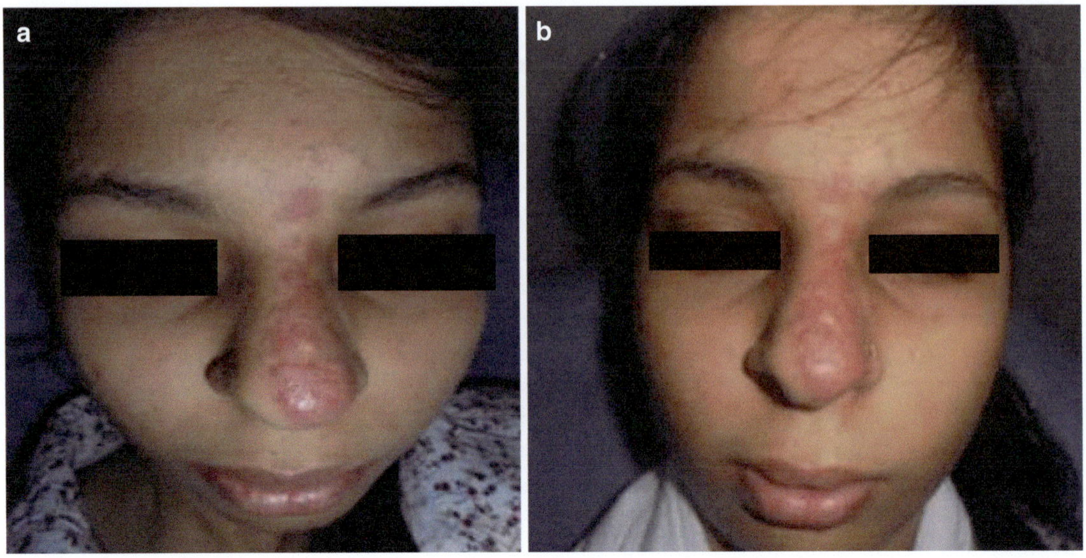

Fig. 8.4 (**a-b**) Pre and post-treatment with PDL in 25 year female with a capillary malformation

crusting, and, rarely, scarring. The hyperpigmentation is usually transient but there is a theoretical risk of permanent hypopigmentation [42].

8.16 Photodynamic Therapy

Photodynamic therapy is based on the use of chromophores. These chromophores once get into the lesion either topically or systemically, photosensitize the lesion. This enhanced sensitivity can be used to target that lesion with a particular wavelength that chromophores absorb. Porphyrin precursors, such as hepatoporphyrin and benzoporphyrin (both have been administered intravenously) and aminolevulinic acid, which is topically administered are most commonly used. Though few studies from China claim excellent results, they could not be reproduced at other centers [43, 44].

8.17 Neodymium:Yttrium-Aluminum-Garnet Laser (Nd:YAG)

The most common resistant CM lesions to PDL are typically thicker, nodular with a deeper extent as it can penetrate only up to 1 mm. To target these, larger wavelength (1064-nm) long-pulsed-Nd:YAG laser that penetrates more deeply has been used effectively. But as it penetrates into deeper tissue, there is also more tissue damage and resultant hypertrophic scar formation. So the long-pulsed Nd:YAG should be reserved for use in the treatment of resistant cases only, as a second-line therapy [45, 46].

8.18 Combined PDL and Nd:YAG Laser Systems

The limitation of PDL in not being able to penetrate deeper and Nd:YAG to cause scarring due to deeper penetration, justifies their combined rational use. New combined modality laser systems, delivers sequential pulses of 595 nm (PDL) followed by 1064 nm (Nd:YAG) separated by 50 to 2000 milliseconds. The initial pulse of 595-nm light (at sub-purpuric doses) induces methemoglobin formation within the treated capillaries. Methemoglobin has a significant absorption peak at approximately 1064 nm, which increases the capillary absorption of the sequentially fired 1064-nm pulse. On one hand, the effectiveness of the lasers is enhanced and on the other, the adverse reactions are minimized by the lower doses of both lasers. This combined 595-nm/1064-nm laser treatment has been shown to result in a greater depth of vascular coagulation. It is also reportedly safe and effective treatment of resistant CM [47, 48].

8.19 Alexandrite Laser

The alexandrite 755-nm laser has a larger penetrating depth making it effective in the deeper vessels of hypertrophic CM [49]. Further, it is absorbed by deoxyhemoglobin as well as oxyhemoglobin which enhances their efficacy in hypertrophic CM. The major adverse effect is a higher risk of significant scarring due to a deeper depth of penetration. This higher risk of scarring warrants an experienced operator and a limited number of sittings in order to prevent extensive deep dermal burns [44].

References

1. Mulliken JB, Glowacki J. Hemangiomas and vascular malformations in infants and children: a classification based on endothelial characteristics. Plast Reconstr Surg. 1982; https://doi.org/10.1097/00006534-198203000-00002.
2. International Society for the Study of Vascular Anomalies. ISSVA classification for vascular anomalies - 2014. Issva. 2014; https://doi.org/10.1542/peds.2014-3673.
3. Sanchez-Carpintero I, et al. Epithelial and mesenchymal hamartomatous changes in a mature port-wine stain: morphologic evidence for a multiple germ layer field defect. J Am Acad Dermatol. 2004; https://doi.org/10.1016/j.jaad.2003.04.002.
4. Smoller BR, Rosen S. Port-wine stains: a disease of altered neural modulation of blood vessels? Arch Dermatol. 1986; https://doi.org/10.1001/archderm.1986.01660140067019.
5. Shirley MD, et al. Sturge–weber syndrome and port-wine stains caused by somatic mutation in GNAQ. N Engl J Med. 2013; https://doi.org/10.1056/NEJMoa1213507.
6. Vural E, et al. The expression of vascular endothelial growth factor and its receptors in port-wine stains. Otolaryngol Head Neck Surg. 2008; https://doi.org/10.1016/j.otohns.2008.07.015.
7. Kaji N, et al. Changes in angiogenic gene expression in a case of expanded capillary malformation: does an expanded capillary malformation grow? Ann Plast Surg. 2005; https://doi.org/10.1097/01.sap.0000162458.88317.99.
8. Mester JL. PTEN hamartoma tumor syndrome. In: Intestinal polyposis syndromes: diagnosis and management; 2016. https://doi.org/10.1007/978-3-319-28103-2_7.
9. Eerola I, et al. Capillary malformation–Arteriovenous malformation, a new clinical and genetic disorder caused by RASA1 mutations. Am J Hum Genet. 2003; https://doi.org/10.1086/379793.
10. Luks VL, et al. Lymphatic and other vascular malformative/overgrowth disorders are caused by somatic mutations in PIK3CA. J Pediatr. 2015; https://doi.org/10.1016/j.jpeds.2014.12.069.
11. Thomas-Sohl KA, Vaslow DF, Maria BL. Sturge-Weber syndrome: A review. Pediatr Neurol. 2004; https://doi.org/10.1016/j.pediatrneurol.2003.12.015.
12. Sudarsanam A, Ardern-Holmes SL. Sturge-weber syndrome: from the past to the present. Eur J Paediatr Neurol. 2014; https://doi.org/10.1016/j.ejpn.2013.10.003.
13. Martínez-Glez V, et al. Macrocephaly-capillary malformation: analysis of 13 patients and review of the diagnostic criteria. Am J Med Genet A. 2010; https://doi.org/10.1002/ajmg.a.33514.
14. Panigrahi I, et al. Macrocephaly-capillary malformation syndrome: three new cases. J Neurol Sci. 2012; https://doi.org/10.1016/j.jns.2011.09.039.
15. Coste K, et al. '[Macrocephaly-capillary malformation. A neonatal case].' Archives de pédiatrie : organe officiel de la Sociéte française de pédiatrie. 2012; https://doi.org/10.1016/j.arcped.2012.06.017.
16. Revencu N, Boon LM, Vikkula M. Capillary malformation/arteriovenous malformation. In: Emery and Rimoin's principles and practice of medical genetics; 2013a. https://doi.org/10.1016/B978-0-12-383834-6.00180-4.
17. Boon LM, Mulliken JB, Vikkula M. RASA1: variable phenotype with capillary and arteriovenous malformations. Curr Opin Genet Dev. 2005; https://doi.org/10.1016/j.gde.2005.03.004.
18. Mulliken JB, Zetter BR, Folkman J. In vitro characteristics of endothelium from hemangiomas and vascular malformations. Surgery. 1982;
19. Revencu N, et al. RASA1 mutations and associated phenotypes in 68 families with capillary malformation-Arteriovenous malformation. Hum Mutat. 2013b; https://doi.org/10.1002/humu.22431.
20. Lamar LM, Farber GA, O'quinn SE. Klippel-Trenaunay-Weber Syndrome. Arch Dermatol. 1965; https://doi.org/10.1001/archderm.1965.01600070064009.
21. Oduber CEU, van der Horst CMAM, Hennekam RCM. Klippel-Trenaunay Syndrome. Ann Plast Surg. 2008; https://doi.org/10.1097/SAP.0b013e318062abc1.
22. Gloviczki P, Driscoll DJ. Klippel-Trenaunay syndrome: current management. Phlebology/Venous Forum of the Royal Society of Medicine. 2007; https://doi.org/10.1258/026835507782655209.
23. Sung HM, et al. Clinical experience of the Klippel–Trenaunay syndrome. Arch Plast Surg. 2015; https://doi.org/10.5999/aps.2015.42.5.552.

24. Happle R. Capillary malformations: a classification using specific names for specific skin disorders. J Eur Acad Dermatol Venereol. 2015; https://doi.org/10.1111/jdv.13147.
25. Dar NR, Ghafoor T, Awan ZI. Cutis marmorata telangiectatica congenita. Journal of the College of Physicians and Surgeons Pakistan. 2003; https://doi.org/10.1111/j.1365-4362.1992.tb03564.x.
26. Mazereeuw-Hautier J, Carel-Caneppele S, Bonafé JL. Cutis marmorata telangiectatica congenita: report of two persistent cases. Pediatr Dermatol. 2002; https://doi.org/10.1046/j.1525-1470.2002.00220.x.
27. Loane M, et al. Paper 3: EUROCAT data quality indicators for population-based registries of congenital anomalies. Birth Defects Research Part A - Clinical and Molecular Teratology. 2011; https://doi.org/10.1002/bdra.20779.
28. Nozaki T, et al. Syndromes associated with vascular tumors and malformations: a pictorial review.' Radiographics : a review publication of the Radiological Society of North America. Inc. 2013; https://doi.org/10.1148/rg.331125052.
29. Lee JW, Chung HY. Capillary malformations (Portwine stains) of the head and neck: natural history, investigations, laser, and surgical management. Otolaryngol Clin N Am. 2018; https://doi.org/10.1016/j.otc.2017.09.004.
30. Lee JW, et al. The natural history of soft tissue hypertrophy, bony hypertrophy, and nodule formation in patients with untreated head and neck capillary malformations. Dermatol Surg. 2015; https://doi.org/10.1097/DSS.0000000000000525.
31. Stier MF, Glick SA, Hirsch RJ. Laser treatment of pediatric vascular lesions: port wine stains and hemangiomas. J Am Acad Dermatol. 2008; https://doi.org/10.1016/j.jaad.2007.10.492.
32. Legiehn GM, Heran MKS. A step-by-step practical approach to imaging diagnosis and interventional radiologic therapy in vascular malformations. Semin Interv Radiol. 2010; https://doi.org/10.1055/s-0030-1253521.
33. Kouba DJ, et al. Topical imiquimod in the treatment of a long-standing capillary malformation [19]. Br J Dermatol. 2007; https://doi.org/10.1111/j.1365-2133.2007.08181.x.
34. Bongiorno MR, Aricò M. Preliminary communication: Imiquimod in mixed capillary/lymphatic malformation. Dermatol Ther. 2008; https://doi.org/10.1111/j.1529-8019.2008.00232.x.
35. Phung TL, et al. Pathological angiogenesis is induced by sustained Akt signaling and inhibited by rapamycin. Cancer Cell. 2006; https://doi.org/10.1016/j.ccr.2006.07.003.
36. Hammill AM, et al. Sirolimus for the treatment of complicated vascular anomalies in children. Pediatric Blood and Cancer. 2011;57(6):1018–24. https://doi.org/10.1002/pbc.23124.
37. Richter GT, Friedman AB. Hemangiomas and vascular malformations: current theory and management. Int J Pediatr. 2012; https://doi.org/10.1155/2012/645678.
38. Lam SM, Williams EF. Practical considerations in the treatment of capillary vascular malformations, or port wine stains. Facial Plast Surg. 2004; https://doi.org/10.1055/s-2004-822962.
39. Van Drooge AM, et al. Port-wine stain progression: is prevention by pulsed dye laser therapy possible? Eur J Dermatol. 2013; https://doi.org/10.1684/ejd.2013.1998.
40. Jasim ZF, Handley JM. Treatment of pulsed dye laser-resistant port wine stain birthmarks. J Am Acad Dermatol. 2007; https://doi.org/10.1016/j.jaad.2007.01.019.
41. Nagore E, et al. Thickness of healthy and affected skin of children with port wine stains: potential repercussions on response to pulsed dye laser treatment. Dermatol Surg. 2004; https://doi.org/10.1111/j.1524-4725.2004.30503.x.
42. Huikeshoven M, et al. Redarkening of port-wine stains 10 years after pulsed-dye–laser treatment. N Engl J Med. 2007; https://doi.org/10.1056/NEJMoa064329.
43. Alexiades-Armenakas M. Laser-mediated photodynamic therapy. Clin Dermatol. 2006; https://doi.org/10.1016/j.clindermatol.2005.10.027.
44. Chen JK, et al. An overview of clinical and experimental treatment modalities for port wine stains. J Am Acad Dermatol. 2012; https://doi.org/10.1016/j.jaad.2011.11.938.
45. Kono T, et al. Long-pulsed neodymium:yttrium-aluminum-garnet laser treatment for hypertrophic port-wine stains on the lips. J Cosmet Laser Ther. 2009; https://doi.org/10.1080/14764170802307940.
46. C.M., G. and S., S. The use of the long-pulsed Nd:YAG laser for venous malformations in the pediatric population. Lasers Med Sci. 2011;
47. Borges da Costa J, et al. Treatment of resistant port-wine stains with a pulsed dual wavelength 595 and 1064 nm laser: a histochemical evaluation of the vessel wall destruction and selectivity. Photomed Laser Surg. 2009; https://doi.org/10.1089/pho.2008.2356.
48. Alster TS, Tanzi EL. Combined 595-nm and 1,064-nm laser irradiation of recalcitrant and hypertrophic port-wine stains in children and adults. Dermatol Surg. 2009; https://doi.org/10.1111/j.1524-4725.2009.01155.x.
49. McGill DJ, MacLaren W, Mackay IR. A direct comparison of pulsed dye, alexandrite, KTP and Nd:YAG lasers and IPL in patients with previously treated capillary malformations. Lasers Surg Med. 2008; https://doi.org/10.1002/lsm.20638.

9 Cystic and Non-Cystic Lymphatic Malformations

Waldemar L. Olszewski and Marzanna T. Zaleska

9.1 Introduction

Lymphatic malformation (LM) results from an error in the embryonic development caused by genetic mutation in the lymphatic system at various body sites. Sprouting lymphatics are not linked with the main lymphatics. Lack of their contacts with the lumen of collecting vessels results either in the formation of cystic lesions filled up with lymph-like fluid or local interstitial fluid accumulation creating foci of circumscribed edema. The cystic lesions are found mainly in head, neck, thorax, and abdominal cavity, whereas, the regions with lack of interstitial fluid outflow appear mainly in the soft tissues of lower parts of the body. The cystic malformations are classified as microcystic and macrocystic or large cysts (Fig. 9.1 a, b, c). Upon puncture, lymph-like fluid can be obtained. There is another group of malformation characterized by non-cystic interstitial accumulation of fluid classically called Milroy's disease. There are no walls separating fluid foci from the adjacent tissue (Fig. 9.1 c, d). Upon puncture, only some few drops of tissue fluid can be harvested. The actual problem in lymphology is whether to include Milroy disease to the malformation group or leave it as has been until now as the so-called "primary lymphedema" This is not only an academic problem, it has practical aspects. Whereas, cystic lesions have to be obliterated or/and be surgically removed, the tissue accumulation of edema fluid should be drained to the sites where it can be absorbed. It can be done either by external compression or formation of flow pathways using surgical methods. Diagnostic differentiation between the two conditions becomes necessary to establish proper therapeutic recommendations.

The large cystic malformations and their therapy will not be analyzed in this chapter as this classic condition has widely been described in a number of articles and textbooks [1]. Ultrasonography, MRI, and computer tomography help to show the topographical location, size, and septal structure of the lesion [1]. Sclerotherapy is the method of choice for large cysts. First, fluid is aspirated, then sclerosing substances are injected [2, 3]. The OK-432, bleomycin, doxycycline, tetradecyl sulfate or 96% ethanol are used. Antibiotics preventing the development of bacterial inflammation should be added. Surgical intervention may be applied only in selected cases depending mostly on the cyst location endangering life functions.

W. L. Olszewski (✉)
Central Clinical Hospital, Department of Vascular Surgery, Ministry of Internal Affairs, Warsaw, Poland

M. T. Zaleska
Department of Applied Physiology, Mossakowski Medical Research Center, Polish Academy of Sciences, Warsaw, Poland

A. K. Khanna, S. K. Tiwary (eds.), *Vascular Malformations*,
https://doi.org/10.1007/978-981-15-9762-6_9

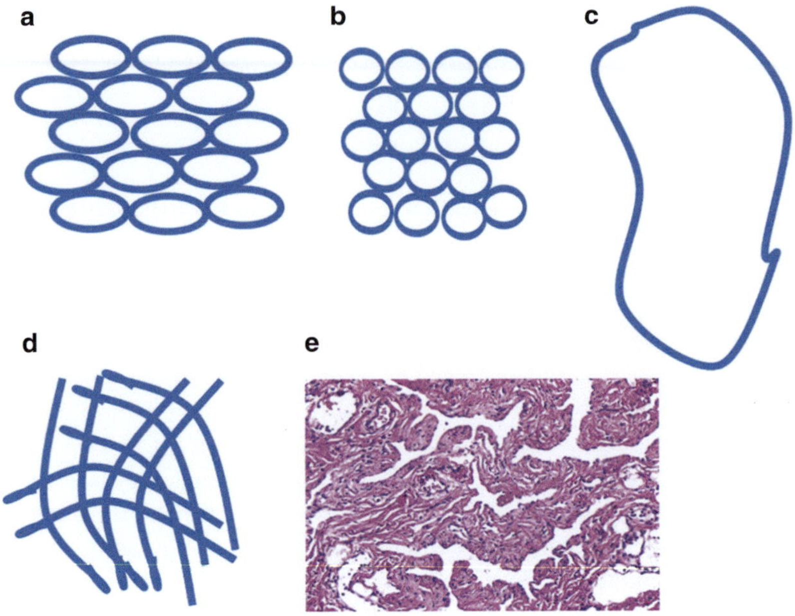

Fig. 9.1 Schematic presentation of cystic and non-cystic malformations: (**a**) microcystic, (**b**) macrocystic, (**c**) large cyst, (**d**) non-cystic, and (**e**) histological picture of noncystic fluid accumulation in the tissue

9.2 Contemporary Problems

The main contemporary problem is the diagnosis of the non-cystic interstitial malformations and specifically their location close to or even penetration of organs, edema fluid accumulation pattern in terms of micro- and macro-lakes, and topographical relation to the lymphatic collectors. The lesions may be formed as a separated tissue mass in the subcutaneous tissue. They may also be bordering to blood vessels and nerves. Lymphoscintigraphy, MRI gadolinium, and indocyanine green lymphography are indispensable. Any of these imaging markers can be injected into the lesion and provide picture of the size of a lesion, penetration to other regions and drainage to the collecting lymphatics and occasionally veins. The knowledge as to whether the lesion has a sponge-like or solid structure is important for the planned compression therapy. Analysis of the indocyanine green pictures is most helpful. It may show a more or less dense network of microchannels filled up with the dye. What would also be important, is the condition of the collecting lymphatics running close to the malformation. The isotope and MRI gadolinium lymphography of the limb or by puncture of the accessible lymph node close to the lesion may show or exclude connection to the lesion. Beside of that, depicted normal collectors would mean that malformation is only a local morphological event.

It should be mentioned, that lymphatic malformations differ between individuals, not only by location, but also by morphological structure, with more or less accumulated interstitial fluid, previous hemorrhagic injuries, inflammatory episodes, and causing functional problems in limbs. This is why diagnostic and therapeutic approach should be strongly individualized. Below we present a series of specific cases of lymphatic malformations encountered in limbs.

9.3 Clinical Cases

9.3.1 A Clinical Case of Cystic Malformation in Hypogastrium with Normal Lymphatic Drainage of the Limb

Lymphangioma was developed in the subcutaneous tissue of the right hypogastrium (Fig. 9.2). Indocyanine green lymphography showed, after the intra-lesion injection, a wide spot delineating

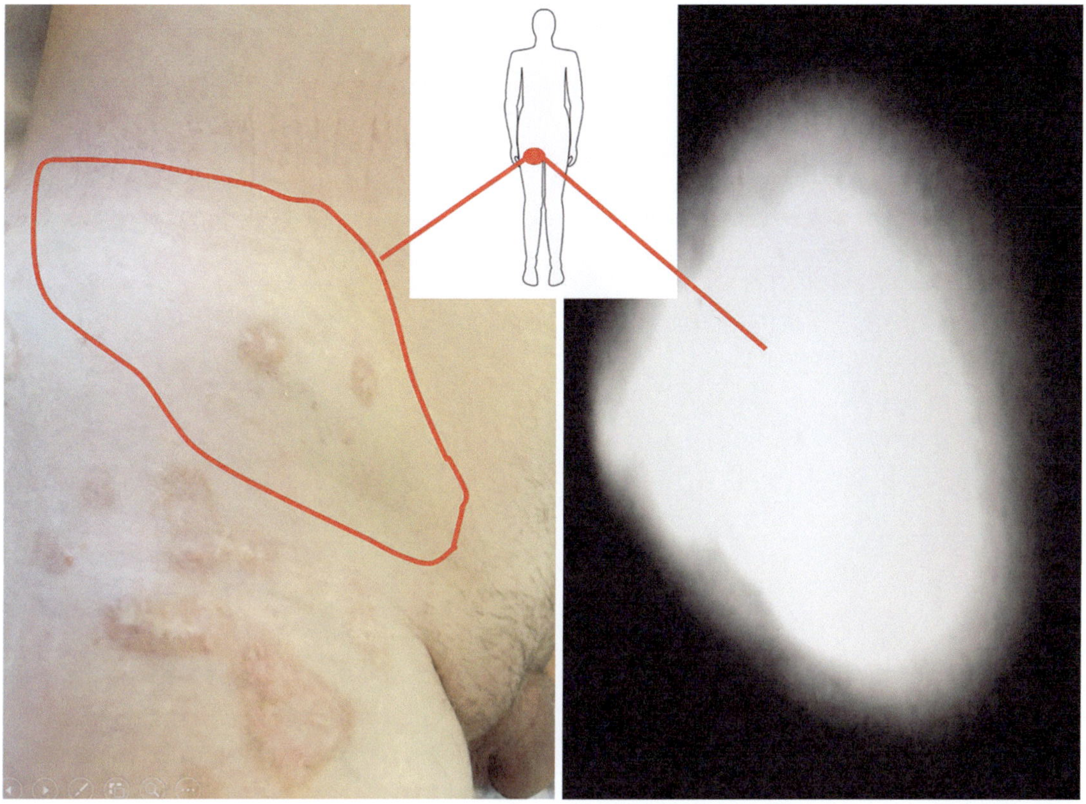

Fig. 9.2 A clinical case of cystic malformation. Lymphangioma localized in the right hypogastrium and accumulation of the ICG dye in this area

the size of the mass, not drained to the local lymphatics (Fig. 9.3). It contained lymph-like fluid on puncture. Obliteration was carried out by 3 injections of bleomycin.

9.3.2 The Most Common Types of Clinical Cases of Limb Lymphatic Non-Cystic Interstitial Malformations-Diagnosis and Therapy Recommendations

9.3.2.1 Inborn Lymphedema of Leg Without Drainage by Collecting Lymphatics

Inborn edema of the lower limb. This type of edema was previously classified as Milroy disease. Mutations in the FLT4 gene have been found in some cases. The FLT4 gene provides instructions for producing the vascular endothelial growth factor receptor 3 (VEGFR-3), which regulates the growth, movement, and survival of the lymphatic endothelial cells. These mutations lead to the development of small or no lymphatic vessels. However, in the majority of patients, this type of mutations is not proved. Nevertheless, these cases should be considered as malformations and not lymphedema. Lymphedema is a condition consisting of the obliteration of developed lymphatics filled with stagnant lymph. In the Milroy disease, there is interstitial accumulation of tissue fluid but not lymph. Lymphoscintigraphy or ICG lymphography shows a dense spot of the marker in the foot dorsum often moving in a retrograde fashion to the toes and plantar tissue (Fig. 9.4). There is usually no free fluid on tissue puncture. Recommended treatment is professionally made compression of foot. Surgical methods for creating edema fluid outflow pathways or plastic reconstructions should be delayed until the age of body growth is stopped.

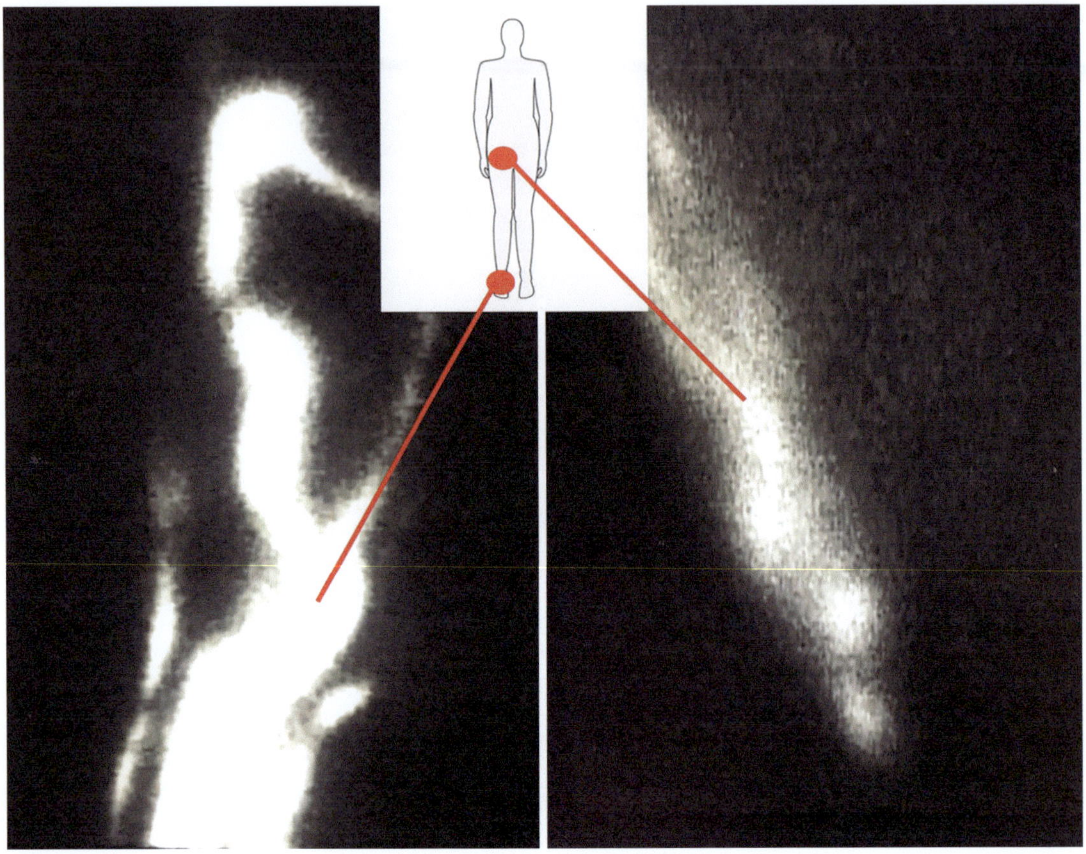

Fig. 9.3 The ICG lymphography shows wide spot of the dye in the foot and in the groin

9.3.2.2 Inborn Lymphedema of Leg with Drainage by Collecting Lymphatics

Inborn leg edema. The ICG dye formed a confluent misty image in the subcutaneous tissue of foot. There is, however, some flow of the dye along the limb forming a confluent accumulation in the groin (Fig. 9.5). The question arises whether it is a local malformation of initial lymphatics in the foot with some patent draining calf collectors and with other malformation in the groin? [4]. The contralateral limb is normal. Recommended treatment is professionally made compression of the whole limb.

9.3.2.3 Inborn Left Hand Edema with Lack of Picture of Forearm and Arm Collectors but Proximal Lymph Drainage

In such case the ICG dye forms a misty image in the hand tissue. There might be some flow of the dye along the limb to the elbow region and axillary lymph node, although collectors have not been depicted (Fig. 9.6). Frequently, it is unilateral with normal lymphatics of the contralateral limb. Under high magnification, a dense micronetwork of spaces filled up with ICG clearly showing the site of tissue fluid accumulation without the link to the initial lymphatics (Fig. 9.7). Recommended treatment is professionally made compression of the whole limb.

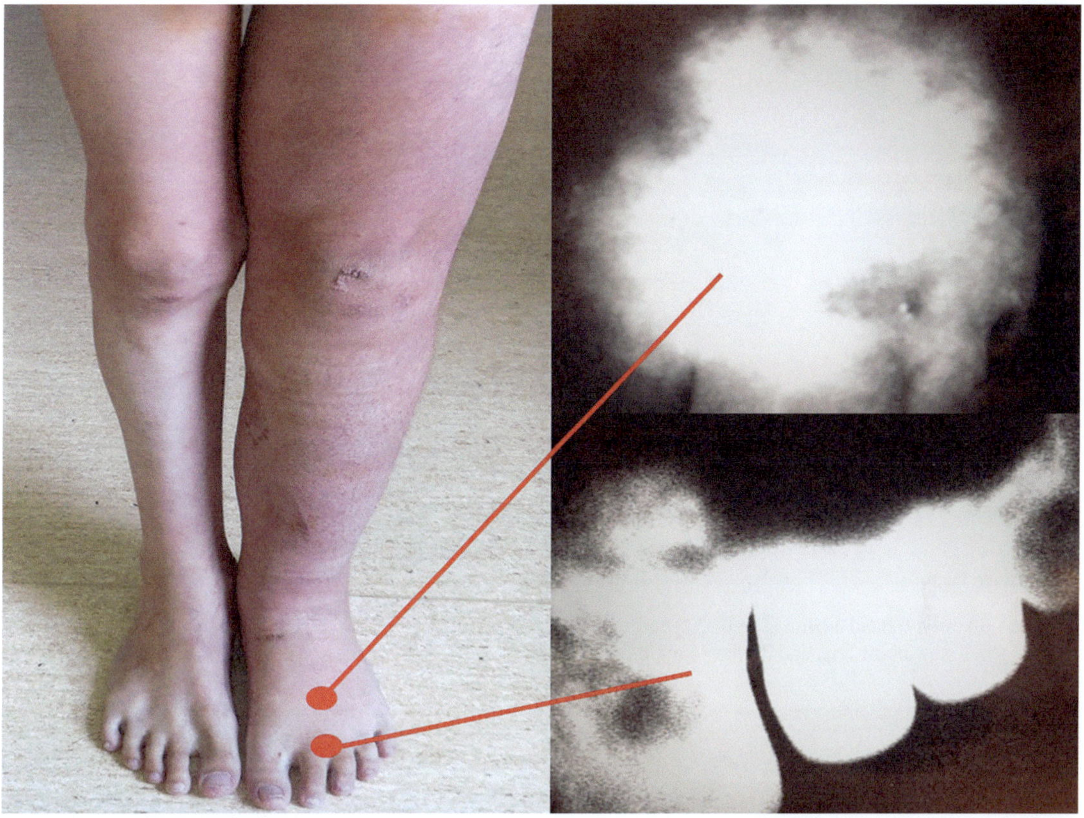

Fig. 9.4 Inborn lymphedema of lower leg. The ICG lymphography shows a dens spot of the dye in the foot dorsum and in the toes on the plantar side

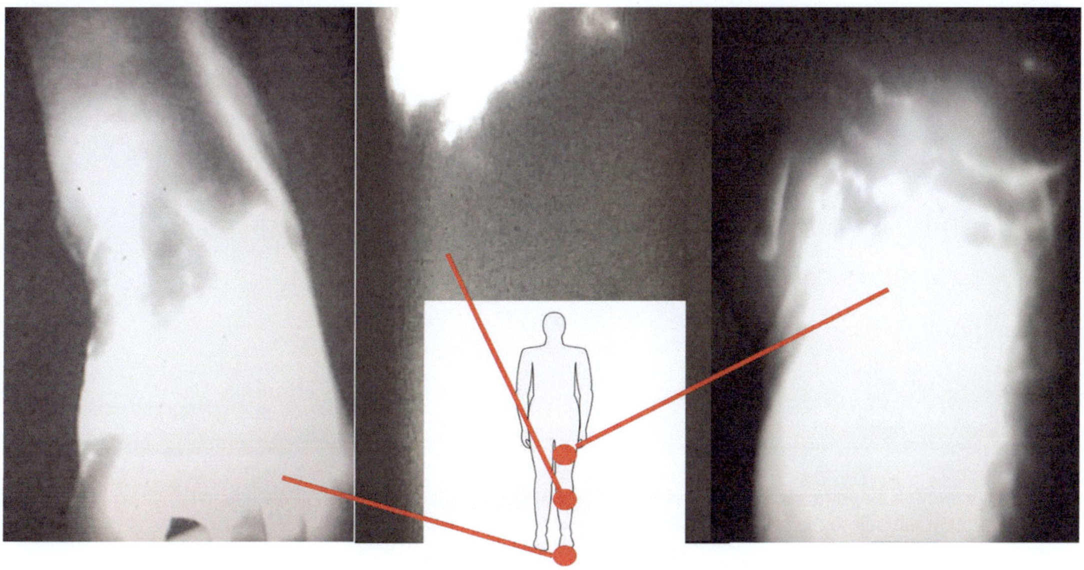

Fig. 9.5 Inborn lymphedema of lower limb. The ICG lymphography shows misty image in the foot, some flow of the dye along the limb and confluent accumulation in the groin

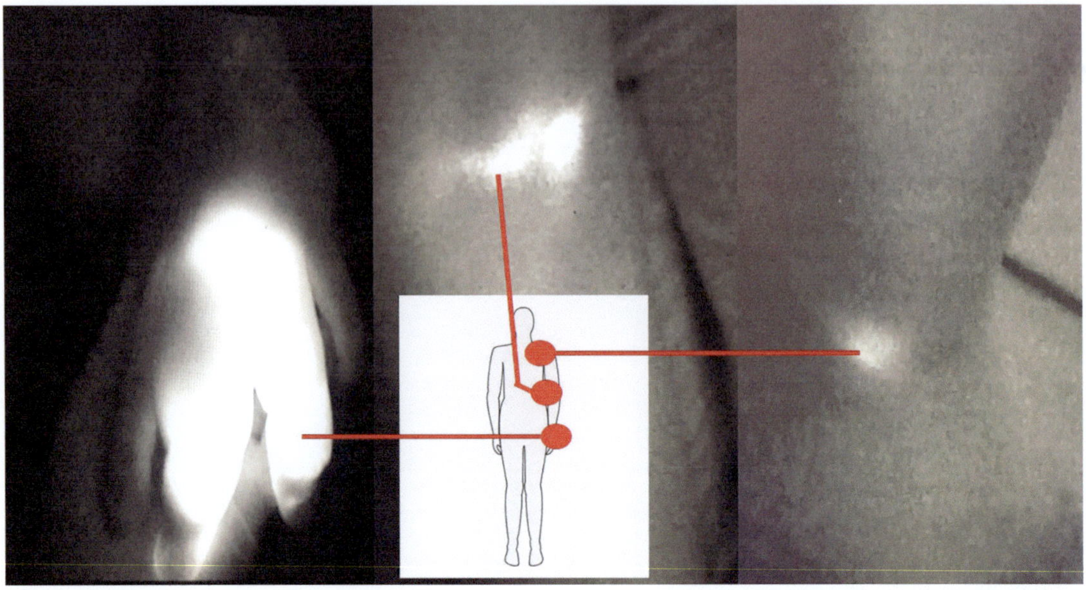

Fig. 9.6 Inborn left hand edema. The ICG lymphography shows a misty image in the hand, some flow of the dye along the forearm to the elbow area and axillary lymph node

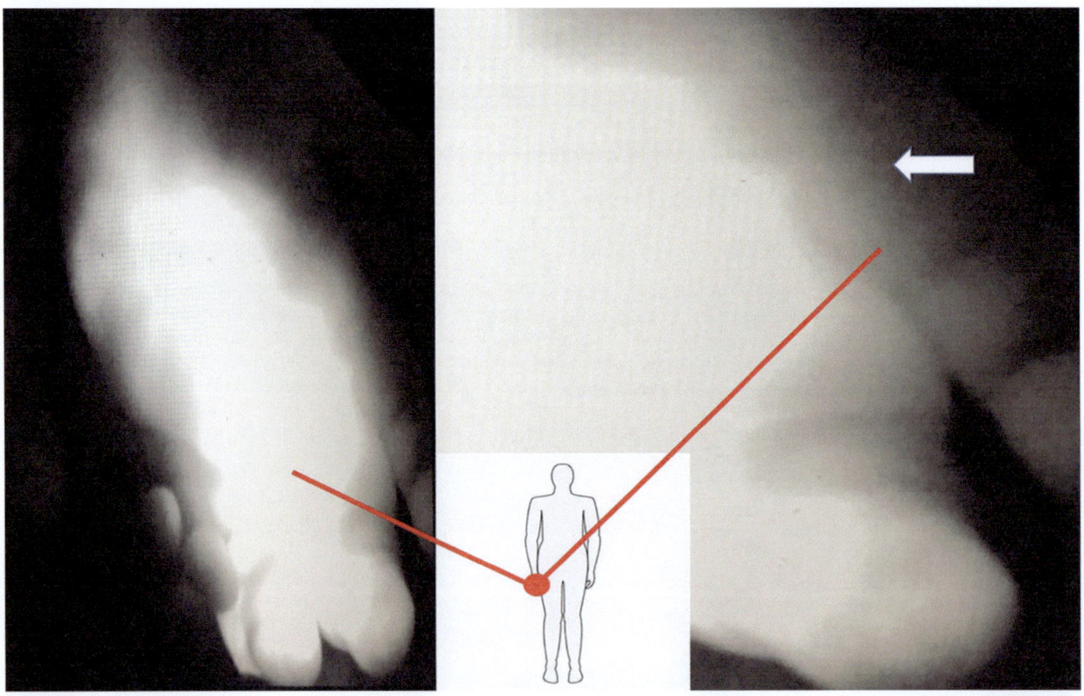

Fig. 9.7 Under high magnification a dens micro-network of speces filled up with the ICG dye in the site of fluid accumulation without the link to the lymphatic can be seen

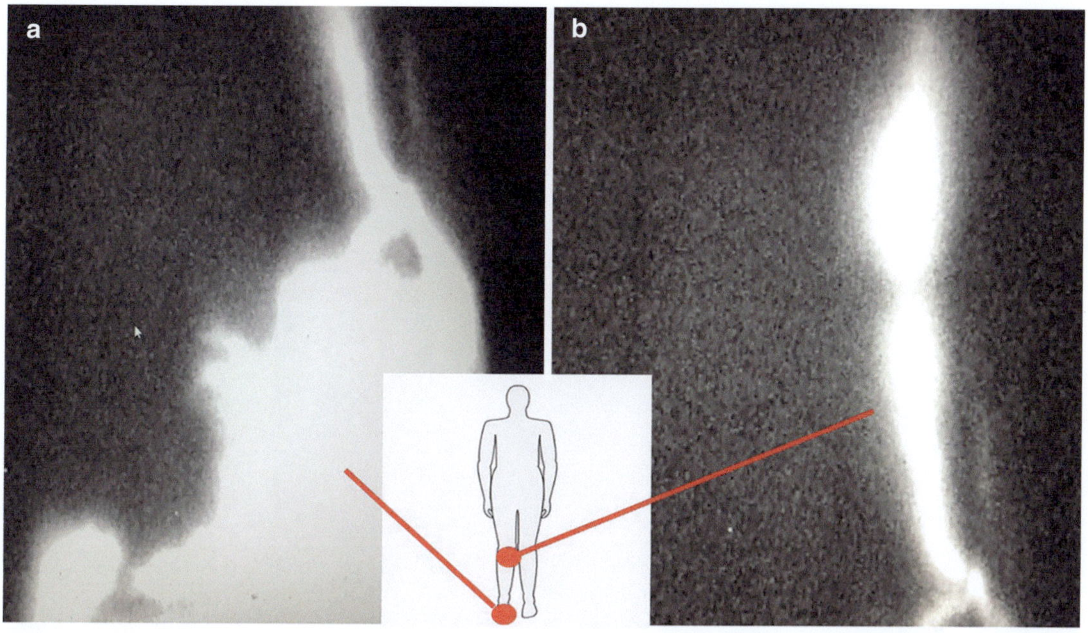

Fig. 9.8 Inborn foot edema. The ICG picture shows a misty image in the foot dorsum (a) and normal collecting lymphatics along the limb (b)

9.3.2.4 Inborn Foot Edema with Lack of Picture of Foot Collectors but Normal Calf Lymphatics

In cases like that dye is forming a misty image in the foot dorsum (Fig. 9.8a). There are normal collecting lymphatics along the limb (Fig. 9.8b). Recommended treatment is professionally made compression of the foot.

Inborn edema of feet with lack of pictures of collecting lymphatics but fast accumulations of dye in the urine.

9.3.2.5 There are cases with foot edema and fast accumulation of the isotop in lymphoscintigraphy or the ICG dye in the urine

isotope or ICG dye in urine (Fig. 9.9). The question arises whether there is drainage of edema fluid from the local lymphatic malformation by blood capillaries or pre-existing lympho-venous communications? A case of inborn foot edema with drainage of edema fluid to a local vein is shown in Fig. 9.10.

9.4 Methods for Diagnosis of Lymphatic Changes in Inborn Edema of Limbs

1. Lymphoscintigraphy of the limb with 99Tc Nanocoll and b. indocyanine green fluorescent lymphography (ICG) of limb, to visualize drainage from the distal parts of the limb either through tissue spaces or by collecting lymphatics.
2. Intra-lesion injection of 99Tc Nanocoll or ICG, to visualize drainage pathways form the lymphangioma or edema region.
3. MRI with the contrast of the limb to depict the exact location and size of the lesion (penetration from the subcutaneous tissue to perivascular and perineural spaces).
4. Collection of fluid from lesion by puncture for a. bacteriology (frequent infections and inflammation), b. cell phenotypes (neoplastic).
5. Biopsy of tissue in cases suspected of neoplastic changes.

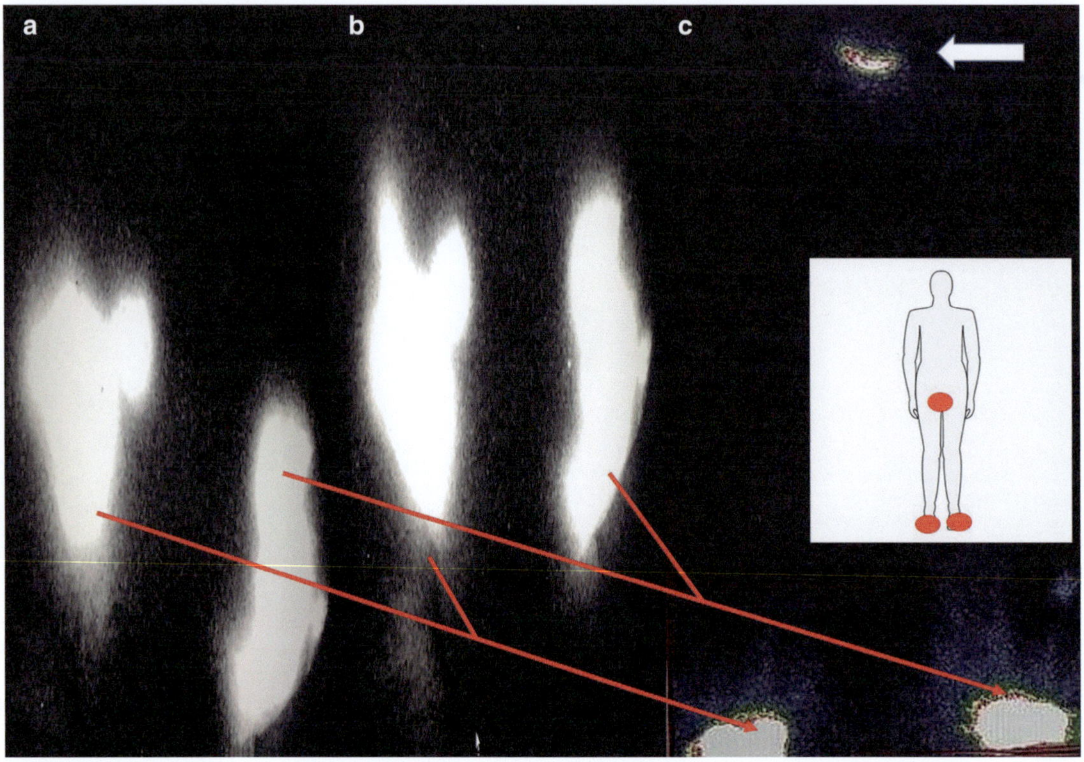

Fig. 9.9 Inborn edema of feet with lack of picture of collecting lymphatics. A misty accumulation of the ICG dye in the feet (**a**, **b**) and fast accumulation of the tracer in the urin on lymphoscintygraphic picture

9.5 Recommended Methods of Therapy

9.5.1 Conservative Therapy

1. Professionally made compression of the affected parts of the limb (manual massage, bandaging, elastic garments.
2. Obliteration procedures. The circumscribed lesions, not drained by lymphatic collectors can be treated by injection of bleomycin, doxycycline, OK-432, tetradecyl sulfate, or ethanol. Lymphoscintigraphic and ICG images should be analyzed before the decision for obliteration not to damage the collecting vessels.
3. Antibiotic therapy should be instituted in cases with recurrent inflammation of the edematous changes.

9.5.2 Surgical Therapy

The surgical therapy as removal of lesions should be limited to: the circumscribed lymphangioma resistant to the obliteration trials and changes developed and gradually enlarging in the life-threatening regions. All other surgical procedures should be postponed until the stop of body growth. Disfigurement and functional disabling of the limb can be a complication of surgery performed at the growth age.

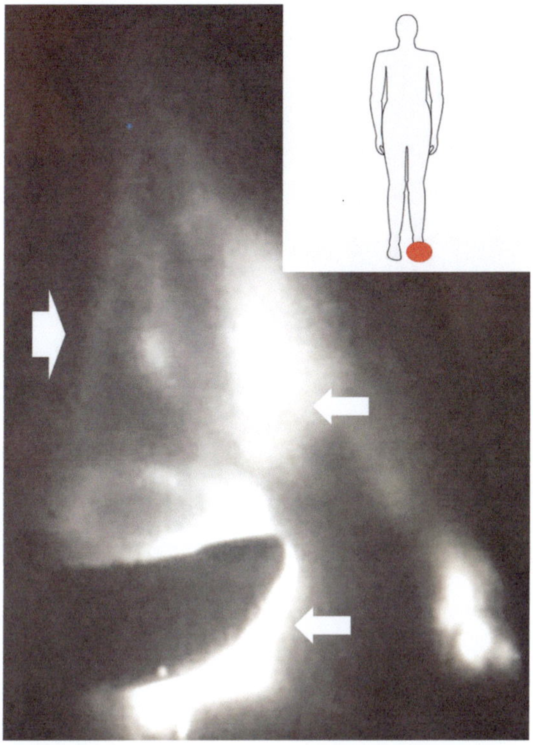

Fig. 9.10 Inborn foot edema. The ICG picture shows the drainage of edema fluid to a local vein

References

1. Defnet AM, Bagrodia N, Hernandez SL, Gwilliam N, Kande JJ. Pediatric lymphatic malformations: evolving understanding and therapeutic options. Pediatr Surg Int. 2016;32:425–33.
2. Greene AK, Sca MM, Perlyn CA, Alomari AI. Management of Lymphatic Malformations. Clin Plastic Surg. 2011;38:75–82.
3. Dubois J, Gilles Soulez F. Common (cystic) lymphatic malformations: current knowledge and management. Tech Vasc Interv Radiol. 2019;22(4):100631.
4. Motoi K, Shoi W, Takuya L, Azusa W. 4.Pattern classification in lymphatic malformations by Indocyanine green Lymphography. Plast Reconstructr Surg. 2019;143:558e–64e.

10 Combined Vascular Malformation

Shantonu Kumar Ghosh

10.1 Combined Vascular Malformation

Combined vascular malformation associates two or more components in one lesion. It can involve any combination of capillary, lymphatic, venous, and arterial channels. Combined vascular malformations may be simple, or malformations of major vessels, or combined. Like single-channel-type vascular malformations, combined lesions are categorized as slow-flow and fast-flow lesions [1]. Often combined malformations constitute an overgrowth syndrome, hypertrophy of soft tissue, and skeletal hypertrophy [2]. Most combined malformations involve limbs, but they can involve any area of the body.

Combined vascular malformations may sometimes associate a cutaneous Capillary Malformation (CM) and an underlying Venous Malformation (VM), Lymphatic Malformation (LM), or Arteriovenous Malformation (AVM), or a VM with an LM (Table 10.1).

Table 10.1 Combined Vascular Malformations

a.	Capillary venous malformation
b.	Capillary-lymphatic malformation
c.	Capillary-arteriovenous malformation
d.	Capillary-lymphatic-venous malformation
e.	Capillary-lymphatic-arteriovenous malformation
f.	Capillary-lymphatic-venous-arteriovenous malformation
g.	Capillary-venous-arteriovenous malformation
h.	Lymphatic-venous malformation

10.1.1 Malformations of Major Named Vessels

These malformations affect veins, arteries, or lymphatics of generally large caliber, often axial or conducting vessels. They consist of anomalies in the origin, course, number, length, diameter (aplasia, hypoplasia, ectasia/aneurysm), or valves. Congenital arteriovenous fistulas and the persistence of embryonic vessels are also included in this group of malformations.

10.1.2 Vascular Malformations Associated with Other Anomalies

Vascular malformations (simple and/or of major named vessels) may be associated with anomalies of bone, soft tissue, or viscera. These nonvascular

S. K. Ghosh (✉)
National Institute of Cardiovascular Diseases and Hospital, Dhaka, Bangladesh

A. K. Khanna, S. K. Tiwary (eds.), *Vascular Malformations*,
https://doi.org/10.1007/978-981-15-9762-6_10

Table 10.2 Vascular Malformations Associated With Other Anomalies

Klippel-Trenaunay syndrome	Capillary-lymphatic-venous malformation with limb overgrowth
Parkes–Weber syndrome:	Capillary malformation, limb overgrowth and AV fistula
Sturge-Weber syndrome:	Facial-leptomeningeal capillary malformation, ocular anomalies with bone and soft tissue overgrowth
Servelle-Martorell syndrome:	Venous malformation of limb with bone undergrowth
Maffucci syndrome:	Venous malformation associated with spindle cell hemangioma and enchondroma
CLOVES syndrome:	Capillary-lymphatic-venous-arteriovenous malformation with lipomatous overgrowth
Proteus syndrome:	Capillary-lymphatic-venous malformation with asymmetric somatic overgrowth
Bannayan–Riley–Ruvalcaba syndrome:	Capillary-venous-arteriovenous malformation and macrocephaly
Microcephaly with capillary malformation	
Macrocephaly with capillary malformation	
Congenital nonprogressive limb hypertrophy with capillary malformation	

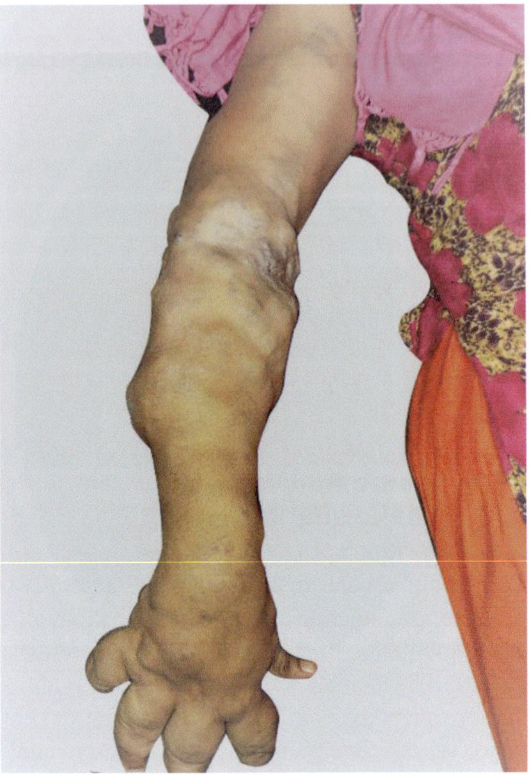

Fig. 10.1 Capillary venous malformation on upper arm

anomalies are often overgrowth of soft tissue and/or bone or, rarely, undergrowth. Most of these syndromes or diseases are listed in Table 10.2 along with their most common associations.

10.2 Slow Flow Malformation

10.2.1 Capillary-Lymphatico-Venous Malformation (Klippel–Trenaunay Syndrome)

The first reports of patients with a slow-flow capillary-lymphatico-venous malformation (CLVM) were published in the nineteenth century by Hilaire, Tre´ lat, and Monod [3, 4]. In 1900 the French physicians, Maurice Klippel and Paul Trenaunay [5] first recognized Klippel–Trenaunay syndrome as a distinct entity [6]. They proposed the syndrome with the main characteristics like localized vascular nevus, congenital, or early infantile varicosities, and hypertrophy of tissue occurring in the same body part. For more than 100 years, the eponym, Klippel–Tre'naunay syndrome, has been used to describe patients with CLVM [1]. Vascular malformations located in the head or pelvis had also been classified as Klippel–Trenaunay syndrome over decades. An international consensus about venous malformations had been done by the International Union of Phlebology (IUP), where Klippel–Trenaunay syndrome was defined as a diffuse venous malformation that involved the whole limb and where a combination of two malformations was present (i.e., truncular or extratruncular venous or lymphatic malformations), without arteriovenous malformations. The consensus also decided that malformations involving only a part of the limb (thigh, calf, or foot) or locations only outside the limbs should not be defined as Klippel–Trenaunay syndrome [7] (Figs. 10.1, 10.2, and 10.3).

10.2.2 Etiology and Genetics

CLVM has an equal gender distribution and occurs sporadically, however, no chromosomal localization or linkage with a causative gene has been identified [6]. Several theories have been proposed as pathogenesis. Klippel and Tre'naunay [5] suggested that the mechanism responsible was a congenital spinal cord abnormality that altered autonomic control of capillaries causing increased blood flow to the skin, soft tissue, and bone with resultant hypertrophy. During the specific stages of embryonic development altered vasculogenesis with localized overgrowth have also been theorized. The angiogenic factor gene, AGGF1, has been suggested as a candidate susceptibility gene [8, 9]. Additional conjectures include paradominant inheritance, genetic mosaicism, and a polygenic hypothesis [6].

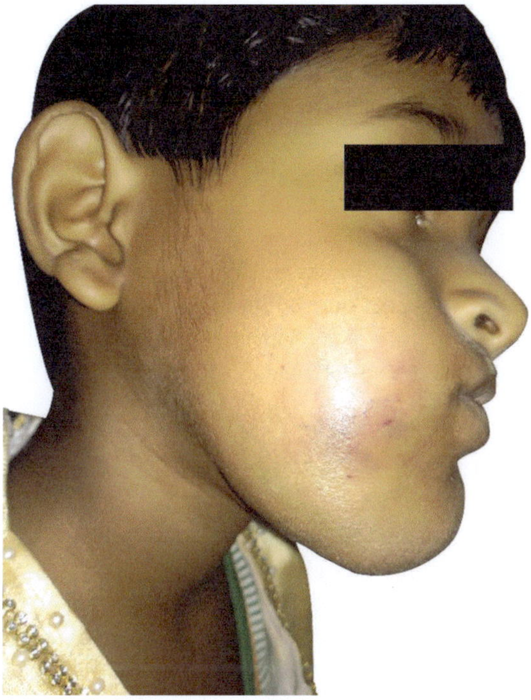

Fig. 10.2 Capillary venous malformation on cheek

10.2.3 Clinical Features

Klippel–Trenaunay syndrome may manifest in the lower limbs with the clinical triad dilated abnormal superficial veins, nevus, and limb length discrepancy due to overgrowth or shortening of the affected limb. However, the nevus may be absent and limb length discrepancies may not be constant (Table 10.2). Bilateral involvement and overgrowth deformity of the foot are also

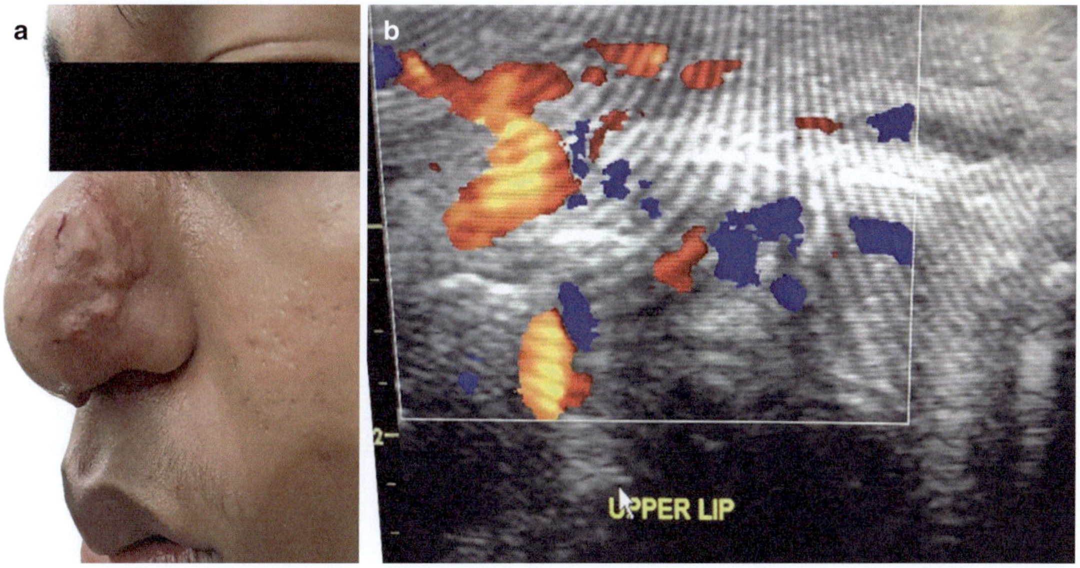

Fig. 10.3 (**a**) Lymphatic-venous malformation on nose. (**b**) Duplex scanning of lymphatic venous malformation on nose

possible. An abnormal, lateral vein, called a marginal vein, is often present. This vein may create stasis, pain, and sometimes, a pulmonary embolism [10]. Patients often complain of heaviness, swelling, and pain, which may be localized to specific areas of the limb. Pelvic involvement including the genitals or the rectum with bleeding is often evident.

10.2.4 Diagnosis

As Klippel–Trenaunay syndrome often appears as a complex of congenital vascular malformations, diagnosis may be difficult. To diagnose the syndrome, a step-by-step procedure is recommended, beginning with the least invasive procedure, as follows:

- Clinical evaluation
- Comparative radiography of the limbs
- Duplex scan
- MRI with and without contrast
- Lymphoscintigraphy
- Other tests, if necessary

The clinical examination should focus on evaluating the extension of the nevus, recognizing and/or excluding differences in limb length, noticing the presence and extension of dilated superficial veins, and checking for signs of arteriovenous malformations, such as abnormal vascular pulsations (ie, thrills). Comparative radiography of the limbs is useful to recognize overgrowth or shortening of the affected limb, presence of phlebolythes (a typical sign of venous malformations), and bone structure anomalies. Duplex scanning provides hemodynamic and morphologic data on congenital vascular malformations. Duplex scanning of the deep and superficial venous systems may demonstrate anomalies of the deep and superficial veins. Vascular masses situated in tissues should be analyzed to determine the type of flow: low flow indicates venous dysplasia; high flow is typical of arteriovenous malformations; and areas with liquid cysts with no flow (i.e., no flow areas) indicate lymphatic extratruncular malformations. Combinations of low flow and no flow vascular areas may coexist. MRI is an excellent diagnostic tool to identify the location and extent of the extratruncular venous and lymphatic malformations, which are often located inside the muscles [11]. Truncular venous malformations have also been well documented. Lymphoscintigraphy is necessary to study the lymphatic drainage system because anomalies are common in Klippel-Tre'naunay syndrome and these cannot be determined using other examinations. A separate study for deep and superficial lymphatic drainage systems is necessary to identify the location and extent of the malformations. Anomalies of the deep lymphatic trunks, such as aplasia or hypoplasia in segments or even the whole vessel, are the most common lymphatic malformations recognized in Klippel–Trenaunay syndrome [12].

10.2.5 Management

Treatment should be planned according to some priorities that include pain; clinical evolution of malformations, such as progression of limb elongation or shortening; risk of complications, such as a pulmonary embolism (ie, in the marginal vein); and esthetic discomfort. Pain mainly occurs due to repeated thrombosis in venous extratruncular masses where blood stasis often occurs. Venous aneurysms in the femoral or popliteal vein may also cause pain due to blood stasis. Progression of limb elongation is often due to the marginal vein, which creates stasis, and due to a slight arteriovenous malformation located in the dysplastic tissues. Limb shortening is due to extensive venous dysplastic masses pressing on bones, which inhibits their growth. Pulmonary embolisms may originate from both large marginal veins and venous aneurysms. Treatment techniques include surgery, sclerotherapy, and laser treatment. Surgery is often the best technique; however, it should be well planned based on a complete recognition of the malformation and the causes of discomfort. Surgical removal of extratruncular masses that cause pain or affect limb growth can considerably improve a patient's condition. However, the best results are obtained with a step-by-step procedure, which avoids extensive single operations that may have complications like infection, difficult wound healing, and thrombosis. Marginal veins should be removed surgically in an open procedure; closed stripping should be avoided due to bleeding complications that can arise from the rupture of larger perforators [10]. This procedure is not indicated for deep vein aplasia because, in this case, the marginal vein is the main draining vessel. For deep hypoplasia, the marginal vein can be resected, as deep veins are able to dilate spontaneously to an almost normal size after resection. Endovascular treatment of marginal veins using laser treatment has been reported [13]. Venous aneurysms can be treated by resection and reconstruction of vein or by resection and substitution with an autologous venous graft. Sclerotherapy of dysplastic veins is an excellent and less invasive technique. However, classic sclerosants like sodium tetradecyl sulfate, polidocanol, etc. are less effective for venous malformations and there is a high incidence of early recurrence. The introduction of alcohol for sclerotherapy has dramatically improved the results because ethanol is the strongest sclerosant that can almost completely occlude the treated vessels. Ethanol is considered the reference sclerosant for venous malformations [7]. Alcohol is best used for the treatment of extratruncular dysplastic venous malformations, whereas truncular malformations are treated better with surgery [14]. For extratruncular vascular masses, laser treatment using an interstitial technique that positions the laser fiber in the mass can be used to occlude dysplastic vessels. Radial fibers may be useful to increase the effect of treatment. Leaking extratruncular lymphatic malformations with repeated inflammation can be treated successfully using laser treatment. Orthopedic techniques are effective if limb length discrepancies develop [15]. During childhood, epiphysiodesis is effective to temporarily block limb growth. The expected growth phase should be accurately predicted to determine when to implant the elongation device. In adults and after growth has stopped, limb elongation of the contralateral extremity is possible using the Ilizarov technique. Osteotomy to shorten the affected limb is performed less frequently. Limb shortening due to venous masses blocking limb growth is the least common condition, which requires occlusion or removal of the dysplastic veins. Correction of a short limb in adults is more complex as limb elongation may be dangerous due to bone fragility and the risk of fracture after removing the elongation device (Figs. 10.4, 10.5, and 10.6).

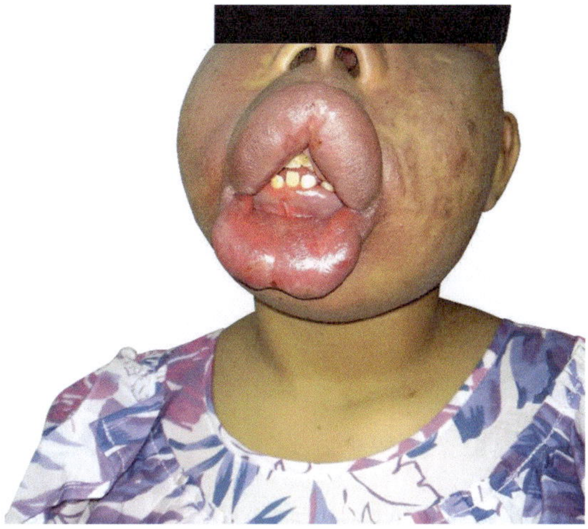

Fig. 10.4 Lymphatic-venous malformation on lips

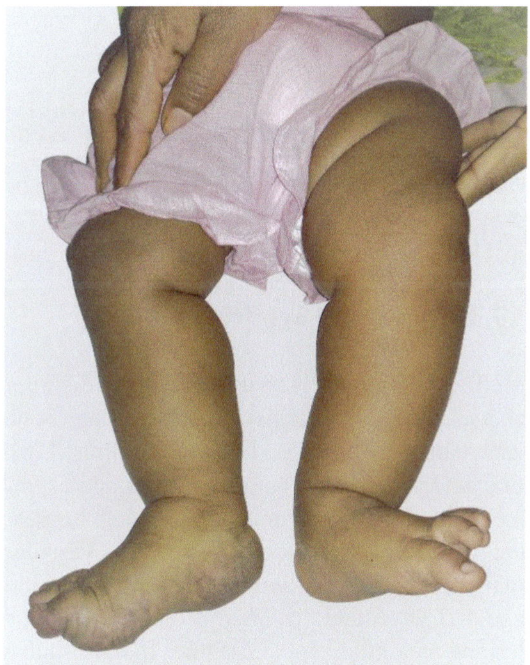

Fig. 10.5 Capillary-lymphatic malformation on leg

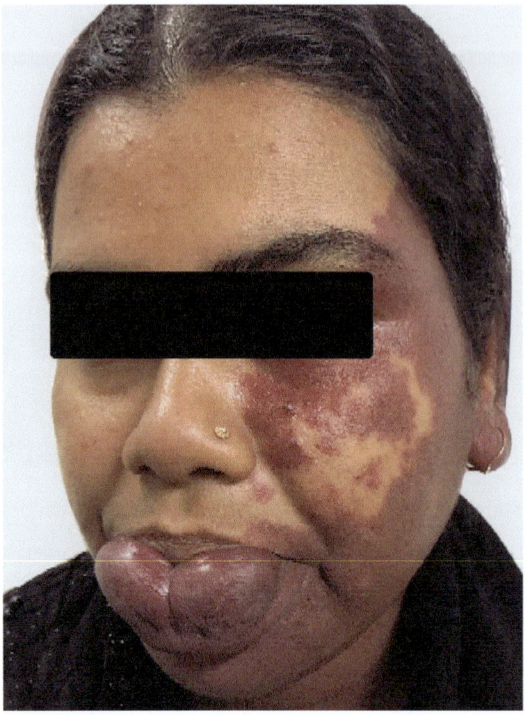

Fig. 10.6 Capillary-lymphatic-venous malformation on face

10.3 Maffucci Syndrome

Maffucci Syndrome is an extremely rare disorder characterized by cutaneous VMs, long bone enchondromas, and skeletal deformities [16]. Enchondromas cause bony distortion and asymmetric growth; it is common for a patient to present with a pathologic fracture. Vascular malformations on the skin usually appear around age 4–5 years and are often progressive. These lesions begin as compressible, round, bluish spots; later they become firm, knotty, and warty, and they often contain phlebolythes. Spindle cell hemangioma often arises in these malformed veins. Patients with Maffucci syndrome are at risk of developing chondrosarcoma and various other malignancies [17].

10.4 Fast Flow Malformation

10.4.1 Capillary-Arteriovenous Malformation and Capillary Arteriovenous Fistulas (Parkes–Weber Syndrome)

Capillary-arteriovenous malformation (CAVM) and capillary-arteriovenous fistulas (CAVFs) correspond to the old eponym Parkes Weber syndrome. This syndrome is characterized by the presence of a confluent or patchy CM with underlying multiple microarteriovenous fistulas in association with soft tissue and skeletal hypertrophy of the affected limb [18, 19]. There is often an associated lymphatic component. The diagnosis may be confirmed at birth, with diffuse enlargement of the involved limb, most commonly a lower extremity. However, sometimes the syndrome is not obvious at birth and becomes apparent during infancy and childhood [20]. The ipsilateral buttock or trunk may also be involved [21]. The stained areas are usually warm; a thrill may be palpable. Auscultation may detect a bruit. Handheld Doppler examination often reveals increased flow and low-resistance runoff when placed over the stained areas (Figs. 10.6 and 10.7).

Mutations in RASA1 have been identified in patients with CAVM who have multifocal CMs [21]. Radiologically, the affected extremity usually has fusiform, subcutaneous, muscular, and bony overgrowth with diffuse micro fistulas. Ultrasonography and color Doppler evaluation of arterial flow may be performed. Generalized arterial and venous dilatations are seen on angiography and venography. Angiography demonstrates discrete arteriovenous shunts, particularly around joint structures [22]. A soft tissue blush is observed involving muscles and subcutaneous fat. Contrast-enhanced T2-weighted MRI sequences reveal vascular flow voids.

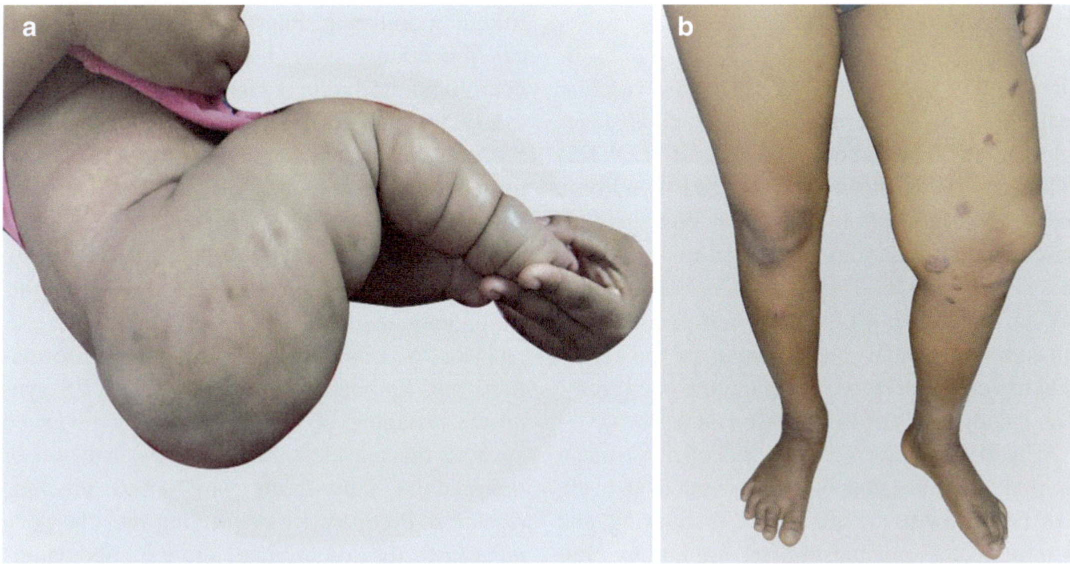

Fig. 10.7 (**a**) Klippel–Trenaunay syndrome in child. (**b**) Klippel–Trenaunay syndrome in adult

Infants and children are followed up annually with monitoring for axial overgrowth, signs of cardiac failure, and cutaneous problems related to ischemia. Treatment is predicated on symptoms. Epiphysiodesis can improve LLDs. Surgical debulking procedures are generally not performed because the micro fistulas frequently permeate the entire extremity. Flow reduction may be accomplished with repetitive superselective embolization which can ameliorate heart failure [23]. For recalcitrant disease, amputation may be required.

10.5 Capillary Malformation-Arteriovenous Malformation

A newly delineated familial disorder, capillary malformation-arteriovenous malformation (CM-AVM) is characterized by single or multiple small (1–2 cm in diameter) pink-to-red, round-to-oval CMs in association with AVM or AVF. Often the small lesions exhibit fast flow on handheld Doppler ultrasound examination. Frequently there is a family history of one or more innocent-appearing capillary stains. There is phenotypic overlap with Parkes Weber syndrome [21, 23].

10.6 Bannayan–Riley–Ruvalcaba Syndrome (PTEN Hamartoma Syndrome)

Bannayan–Riley–Ruvalcaba Syndrome, also known as PTEN hamartoma syndrome, is characterized by macrocephaly, multiple lipomas, hamartomatous polyps of distal ileum and colon, Hashimoto thyroiditis, pigmented penile macules, and vascular anomalies including CM, VM, and AVM [24]. Affected patients have an increased risk of malignancy, particularly of the thyroid and breast. About 31% of patients develop multinodular goiter, thyroid adenoma, or thyroid cancer [25]. Bannayan–Riley–Ruvalcaba syndrome is an autosomal dominant disorder caused by a mutation in tumor suppressor gene PTEN.

10.7 Cloves Syndrome

Congenital lipomatous overgrowth, vascular malformations, epidermal nevi, and spinal/skeletal anomalies and/or scoliosis (CLOVES) syndrome is a newly recognized syndrome mainly presents with truncal lipomatous masses, vascular malformations, and acral/musculoskeletal anomalies [26, 27]. Like CLVM and Parkes Weber syndrome, CLOVES syndrome may be suspected antenatally because many of the abnormalities can be seen on prenatal ultrasonography. The pathogenesis of the disease is unknown.

The key feature is the presence of a truncal lipomatous mass that is usually noted at birth. The fatty growths are often large, disfiguring, and painful. The lipomatous masses are hypervascular and exhibit rapid post-resection recurrence. These masses are also infiltrative and frequently extend from the trunk into adjacent areas such as the retroperitoneum, mediastinum, and thoracic cavity. Many of the lipomatous growths involve the spinal column and extend into the epidural space; causing compression of the cord, thecal sac, and nerve roots. Vascular malformations are also a distinguishing characteristic of CLOVES syndrome, may be either slow-flow or fast-flow. MRI with venous and arterial sequences early in life can determine the presence, location, and extent of the fast-flow lesions. Occasionally, neurologic monitoring, interventional, and/or surgical procedures may be required to prevent neurologic morbidity. Embolization may be necessary to manage the fast-flow malformations. Musculoskeletal abnormalities in CLOVES syndrome most commonly involve the feet and hands. Acral deformities include large, wide feet and hands, macrodactyly, and a wide sandal gap. Scoliosis has also been observed. Skeletal stabilization may be required in these patients.

Prior to debulking the slow-flow malformations and lipomatous masses in CLOVES syndrome, imaging should be carefully reviewed because the muscles are frequently involved or replaced by fatty tissue which may preclude resection. Preoperative counseling must be done regarding the recurrence of the lipomatous masses and the risk of DVT and PE. The use of LMWH and/or retrievable IVC filters and superior vena cava filters in the perioperative period potentially reduces the risk of PE (Figs. 10.8, 10.9, and 10.10).

Summary Proper diagnosis is essential for patients affected by complex combined vascular malformations. These patients benefit from an interdisciplinary approach involving many medical and surgical specialists. Interventions must be tailored to the specific needs and symptoms of the patient. Outcomes are optimized with careful preoperative planning, identification of comorbidities, and realistic expectations on behalf of both the patient and surgeon.

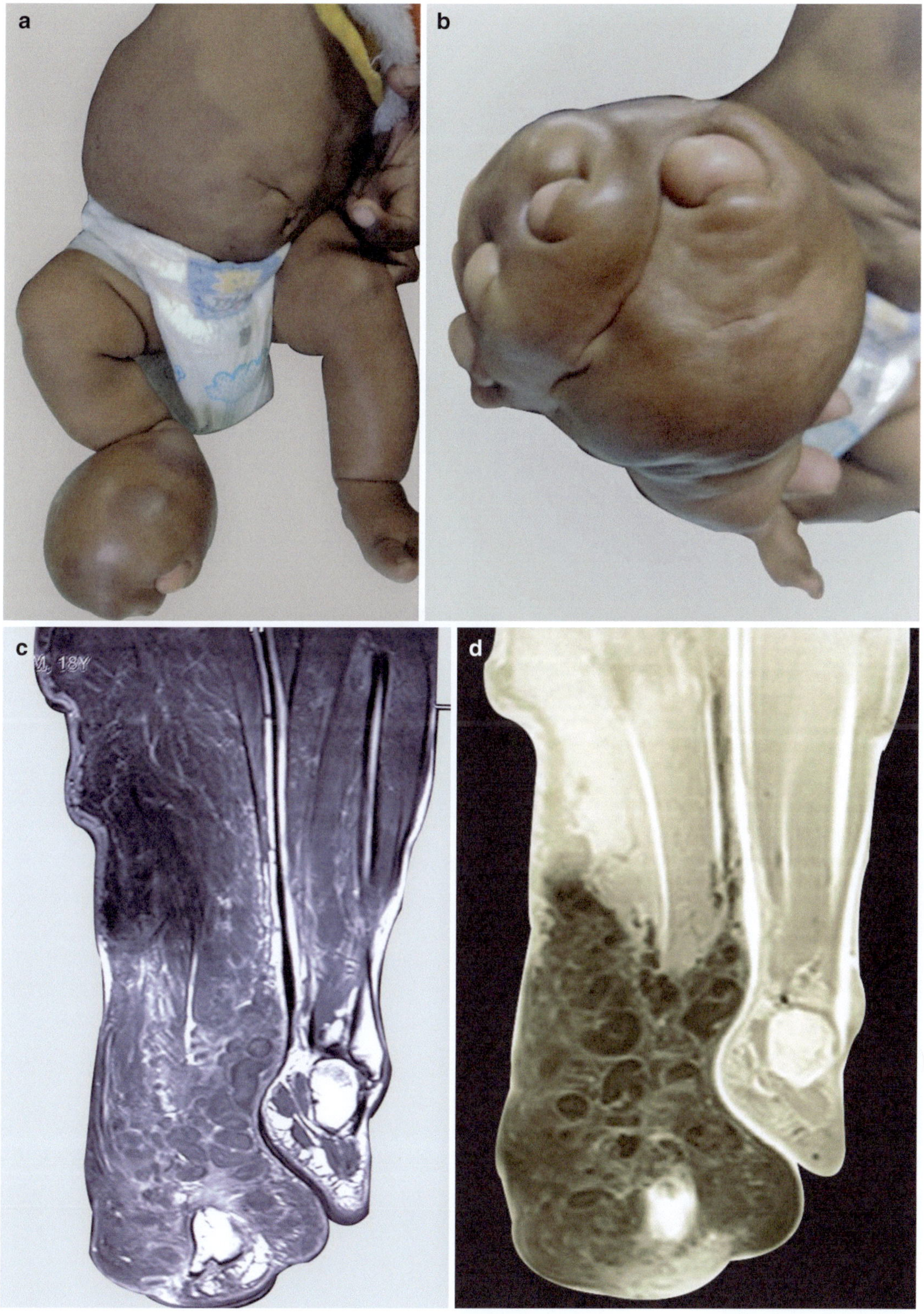

Fig. 10.8 (**a**) CLOVES syndrome newborn. (**b**) CLOVES syndrome newborn foot. (**c**) CLOVES syndrome newborn MRI scan. (**d**) CLOVES syndrome newborn MRI scan

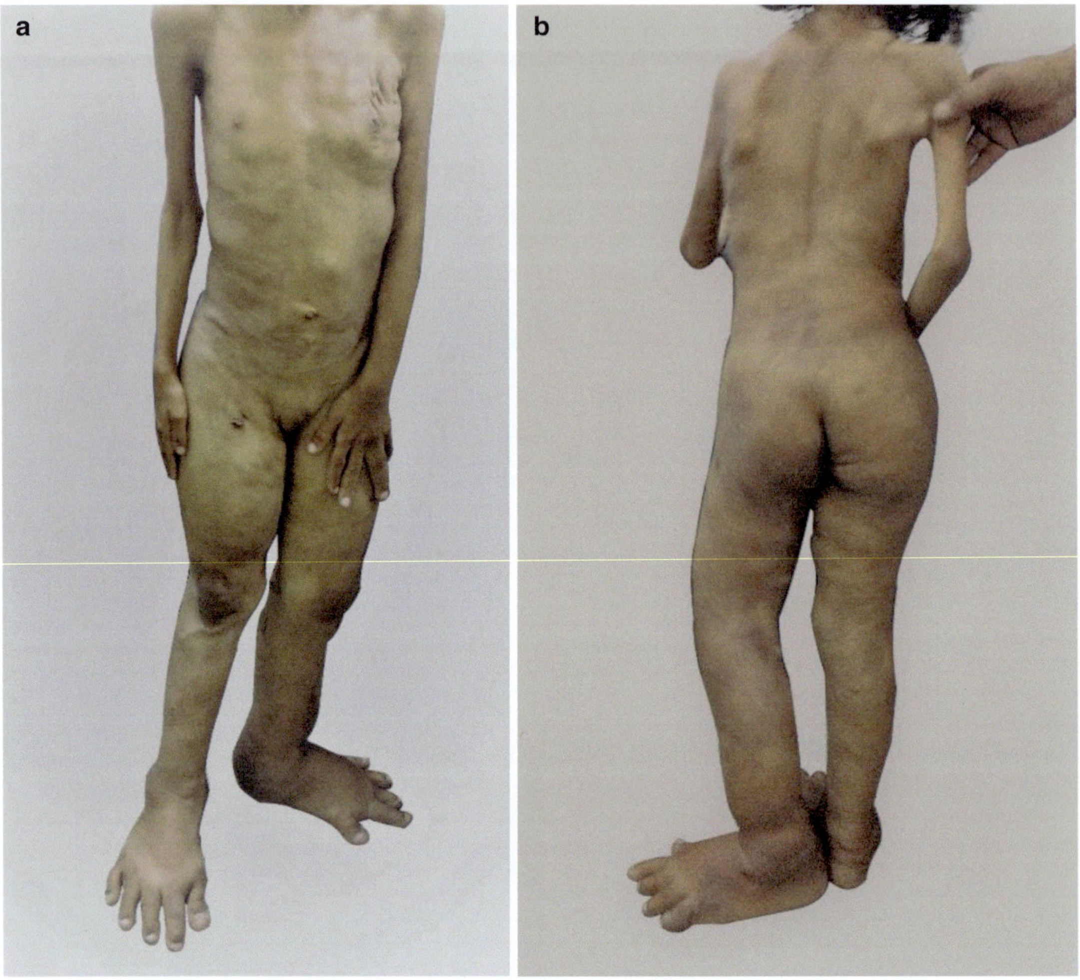

Fig. 10.9 (**a**) CLOVES syndrome young adult. (**b**) CLOVES syndrome young adult

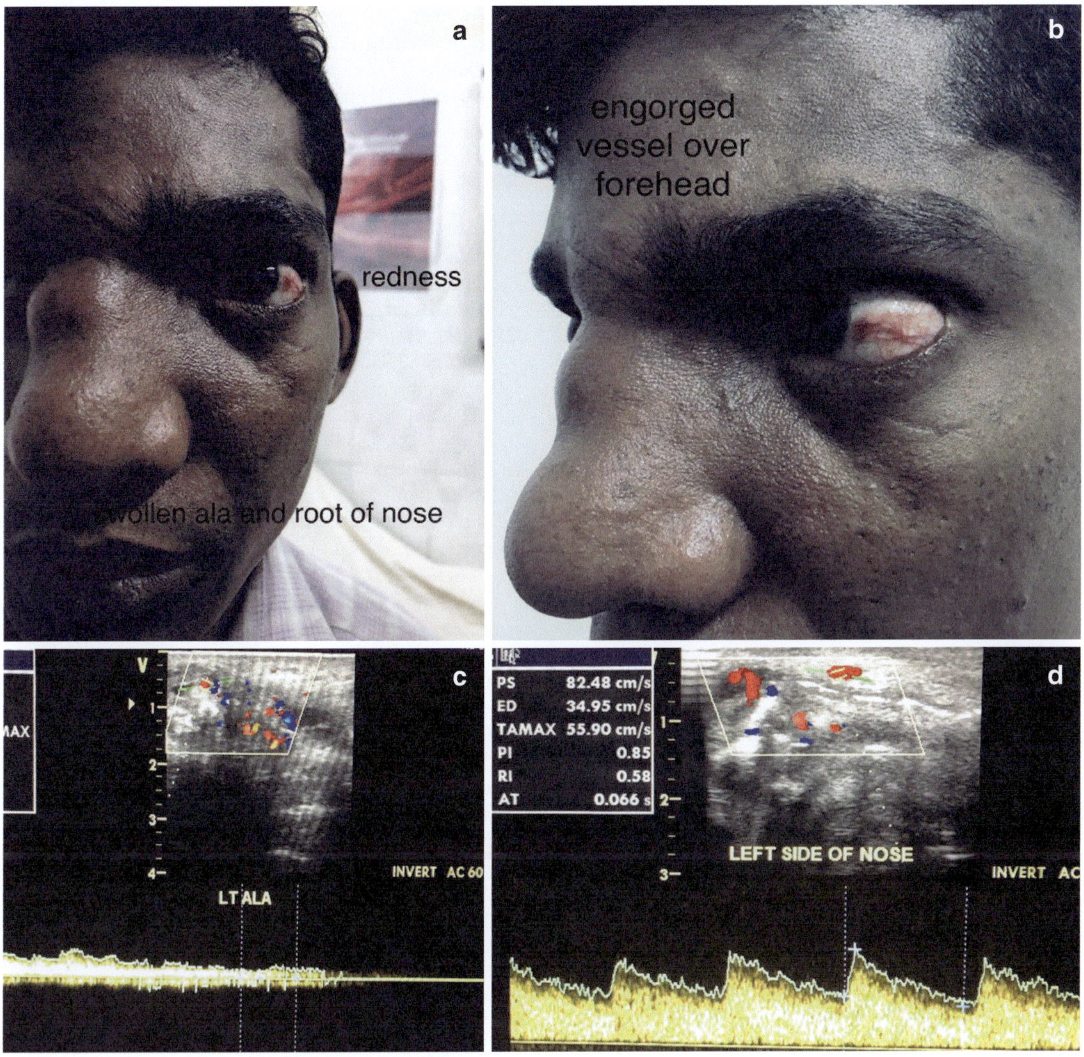

Fig. 10.10 (**a**) Arteriovenous malformation on nose and forehead. (**b**) Arteriovenous malformation on nose and forehead. (**c**) Duplex scanning of venous component of AVM nose. (**d**) Duplex scanning of arterial component of AVM nose

References

1. Kulungowski AM, Fishman SJ. Management of combined vascular malformations. Clin Plastic Surg. 2011;38:107–20.
2. Rogers CR, Mulliken JB. Classification and natural history of vascular anomalies. In: Rutherford's vascular surgery. 8th ed. Philadelphia, PA: Elsevier Saunders; 2014. p. 1044–50.
3. Hilaire GS. Histoire generale et particuliere des anomalies de l'organisation chez l'homme et les animaux. Paris: Tome I; 1832. p. 328e33. [in French
4. Trelat U, Monod A. De l'hypertrophie unilaterale partielle ou totale du corps. Arch Gen Med. 1869;13:536e8. in French
5. Klippel M, Tre'Naunay P. Memoires originaux: du noevus variquex osteo-hypertrophique. Arch Gen Med. 1900;185:641e72. in French
6. Oduber CE, et al. Klippel-Trenaunay syndrome: diagnostic criteria and hypothesis on etiology. Ann Plast Surg. 2008, Feb;60:217–23.
7. Lee BB, et al. Guideline: diagnosis and treatment of venous malformations. Consensus document of the International Union of Phlebology (IUP): updated-2013. Int Angiol. 2014 Jun 10; (Epub ahead of print)

8. Fan C, et al. Novel roles of GATA1 in regulation of angiogenic factor AGGF1 and endothelial cell function. J Biol Chem. 2009;284(35):23331–43.
9. Hu Y, et al. Identification of association of common AGGF1 variants with susceptibility for Klippel-Tre'naunay syndrome using the structure association program. Ann Hum Genet. 2008;72:636–43.
10. Mattassi R, Vaghi M. Management of marginal vein: current issues. Phlebology. 2007;22(6):283–6.
11. Dubois J, Alison M. Vascular anomalies: what a radiologist needs to know. Pediatr Radiol. 2010;40:895–905.
12. Dentici R, Mattassi R. Nuclear medicine diagnostics. In: Mattassi R, et al., editors. Hemangiomas and vascular malformations: an atlas of diagnosis and treatment. 2nd ed. Milan, Italy: Springer; 2015. p. 223–36.
13. King K, et al. The use of endovenous laser treatment in toddlers. J Vasc Interv Radiol. 2013;24(6):855–8.
14. Mattassi R. Management of combined venous and lymphatic malformations. Phlebolymphology. 2016;23(2):112–20.
15. Hauert J, Loose DA. Orthopedic problems. In: Mattassi R, et al., editors. Hemangiomas and vascular malformations: an atlas of diagnosis and treatment. 2nd ed. Milan, Italy: Springer; 2015. p. 369–78.
16. Pansuriya TC, et al. Somatic mosaic IDH1 and IDH2 mutations are associated with enchondroma and spindle cell hemangioma in Ollier disease and Maffucci syndrome. Nat Genet. 2011;43:1256–61.
17. Verdegaal SH, et al. Incidence, predictive factors, and prognosis of chondrosarcoma in patients with Ollier disease and Maffucci syndrome: an international multicenter study of 161 patients. Oncologist. 2011;16:1771–9.
18. Mulliken JB, Young AE. Vascular birthmarks: hemangiomas and malformations. Philadelphia: Saunders; 1988.
19. Weber FP. Hemangiectatic hypertrophy of limbs: congenital phlebarteriectasias and so-called congenital varicose veins. Br J Child Dis. 1918;15:13–7.
20. Enjolras O, et al. Vascular anomalies and the growth of limbs: a review. J Pediatr Orthop B. 2004;13:349–57.
21. Revencu N, et al. Parkes Weber syndrome, vein of Galen aneurysmal malformation, and other fast-flow vascular anomalies are caused by RASA1 mutations. Hum Mutat. 2008;29:959–65.
22. Marler JJ, Mulliken JB. Vascular anomalies. In: Mathes SJ, Hentz VR, editors. Plastic surgery. 2nd ed. Philadelphia: Elsevier; 2009. p. 19–68.
23. Mulliken JB, et al. Vascular anomalies. Curr Probl Surg. 2000;37:517–84.
24. Eerola l, et al. Capillary malformation-arteriovenous malformation, a new clinical and genetic disorder caused by RASA1 mutations. Am J Hu Genet. 2003;73:1240–9.
25. Cohen MM Jr. Bannayan-Riley-Ruvalcaba syndrome: renaming three formerly recognized syndromes as one etiologic entity. Am J Med Genet. 1990;35:291–2.
26. Alomari AI. Characterization of a distinct syndrome that associates complex truncal overgrowth, vascular, and acral anomalies: a descriptive study of 18 cases of CLOVES syndrome. Clin Dysmorphol. 2009;18:1–7.
27. Sapp JC, et al. Newly delineated syndrome of congenital lipomatous overgrowth, vascular malformations, and epidermal nevi (CLOVE syndrome) in seven patients. Am J Med Genet A. 2007;143:2944–58.

11 Investigations in Vascular Malformations

Satyendra K. Tiwary

Vascular malformation is a complex clinical condition with myriad manifestations resulting from a variety of vascular lesions due to proliferative endothelium resulting from embryonic dysmorphogenesis. Clinical evaluation (Fig. 11.1) without imaging modality is never sufficient to classify categorically for complete diagnosis and guiding the treatment plan. Vascular endothelial lining of veins, arteries, lymphatics, or combined structures in skin, subcutaneous tissue, muscles, bones, or deep inside abdominal viscera may give rise to vascular malformations in various forms which need imaging evaluation (DUS, CT, MRI) always for complete diagnosis and treatment. The commonest location in the body is the head and neck region (40%), followed by extremities (40%) and trunks (20%) [1]. Prevalence of vascular malformations is about 4.5% with peripheral vascular malformations in population 0.8–1% [2, 3].

Investigations are essential for definite diagnosis in detail and imaging is a central component with first and foremost being non-invasive evaluation with DUS, CT, and MRI. The first diagnostic tool after the clinical evaluation is duplex ultrasonography (DUS) examination which is widely used for initial screening, but essential in all cases for planning treatment and further imaging assessment with B-mode for morphologic study and spectral, color, and power Doppler to find out flow characteristics [4].

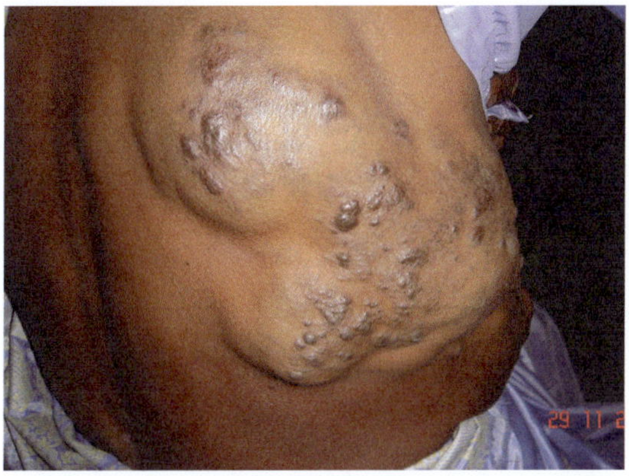

Fig. 11.1 Vascular malformation chest wall

The second line investigations are MRI and CT without or with contrast which allow a better morphologic study and lucid hemodynamic data and either of the above combined with DUS in most cases.

The third group in the line of examinations includes different tests performed mainly after the former two, decided by the data derived. It includes lymphoscintigraphy, whole blood pool scintigraphy, transarterial lung perfusion scintigraphy, bone scanogram.

The fourth and last panel is the invasive tests group, including catheter angiography which is used during the therapeutic session rather than

S. K. Tiwary (✉)
Department of Surgery, Institute of Medical Science, Banaras Hindu University, Varanasi, India

A. K. Khanna, S. K. Tiwary (eds.), *Vascular Malformations*,
https://doi.org/10.1007/978-981-15-9762-6_11

diagnostic tool, phlebography, and lymphography which are used rarely nowadays.

11.1 Non-Invasive Diagnostic Tools

11.1.1 Duplex Ultrasound (DUS)

In the diagnostic dilemma of vascular malformations, duplex ultrasound remains basic, screening, most widely used and primary investigation practiced in all cases. The role of DUS is more and more due to the large scale availability of the equipment, low cost, lack of radiation exposure, lack of invasiveness, and the real-time investigation. Assessment of morphology and hemodynamic features are two outcomes after duplex study helping to plan further investigations or final therapeutics. Size of the vascular malformation can be derived always. The limiting point in the investigation is the limited special resolution. Very high temporal resolution facilitates real-time examinations and an accurate hemodynamic assessment. Limiting factors in DUS is the dependency on the operator, and finding in the investigation are related to knowledge of anatomy and pathology in addition to technical skills. There is some agreement for the necessity to standardize the examination and to perform it according to different depths [5].

Ultrasound is a good screening tool but it has limitations in defining the extent of lesions not located in the extremities and it is essential to supplement ultrasound assessment with MRI evaluation. Deep intramuscular lesions are best detected by MRI which may help in locating the lesion on ultrasound. The biggest challenge in Ultrasound investigations is examination in presence of air (e.g., lungs) or when lesions are located within bones. CT has an upper edge in the evaluation of Bony anomalies which may be the imaging modality of choice for lesions inside the bones. Limitations in the hemodynamic evaluation of venous status with USG can be compensated with intravascular pressure measurement and/or intravascular ultrasound (IVUS). However, it is always a rule to do IVUS or invasive pressure measurements only in selective cases and preferred with definitive intervention only but not as a routine procedure.

11.2 Duplex Ultrasound (DUS) Examination Procedure

Basic Principles

Clinical presentations should be in the background briefly with the time of onset, family history, and rate of progression before evaluating and interpreting ultrasound findings. Contralateral side should be examined to search occult malformations and to compare the morphology and hemodynamics. In unilateral lesions, complete clinical examination of contralateral side and Duplex USG comparison of both sides to identify normal size and structures is the key principle. Limbs should be examined both in erect and supine positions in all case with the recording of and the difference in size of the vessels.

Continuous Wave(CW)-Doppler Localization: First assessment with CW-Doppler is recommended:

(a) To localize the lesion
(b) To determine the basic flow characteristics and
(c) To guide the duplex examination

Probe Selection

Most superficial lesions are assessed with linear probe of high frequency and pressure applied by probe should be minimum over the thick layer of ultrasound gel to avoid distortion and compression of the lesion. The advantage with using broadband transducers should be optimized to obtain the best image. When assessing facial lesions or anomalies in neonates and small children, a "hockeystick" probe may be selected. In case of superficial lesions, minimum pressure should be applied to the probe using a thick layer of ultrasound gel to prevent excessive compression on the lesion.

Salient Evaluation

The ultrasound examination should aim to achieve the following four key procedural outcomes [6, 7]:

1. Lesion: Diagnosis, Dimension, and Definite Classification
2. Localization and relationship with regional structures
3. Location: Compete mapping pre-operatively
4. Long term outcome: Post-intervention follow-up studies

11.2.1 Define the Lesion: Diagnosis, Dimension, and Definite Classification

Aims

(a) To recognize the presence of a vascular anomaly
(b) To differentiate between vascular tumor and malformation
(c) To classify as a high flow (AVM), low flow (VM), or no flow (LM) lesions
(d) To document the dimensions of the lesion and flow characteristics

B-Mode

First-hand tool in Duplex Study is the B-mode examination and it should be done before the Doppler examination. Initial assessment with B-Mode identifies either collection of vessels or cystic spaces or soft tissue mass or adjacent structures like nerve trunks. Compressibility on B-mode differentiate

(a) VM (compressible).
(b) Thrombosed or sclerosed VM (non-compressible).
(c) LM (non-compressible cystic spaces) and.
(d) AVMs (partially compressible).

B-mode will help in the evaluation of axial trunks and its patency, duplication, aplasia, hypoplasia, hyperplasia, valves in whole length, or in the localized segment. Outside the vessel, information about surrounding structures regarding echogenicity, regularity, the plane of separation may be obtained [8].

11.2.1.1 Doppler Mode (Color Doppler and Spectral Analysis)

Doppler assessment determines either flow within the lesion (active tumors, AVMs, VMs) or no flow at all (LMs, involuted tumors, thrombosed/sclerosed VMs). Flow within the lesion may be either induced (VMs) or spontaneous (AVMs). The examination includes both Color Doppler and Spectral analysis. For examination in the color mode examination, the pulse repetition frequency (PRF) is set to the flow velocity of the target vessel, i.e., PRF is increased for arterial flow and decreased for venous flow in VMs. Assessing high flow malformations, the setting of the color Doppler should be set on real time always without delay. Low amplitude flows better detected in Power Doppler as it is more sensitive than Color Doppler.

Spontaneous and augmented blood flow are detected in spectral analysis with Peak velocity and the Resistive Index (RI) in arterial vessels ([peak systolic velocity–end diastolic velocity] / peak systolic velocity) documentation always.

Reflux time is the key finding in venous Doppler examination and should be included always in venous examination mapping of the veins in the lower limb.

11.2.1.2 Diagnosis and Definite Classification

B-Mode and Doppler Mode study should be combined for a definite diagnosis and complete classification.

11.2.1.3 Dimension

The lesion should be measured and documented in all dimensions with an adequate number of B-mode images and definite morphology must be derived after demonstrating the basic features in the lesion should be obtained. Size, number, flow, and the hemodynamic characteristics of the lesion are recorded to monitor the course of the disease in terms of progression, the natural evolution, outcome either with success or failure of the treatment [9].

11.2.2 Localization and Relationship with Regional Structures

Localization of the lesion with documentation of the relationship with the regional blood vessels, nerves, muscles, and fascia (Fig. 11.2). Derived data should be a guiding factor for further investigations like MRI or CT. Both clinical and ultrasound examination should be combined for localization of the lesion with documentation of important landmarks in adjoining tissue structures.

Structures in the vicinity to the lesion should be identified ideally, assessed adequately with all vessels including arterial, venous, lymphatic along with adjoining structures including nerves, fascia, tendons, and muscles should be included in documentation. Nearby normal vascular structures along with normal opposite side examination is essential for evaluation of the size and flow of the vascular malformation. Architectural triad (Fig. 11.3) in VMs Afferent arterial "feeders," Efferent "draining" veins, and connecting central nidus should be delineated [10–12]). Ultrasound findings should guide further investigations like MRI in selected lesions only for complete diagnosis and subsequent therapeutic plan, protocol, and procedure.

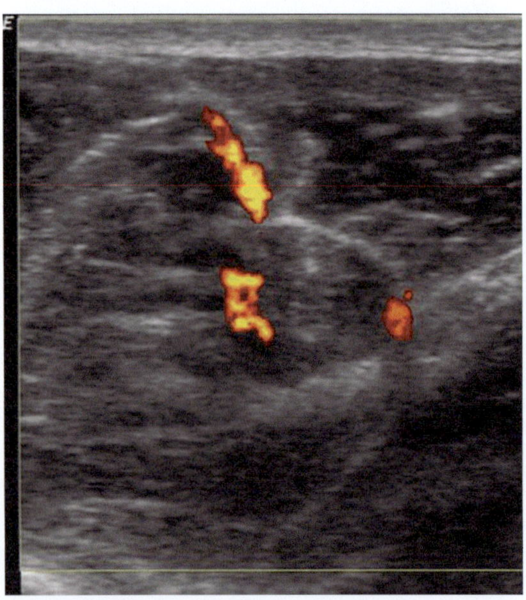

Fig. 11.2 Tiny serpentine anechoic channels (venous malformations) are noted in duplex scan involving posterior fibers of the deltoid muscle. Few echogenic foci are noted within phleboliths. Low-flow signals are noted

11.2.3 Location: Complete Pre-Operative Mapping

Therapeutic approach to target the lesion is always guided by complete pre-operative mapping with identification and marking of all important adjoining structures like arteries, veins, nerves, tendons, ligaments, muscles with proper identification of feeding arteries and draining veins and any other communications with the vascular system.

Complete and comprehensive duplex assessment should be complemented by surface markings over the skin to guide the site of vascular approach and plan of treatment. Significant surrounding structures should be documented and marked on the skin. Neural protection should be in each and every case with the identification of nerve trunks before intervention as damage to the nerve may be devastating which is a dreaded complication of endovascular or surgical procedures performed for vascular malformations. Direct puncture, the direct effect of therapeutic agents like sclerosant or embolic agent, or diffuse edema after intervention leading to compartment syndrome may cause nerve damage.

11.2.4 Long Term Outcome (Follow-Up Studies): Complications/Success/Failure

Follow-up study to analyze outcome in terms of complications, success, or failure of therapy is screened always by ultrasound in almost all cases. Residual and recurrent disease is the most significant phenomenon associated with vascular malformations which are detected during follow-up with the use of ultrasound. Early complications like DVT develops within days and to detect it earliest USG is advised within the first week of intervention.

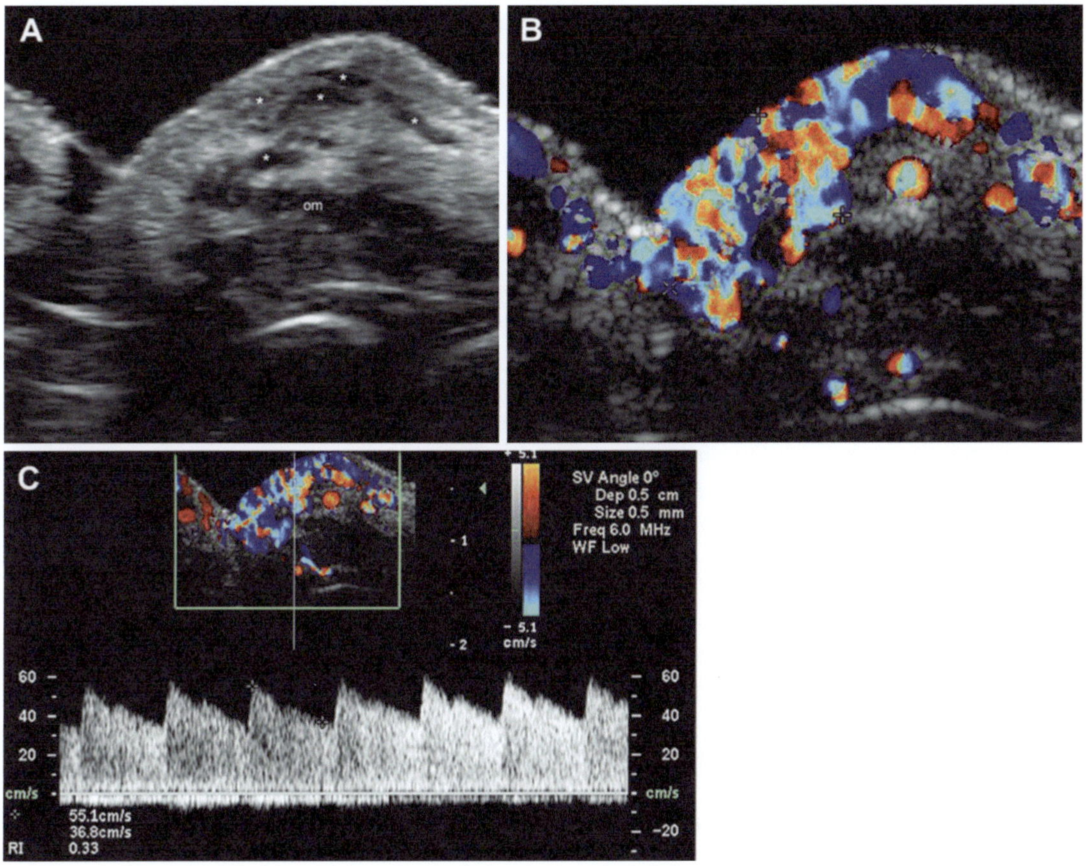

Fig. 11.3 High-flow-arterial-vascular-malformation-lower-lip-A-Gray-scale-longitudinal-view

Ultrasound examinations during long term follow-up should follow the same protocol as for the initial assessment,

This should include:

(a) B-mode images of lesion
(b) Measurements of the size and
(c) Flow
(d) Transverse dual image of the lesion to assess for compressibility
(e) Color Doppler images of the lesion and
(f) Sample spectral traces in associated vessels and nidus

11.2.4.1 Success/Failure of Endovascular Interventions

Compressibility is the key parameter in USG examination for evaluation of the vascular malformations but it loses its importance after endovascular intervention as it has a limitation in assessing the success of the therapy. Treated lesions are sclerosed or thrombosed and may not be compressible despite residual flow containing lesions which is assessed by Color Doppler study.

11.3 Venous Malformation (VM): Key Points

Venous Malformations (VMs) are anomalies of the venous system classified as truncular or extra-truncular [11, 12]. It is either isolated or may be associated with other malformations like Lymphatic(LM), Capillary(CM), Arteriovenous(AVM), or generalized syndromes(KTS).

11.4 Lymphatic Malformations (LM): Key Points

LMs are classified in truncular malformations and extratruncular lesions. LMs may be isolated or combined with others like CMs, VMs, and AVMs or as part of a generalized syndrome-like KTS.

Truncular LMs are may be due to agenesis, aplasia, hypoplasia, or hyperplasia/dilatation of the lymphatic vessels. Clinically presentation of truncular LMs manifests as primary lymphedema while Extratruncular lesions present as macrocytic or microcystic lesions. Division in macrocystic and microcystic is based on size which is less than 2 cm for microcystic and more than 2 cm for macrocystic. Fluid overload in soft tissues is always present in truncular lesion causing lymphedema [13, 14].

Central and key tool in the assessment of LMs remains Ultrasound which may be supplemented with lymphoscintigraphy(LSG). LSG is the gold standard in the study of the lymphodynamics in truncular lymphatic malformations. Ultrasonography in LMs is comparable with the information revealed by MRI.

Skin thickness measurement is the most important parameter in LMs to assess and evaluate the response of the treatment or progression of the disease which may be done by USG/CT/MRI. Skin elasticity and subcutaneous tissue thickness (Suprafascial and subfascial)may be assessed by the USG transducer to detect the progression of lymphedema [15–17].

Ultrasound evaluation of subcutaneous tissue thickness is a useful parameter to evaluate lymphedema and its response to treatment. These are measurements allow periodic evaluation of the response to therapy and serve the purpose of monitoring the progression of LMs and predicting prognosis [18, 19].

Thickening of all 3 components: cutaneous, epifascial, and subfascial with high-frequency USG (20 MHZ) is observed always to identify and classify lymphedema with fluid localization in various types of edema. Ultrasound is used for the diagnostic purpose as well as therapeutic monitoring.

11.5 Arterio-Venous Malformations (AVM): Key Points

AVMs are congenital anomalies comprising both arterial and venous systems. They are classified as truncular or extratruncular and may be associated with other CVMs such as VMs, LMs, and CMs or may be part of a generalized syndrome like the Parkes–Weber syndrome (PWS).

Duplex ultrasound is the first choice investigation amongst noninvasive modalities in clinical assessment and subsequent follow-up of AVMs either after intervention or after observation for a long time.

11.6 Arterial Malformations: Key Points

There are two variants for sciatic artery malformation. Either the sciatic artery coexists with normal iliac-femoral arteries or it may be accompanied and compensates for an aplasia of the iliac-femoral arteries. Both the conditions are easily identified by ultrasound. The symptoms manifest due to the compression of the sciatic nerve, distal embolization, and acute ischemia secondary to the thrombosis of the aneurysmal sac [20, 21]. The role of investigations should be appraisal of these finding apart from sciatic artery malformation.

11.7 Magnetic Resonance Imaging (MRI)

Almost all forms of vascular malformations need ultrasound evaluation for the assessment of the lesion initially as during the intervention or evolution phase but the investigation of choice in most vascular malformations remains MRI. Better spatial resolution/definition and a wider field of view give MRI always an edge over the ultrasound. The biggest advantage is the capability to visualize blood flow and characteristics of tissues without risks of ionizing radiation [22, 23]. However, both USG and MRI have the possibility of multiplanar acquisition (Fig. 11.4).

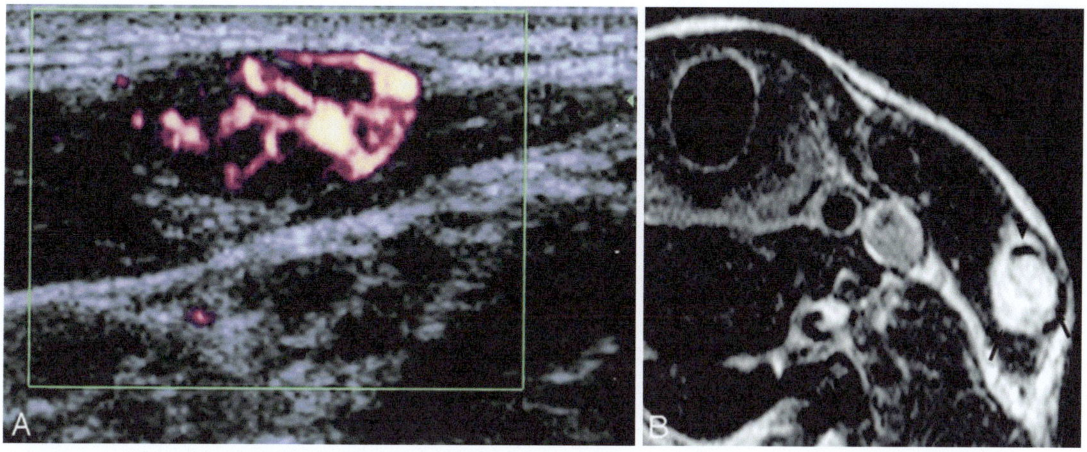

Fig. 11.4 Sonographic and MR images obtained in a vascular malformation of the left external jugular vein

Vascular malformations should be investigated with equipment of high power (at least 1.5 Tesla) to have better contrast and spatial resolution which identifies and detects even small anomalies [24]. Some of the drawbacks of MRI are that longer duration in the examination, noise above normal level, and claustrophobic feelings leading to fear and difficulty mostly in the examination for the children with the requirement of sedation and risks subsequently [22].

Each vascular anomaly has a unique MRI feature as summarized in Table 11.1 [25].

A typical Vascular malformation (VM) imaging protocol consists of spin echo (SE) or fast spin echo (FSE) in T1weighted sequences axial to the lesion generally with fat suppression in order to highlight the lesion. Later on images obtained after gadolinium contrast injection are useful to distinguish LMs and VMs which have similar images in the normal and angiographic acquisition. SE sequences can also identify signal voids representing arterial feeders [26].

T2-weighted images (FSE with fat suppression or in alternative short tau inversion recovery—STIR—images) in at least two planes are most sensitive and specific for identification of the extent and depth of the lesion because of a generally bright signal intensity lesion over a low signal intensity fat, muscle, and bone background. These sequences can also show the content of the malformation [22, 27].

The presence of signal voids on T2-weighted images is highly suggestive for hemosiderin, dystrophic calcification, or phleboliths which are typical findings for venous malformations [23].

Magnetic resonance angiography (MRA) techniques are complementary to the conventional MRI once definitive intervention is planned in vascular malformations and it is termed as contrast-enhanced MRA (CE-MRA) [28] which uses 3D T1-weighted sequences with fat suppression: the contrast medium (gadolinium chelates) is injected in a peripheral vein causing a shortening of T1 relaxation times [23].

CE-MRA can be done by a variety of techniques, but time-resolved 3DMR digital subtraction angiography is the Gold standard for evaluating vascular anomalies. In this technique, a serial acquisition of images of less than or equal to 10 second duration is performed in rapid succession. At least one acquisition will certainly coincide with the arterial phase and at least one will coincide with the venous phase of enhancement. Of course for optimal visualization, the temporal resolution must be maximized. Improvement of data processing techniques can generate 3D images every 2 seconds [23].

Multiplanar reconstructions, no use of ionizing radiation, non-invasive modality are definite advantages of CE-MRA over the conventional MR angiography. The drawbacks of CE-MRA are usually are identified that spatial resolution and the area of interest are influenced by a high

Table 11.1 MRI Imaging features of vascular anomalies

Vascular pathology	MRI Imaging features
Hemangioma of infancy (HOI)	In the proliferating phase appearance of a well-lobulated mass with low signal intensity on T1W images and high intensity in T2W images, presence of flow voids in SE T1W images, no perilesional edema, and early homogeneous enhancement Involuting phase: Fat replacement with high signal T1W images and decreased enhancement
Venous malformations (extratruncular)	Lobulated sometimes septated mass with low sig intensity in T1W images, high intensity in T2W images, flow voids in T2W fat saturation images (phleboliths), slow gradual enhancement in delay with contrast media
Lymphatic malformations (extratruncular)	The same characteristics of the venous malformations. No enhancement in microcystic malformations. Septal and rim enhancement in macrocystic malformations
Capillary	Skin thickness lesion
Arterio-venous malformations (extratruncular)	Enlarged feeding arteries and draining veins. Flow voids in T1W SE se-quences; early enhancement of arteries nidus and draining veins

time resolution selectivity is not associated to limit its role in selective catheterization [29].

In summary, MR imaging (MRI) is a major noninvasive test together with the Duplex ultrasonographic (DUS) evaluation. Better spatial resolution is the best parameter with MRI covering a wider field of examination which allows to highlight layer-wise different anatomic components decided by magnetic stimulation of the organs. The best evaluation tool for organ involvement in vascular malformation is definitely MRI.

11.7.1 Extratruncular Venous Malformations (VM)

MRI along with MR venography (MRV) are complete tools for evaluation of venous malformations. The Extension, type of the VM, feeding and draining vessels, adjoining soft tissue (muscle, fascia, fat), the vascular structures (arteries, veins), and nerve trunks can be identified easily. MRI and MRV are therefore, essential imaging modality to provide a highly accurate diagnosis before performing interventions on VMs [30].

MRI findings of the VMs including the typical appearance of VMs as a collection of serpentine structures and its relationships with adjacent tissue/structures were thoroughly described in the diagnostic section of the VM. They usually show low to intermediate signal in T1-weighted sequences and high contrast in FSE.

T2weighted or STIR sequences, where the vascular malformation is highlight from the surrounding fat (Fig. 11.5). In case of thrombosis or hemorrhage heterogeneous signals are seen in T1-weighted images. VM lesions may be localized or diffuse or have lobulated margins.

A slow filling of the malformation is visible with the use of contrast medium [28]. This characteristic of the VMs is important in the differentiation with the LMs and other cystic lesions which do NOT have any contrast enhancement after gadolinium injection.

The morphological features of VMs correlate with the success of the sclerotherapy [29]. Well-defined margins and dimensions less than 5 cm are predictive of good results after ethanol therapy.

11.7.2 Extratruncular Lymphatic Malformations (LM)

MRI findings in microcystic LMs are usually diffuse areas with low signal intensity with T1-weighted and high signal intensity in T2-weighted imaging sequences [29]. Small cysts in microcystic LMs are difficult to be individually identified on MRI and they are no flow lesions with complete avascularity or only mild enhancement.

On the other hand, the macrocystic LMs are easily identified for the presence of cysts and well-defined septa (Fig. 11.6). Low signal intensity on T1-weighted sequences and appear markedly hyperintense on T2weighted images

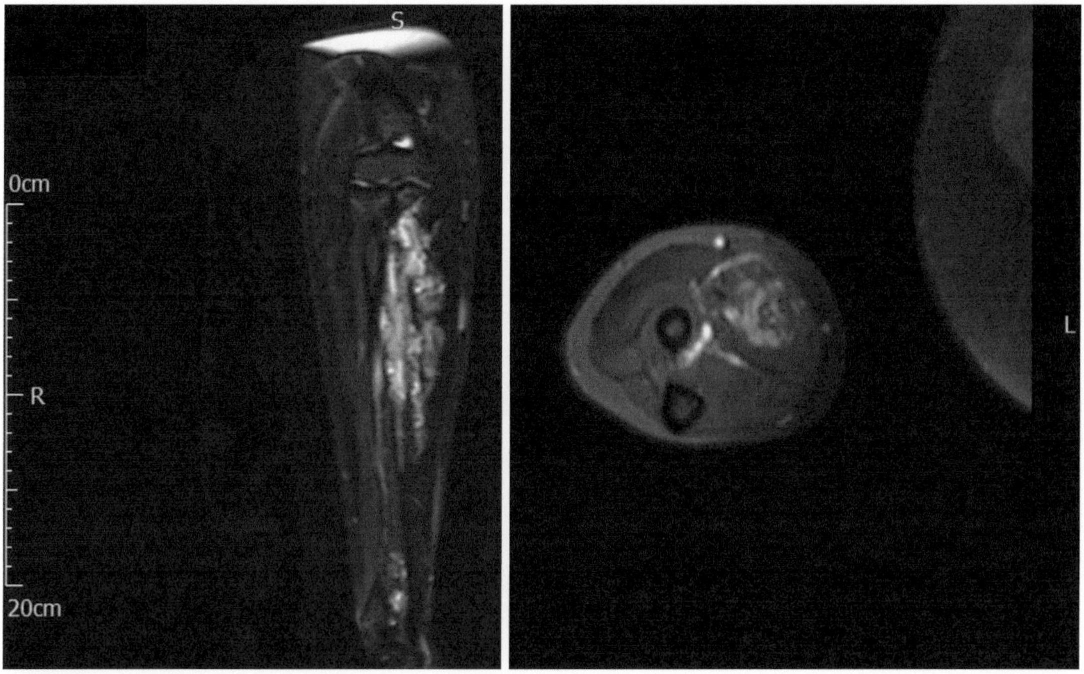

Fig. 11.5 MRI with Coronal STIR and Axial T1 weighted images of a low-flow venous malformation showing Typical high signal and enhancing venous spaces

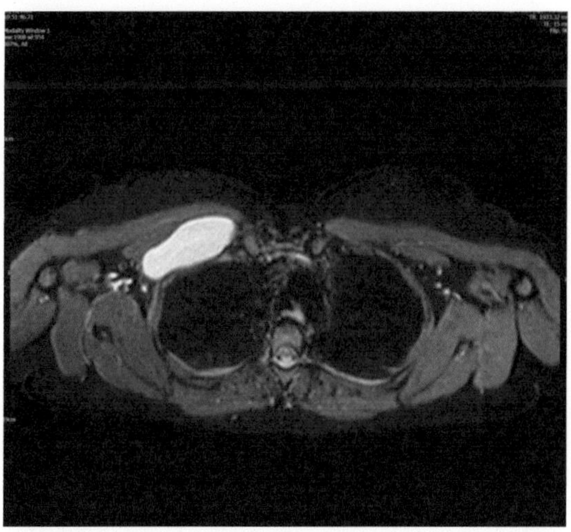

Fig. 11.6 Axial T2 weighted chest MRI with a large bright left side anterior chest wall macrocystic malformation

are characteristic features in macrocystic LMs. Fluid–fluid level within the cyst is identified, due to the presence of blood or proteins.

The septa and the walls of the cyst after injection of contrast present a Mild enhancement in the septa and the walls of the cysts after contrast injection which is never in cystic spaces. Mild enhancement in cystic spaces is finding with venous malformations. An enhancement of the cyst can be recognized after treatment sometimes or in the case of associated mixed malformations (LVM) [29].

11.7.3 Arteriovenous Malformations (AVM)

The blood vessels in AVMs cause Linear or rounded signal voids are identified as blood vessels in AVM in the T1weighted SE sequences which correlates with signal hyperintensity in the GRE sequences [23, 29]. Nidus is characterized by heterogeneous tangle of multiple empty signal in T1-weighted sequences in association with dysplastic veins, well identified in the T2-weighted sequences [27]. Thickened skin, increasing fat tissue, and reduced muscle mass are in associated findings with AVM. The AVM can affect Bone may be affected causing hypo-

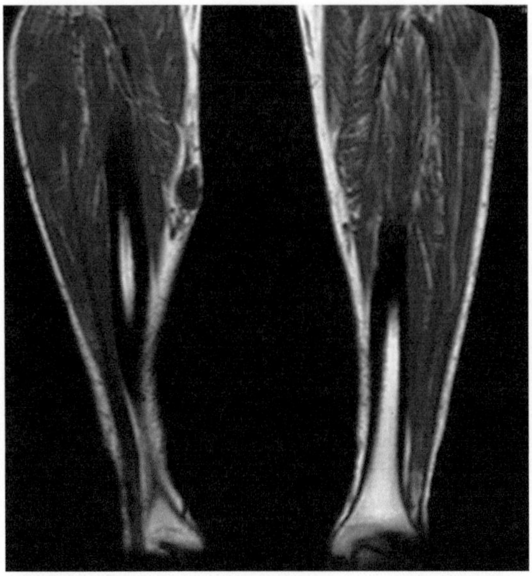

Fig. 11.7 MRI STIR both legs show arteriovenous malformation at the right leg medial side

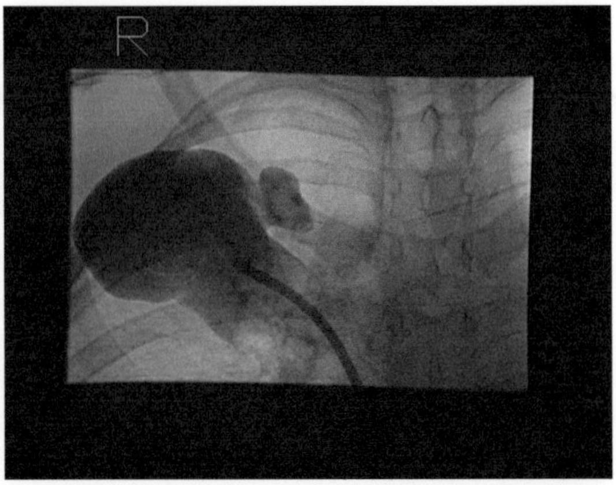

Fig. 11.8 Percutaneous sclerotherapy of a large right-side anterior chest wall lymphatic macrocystic malformation. Contrast injected under fluoroscopic guidance opacity macrocystic lymphatic space

plasia, cortical thinning and demineralization, or direct involvement of the bone which is identified by the presence of intraosseous high flow vessels [23, 27, 31].

Altered signals in surrounding tissue may be indicative of edema which can be detected with MRI examination (Fig. 11.7). The differential diagnosis between an AVM and a vascular tumor (rhabdomyosarcoma, hemangiopericytoma, angiosarcoma) can be very difficult and useful parameters in the diagnosis of AVM are the presence of fat within the lesion, muscle atrophy, and absence of surrounding edema [1].

CE-MRA is used to identify a dilation of arteries, dilatation of veins, early identification of the draining veins, detailed demarcation of vascular anatomy which is useful for the treatment or further work-up angiography [23].

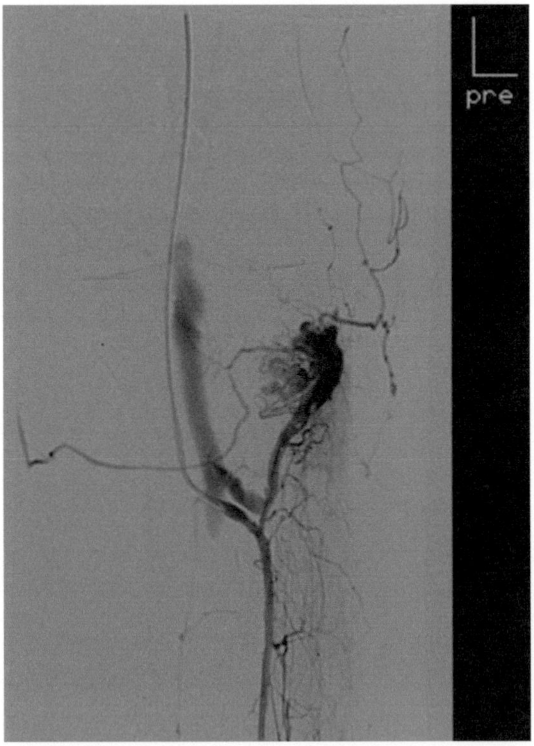

Fig. 11.9 Left knee arteriovenous malformation embolization and sclerotherapy

11.7.4 Follow-Up Studies

Treatment success with vascular malformation in follow-up studies may be identified with reduction in size or reduced flow. Response after percutaneous sclerotherapy (Fig. 11.8) or surgical excision (low-flow malformations), transarterial embolization (high flow malformations) are assessed with contrast injection of gadolinium (Fig. 11.9) always during follow-up studies which allows detection of the perfused area [32].

11.8 Computed Tomography (CT)

Preferred investigation after basic duplex scanning is MRI in vascular malformations but sometimes CT may be either a substitute or complementary to MRI in some selected cases. CT is an alternative investigation to MRI in those group of patients who are at high risk or with fragile health due to respiratory or cardiac as the images acquisition is very fast in CT as compared to MRI. Another situation where it is useful in patients who have contraindications to sedation with MRI and is preferable to MRI in imaging vascular anomalies of bowels and lungs [22].

Fewer artifacts are always with CT as compared to MRI in patients with embolization coils or metallic clips. Apart from less artifacts, CT better defines bone, calcifications, and phleboliths [27]. In bony involvement with high flow vascular malformations, CT may provide more information as compared to MRI.

The adverse effects are always more with CT and exposure to ionizing radiation and subsequent risk of malignancy especially for pediatric populations and risks increase more in vascular malformations due to the necessity of the use of contrast to visualize the vessels.

Venous Malformations (VMs) usually appear as hypodense or heterogeneous lesions which enhance slowly from the periphery after the injection of contrast [32].CT venography is an excellent tool for evaluation of obstructed, anomalous, atretic, absent veins along with and other anomalies of large veins in the chest, abdomen, or pelvis. Identifies the underlying pathology, confirming venous obstruction or extrinsic compression, delineating anatomic variations and the extent of venous thrombosis are best assessed with CT venogram [33, 34].

Low-attenuation masses occasionally with fluid–fluid levels and peripheral contrast enhancement of the wall are characteristic in lymphatic malformations (LMs) [32].

CECT of AVMs usually done, with bolus tracking technique (CT-angiography:CTA) to get an optimal study of arterial vessels, including enlarged feeding arteries and rapid shunting of contrast into enlarged draining veins without significant intervening tissue enhancement which is usual within a normal capillary network. Best use of Contrast-enhanced CT is possible with AVMs which is significantly more informative as compared to other vascular malformations because it provides a distinct three-dimensional data set for accurate mapping and measurement of arterial, nidal, and venous structures and assessment of flow patterns for interventional radiologic or surgical planning which is possible especially due to the many post-processing options [35].

CT with intravenous contrast enhancement has been used for the differential diagnosis of hemangiomas and VMs [36].

Standard MRI is not a good technique for precisely demonstrating the nidus or arteriovenous connection. Instead, CTA provides much better anatomical information, sometimes showing the arterial and venous anatomy in excellent detail, but is inferior in all aspects to the newer technique of CEMRI [1].

Even considering that CTA may give more precise anatomical detail than MRI, particularly in small blood vessels, the benefits of clinically justified CT examinations should always outweigh the risks for an individual child, and referral to a center that performs CE-MRI should be considered as well.

MRI should remain as the option of choice in the diagnosis of high flow vascular anomalies for this special group. Only when dealing with a specific AVM in a critical area difficult to treat, CT is indicated, though extremely rare [1].

CT scan is a useful test in association with the contrast medium providing excellent spatial and temporal resolution. Thoracic and visceral malformations as well as AVM with bone involvement are assessed better with contrast-enhanced CT.

11.8.1 Radiography

Plain X-ray films are of limited use as low soft tissue contrast resolution is not much helpful. It is most useful in demonstrating soft tissue overgrowth, bony hypertrophy, bony erosion, periosteal reaction, pathological fracture, limb length discrepancy, and phleboliths. The presence of phleboliths in soft tissues is suggestive of a low-flow venous malformation (Fig. 11.10).

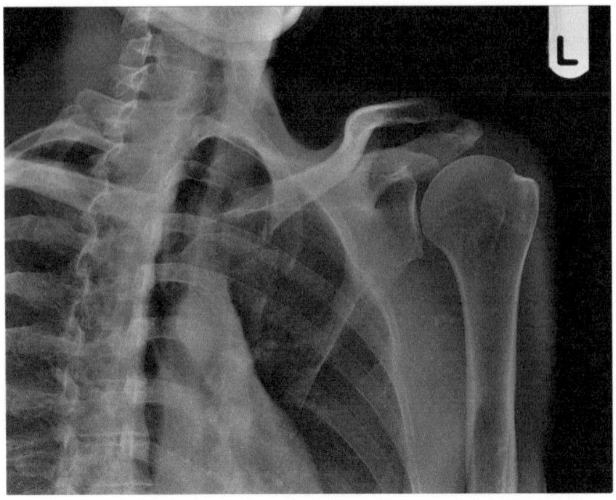

Fig. 11.10 Few tiny calcification foci (Phlebolith) in soft tissue at the level of proximal shaft of humerus

Scanograms are long bone radiographs that provide accurate measurement of the long bone length of the upper and lower limbs. Scanograms are needed to assess any bone length discrepancy between the limbs. This document would become objective criteria for further management [37].

Conventional radiologic techniques are addressed to discover bone involvement in CVMs. Bones may be elongated, shortened, deformed, thickened, or thinned because of osteolysis [22]. The pathological cause is related to ischemia of the osteoblasts representing a growth stimulation or to compression of the bone by the surrounding structures or vein and lymph stasis.

Calcification in the soft tissues is a hallmark of VMs. Multiple enchondromas are typical of Maffucci syndrome and they have the tendency to progress to malignancy.

Plain X-rays are an essential test in detecting basic bone pathology including lengthening, shortening, enchondromas, and vanishing bone syndrome. These images are also useful in detecting calcifications (phleboliths) in soft tissues which is diagnostic feature of VMs.

11.9 Invasive Diagnostic Evaluation

- Venography/phlebography (ascending/descending/segmental)
- Arteriography (standard/segmental)
- Percutaneous direct puncture angiography: arteriography, phlebography, varicography, lymphography

"Invasive" tests are rarely required needed to establish the diagnosis of the Vascular Malformations as Non- invasive tests are sufficient enough to establish the diagnosis most of the time as invasive tests should be deferred until intervention is planned. The role of invasive tests is limited as it is required for treatment planning either surgical or endovascular. However, invasive tests may be required for diagnosis when non- to minimally invasive tests (e.g., CT and/or MRI) fail to confirm the diagnosis or to delineate important diagnostic details which are important for options of treatment [10].

Ascending phlebography combined with intravascular ultrasound (IVUS) for identification of lesion and proper therapeutic planning in case like truncular lesions along iliac vein is ideal tool studies is essential for proper management. The role of descending phlebography is an integral component for the assessment of deep venous reflux along the pelvic veins and/or sciatic veins. Any embolotherapy intervention must be preceded by phlebography for better planning and identification of the lesion for therapeutic intervention.

Direct puncture phlebography is also very useful to identify a large efferent vein of extratruncular lesions [38, 39]. These veins can be treated in advance to allow more effective therapy with reduced risk of recurrence, with subsequent embolotherapy or sclerotherapy [1, 25].

Angiography should be reserved only in AVM as a road map to further define the lesion and plan proper treatment. To minimize radiation exposure, these techniques are usually performed at the time of treatment in young patients [40].

These studies include:

- Selective and superselective arteriography
- Percutaneous direct puncture phlebography

Therefore, once the intervention is decided, complete pretherapeutic mapping of the lesion is essential including the angiographic classification of extratruncular VMs (Table 11.2) and also AVMs (Flow Diagram 1) proposed by Puig and YS Do et al., respectively [41, 42]. These classifications have a great importance as predictive measurement for the results of intravascular therapy.

Table 11.2 Angiographic classification of Venous Malformation [41]

Description	
Type 1	isolated malformation without peripheral drainage
Type 2	malformation that drains into normal veins
Type 3	malformation that drains into dysplastic veins
Type 4	malformation that represents a ectasia

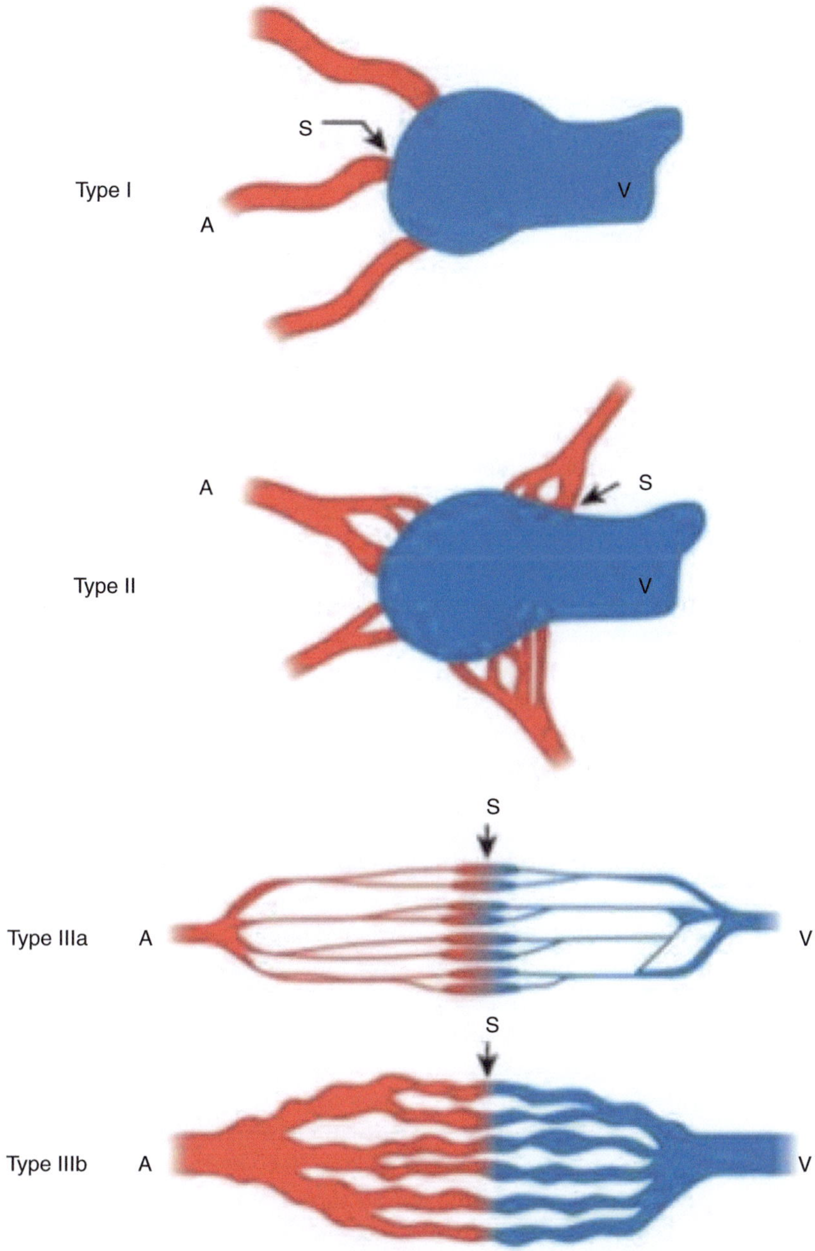

Flow Diagram 1. Arteriographic classification of AV Malformation [42]. Type I (arteriovenous fistulae): at most three separate arteries shunted to a single draining vein. Type II (arteriovenous fistulae): multiple arterioles shunted into a single draining vein. Type III (arteriovenous fistulae): multiple shunts between the arterioles and venules

Phlebography

Hemodynamic characteristics and classification of vascular malformation are best assessed with phlebography as anatomy is best derived along with communication pattern and draining venous system Based on the appearance of the VMs and the draining venous system during phlebography all VMs can be classified into four distinct groups: Type I (isolated VMs without phlebographically appreciable venous drainage), Type II and Type III VMs (demonstrate normal sized and enlarged venous drainage, respectively) and Type IV VMs (characterized by essentially ecstatic dysplastic veins) [41, 43].

From a diagnostic work-up, phlebographic evaluation of patency and anatomic variations of the deep venous system deserves special consideration in addition to phlebographic classification of the VM. Although above mentioned phlebographic classification does not provide information regarding the location of the VMs or the involvement of surrounding anatomical structures it provides useful data for treatment planning, especially when the sclerotherapy is considered as a treatment option [1].

Ascending phlebography is of limited use only for the diagnosis of truncular venous disease and in particular of superficial veins and hypoplasia or aplasia of deep veins according to the noninvasive investigations [38, 39]. Technical skills are required to avoid incorrect results of phlebography, as preferred abnormal outflows may sometimes simulate absence or main vein stenosis.

The main advantage of this procedure is that the imaging can be performed in orthostatism [25]. Descending phlebography is indicated in pelvic, sciatic, and visceral malformations. Direct puncture venography is related to the treatment of extratruncular VM lesions. With this procedure, it is possible to visualize the outflow drainage of the malformation and it is possible to distinguish four types according to the drainage veins.

Direct puncture phlebography is used for the evaluation of the venous outflow of the lesion. It helps in understanding the success probability of a vascular surgical procedure or sclerotherapy. Retrograde phlebography is useful to evaluate deep venous incompetence in the lower limbs, visceral and pelvic malformations.

Arteriography

Arteriography is now almost obsolete with the availability of MRI and CT scans for the management of the vascular malformations in general but it still remains as the gold standard for the precise assessment for the AVMs and warranted for the planning of the treatment of an AVM which were already studied with non-invasive diagnostic tools.

It is necessary to have panoramic and superselective pictures in order to highlight the feeding arteries to lead to the nidus. It is possible to adopt an arteriographic classification of AV shunts in order to guide the therapy as mentioned in detail above [42].

Atreriography is an invasive investigation and used only for the patients who need a therapy and it should be performed at the centers which deliver the therapy.

Lymphography

In evaluations of LMs, Invasive tests are rarely required for the diagnosis but occasionally needed for differential diagnosis as well as sometimes for confirmation of the diagnosis [43]. The usual protocol is to defer the invasive tests. Direct puncture percutaneous lymphangiography can be generally deferred to later stages if there is a need for refining the diagnosis or if surgical or other invasive therapeutic measures are considered. It is reserved for road-mapping in subsequent therapy if needed.

Conventional oil contrast lymphangiography when combined with CT scan, is very informative in selected patients with chylous dysplasia and gravitational reflux disorders in order to define more clearly the extension of the pathologic alterations and sites of lymphatic and chylous leakage. These are the only diagnostic investigations that can clearly demonstrate pathologies of chylous vessels, chylous cyst, and thoracic duct in cases of chylothorax, chylous ascites, protein-losing enteropathy, etc. [19, 44, 45].

Lymphography has been substituted by lymphoscintigraphy for the diagnosis of lymphedema. There is a revival in the use of lymphography in case of lymphoceles, and pathology of chylous reflux. In this case, a direct puncture of inguinal nodes is made under ultrasound and lipiodol infused. The procedure causes the inflammation of the lymphatic pathways and may be curative [46, 47].

11.10 Nuclear Medicine Evaluation

11.10.1 Whole Body Blood Pool Scintigraphy (WBBPS)

The presence of a vascular malformation is detected by WBBPS using Tc99. The advantage lies with a single examination detecting the presence of any vascular malformation in the whole body. The main strength associated with WBBPS, is the ability to investigate all anatomic structures in one examination. It gives Some quantitative data on the blood trapping of the lesion can be derived easily which calculates the possibility to assess the results of treatment [48, 49].

WBBPS is an screening test used sometimes in multiple VM lesions which are scattered in the whole body. It allows qualitative and quantitative evaluation of the VM lesion especially during multisession sclerotherapy as a cost-effective measure. It is an excellent tool for routine follow-up and the evaluation of therapy to assess the progress of treatment and the natural course of the VM lesion with some numerical values. It can exclude the LM where the absence of an abnormal blood pool over the lymphatic lesion is the typical finding [1].

WBBPS is also an excellent optional test for the AVM evaluation as well. But it is rather more useful for the screening of hidden CVM lesions throughout the body and for a qualitative analysis of the AVM lesion along the course of the multisession therapy as a cost-effective measure. It is an excellent tool for the routine follow-up on the progress of treatment and its natural course as well when TLPS is not feasible/available [50, 51].

Whole body blood pool scintigraphy as a very useful tool to detect the presence of a vascular malformation throughout the body.

11.10.2 Transarterial Lung Perfusion Scintigraphy (TLPS)

An essential examination is scintigraphy which is necessary for the diagnosis of AVM and CVM in general but it remains an option as a secondary investigation only in few selected cases. TLPS has a unique role in determining the degree of AV shunting by the AVM lesion within an extremity [52, 53].

TLPS has a special role to detect and assess a micro-AV shunting lesion, which is often difficult with conventional techniques. Micro-AVMs frequently exist in the combined form of CVM, the hemolymphatic malformation (HLM), and its delayed or overlooked diagnosis with subsequent progress beyond the optimum time for the interception can be avoided with TLPS alone [52–54].

TLPS allows not only to quantify the AV shunt present in a malformation but also provides quantitative measurement of the shunting status during therapy [55]. TLPS may replace the substantial role of traditional arteriography as a follow-up assessment tool for extremity AVMs. TLPS is not indicated for evaluation of the VM lesion but its major function is to rule out the presence of a combined AVM lesions [54]. Transarterial lung perfusion scintigraphy should be used to quantify the AV shunt in an AVM only in indicated cases.

11.10.3 Radionuclide Lymphoscintigraphy (LSG)

LSG is basically a physiological and functional study which complements the anatomical information provided by lymphangiography. There are no standardizations nor is there a gold standard as of yet [13, 19]. It is performed with injection of 99mTclabeled human serum albumin or 99mTc-labeled Sulphur Colloid subcutaneously into the first and second webspace of the toes or fingers, is the test of choice to confirm or exclude lymph vessel pathology as the cause of chronic limb swelling [13, 19].

Movement of the colloid from the injection site, the transition time to the knee, groins or axilla, absence or presence of major lymphatic collectors, number and size of vessels and nodes (e.g., popliteal nodes), the presence of collaterals and reflux, symmetric activity with the opposite side are recorded and used for interpretation. Semi-quantitative assessment has been reported, and most recently, the technique of quantitative assessment of transit time from the foot to the knee was also validated [56, 57].

LSG represents the main examination to evaluate the lymph dynamics of the limbs. This will be recorded in rest, after exercise, and 1 h of daily activity. With this examination, it is possible to detect the presence of deep and superficial lymphatic vessels and the presence or absence of reflux. In patients with genital and abdominal lymph leakage, there is an indication for SPECT examination to visualize the intraabdominal lymph node status [25].

LSG is essential to rule out lymphatic dysfunction especially due to the presence of a truncular LM known as primary lymphedema, which often exists with the VM lesion (e.g., KTS) [58, 59].

LSG remains the gold standard for lymphatic function evaluation since the LSG is the only test that can clearly indicate lymphatic function. Radionuclide lymphoscintigraphic findings provide the proper clinical and/or laboratory staging that may be essential for proper clinical management.

LSG, along with clinical evaluation, is the most essential component for the diagnosis of chronic lymphedema.

LSG is extremely useful for identifying the specific lymphatic abnormality and has largely replaced conventional oil contrast lymphography for visualizing the lymphatic network. LSG can easily be repeated with minimal risk. Data and images obtained from the study identify lymphatic (dys)function, based on visualization of lymphatics, lymph nodes, and dermal backflow as well as semi-quantitative data on radiotracer (lymph) transport.

However, the LSG has not been standardized with regard to the various radiotracers and radioactivity doses, different injection volumes, intracutaneous vs. subcutaneous injection site, epi-or subfascial injection, number of injections, different protocols of passive and active physical activity, varying imaging times, static and/or dynamic techniques.

Lymphoscintigraphy is the most essential non-invasive test for a morphodynamic evaluation of the lymphatic circulation.

11.11 Laboratory Tests

Coagulation disorders usually associated with high frequency in patients with extensive VMs and may result in potentially severe thromboembolic events and hemorrhagic complications [1]. Extensive VMs usually leads to "localized intravascular coagulopathy" (LIC). LIC results due to stagnant flow in extratruncular lesions leading to a cycle of ongoing intravascular thrombosis and fibrinolysis. Secondary hypofibrinogenemia is the end point spontaneous hemorrhage.

Currently, there are no evidence based guidelines to advocate screening for coagulopathy in patients with potentially lifethreatening VMs. It is important to follow an accurate diagnostic algorithm for coagulopathies associated with especially extensive VMs involving large surface areas, muscle involvement, and/or palpable phleboliths [1].

Assessment of the coagulation profile and D-dimer levels is indicated in patients with extensive VMs. D-dimer (a degradation product of crosslinked fibrin) measured with rapid enzyme-linked fluorescent immunoassay is being increasingly utilized in the assessment of VM patients and is the biochemical gold standard for ruling out an episode of thrombophlebitis or thromboembolic events.

D-dimer can detect a sign of consumptive coagulopathy which is common among VMs [60, 61].

Elevated D-dimer among the symptomatic VMs has a unique value for the clinical assessment of the severity of the VM lesions although D-dimer in general is highly non-specific. D-dimer levels may also assist in the diagnosis of occult lesions and help differentiate GVMs and LMs (normal D-dimer levels) from other multifocal venous lesions.[237] Therefore, in addition to imaging studies, plasma Ddimer representing a direct measurement of endogenous fibrinolysis as a biological marker should be evaluated in the diagnosis and followup of VMs.

Patients with *extensive* VMs or *high-risk* lesions, in particular, should undergo the following laboratory tests

- Full blood count including hemoglobin levels and platelet count
- Ddimer-quantitative assay
- Fibrinogen
- PT, APTT
- Thrombophilia screening

D-dimer measurements to detect elevated values linked to the presence of VMs, platelet count, and fibrinogen levels in Kasabach Merritt syndrome often associated with kaposiform hemangioendotheliomas.

11.11.1 Histology

Biopsy should be reserved to make an accurate diagnosis and is mostly required when the lesion is suspected to be a tumor. Biopsy may be required to differentiate between AVMs, NICH, and vascular sarcomas. Histologic differentiation between HOI and congenital hemangiomas may be required and can be facilitated by GLUT1 staining of HOI which persists also after regression. Biopsy may also be required to differentiate between GVM and BRBNS.

Recently, immunohistochemistry has been used in the study of hemangiomas and supports a new classification of the pediatric liver vascular tumors based on the expression of GLUT1 as a substitution of the old and confusing term of hepatic infantile hemangioendothelioma.

GLUT1 positive expression is usually demonstrated in multifocal, and diffuse hepatic infantile hemangioma which shares clinical and morphological features with cutaneous infantile hemangioma. Diffuse neonatal hemangiomatosis is a disorder characterized by multiple cutaneous and hepatic hemangiomas [62].

Therefore, timely identification of GLUT-1 expression is crucial for children with hepatic hemangiomas in view of improved management before reaching the liver transplantation. In the last 5 years, propranolol has dramatically changed the scope of children with hepatic hemangiomas. Prognosis is currently considered as favorable and those previously considered as unfortunate patients are not any more candidates for liver transplantation.

Biopsy should be recommended only for unclear cases.

11.11.2 Endoscopic Evaluation

Endoscopic examinations are recommended when vascular anomalies are suspected to involve intracavity organs. This is usually performed when investigating the causes of occult bleeding.

CVMs located on the face and neck often require early pharyngolaryngotracheoscopy as the possible associated mucosal involvement may result in bleeding, infection, or respiratory complications. Conventional imaging techniques may not be precise enough to detect such lesions. Endoscopic identification and destruction of the lesion may be achieved during the same session.

Malformations located in the pelvic cavity and lower extremities often need proctosigmoidoscopy, urethrocystoscopy, and/or vaginoscopy (colposcopy) for early detection before bleeding occurs. This is especially true in patients with KTS which accompanies a high incidence of gastrointestinal and genitourinary involvement.

Arthroscopy is indicated to assess lesions involving the knee as small lesions are frequently not detected by conventional imaging techniques. Accurate assessment is required for subsequent laser coagulation.

Patients with BRBNS need regular esophago-gastro-duodenoscopy and complete colonoscopy due to the high risk of gastrointestinal mucosal involvement that can cause severe bleeding.

11.11.3 Genetic Testing and Family Screening

Germline and somatic mutations have been identified in a few vascular anomalies. Germline mutations were identified when practitioners observed a familial occurrence of some vascular lesions, and blood samples from these individuals enabled researchers to identify these mutations. Sporadic syndromes are thought to occur due to the mosaic distribution of somatic mutations that are detected from studies of affected tissue [63–67].

However, certain vascular anomalies occur with variable penetrance, such that parents of the proband patient may harbor a genetic mutation without overt expression of the disorder (e.g., GVM). If these parents are interested in further offspring (and the genetic mutation has been identified), prenatal genetic testing can be offered.

Options include chorionic villus sampling, amniocentesis, or pre-implantation genetic testing with in vitro fertilization of an unaffected embryo. Identification of the PTEN mutation requires counseling regarding the necessity for early and consistent surveillance for early detection of malignancies. Additionally, affected patients can be educated about their chances of having affected offspring.

Identification of somatic mutations may have implications for new therapies. In many cases, discussion with a specialist in human genetics and/or genetic counselor is recommended. In the USA, many insurance plans require prior authorization for this testing, which may be costly. Some research laboratories are interested in patient/family blood and/or tissue samples for genetic studies.

11.11.4 FollowUp Assessment

Follow-up is essential to evaluate the natural evolution of the disease even without treatment or with treatment in terms of pathology and/or the therapy results. The follow-up assessment tools are non-invasive investigations usually (MRI and ultrasound). A transient increase in size after endovascular intervention is usually observed most of the times. Using WBBPS, scattered or multiple vascular malformations can be usually identified during follow-up .

Follow-up evaluation to evaluate the natural evolution of the pathology and/or the therapy results. The follow-up shall be based on non-invasive investigations (MRI and ultrasound) mostly and sometimes invasive investigation like WBBPS.

References

1. Dubois J, Soulez G, Oliva VL, et al. Soft-tissue venous malformations in adult patients: imaging and therapeutic issues. Radiographics. 2001;21:1519–31.
2. Greene AK, Kim S, Rogers GF, et al. Risk of vascular anomalies with down syndrome. Pediatrics. 2008;121:e135–40.
3. Tasnádi G. Epidemiology and etiology of congenital vascular malformations. SeminVasc Surg. 1993;6:200–3.
4. Dubois J, Garel L. Imaging and therapeutic approach of hemangiomas and vascular malformations in the pediatric age group. Pediatr Radiol. 1999;29:879–93.
5. Laroche JP, Becker F, Khau-Van-Kien A, Baudoin P, Brisot D, Buffler A, Coupé M, Jurus C, Mestre S, Miserey G, Soulier-Sotto V, Tissot A, Viard A, Vignes S, Quéré I. Quality standards for ultrasonographic assessment of peripheral vascular malformations and vascular tumors. Report of the French society for vascular medicine. J Mal Vasc. 2013;38(1):29–45.
6. McCafferty IJ, Jones RG. Imaging and management of vascular malformations. Clin Radiol. 2011;66:1208–18.
7. Offergeld C, Schellong SM, Daniel WG, Huttenbrink KB. Value of color–coded duplex ultrasound in interstitial laser therapy of hemangiomas and vascular malformations. Laryngorhinootologie. 1998 Jun;77(6):342–6.
8. Gloviczki P, Stanson AW, Stickler GB, Johnson CM, Toomey BJ, Meland NB, Rooke TW, Cherry KJ Jr. Klippel–Trenaunay syndrome: the risks and benefits of vascular interventions. Surgery. 1991 Sep;110(3):469–79.
9. Park KB, Do YS, Lee BB, Kim DI, Wook Kim Y, Shin BS, et al. Predictive factors for response of peripheral arteriovenous malformations to embolization therapy: analysis of clinical data and imaging findings. J Vasc Interv Radiol. 2012 Nov;23(11):1478–86.

10. Lee BB, Laredo J. Chapter 63. Venous Malformation and Tumors: Etiology, Diagnosis, and Managment. Part V. Congenital Venous Abnormalities. Page 541-548, The Vein Book. John J. Bergan and Nisha Bunke-Paquette (Eds), 2014, 2nd Edition, Oxford University Press, New York, NY, USA.
11. Lee BB, Laredo J. Editorial. Venous malformation: treatment needs a bird's eye view. Phlebology. 2013;28:62–3.
12. Lee BB, Baumgartner I. Contemporary diagnosis of venous malformation. J Vasc Diagnostics. 2013;(1):25–34.
13. Lee BB: Lymphedema–diagnosis and treatment. Tredbar, Morgan, Lee, Simonian, Blondeau (eds). Lymphatic malformation, pages 3142. SpringerVerlag London 2008.
14. Lee BB, Laredo J, Neville R. Primary lymphedema as a truncular lymphatic malformation. Chapter 51, section XI lymphedema and congenital vascular malformation. In: Lee ByungBoong, Bergan J, Rockson SG, editors. LYMPHEDEMA: a concise compendium of theory and practice. 1st ed. London, UK: Springer-Verlag; 2011. p. 419–26.
15. Antignani PL, Benedetti Valentini F, Aluigi L, baroncelli T, et al. Guidelines of Italian society for vascular investigation. Int Angiol. 2012;5:1–78.
16. Gniadecka M. Localization of dermal edema in lipodermatosclerosis, lymphedema and cardiac insufficiency: high–frequency ultrasound examination of intradermal echogenicity. J Am Acad Dermatol. 1996;35:37–41.
17. Szuba A, Rockson SG. Lymphedema: classification, diagnosis and therapy. Vasc Med. 1998;3(2):145–56.
18. Lee BB, Baumgartner I, Berlien HP, Bianchini G, Burrows P, Do YS, Ivancev K, Kool LS, Laredo J, Loose DA, Lopez-Gutierrez JC, Mattassi R, Parsi K, Rimon U, Rosenblatt M, Shortell C, Simkin R, Stillo F, Villavicencio L, Yakes W. Consensus document of the International Union of Angiology (IUA)-2013. Current concept on the management of arterio-venous malformation. Int Angiol. 2013 Feb;32(1):9–36.
19. Lee BB, Andrade M, Antignani PL, Boccardo F, Bunke N, Campisi C, Damstra R, Flour M, Forner-Cordero J, Gloviczki P, Laredo J, Partsch H, Piller N, Michelini S, Mortimer P, Rabe E, Rockson S, Scuderi A, Szolnoky G, Villavicencio JL. Diagnosis and treatment of primary lymphedema. consensus document of the International Union of Phlebology (IUP)–2013. Int Angiol. 2013;32(6):541–74.
20. Wang B, Liu Z, Shen L. Bilateral persistent sciatic arteries complicated with chronic lower limb ischemia. Int J Surg Case Rep. 2011;2(8):309–12.
21. Patel MV, Patel NH, Schneider JR, Kim S, Verta MJ. Persistent sciatic artery presenting with limb ischemia. J Vasc Surg. 2013 Jan;57(1):225–9.
22. Legiehn GM, Heran MK. Classification, diagnosis, and interventional radiologic management of vascular malformations. Orthop Clin North Am. 2006;37(3):435–74.
23. Konez O, Hopkins KL, Burrows PE. Pediatric techniques and vascular anomalies. In: Rubin GD, Rofosky NM, editors. CT and MR angiography: Lippincott; 2009. p. 1118–87.
24. Navarro OM, Laffan EE, Ngan BY. Pediatric soft tissue tumors and pseudotumors: MR imaging features with pathologic correlation. I. Imaging approach, pseudotumors, vascular lesions, and adipo–cystic tumors. Radiographics. 2009;29(3):887–906.
25. Lee BB, Antignani PL, Baraldini V, Baumgartner I, Berlien P, Blei F, Carrafiello GP, Grantzow R, Ianniello A, Laredo J, Loose D, Lopez Gutierrez JC, Markovic J, Mattassi R, Parsi K, Rabe E, Roztocil K, Shortell C, Vaghi M. ISVI-IUA consensus document diagnostic guidelines of vascular anomalies: vascular malformations and hemangiomas. Int Angiol. 2015 Aug;34(4):333–74.
26. Moukaddam H, Pollak J, Haims AH. MRI characteristics and classification of peripheral vascular malformations and tumors. Skelet Radiol. 2009;38(6):535–47.
27. Rak KM, Yakes WF, Ray RL, Dreisbach JN, Parker SH, Luethke JM, Stavros AT, Slater DD, Burke BJ. MR imaging of symptomatic peripheral vascular malformations. AJR Am J Roentgenol. 1992;159(1):107–12.
28. Stepansky F, Hecht EM, Rivera R, et al. Dynamic MR angiography of upper extremity vascular disease: pictorial review. Radiographics. 2008;28:e28.
29. Goyal M, Causer PA, Armstrong D. Venous vascular malformations in pediatric patients: comparison of results of alcohol sclerotherapy with proposed MR imaging classification. Radiology. 2002;223(3):639–44.
30. Lee BB, Bergan J, Gloviczki P, Laredo J, Loose DA, Mattassi R, Parsi K, Villavicencio JL, Zamboni P. Diagnosis and treatment of venous malformations – consensus document of the International Union of Phlebology (IUP)-2009. Int Angiol. 2009 December;28(6):434–51.
31. Meyer JS, Hoffer FA, Barnes PD, Mulliken J. Biological classification of soft–tissue vascular anomalies:MR correlation. AJR Am J Roentgenol. 1991;157:559–64.
32. Barnes PD, Burrows PE, Hoffer FA, et al. Hemangiomas and vascular malformations of the head and neck: MR characterization. AJNR Am J Neuroradiol. 1994;15(1):193–5.
33. Elsayes KM, Menias CO, Dillman JR, Platt JF, Willatt JM, Heiken JP. Vascular malformation and hemangiomatosis syndromes: spectrum of imaging manifestations. Am J Roentgenol. 2008 May;190(5):1291–9.
34. Rauch RF, Silverman PM, Korobkin M, et al. Computed tomography of benign angiomatous lesions of the extremities. J Comput Assist Tomogr. 1984;8:1143–6.
35. Konez O, Burrows PE. An appropriate diagnostic workup for suspected vascular birthmarks. Cleve Clin J Med. Jun 2004;71:505–10.
36. Lidsky M, Spritzer C, Shortell C. The role of dynamic contrast–enhanced magnetic resonance imaging in the

diagnosis and management of patients with vascular malformations. J Vasc Surg I. 2011;53(1):131–7.
37. Belov S. Correction of lower limbs length discrepancy in congenital vascular–bone diseases by vascular surgery performed during childhood. Semin Vasc Surg. 1993 Dec;6(4):245–51.
38. Rutherford RB. Congenital vascular malformations: diagnostic evaluation. Semin Vasc Surg. 1993;6:225–32.
39. Weber J, Daffinger N. Congenital vascular malformations: the persistence of marginal and embryonal veins. Vasa. 2008;35:67–77.
40. Puig S, ArefH CV, Bonin B, Brunelle F. Classification of venous malformations in children and implications for sclerotherapy. Pediatr Radiol. 2003;33:99–103.
41. Puig S, Casati B, Staudenherz A, Paya K. Vascular low–flow malformations in children: current concepts for classification,diagnosis and therapy. Eur J Radiol. 2005 Jan;53(1):35–45.
42. Park KB, Do YS, Lee BB, Kim DI, Wook Kim Y, Shin BS, et al. Predictive factors for response of peripheral arteriovenous malformations to embolization therapy:analysis of clinical data and imagin findings. J Vasc Interv Radiol. 2012 Nov;23(11):1478–86.
43. Dubois J, Patriquin HB, Garel L, Powell J, Filiatrault D, David M, Grignon A. Soft–tissue hemangiomas in infants and children: diagnosis using Doppler sonography. AJR Am J Roentgenol. 1998 Jul;171(1):247–52.
44. Boccardo F, Bellini C, Eretta C, Pertile D, Da Rin E, Benatti E, Campisi M, Talamo G, Macciò A, Campisi C, Bonioli E, Campisi C. The lymphatics in the pathophysiology of thoracic and abdominal surgical pathology: immunological consequences and the unexpected role of microsurgery. Microsurgery. 2007;27(4):339–45.
45. Nadolski GJ, Itkin M. Feasibility of ultrasound–guided intranodal lymphangiogram for thoracic duct embolization. J Vasc Interv Radiol. 2012 May;23(5):613–6.
46. Rajebi MR, Chaudry G, Padua HM, Dillon B, Yilmaz S, Arnold RW, Landrigan-Ossar MF, Alomari AI. Intranodal lymphangiography: feasibility and preliminary experience in children. J Vasc Interv Radiol. 2011 Sep;22(9):1300–5.
47. Dentici R, Mattasi R, Vaghi M. La diagnostica per immagini in medicina nucleare. Capitolo 19. In: Mattassi BS, Loose DA, Vaghi M, editors. Malformaziono vascolari ed emangiomi. Testo–atlantie di diagnostica e terapia. Milano, Italy: Springer-Verlag. p. 32–9.
48. Fukuda Y, Murata Y, Umehara I, Yamashita T, Ono C, Iwai T, Shibuya H. Perfusion and blood pool scintigraphy for diagnosing soft–tissue arteriovenous malformations. Clin Nucl Med. 1999 Apr;24(4):232–4.
49. Lee BB, Kim BT, Choi JY, Cazaubon M. Prise en charge des malformations vasculaires congénitales (MVC) en 2003: rôle de la scintigraphy corps entier dans las surveillance évolutive. Angeiologie. 2003;55(3):17–26.
50. Inoue Y, Wakita S, Ohtake T, Ohkubo T, Hayashi N, Nishikawa J, Sasaki Y. Use of whole–body imaging using Tc–99m RBC in patients with soft–tissue vascular lesions. Clin Nucl Med. 1996 Dec;21(12):958–9.
51. Vaisnyte B, Vajauskas D, Nevidomskyte D, Misonis N, Palionis D, Kurminas M, Mataciunas M. Arteriovenous malformations treatment strategies based on transarterial lung perfusion scintigraphy(TLPS) communication at the 19th Int. workshop on vascular anomalies, June 16–19. Malmö Sweden; 2012.
52. Pecking AP, Alberini JL, Wartski M, Edeline V, Cluzan RV. Relationship between lymphoscintigraphy and clinical findings in lower limb lymphedema: towards a comprehensive staging. Lymphology. 2008;41:1–10.
53. Lee BB, Mattassi R, Kim BT, Park JM. Advanced management of arteriovenous shunting malformation with Transarterial lung perfusion Scintigraphy (TLPS) for follow up assessment. Int Angiol. 2005;24(2):173–84.
54. Lee BB, Lardeo J, Neville R. Arterio–venous malformation: how much do we know? Phlebology. 2009;24:193–200.
55. Lee BB, Villavicencio JL. Primary lymphedema and lymphatic malformation: are they the two sides of the same coin? Eur J Vasc Endovasc Surg. 2010;39:646–53.
56. Solari N, Gipponi M, Stella M, Queirolo P, Somma d, et al. Predictive role of preoperative lymphoscintigraphy on the status of the sentinel lymph node in clinically node–negative patients wit cutaneous melanoma. Melanoma Res. 2009;19(4):243–51.
57. Gloviczki P, Calcagno D, Schirger A, et al. Noninvasive evaluation of the swollen extremity: experiences with 190 lymphoscintigraphy examinations. J Vasc Surg. 1989;9:683–90.
58. Lee BB, Bergan JJ. New clinical and laboratory staging systems to improve Management of Chronic Lymphedema. Lymphology. 2005;38(3):122–9.
59. Lee BB, Laredo J. Classification: Venous–Lymphatic Vascular Malformation. Chapter 21, Part 3. In: Antignani PL, Kalodiki E, editors. News in Phlebology, C. Allegra. Turin, Italy: Edizioni Minerva Medica; 2013. p. 91–4.
60. Dompmartin A, Ballieux F, Thibon P, et al. Elevated D–dimer level in the differential diagnosis of venous malformations. Arch Dermatol. 2009;145:1239–44.
61. Dompmartin A, Vikkula M, Boon M. Venous malformation: update on aetiopathogenesis, diagnosis and management. Phlebology. 2010;25:224–35.
62. Patiño-Seijas B, Lorenzo-Franco F, Rey-Sanjurjo JL, González-Cuesta M, Cembranos JLL-C. Vascular lesions: GLUT–1 expression as a diagnostic tool to discriminate tumors from malformations. J Oral Maxillofac Surg. 2012 Oct;70(10):2333–42.
63. Shirley MD, Tang H, Gallione CJ, Baugher JD, Frelin LP, Cohen B, et al. Sturge–Weber syndrome and port–wine stains caused by somatic mutation in GNAQ. N Engl J Med. 2013;368(21):1971–9.
64. Lindhurst MJ, Wang JA, Bloomhardt HM, Witkowski AM, Singh LN, Bick DP, et al. AKT1 gene mutation

levels are correlated with the type of dermatologic lesions in patients with Proteus syndrome. J Invest Dermatol. 2013;134(2):543–6.
65. Blumenthal GM, Dennis PA. PTEN hamartoma tumor syndromes. European Journal of Human Genetics: EJHG. 2008;16(11):1289–300.
66. Eerola I, Boon LM, Mulliken JB, Burrows PE, Dompmartin A, Watanabe S, et al. Capillary malformation–arteriovenous malformation, a new clinical and genetic disorder caused by RASA1 mutations. Am J Hum Genet. 2003;73(6):1240–9.
67. Wouters V, Limaye N, Uebelhoer M, Irrthum A, Boon LM, Mulliken JB, et al. Hereditary cutaneomucosal venous malformations are caused by TIE2 mutations with widely variable hyper–phosphorylating effects. European Journal of Human Genetics: EJHG. 2010;18(4):414–20.

12 Medical Management of Vascular Malformations

Shanmugavelayutham Chitravelu and Ajay K. Khanna

12.1 Introduction

The International Society for the Study of Vascular Anomalies (ISSVA) classification [1] of vascular anomalies is the most widely used classification for vascular anomalies.as per this classification.

Vascular anomalies are broadly divided into vascular tumors and vascular malformations.

Vascular tumors are endothelial neoplasms characterized by increased endothelial turnover. Infantile hemangioma is the most common in this category. Other examples are congenital hemangioma, hemangioendotheliomas, tufted angioma, hemangiopericytomas, angiosarcoma, and pyogenic granuloma. They are often characterized by a periods of growth and involution.

Vascular malformations can further be subdivided into groups based on vessel type and flow characteristics [2]. Capillary, venous, and lymphatic malformations are slow-flow lesions, while arteriovenous malformations and fistulae are fast-flow lesions. Vascular malformations are often recognized at birth and grow proportionately with the child and become prominent in the second decade of life. Vascular malformations do not involute.

In this chapter we shall discuss the medical management (topical/systemic/intralesional) of both these types of vascular anomalies, the management would vary depending upon the nature of the specific type of vascular anomaly (lymphatic, capillary, venous, arterial, mixed arteriovenous).

While lymphatic and venous malformations are mainly slow-flow, arterial, and mixed arteriovenous malformations are generally high flow lesions. Mixed malformations like arteriovenous varieties are the most challenging lesions and they require a multidisciplinary approach.

Lesions that are located near the vital structure and those in the head and neck areas are very challenging to treat and in this subset of patients, medical management forms a significant part of management.

The conservative treatment by far is compression therapy of vascular malformations. Adequate compressive treatment can possibly minimize symptoms and also prevent complications. Further Conservative approaches are proper skin and wound care. Lifestyle modification like reducing body weight, etc. and physical treatments like orthopedic footwear would improve the quality of life and limb. Further many patients have lot of anxiety problems so that have to be taken care properly.

S. Chitravelu
Vascular Surgery, Govt. Stanley Medical College, Chennai, India

A. K. Khanna (✉)
Department of Surgery, Institute of Medical Science, Banaras Hindu University, Varanasi, India

A. K. Khanna, S. K. Tiwary (eds.), *Vascular Malformations*,
https://doi.org/10.1007/978-981-15-9762-6_12

12.2 Medical Treatment

Medical therapies can be of some use in the management of Vascular malformations. They can control cellular proliferation and abnormal growth of tissue. There is very few medical treatment which can really arrest the growth of vascular malformations They are also helpful in avoiding bleeding, pain, infection which are the complications of vascular malformation. Venous malformations (VMs) are associated with an increased risk for thrombosis as well as bleeding. Patients with VM frequently suffer from painful episodes of local thrombosis. These can be treated with Low Molecular weight heparin or oral anticoagulants [3]. Patients with lymphatic malformations especially are associated with recurrent infections, a long-term antibiotic prophylaxis can be prescribed. A study on "Prophylactic Antibiotics for the Treatment of Cellulitis at Home" (PATCH) group have confirmed the use of antimicrobial prophylaxis especially Penicillin [4].

Medical treatment for Vascular malformations can be divided into three groups: Topical, systemic, Intralesional.

12.3 Topical

Topical agents are mainly used in the management of infantile hemangiomas.

12.3.1 Timolol

0.5% gel (topical) is a non-selective beta-blocker used for the treatment of glaucoma. 1 drop three times a day is directly applied to the hemangioma, and carefully spread over the lesion. The duration of treatment is from 6 months to a year. Adverse effects are mainly due to systemic absorption and include bradycardia, hypotension, bronchospasm, peripheral vasoconstriction, weakness and fatigue, alopecia, rash, sleep disturbance, and hypoglycemia. Response rates in the individual studies of topical timolol ranged from 47% to 100%, with the met estimate being 83% (95% CI 65% to 93%) [5]. This drug is contraindicated in reactive airway disease including asthma severe chronic obstructive pulmonary disease; sinus bradycardia, sick sinus syndrome sinoatrial block, second- or third-degree atrioventricular block, overt cardiac failure, and cardiogenic shock.

12.3.2 Imiquimod 5% Cream

It is an immune response modifier with antiangiogenic and pro-apoptotic properties. It is directly applied to the hemangiomatous lesion on alternate days at bedtime and left for 8 h, it is washed with mild soap the next morning. The duration of therapy is about 4 months [6, 7] Severe inflammatory reactions may occur with the application of imiquimod.

12.4 Systemic

12.4.1 Propanolol

It is a non-selective beta-blocker used as antihypertensive. The mechanism of action of propranolol on IHs is vasoconstriction; decreased expression of vascular endothelial growth factor (VEGF) and basic fibroblast growth factor (bFGF) genes through downregulation of the RAF/mitogen–activated protein kinase pathway; and apoptosis of capillary endothelial cells. The dose of propranolol is 1 mg/kg/day in three divided doses to start with and increased to 2 mg/kg/day at 1 week if it is well tolerated [8]. Approximately 90% of tumors will regress or caese to grow. Risks (<3%) include bronchospasm, bradycardia, hypotension, hypoglycemia, seizures, and hyperkalemia.

12.4.2 Prednisolone

Corticosteroids are the commonly accepted first-line treatment in venous malformations. Steroids are most effective in the early proliferative phase. They have an inhibitory effect on the production of vascular endothelial growth factor A (VEGF-A) by stem cells in hemangiomas. Administration of prednisone, more than 2 to 3 mg/kg per day, resulted in a 75% response (>3 mg/kg per day resulted in a 94% response but greater adverse effects). Lesser dosing (≤2 mg/kg per day) resulted in fewer responses and adverse effects reported, but rebound occurred in 70% of patients [9]. Patients are given prednisolone 3 mg/kg per day for 1 month; the drug is then tapered by 0.5 mg every 2–4 weeks until it is discontinued between 10–12 months of age when the tumor is no longer proliferating. Satisfactory results are reported in only 30% of cases. Numerous side effects are reported with steroid treatment in infants, including irritability, hypertension, immunosuppression, growth retardation, and osteoporosis. Most of these are reversible following cessation of treatment.

12.4.3 Vincristine

It is a chemotherapeutic agent. There are anecdotal reports of vincristine being used for the treatment of life-threatening, steroid resistant hemangiomas in cases associated with Kasabach–Merritt syndrome or thrombocytopenia [10]. It has also been used for the treatment of hemangiomas causing respiratory distress. Vincristine (1.5 mg/m^2) once weekly is given till signs of resolution. Adverse reactions are acute neurotoxicity in adults manifesting as constipation, abdominal pain, and ileus. It also causes bone pain, particularly in the jaw.

12.4.4 Interferon Alpha 2 Alpha

It is used for corticosteroid resistant hemangiomas [11], but limited by side effects as fever, neutropenia, and anemia. Neurotoxicity is an important long-term side effect (20% develop spastic diplegia).

12.4.5 Doxycycline

Is a matrix metalloproteinase inhibitor with mild antiangiogenesis effects that has been used to treat brain AVMs.

12.4.6 Thalidomide

Has also been used to treat symptomatic AVMs. Unfortunately, the AVM usually does not diminish with this medication. Thalidomide reduces bleeding in hereditary hemorrhagic telangiectasia, probably by promoting vessel maturation [12]. The drug also has antiangiogenic effect by suppression of endothelial growth factor. Combination of thalidomide and interferon has also been used in extensive CVM with acceptable results. Side effects of thalidomide are neutropenia, peripheral neuropathy, somnolence, constipation, macular rash [13].

12.4.7 Sildenafil

Selectively inhibits phosphodiesterase- 5 and prevents the breakdown of cyclic guanosine monophosphate. Inhibition of phosphodiesterase-5 decreases the contractility of vascular smooth muscle thereby produces vasodilation. This drug has been used for complex lymphatic malformations with good outcome [14].

12.4.8 Sirolimus

Angiogenesis Inhibitors(Rapamycin) is a macrolide produced by the bacteria Streptomyces hygroscopicus.Sirolimus (Rapamune) is a specific and potent inhibitor of mTOR, a serine/threonine kinase in the phosphoinositide-3- kinase (PI3K)/Akt pathway which regulates numerous cellular processes including cellular catabolism and anabolism, cell motility, angiogenesis, and cell growth. (Rapamycin) is a macrolide produced by the bacteria Streptomyces hygroscopicus. It was originally developed as an antifungal agent but it was found to be having an immunosuppressive and antiproliferative effect so it was used as an immunosuppressant in transplant. Further, it has been coated on the stents for use of coronary bypass. This drug has also been used in vascular malformations especially of lymphatic type [15, 16]. In recent years, several studies have demonstrated that sirolimus inhibits lymphatic vessel regeneration and invasion. Although prospective clinical trials have been limited, numerous reports have been published on the efficacy of sirolimus treatment for macrocystic and microcystic lymphatic malformations as well as combined malformations with a lymphatic component.

12.4.9 Angiogenesis Inhibitors

Small number of studies in animal models have also demonstrated that the blockade of VEGF and other chemokines involved in angiogenesis can prevent progression of AVMs.Bevacizumab (Avastin) is a recombinant humanized monoclonal antibody that binds to VEGF receptors on endothelial cells and serves as a competitive antagonist. Although highly specific for angiogenesis, it remains unclear whether VEGF-targeted therapy is a useful treatment for bleeding of preexisting vascular malformations.

12.5 Intralesional Sclerosants

There are several sclerosing agents, including sodium morrhuate, ethanol amine oleate, ethanol, bleomycin, STS 3% foam preparation, and hypertonic saline. Sclerosants destroy the vascular endothelium by various mechanisms as: iodine and alcohol are chemical agents, Salicylates and Hypertonic saline are osmotic agents while morrhuate sodium, sodium tetradecyl sulfate, polidocanol, and diatrizoate sodium are detergents, which change the surface tension of the cell, producing tissue maceration. They work by destroying the endothelial cells, accelerating protein coagulation in the blood of the lesions, promoting platelet adhesion to the vascular wall during thrombosis formation, and causing thrombosis of the vessels.

12.5.1 Sodium Tetra Decyl Sulfate (STS)

Can be used as liquid or foam sclerotherapy. 0.1 ml of sodium tetradecyl sulfate injection (STS) (3%) is administered directly into skin/mucosa. Manual compression is applied for 15 to 20 minutes. The total dose should not exceed 2.0 ml. It can be used as *Foam sclerotherapy.* 2 ml of 3% sodium tetradecyl sulfate Sclerosant is mixed with a certain amount of air (the most commonly used liquid-to-air ratio is 1: 4) as sclerosing foam using Tessari technique (oscillated vigorously between the two syringes about 10–20 times. The foam thus created will be stable for about 2 minutes after preparation. It reduces the dosage and concentration of the sclerosants, the selectivity of action on the endothelium of the foam reduces the risk of tissue damage while the sclerosant runs off the vessels. The rate of relapse after treatment with sclerosing foam is higher compared with liquid sclerosants. Sodium tetradecyl sulfate is the most commonly used sclerosant for venous malformations. The most common local complication is skin ulceration. (Figs. 12.1 and 12.2).

Other complications include muscle atrophy and contracture from extravasation, compartment compression, hemolysis, hemoglobinuria, and DIC. The specific complication that may occur is embolization stroke by flowing foam bubbles going through patent ductus arteriosus (PDA) [17, 18].

12.5.2 Absolute Alcohol (99% Ethanol)

The venous malformation is punctured using a scalp vein set under ultrasound guidance. The needle is adjusted till a free flow of blood through the connecting tube of the butterfly needle. The contrast medium is then injected until the draining veins are demonstrated. The dosage of absolute ethanol is approximately 1/2 to 2/3 of the amount of the contrast used. For large venous malformations involving multiple anatomical sites, the injection can be done simultaneously in different areas. The cumulative total dose of ethanol should not exceed 1 ml ethanol/kg body weight. It is especially useful for head and neck regions, trauma prone regions (joints), potential life-threatening areas, vascular bone syndrome. Complications include superficial

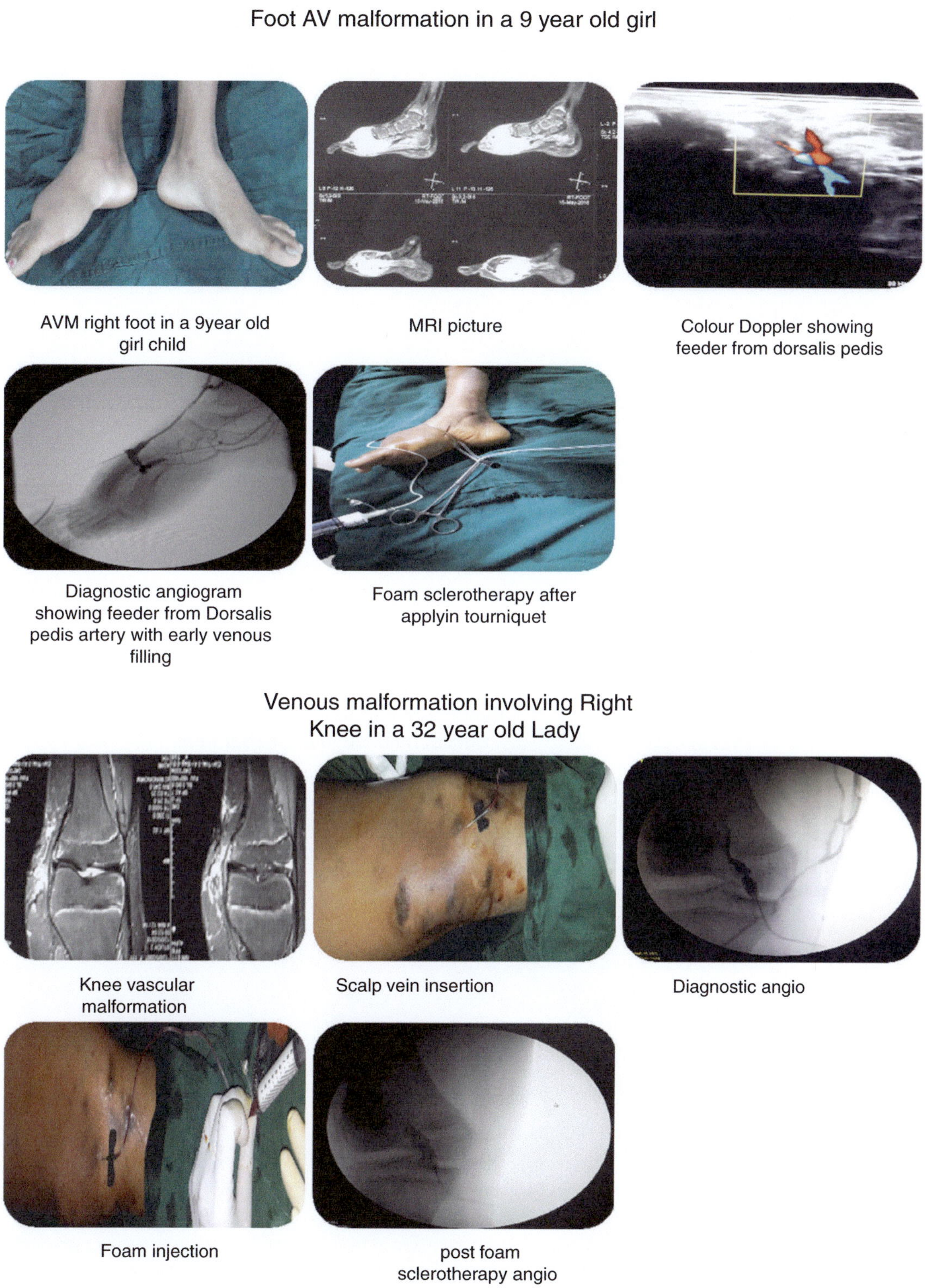

Fig. 12.1 (**a**) Foot AV malformation in a 9 year old girl. (**b**) Venous malformation involving Right Knee in a 32year old Lady. (**c**) Chest wall Venous malformation in a 22 year lady

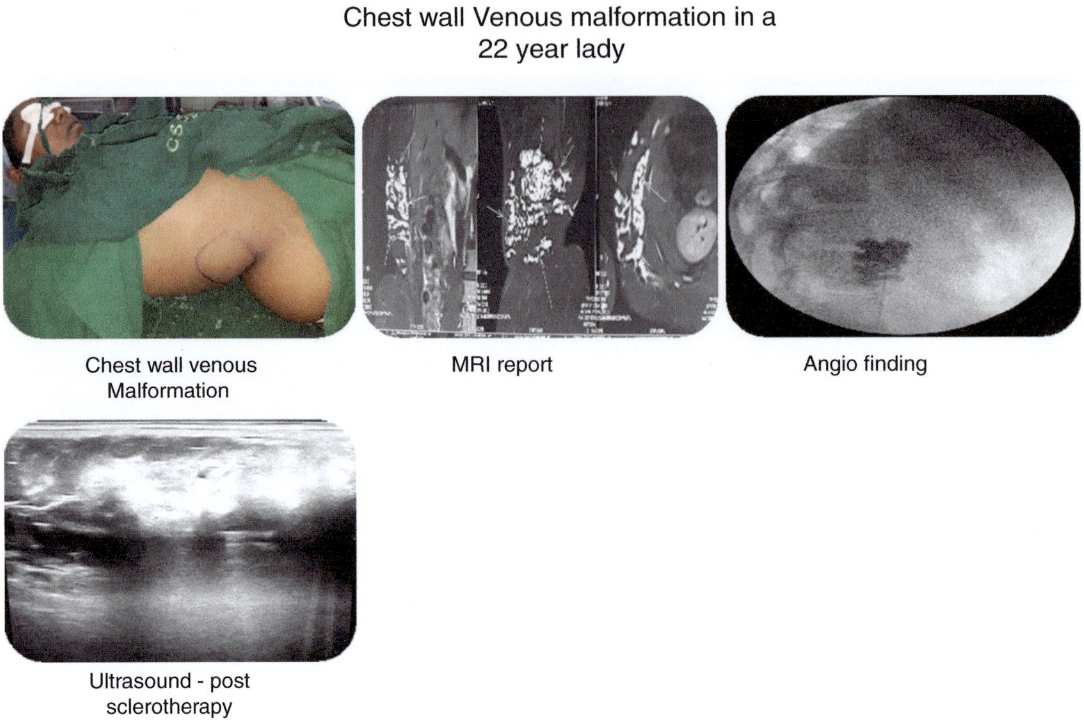

Fig. 12.1 (continued)

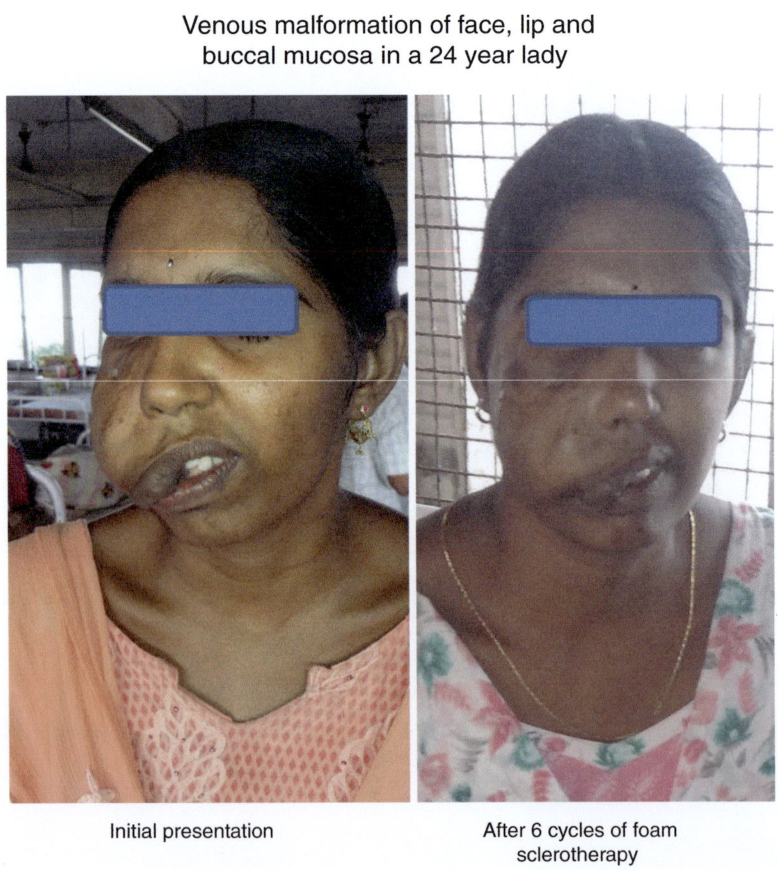

Fig. 12.2 Venous malformation of face, lip and buccal mucosa in a 24 year lady

ischemic bullae formation, tissue fibrosis, tissue necrosis, deep vein thrombosis of the lower extremity, pulmonary embolism, nerve palsy (temporary and permanent), and transient pulmonary arterial pressure elevation during the procedure.

12.5.3 Polidocanol

95% hydroxypolyethoxydodecane and 5% ethyl alcohol is a moderate form of ethanol most commonly used in European countries. It has a low risk of complications. The total dosage is determined by the location and size of the lesions and the patient's age, with no more than 3 ml at each injection (less than 1 ml for children). For patients with lesions that fail to have a complete response, injection is repeated at an interval of 1 to 2 weeks but not more than 5 consecutive sessions. it has a definite anesthetic effect; the injection is painless and well tolerated by the patients. Allergic reactions are rare, and hemolysis seldom occurs, which largely reduces the possibility of pigmentation. Therefore, it is suitable for treating head and neck venous malformations. The main disadvantage is tissue necrosis and ulceration which may occur if the solution leaks out into the skin or mucosa. The concentration used to produce foam sclerosing agent is 0.25% to 4%, depending on the size of the malformation and hemodynamic characteristics of the lesions. A higher concentration (3% to 4%) is used for intramuscular venous malformations and lower concentrations (0.25% to 0.5%) for the peripheral portions of huge venous malformations. 1% to 2% is chosen for residual lesions after treatment [19].

12.5.4 Bleomycin

Offers control of symptoms in patients with VMs when used as a sclerosing agent. It is effective and safe with minimal side effects. The big concern with bleomycin is pulmonary fibrosis, a major complication when using bleomycin as seen in cancer patients [20].

12.6 Conclusion

Medical treatment of Vascular malformations is mainly to restrict the growth of tissue and for the complications. Intralesional sclerotherapy is of tremendous use and usually always a part of the combined modality of vascular malformations.

References

1. Enjolras O, Mulliken JB. Vascular tumors and vascular malformations (new issues). Adv Dermatol. 1997;13:375–423.
2. Huang JT, Liang MG. Vascular malformations. Pediatr Clin N Am. 2010;57(5):1091–110.
3. Lee BB, Baumgartner I, Berlien P, Bianchini G, Burrows P, Gloviczki P, Huang Y, Laredo J, Loose DA, Markovic J, Mattassi R, Parsi K, Rabe E, Rosenblatt M, Shortell C, Stillo F, Vaghi M, Villavicencio L, Zamboni P. Diagnosis and treatment of venous malformations consensus document of the international union of phlebology (IUP): updated 2013. Int Angiol. 2015;34(2):97–149.
4. Chlebicki MP, Oh CC. Recurrent cellulitis: risk factors, etiology, pathogenesis and treatment. Curr Infect Dis Rep. 2014;16(9):422–32.
5. Anon, Infantile haemangioma: topical timolol. Guidance and guidelines. NICE. Accessed November 23, 2018, from https://www.nice.org.uk/advice/esuom47/chapter/full-evidence-summary
6. Martinez MI. Infantile Hemangioma. Arch Dermatol. 2002;138(7):881.
7. A Gaspari A, Tyring SK, Rosen T. Beyond a decade of 5% imiquimod topical therapy. J Drugs Dermatol. 2009 May;8(5):467–74.
8. McGee P, Miller S, Black C, Hoey S. Propranolol for infantile haemangioma: A review of current dosing regime in a regional Paediatric hospital. Ulster Med J. 2013;82(1):16–20.
9. Greene AK, Mulliken JB. Plastic surgery: volume 3: craniofacial, head and neck surgery and pediatric plastic surgery, vol. 39. p. 866–87.
10. Soni H, Pimpalwar S, Margolin J. Medical therapy for pediatric vascular anomalies. Semin Plast Surg. 2014;28(02):079–86.
11. Greinwald JH, et al. An update on the treatment of Hemangiomas in children with interferon Alfa-2a. Archives of Otolaryngology–Head & Neck Surgery. 1999;125(1):21.
12. Lebrin F, Srun S, Raymond K, Martin S, van den Brink S, Freitas C, Bréant C, Mathivet T, Larrivée B, Thomas JL, Arthur HM, Westermann CJ, Disch F, Mager JJ, Snijder RJ, Eichmann A, Mummery CL. Thalidomide stimulates vessel maturation and reduces epistaxis in individuals with hereditary hemorrhagic telangiectasia. Nat Med. 2010;16(4):420–8.

13. Molloy FM, Floeter MK, Syed NA, Sandbrink F, Culcea E, Steinberg SM, Dahut W, Pluda J, Kruger EA, Reed E, Figg WD. Thalidomide neuropathy in patients treated for metastatic prostate cancer. Muscle Nerve. 2001;24:1050–7.
14. Danial C, Tichy AL, Tariq U, Swetman GL, Khuu P, Leung TH, Benjamin L, Teng J, Vasanawala SS, Lane AT. An open-label study to evaluate sildenafil for the treatment of lymphatic malformations. J Am Acad Dermatol. 2014;22(14):01119.
15. Hammill AM, Wentzel M, Gupta A, Nelson S, Lucky A, Elluru R, Dasgupta R, Azizkhan RG, Adams DM. Sirolimus for the treatment of complicated vascular anomalies in children. Pediatr Blood Cancer. 2011;57(6):1018–24.
16. Curry S, Logeman A, Jones D. Sirolimus: a successful medical treatment for head and neck lymphatic malformations. Case Rep Otolaryngol. 2019 Mar 24;2019:2076798. https://doi.org/10.1155/2019/2076798.
17. Behravesh S, Yakes W, Gupta N, Naidu S, Chong BW, Khademhosseini A, et al. Venous malformations: clinical diagnosis and treatment. Cardiovasc Diagn Ther. 2016;6:557–69.
18. Ahmad S. Efficacy of percutaneous Sclerotherapy in low flow venous malformations - A single center series. Neurointervention. 2019 Mar;14(1):53–60. https://doi.org/10.5469/neuroint.2019.00024.
19. Zheng JW, Mai HM, Zhang L, et al. Guidelines for the treatment of head and neck venous malformations. Int J Clin Exp Med. 2013;6(5):377–89.
20. Spence J, Krings T, terBrugge KG, da Costa LB, Agid R. Percutaneous sclerotherapy for facial venous malformations: subjective clinical and objective MR imaging follow-up results. AJNR Am J Neuroradiol. 2010;31:955–60.

13 Surgical Treatment in Vascular Malformations

Dong-Ik Kim and Je Hoon Park

13.1 Introduction

Congenital Vascular malformations (CVMs) are subgrouped based on the histology of the lesion and hemodynamics of the lesion["high flow" or "low flow"]. The "high flow" CVMs are characterized by a direct communication between arterial and venous vessels without an intervening capillary bed such as arteriovenous malformations (AVMs) and arteriovenous fistulas (AVFs) and the "low-flow" CVMs are comprised of capillary malformations (CMs), venous malformations (VMs) and lymphatic malformations (LMs) [1].

Generally one should take into account some component before the treatment, such as (1) necessity to treat or observe, (2) result of an expected natural course of CVM lesion, (3) optimal timing for the treatment, (4) important structures around the CVM lesion, (5) the method of treatment approach including tissue or organ damage, and (6) rates of recurrence and treatment-associated complications [2].

CVMs have a different natural course and prognosis, thus these are not always needed the treatment or equally treated. Also, the depth of CVM involvement and anatomical location of the CVM lesion are important to determine an optional treatment strategy. The treatment plan can be decided according to treatment-associated cosmetic or functional complications.

Currently, the basic treatment concept for the CVMs mainly depends on endovascular treatment, especially for patients with surgically inaccessible CVM lesion such as diffuse infiltrating type extratruncular CVM lesions involving extensive regions of tissues [3].

Surgery for CVMs has been recommended only for limited and selected patients because of the risk of intraoperative massive bleeding, unavailability to remove all vascular malformation lesions, and high complication and recurrence rates. Surgical excision of limited and localized CVM lesion can be adopted as long as complete excision of the lesion is available with an acceptable risk of complication. Additionally, it is reported that certain CVM lesions can be aggravated by incomplete surgical removal or feeding artery ligation resulting in rapid collateralization from adjacent arteries and further limit access to the nidus for future treatment [4].

D.-I. Kim (✉)
Division of Vascular Surgery, Samsung Medical Center, Sungkyunkwan University, Seoul, Korea
e-mail: dikim@skku.edu

J. H. Park
International St. Mary's Hospital, Korea

A. K. Khanna, S. K. Tiwary (eds.), *Vascular Malformations*,
https://doi.org/10.1007/978-981-15-9762-6_13

13.2 Indications for Surgery

13.2.1 Arteriovenous Malformation (AVM)

AVMs are an active lesion, and they have a high tendency to progress and to worsen and to reexpand after treatment. Thus these are very challengeable especially in extratruncular type [5]. Treatment of an AVM is based on the concept of obliteration of the nidus which is thought to be responsible for the growth of the lesion. Sclerotherapy and embolization treatment remain first-line options to allow for safer intraoperative resection with less blood loss [6]. Ligation of feeding vessels should never be done because this results in the rapid recruitment of collaterals and enriches vascularity. When considering resection of an AVM, it is important to realize that these lesions are rarely curable, but rather one should focus on disease control.

There are various symptoms and signs in extratruncular AVMs such as cosmetic problem, thrill and pulsation, pain, heating sensation, skin ulcer, port-wine stain, bleeding, tingling sensation, functional limitation, and fracture. Indications for intervention include ischemic pain, recurrent ulcerations/bleeding, or cardiac dysfunction [7]. Surgical indications include necrosis, major bleeding, functional loss, and so on [5].

13.2.2 Venous Malformation (VM)

Treatment options for VM depend on both the extent of the lesion and the location. Limited intramuscular or extramuscular VM are can be removed by surgery, but diffuse, intramuscular infiltrating VM and VM in the head can be treated often by nonsurgical treatment [8]. And surgery may be selected in some situations, such as (1) to ligate efferent veins to improve the sclerotherapy result, (2) to remove residual VM after sclerotherapy, (3) to remove lesion resistant to sclerotherapy, or (4) localized lesion amenable to complete excision [9]. Also, surgical treatment can be an option in patients with VMs, especially with symptoms that cannot be managed with conservative therapy or sclerotherapy.

After excisional or debulking surgery in patient with VMs, remission or improvement can be observed in 75% [10]. Recent study shows that approximately half (54%) of slow-flow VM patients were able to undergo surgery, and around half (44%) of those patients were able to fully recover after total excision. And high satisfaction after surgery was found and relatively few complications were reported [11].

13.2.3 Lymphatic Malformation (LM)

LMs may be classified into truncular and extratruncular types. Truncular LMs arise at later stages (>3 weeks) of embryogenesis and hence involve mature lymphatic vessels, thus presenting with primary lymphedema. Extratruncular LMs arise earlier (<3 weeks) than truncular LMs during the reticular phase of vasculogenesis and result in cystic deformities. These types of LMs are further classified into macrocystic (cysts >1 cm), microcystic (cysts <1 cm), or mixed cystic lesions. There are various treatment modalities including conservative measures, medical treatments, percutaneous drainage, sclerotherapy, laser therapy, radiofrequency ablation, and surgery.

Surgical resection of LMs can be associated with significant morbidity including major bleeding, iatrogenic injury, and deformity. The goals of resection focus on gross debulking of defined anatomic field, limiting blood loss, and minimizing damage to surrounding structures [9]. Surgical resection is indicated as follows: (1) lesions larger than 3 cm, (2) patients with airway compromise, dyspnea, dysphagia, bone erosion, or significant deformity [12] (3) lesions suitable for a complete excision such as well-circumscribed macrocystic LMs of the neck (cystic hygroma) or localized microcystic lesions, and (4) after failed sclerotherapy [13].

Localized microcystic lesions of the head and neck can be removed completely. But complete resection is impossible for extensive and diffuse ones, because of (1) severe cosmetic and functional complications due to massive tissue defects by complete removal, especially in the lesion involving the lip, cheek, and tongue; (2) the poorly demarcating lesions; (3) thin and friable walls of lymphatic vessels of LMs; (4) tendency to the involvement of important structures such as the cranial nerves or vital blood vessels, making complete removal more difficult; (5) more common challenging because of the potential complications, such as facial nerve damage, Horner's syndrome, postoperative lymphatic leakage, seroma, and poor wound healing; and (6) common incidence of tissue defects, heavy bleeding and infection after total excision (3.1%, 1.6%, and 2.5%, respectively) [14].

The choice of treatment should be individualized and based on several factors such as the hyoid level, bilaterality, age of onset, growth rate, type, depth, extent, anatomical location, potential deformity or dysfunction of LMs [15]. There is no difference in complications and clinical outcomes between primary surgery and primary sclerotherapy for head and neck LMs [16].

13.3 Tips for Surgery

Vascular surgical treatment is indicated for the five main types of peripheral vascular malformations which cause vascular insufficiency, cardiac overload and limb length discrepancy, disfiguration, and dysfunction. The bases of this treatment are six different therapeutic strategies; reconstructive vascular surgery, operations to remove the vascular defect, operations to reduce the hemodynamic activity of the vascular defects, combined treatment, unconventional surgical methods, and multidisciplinary treatment [17].

13.3.1 Arteriovenous Malformation (AVM)

Management of AVM includes embolization alone or in combination with surgical excision. Various surgical reconstructive options are applied such as free flaps, local or regional flaps, tissue expansion, tendon recession, tendon transfer, osseo-integration, and skin grafting [7]. After preoperative embolization of the nidus, surgical resection should be done within 2 to 3 days, since rapid expansion can occur during the period between embolization and resection [18–20]. Sometimes a two-staged surgical approach may be a good option in selective patients [21].

The proximal surgical ligation of feeding arteries without resection (and endovascular coiling of feeder arteries) is doomed to failure and must be avoided as it does not cure the nidus which allows the AVM to grow. Furthermore, these procedures make a subsequent access and therapeutic embolization difficult [22]. Large excisions incapable of primary closure can be managed with vacuum-assisted closure devices or tissue transfer techniques. For difficult extremity, AVM, particularly those with loss of function, amputation can be done.

AVM of the thoracic and abdominal cavity including gastrointestinal tract, spleen, pancreas, and liver are managed with a combination of sclerotherapy and open resection [19].

Infiltrating AVM very often cannot be treated by direct puncture or by catheter embolization techniques [23]. In this situation, the surgical technique of Belov can be applied: clamping of the infiltrated part of the tissue followed by a continuous Blalock suture and resection of the overcoming part of the AVM. The advantage of this technique is that a cutdown of the infiltrated tissues with massive bleeding can be avoided [24].

13.3.2 Venous Malformation (VM)

Preoperative ethanol sclerotherapy can be emphasized for the prevention of massive bleeding during the surgical resection. Roh et al. [10] reported the good result of surgery of VMs with preoperative ethanol sclerotherapy. After ethanol sclerotherapy, unresectable lesions became resectable, and these were excised radically only with minimal complications. With preoperative glue embolization, there was no perioperative blood loss requiring transfusion. When lesions involve the dermis or are just below the dermis, flaps should be made as thinly as possible without devascularization of the skin. One should take into account the preservation of nerves, tendons, and joint cavities; and closed-suction drains are placed in the flap. Large resection areas can be covered by local or distant flaps or skin grafts [19].

13.3.3 Lymphatic Malformation (LM)

The principal goal of surgical LM management is lesion excision with the restoration of functional and esthetic integrity. The operative approach must consider that this is a benign disease process that warrants the preservation of vital structures [25]. Incomplete or partial excision does not absolutely imply recurrence requiring additional therapeutic intervention.

13.4 Complications Related with Surgery

Maftei et al. [26] reported significantly higher blood loss was associated with debulking surgery and with the previous history of major hemorrhage during CVM surgery. Predictors of significant blood loss during surgery include high flow AVM, inability to use tourniquet, debulking surgery, and low platelet count [26]. Vascular malformations, including VM and LM, of the head and neck are effectively treated by percutaneous sclerotherapy with an excellent result in most patients. Minor complications related to treatment occur in 10–12% of patients treated with detergent sclerosants and in up to 50% of patients when absolute ethanol is used. Also, major complications are more common with the use of absolute ethanol rather than of detergent sclerosants [27].

Visser et al. reported a recurrence rate of 8.7% following definitive surgery for AVM. Surgical complications are variously reported such as deep vein thrombosis with pulmonary embolism, wound breakdown, hematoma, and nostril stenosis requiring release and cartilage grafting [7].

VM have fragile, dysplastic vessels and permeate into surrounding tissues, which can result in significant blood loss with dissection [28]. Cutting through a VM produces a surface resembling a sponge, and bleeding is difficult to control with electrocautery, clamps, or sutures.

The higher the clinicoradiologic stage, the greater the risk of intra- and postoperative complications [29, 30]. Surgery for LMs has been reported with complication rate 19–33%, a mortality rate 6%, and a recurrence rate of up to 53% [31]. According to the LM location, there is a potential operative risk to cranial nerves VII, IX, X, and XII [32]. Postoperative seroma or lymphocele is very common, with a resultant risk of wound infection. Postoperative suction drainage is needed, and prolonged lymphorrhea may require medical management [25]. There are various complications such as major bleeding, iatrogenic injury, and deformity [14]. Emery et al. [32] reported that the incidence of facial palsy after surgical removal was 5.9–33%; Hancock et al. [33] demonstrated seromas in 9.8% of wounds with local drains and 3.6% of the wounds without drains. The dermal LM is recommended for wide local excision as the standard care [34]. Even with surgery, recurrence rates range from 17% to 25% for macroscopically complete excision and 40% for incomplete excision [35]. In a series of 65 patients with dermal LM, the recurrence rate was 75% for lesions greater than 1 cm^2 [36]. Nearly all recurrences were within 14 months of the initial resection, with 54% recurring within 3 months [37]. These recurrences may be continuously problematic and difficult to manage [38].

13.5 Cases of Surgery

To help readers understand, the author prepared interesting surgical cases according to the subgroup of congenital vascular malformation (Figs. 13.1, 13.2, 13.3, 13.4, 13.5, 13.6, 13.7, 13.8, 13.9, 13.10, 13.11, 13.12, 13.13, 13.14, 13.15, 13.16, 13.17, 13.18, 13.19, 13.20, 13.21, 13.22, 13.23, 13.24, 13.25, 13.26, 13.27, 13.28, 13.29, 13.30, 13.31, 13.32, 13.33, and 13.34).

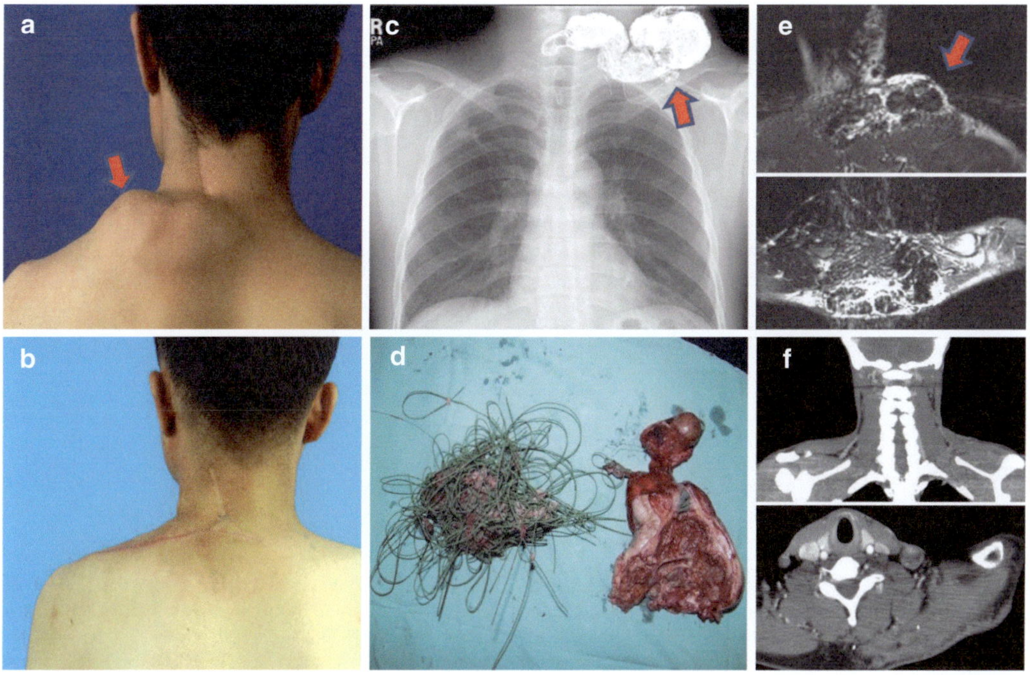

Fig. 13.1 CC: pulsating mass on the left lower neck. Dx: Arteriovenous malformation. (**a**) preop picture. (**b**) postop picture. (**c**) coil embolization. (**d**) op finding: AVM mass and coil within the mass. (**e**) preop MRI. (**f**) postop CTA

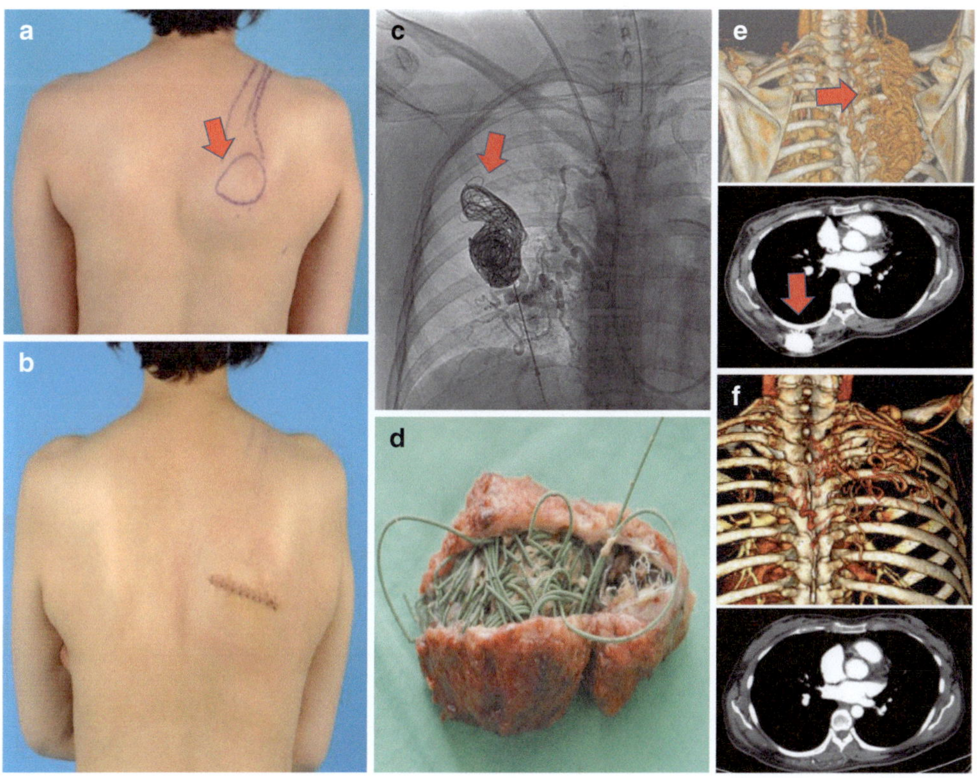

Fig. 13.2 CC: pulsating mass on back. Dx: Arteriovenous malformation. (**a**) preop picture. (**b**) postop picture. (**c**) coil embolization. (**d**) op finding: AVM mass and coil within the mass. (**e**) preop CTA. (**f**) postop CTA

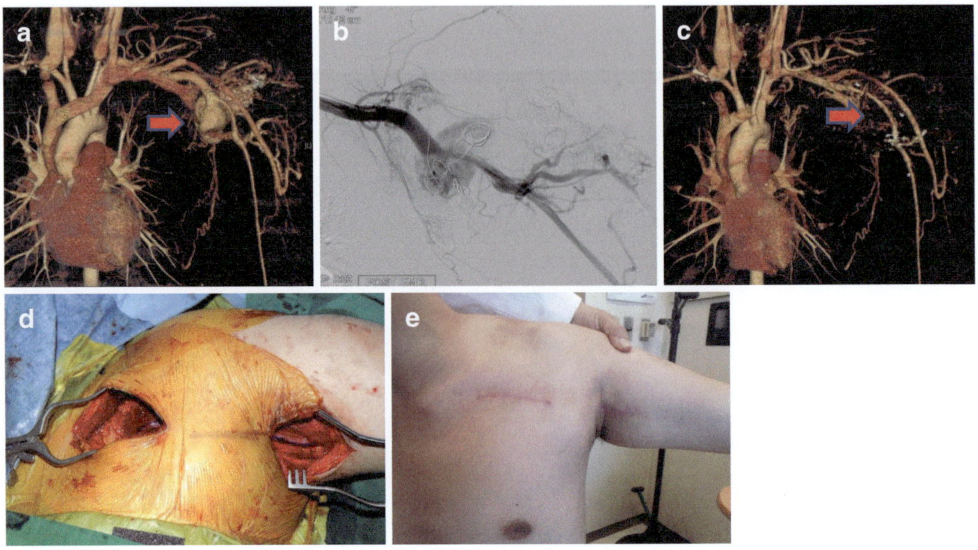

Fig. 13.3 CC: pulsating mass on left sub-clavicular and axillary area. Dx: Arteriovenous malformation. (**a**) preop CTA: AVM involving left subclavian and axillary artery. (**b**) preop coil embolization. (**c**) postop CTA: bypass between subclavian and axillary artery. (**d**) op finding: excision of main AVM mass and subclavian to axillary artery bypass with saphenous vein interposition. (**e**) postop picture

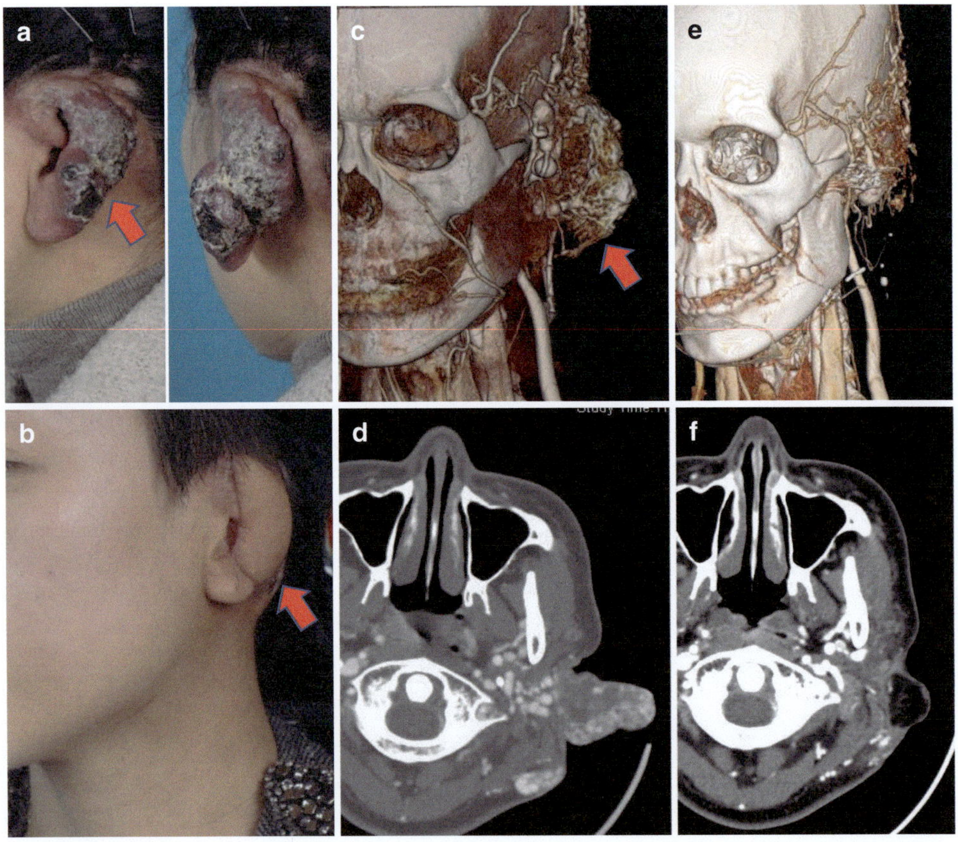

Fig. 13.4 CC: pulsating mass and tissue necrosis on ear. Dx: Arteriovenous malformation. (**a**) preop picture. (**b**) postop picture: excision of AVM mass including upper 2/3 part of ear and ear reconstruction with myo-cutaneous free flap. (**c** and **d**) preop CTA. (**e** and **f**) postop CTA

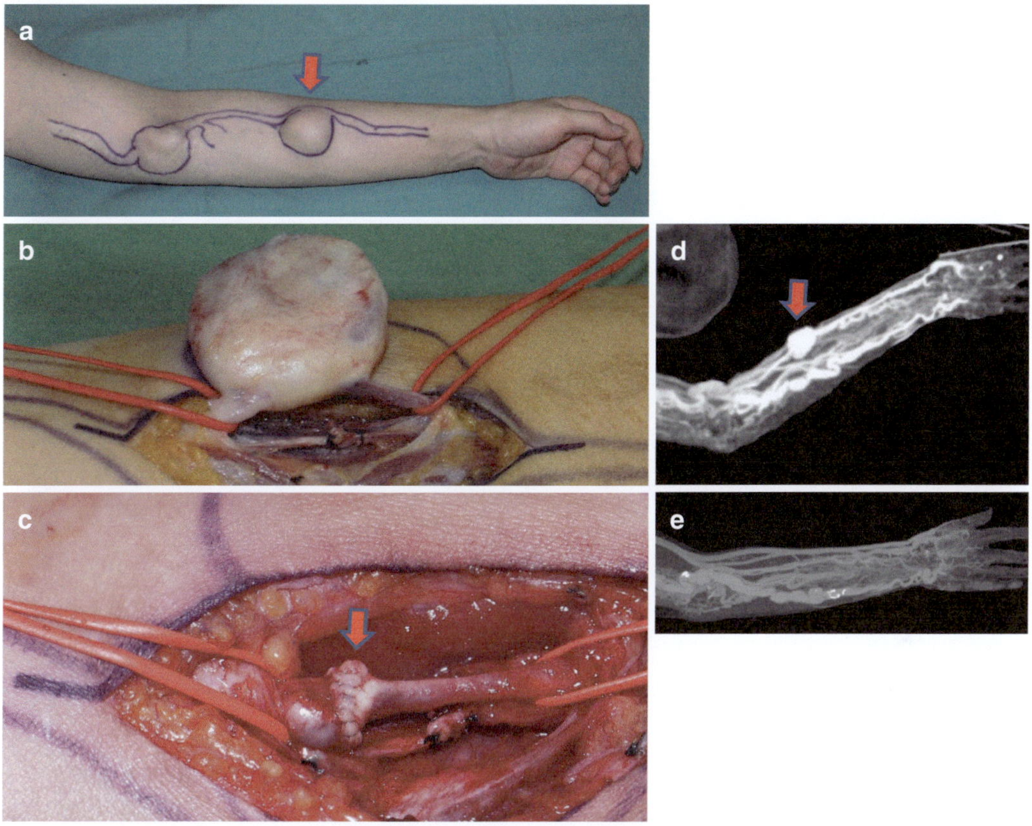

Fig. 13.5 CC: pulsating mass on forearm. Dx: Arteriovenous malformation. (**a**) preop picture. (**b** and **c**) op finding: AVM resection and end to end anastomosis. (**d**) preop CTA. (**e**) postop CTA

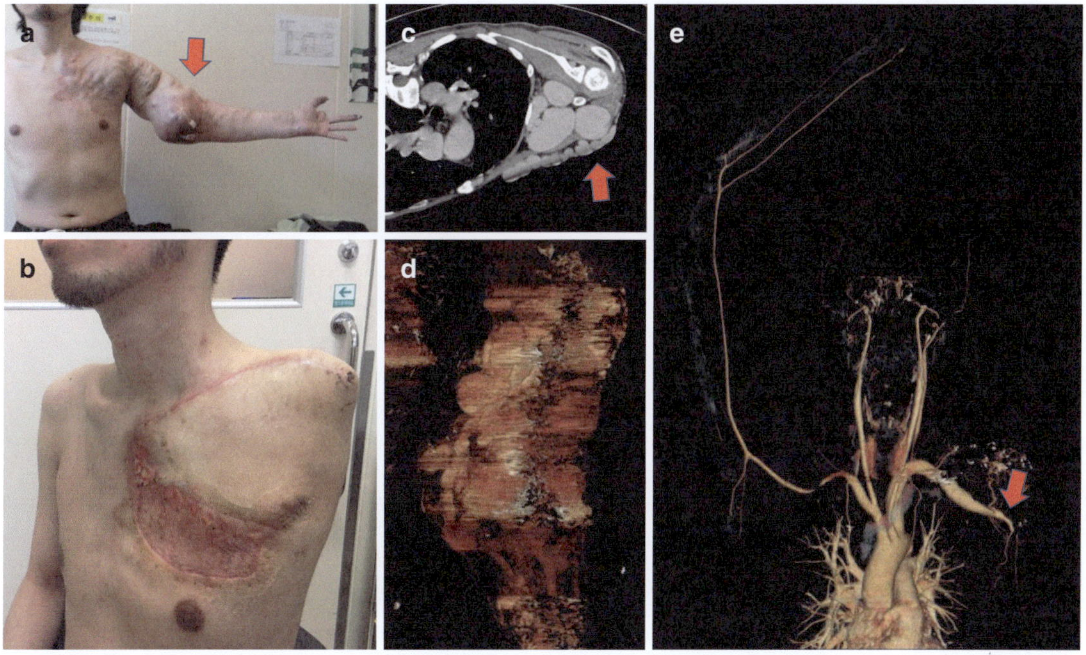

Fig. 13.6 CC: pulsating mass on left forearm and chest wall. Dx: Arteriovenous malformation. (**a**) preop picture. (**b**) post op picture: left arm disarticulation. (**c** and **d**) preop CTA. (**e**) postop CAT

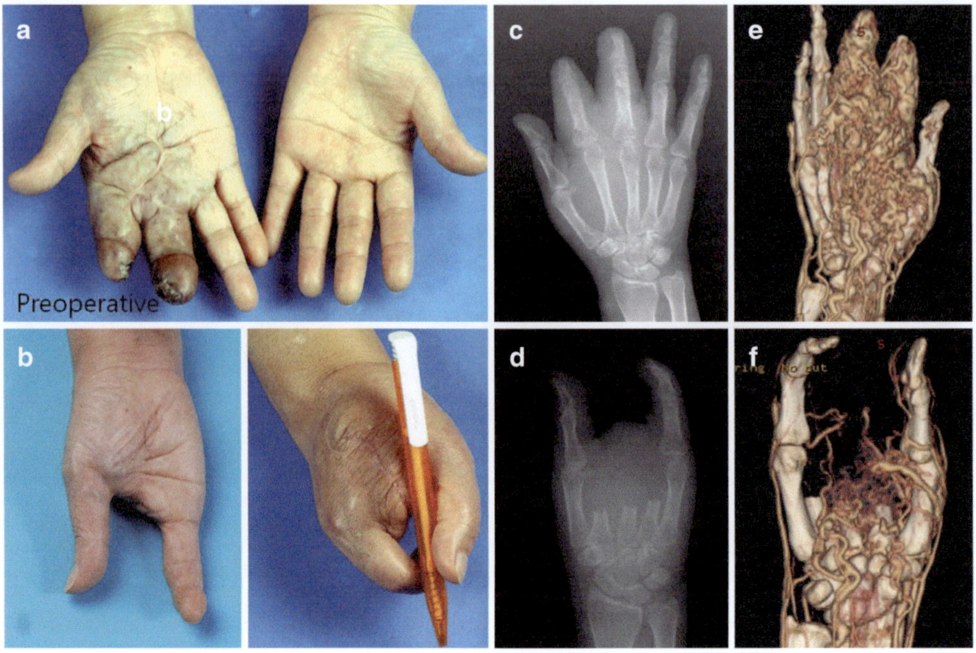

Fig. 13.7 CC: finger necrosis . Dx: Arteriovenous malformation. (**a**) preop picture. (**b**) postop picture: she can hold materials. (**c**) preop bone X-ray. (**d**) post-bone X-ray. (**e**) preop CTA. (**f**) postop CTA

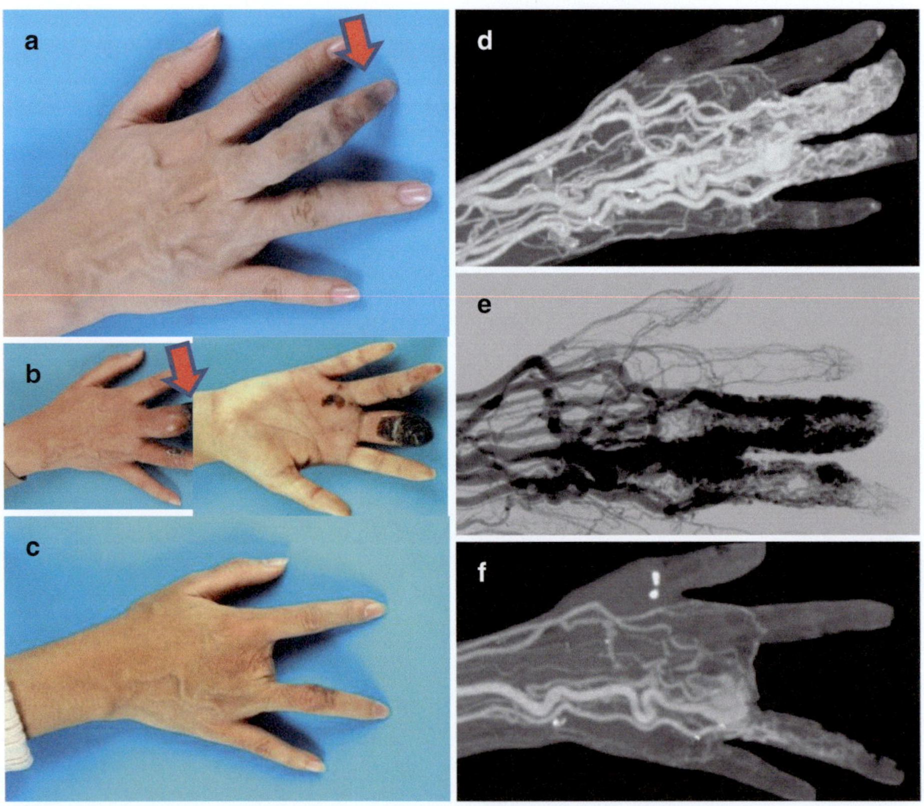

Fig. 13.8 CC: finger necrosis after alcohol injected sclerotherapy. Dx: Arteriovenous malformation. (**a**) pre-sclero picture. (**b**) third finger necrosis after sclerotherapy. (**c**) postop picture: third finger amputation. (**d**) pre-sclero CTA. (**e**) angiogram during alcohol injected sclerotherapy. (**f**) postop CTA

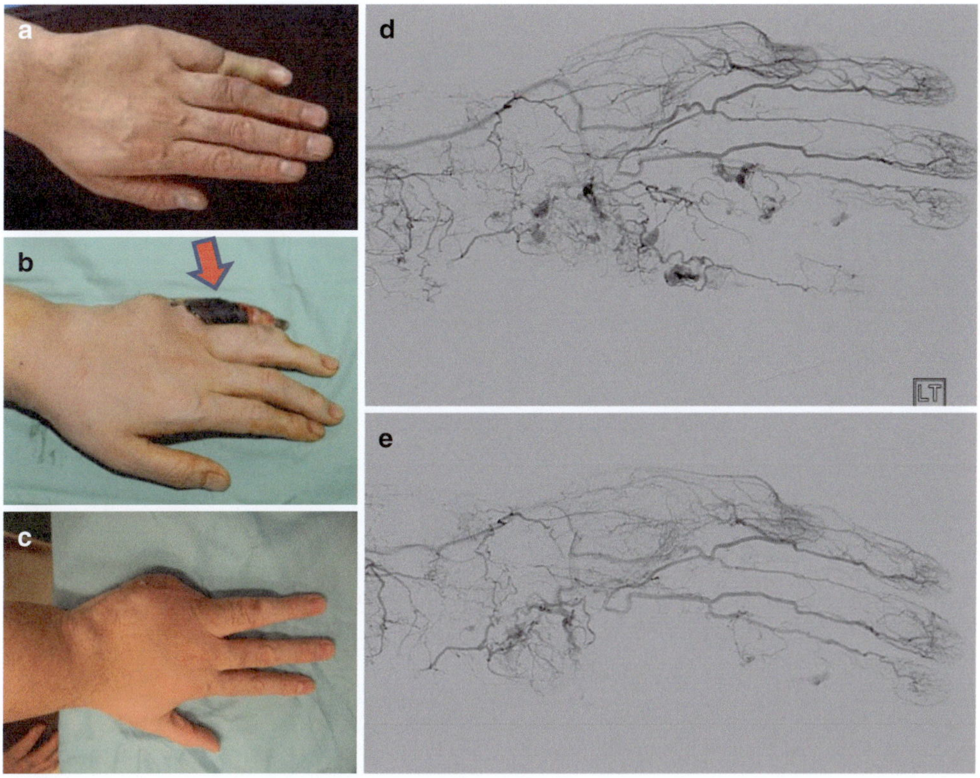

Fig. 13.9 CC: finger necrosis after alcohol injected sclerotherapy. Dx: Arteriovenous malformation. (**a**) pre-sclero picture. (**b**) fifth finger necrosis after sclerotherapy. (**c**) postop picture: fifth finger amputation. (**d**) pre-sclero angiogram. (**e**) alcohol injected sclerotherapy

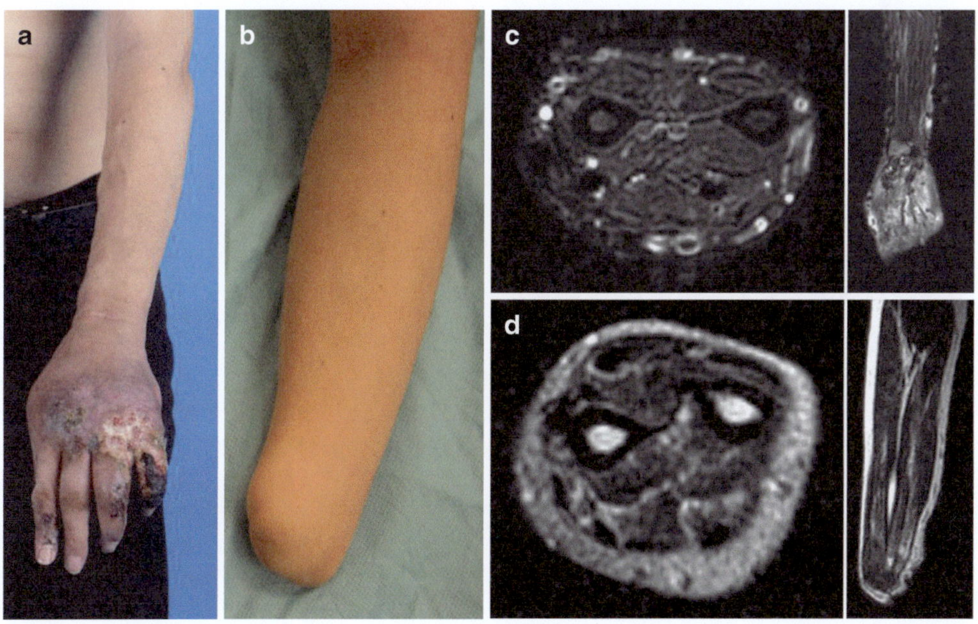

Fig. 13.10 CC: hand necrosis. Dx: Arteriovenous malformation. (**a**) preop picture. (**b**) postop picture: hand amputation. (**c**) preop MRI. (**d**) postop MRI

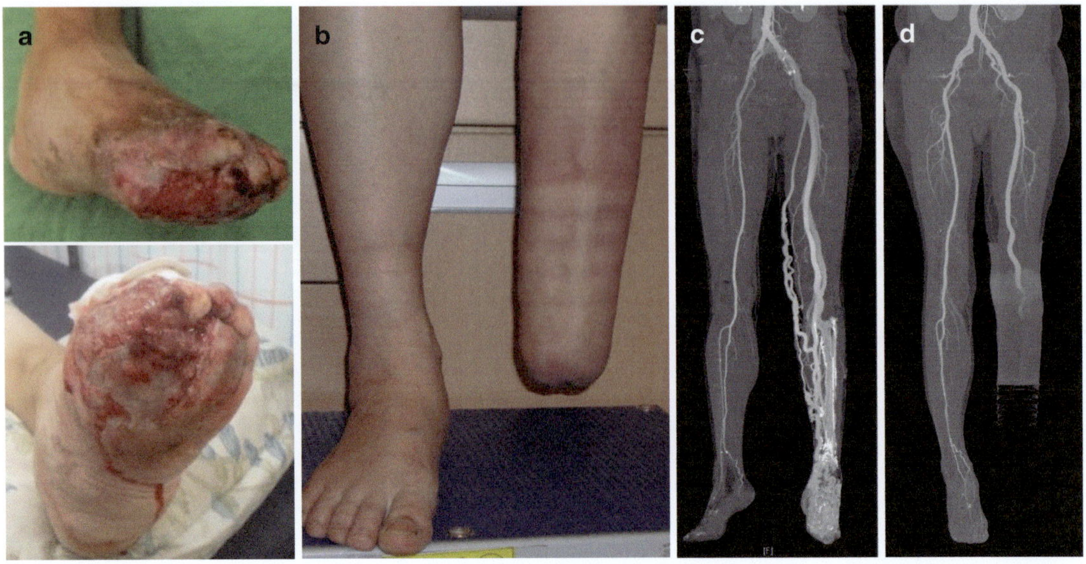

Fig. 13.11 CC: left foot necrosis. Dx: Arteriovenous malformation. (**a**) preop picture. (**b**) postop picture: left leg amputation. (**c**) preop CTA. (**d**) postop CTA

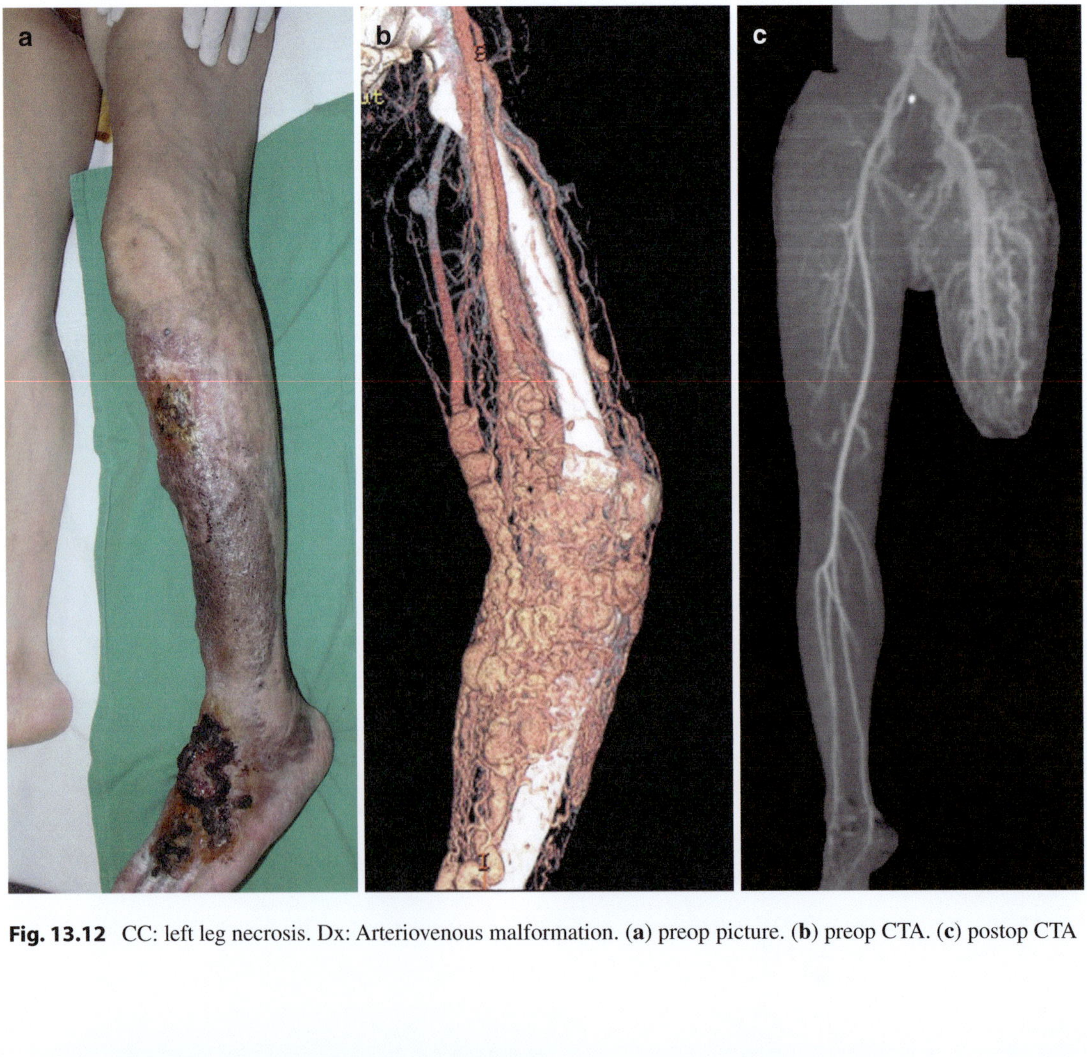

Fig. 13.12 CC: left leg necrosis. Dx: Arteriovenous malformation. (**a**) preop picture. (**b**) preop CTA. (**c**) postop CTA

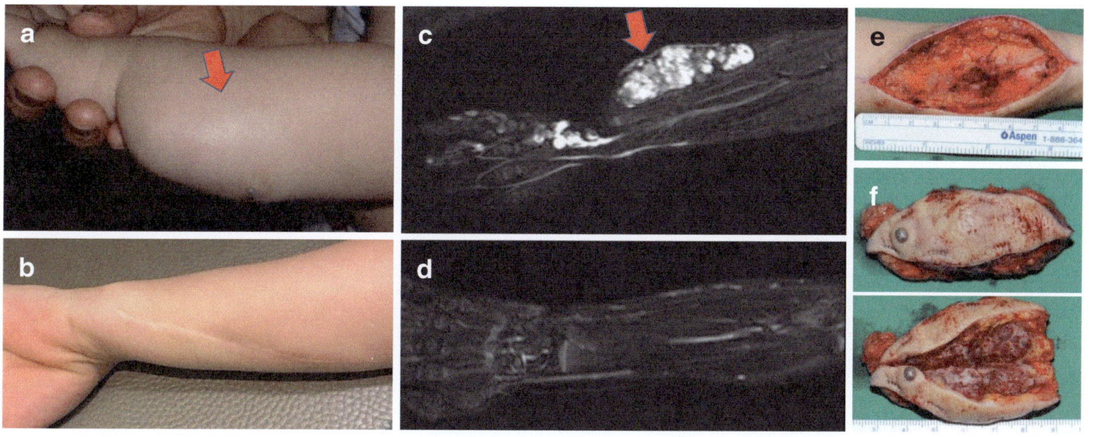

Fig. 13.13 CC: mass on forearm. Dx: Venous malformation. (**a**) preop picture. (**b**) postop picture. (**c**) preop MRI. (**d**) postop MRI. (**e**) op finding. (**f**) op specimen: excision of VM mass

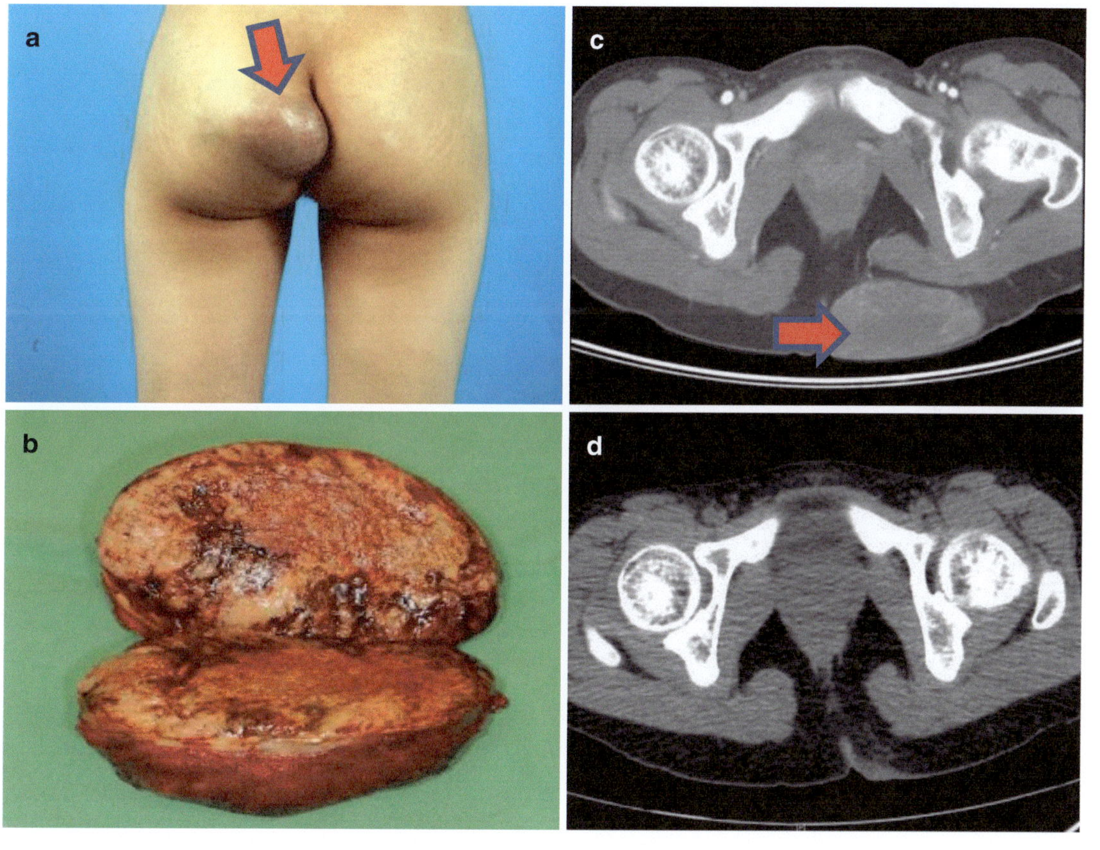

Fig. 13.14 CC: mass on buttock. Dx: Venous malformation. (**a**) preop picture. (**b**) op specimen: excision of VM mass. (**c**) preop MRI. (**d**) postop MRI

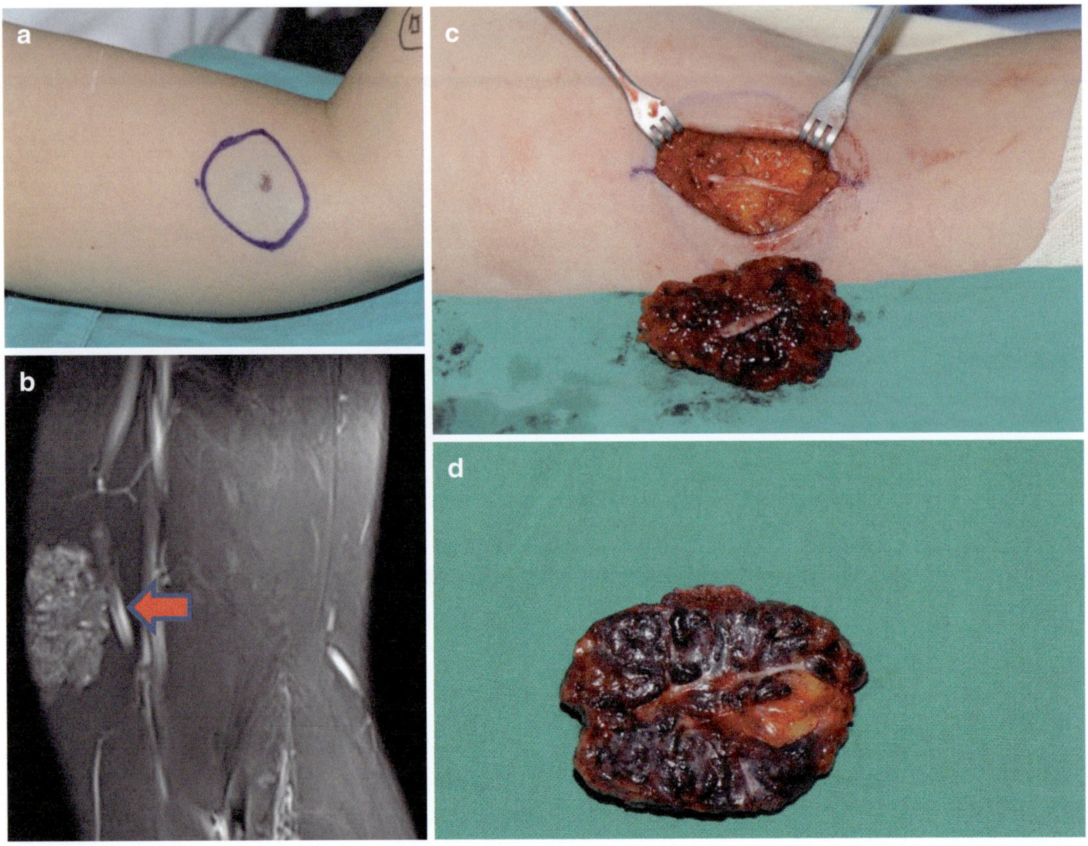

Fig. 13.15 CC: mass on upper arm. Dx: Venous malformation. (**a**) preop picture. (**b**) preop MRI. (**c**) op finding: excision of VM mass. (**d**) op specimen

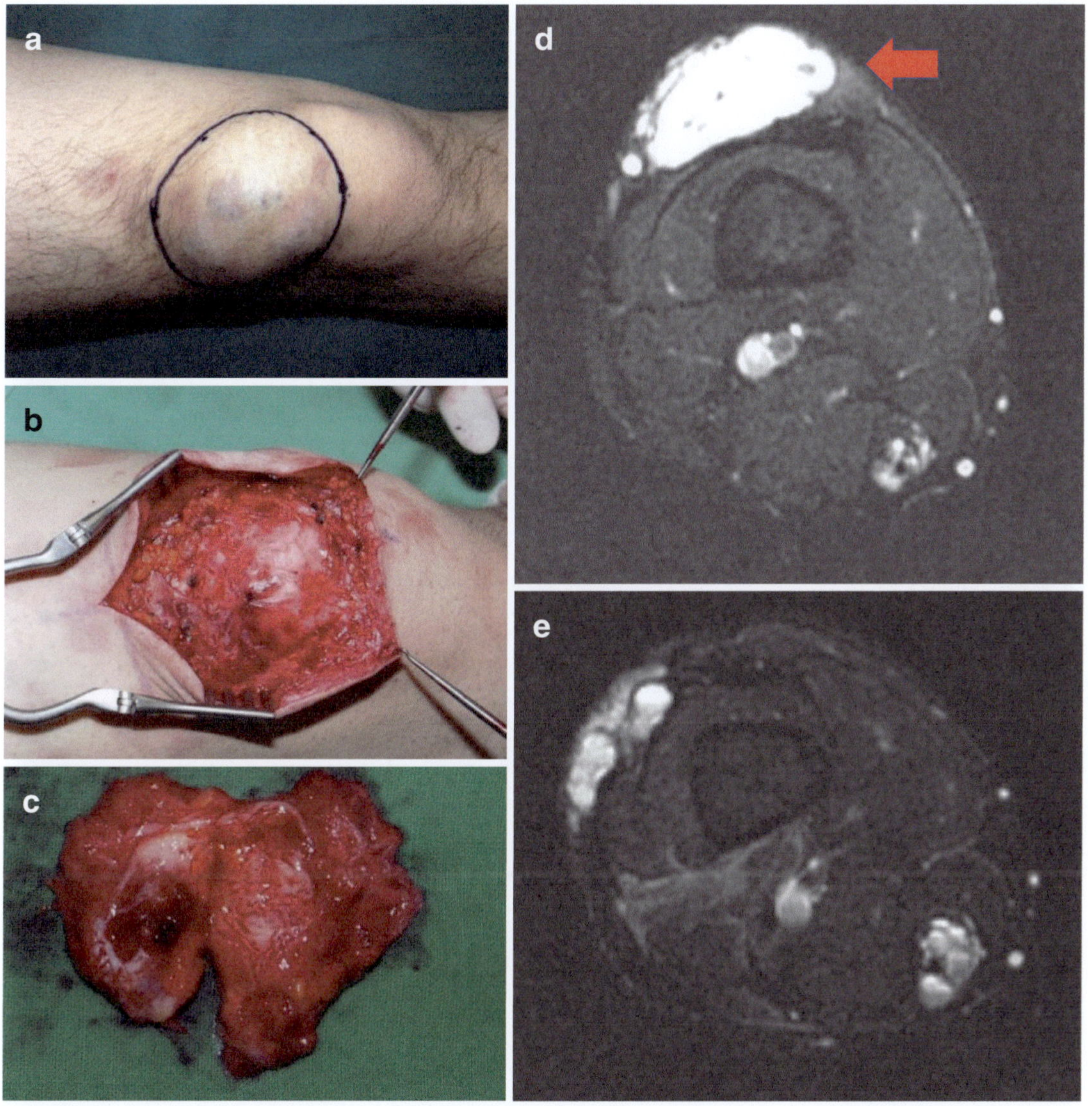

Fig. 13.16 CC: mass on knee. Dx: Venous malformation. (**a**) preop picture. (**b**) op finding: excision of VM mass. (**c**) op specimen. (**d**) preop MRI. (**e**) postop MRI

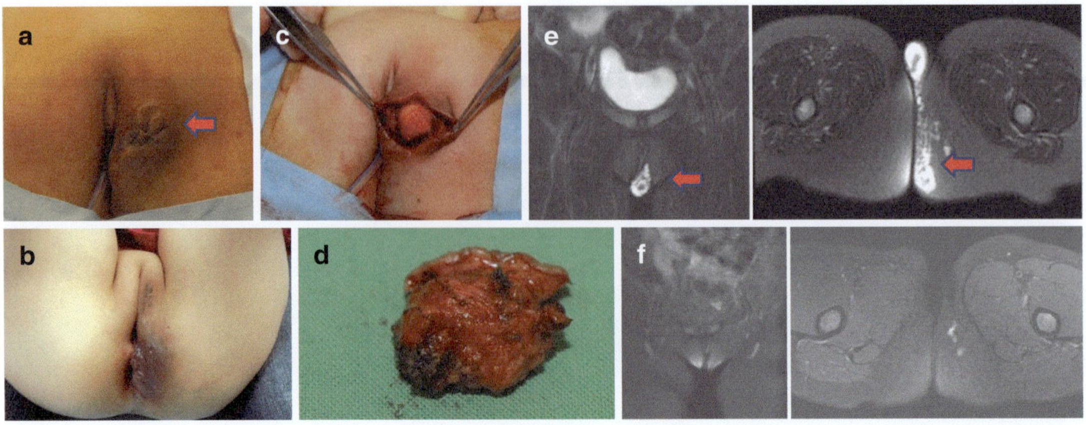

Fig. 13.17 CC: mass on vulva. Dx: Venous malformation. (**a**) preop picture. (**b**) postop picture. (**c**) op finding: excision of VM mass. (**d**) op specimen. (**e**) preop MRI. (**f**) postop MRI

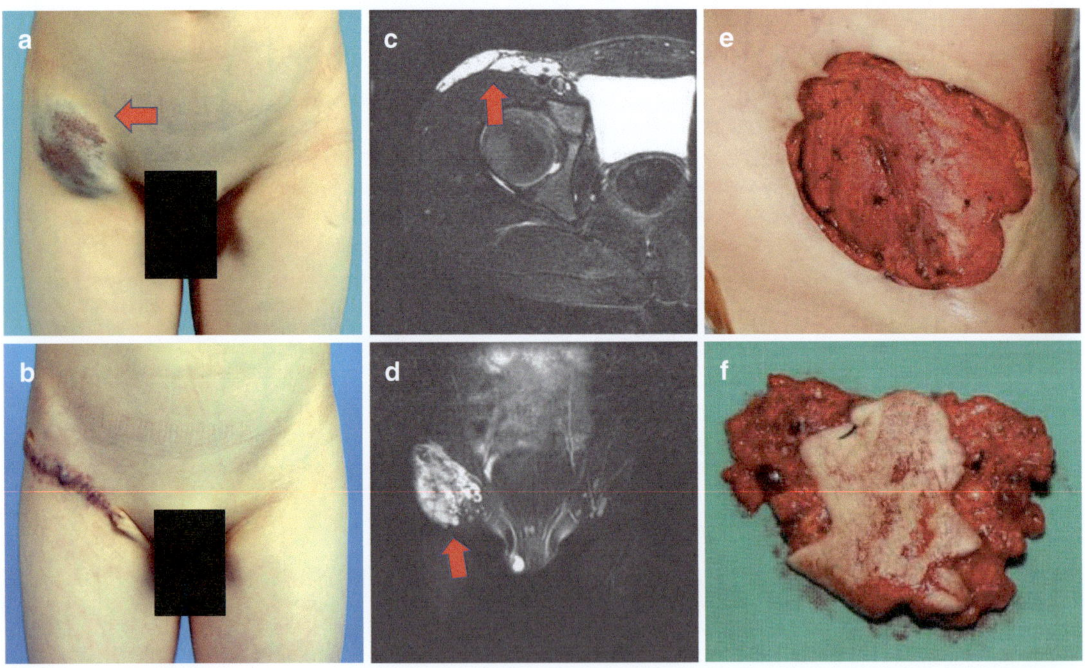

Fig. 13.18 CC: mass on inguinal area. Dx: Venous malformation. (**a**) preop picture. (**b**) postop picture. (c and d) preop MRI. (**e**) op finding: excision of VM mass. (**f**) op specimen

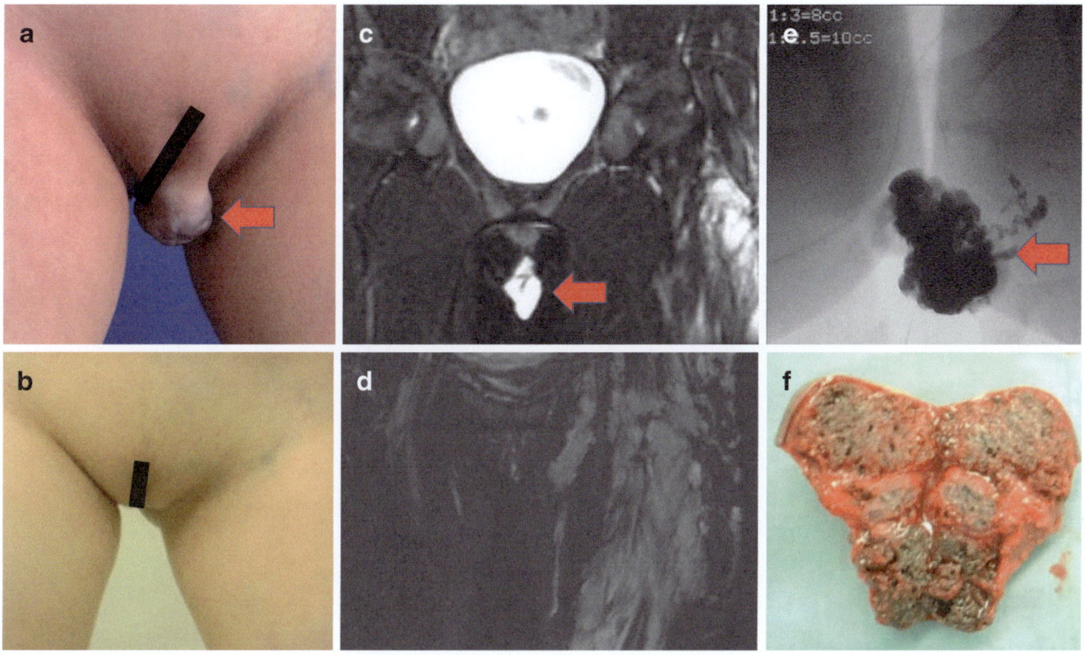

Fig. 13.19 CC: mass on vulva. Dx: Venous malformation. (**a**) preop picture. (**b**) postop picture. (**c**) preop MRI. (**d**) postop MRI. (**e**) preop glue embolization. (**f**) op specimen

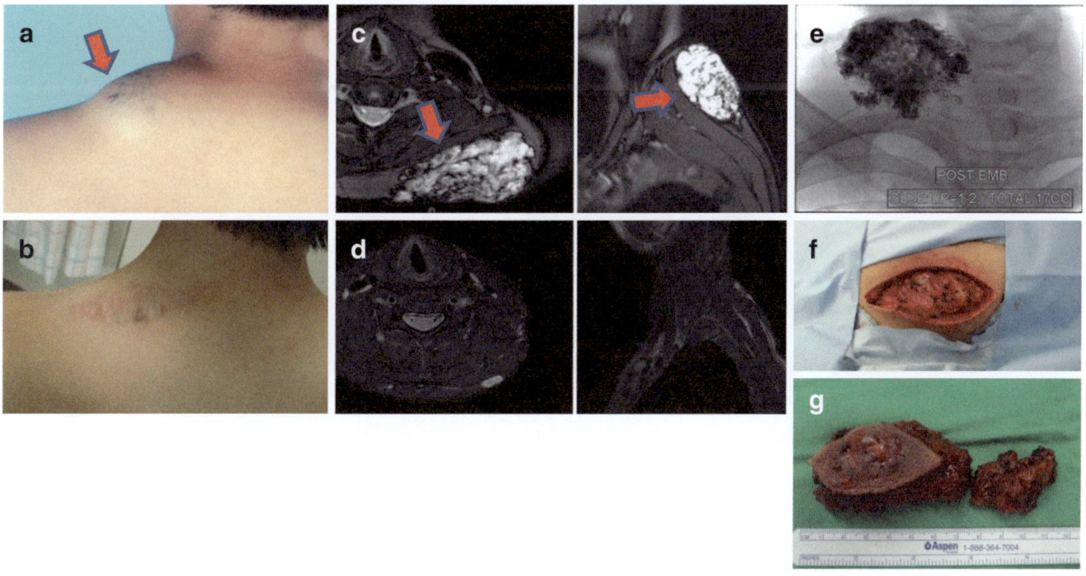

Fig. 13.20 CC: mass on left shoulder. Dx: Venous malformation. (**a**) preop picture. (**b**) postop picture. (**c**) preop MRI. (**d**) postop MRI. (**e**) preop sclerotherapy: glue embolization. (**f**) op finding: excision of VM mass. (**g**) op specimen

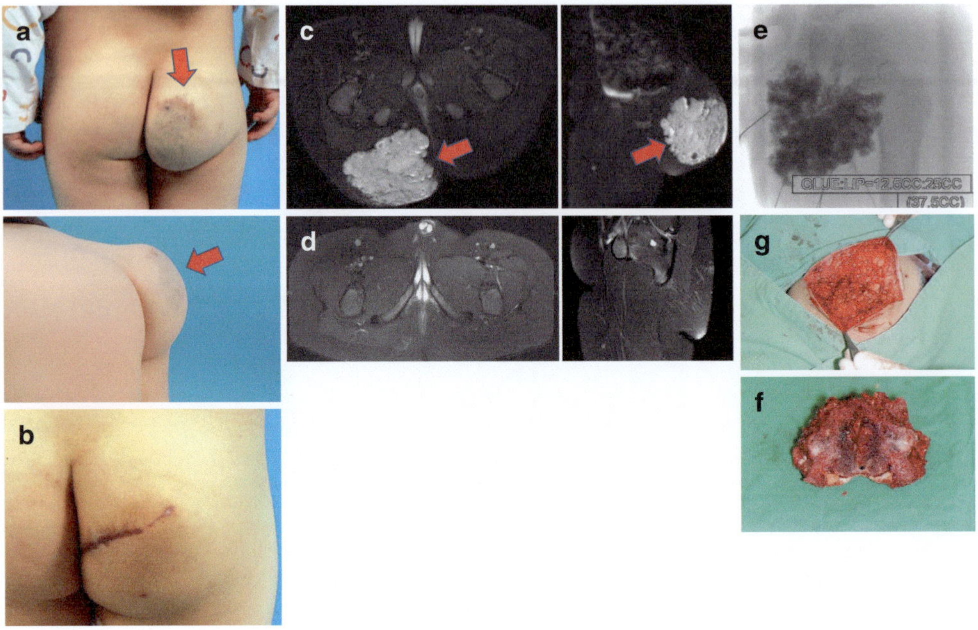

Fig. 13.21 CC: mass on right buttock. Dx: Venous malformation. (**a**) preop picture. (**b**) postop picture. (**c**) preop MRI. (**d**) postop MRI. (**e**) preop glue embolization. (**f**) op finding: excision of VM mass. (**g**) op specimen

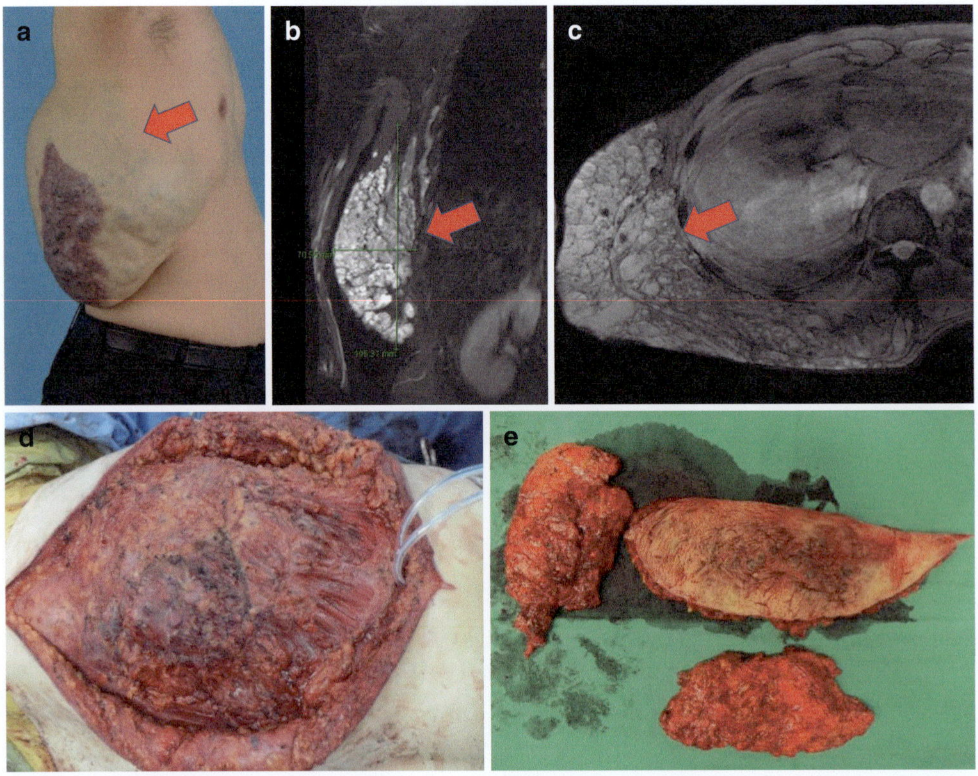

Fig. 13.22 CC: mass on chest. Dx: Venous malformation. (**a**) preop picture. (**b** and **c**) preop MRI. (**d**) op finding: excision of VM mass. (**e**) op specimen

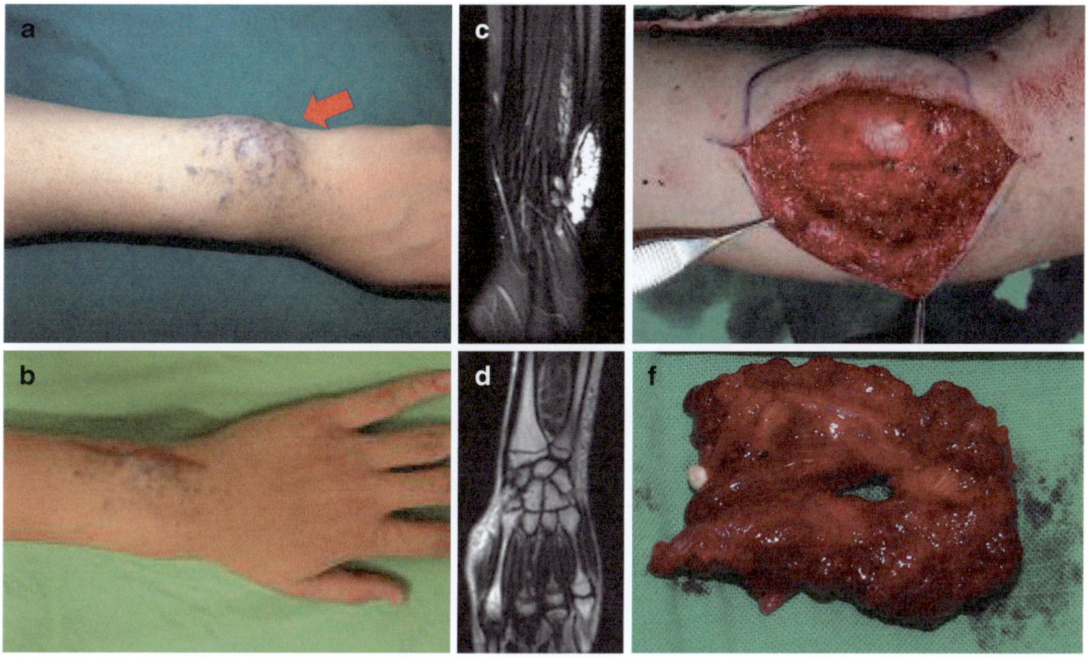

Fig. 13.23 CC: mass on wrist. Dx: Venous malformation. (**a**) preop picture. (**b**) postop picture. (**c**) preop MRI. (**d**) postop MRI. (**e**) op finding: excision of VM mass. (**f**) op specimen

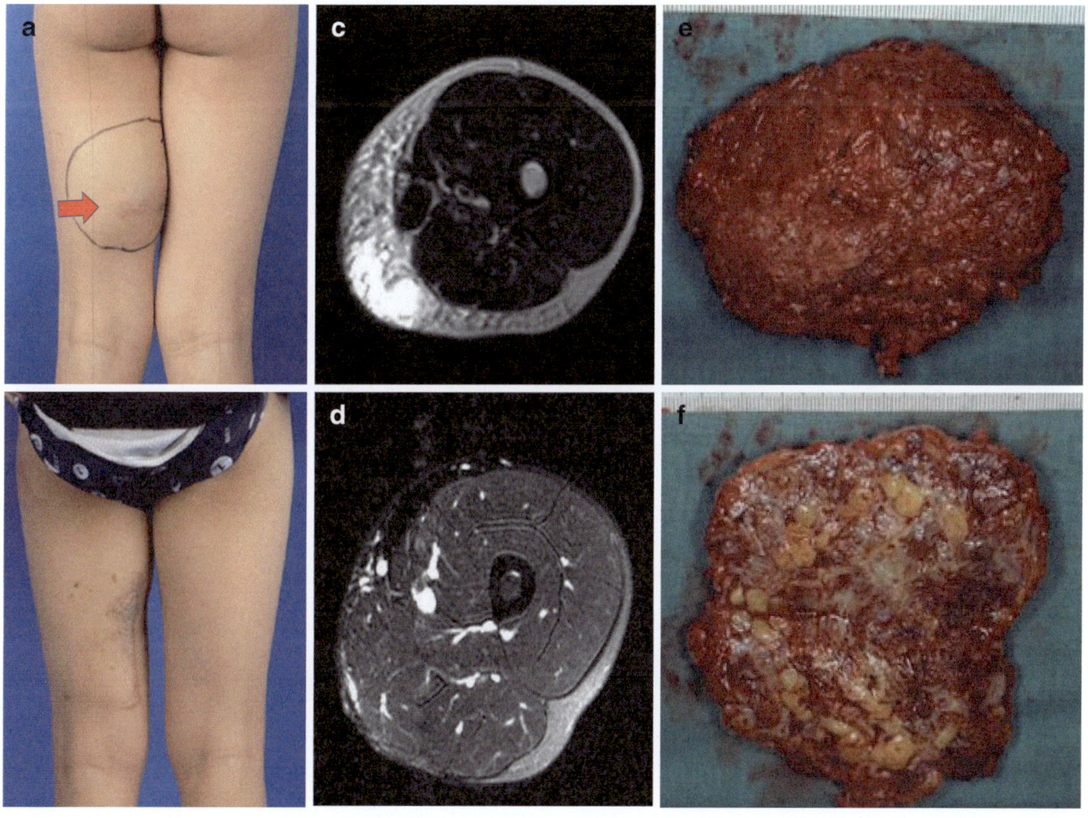

Fig. 13.24 CC: mass on left thigh. Dx: Venous malformation. (**a**) preop picture. (**b**) postop picture. (**c**) preop MRI. (**d**) postop MRI. (**e** and **f**) op specimen

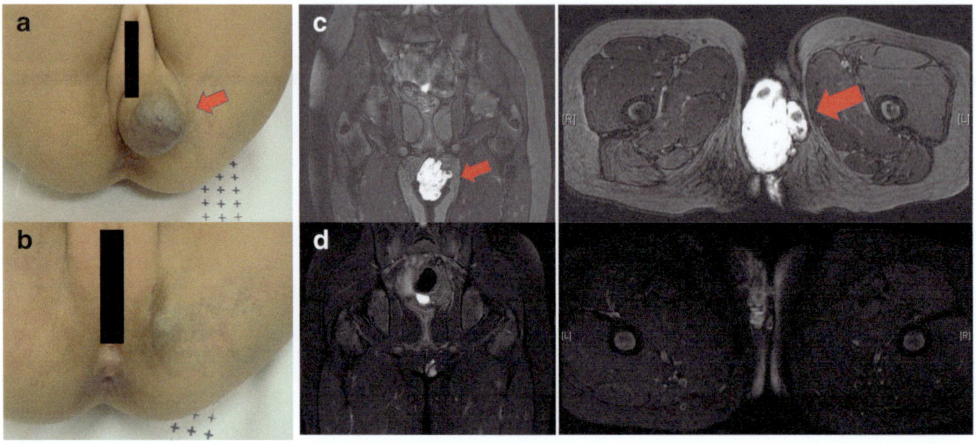

Fig. 13.25 CC: mass on vulva. Dx: Venous malformation. (**a**) preop picture. (**b**) postop picture. (**c**) preop MRI. (**d**) postop MRI

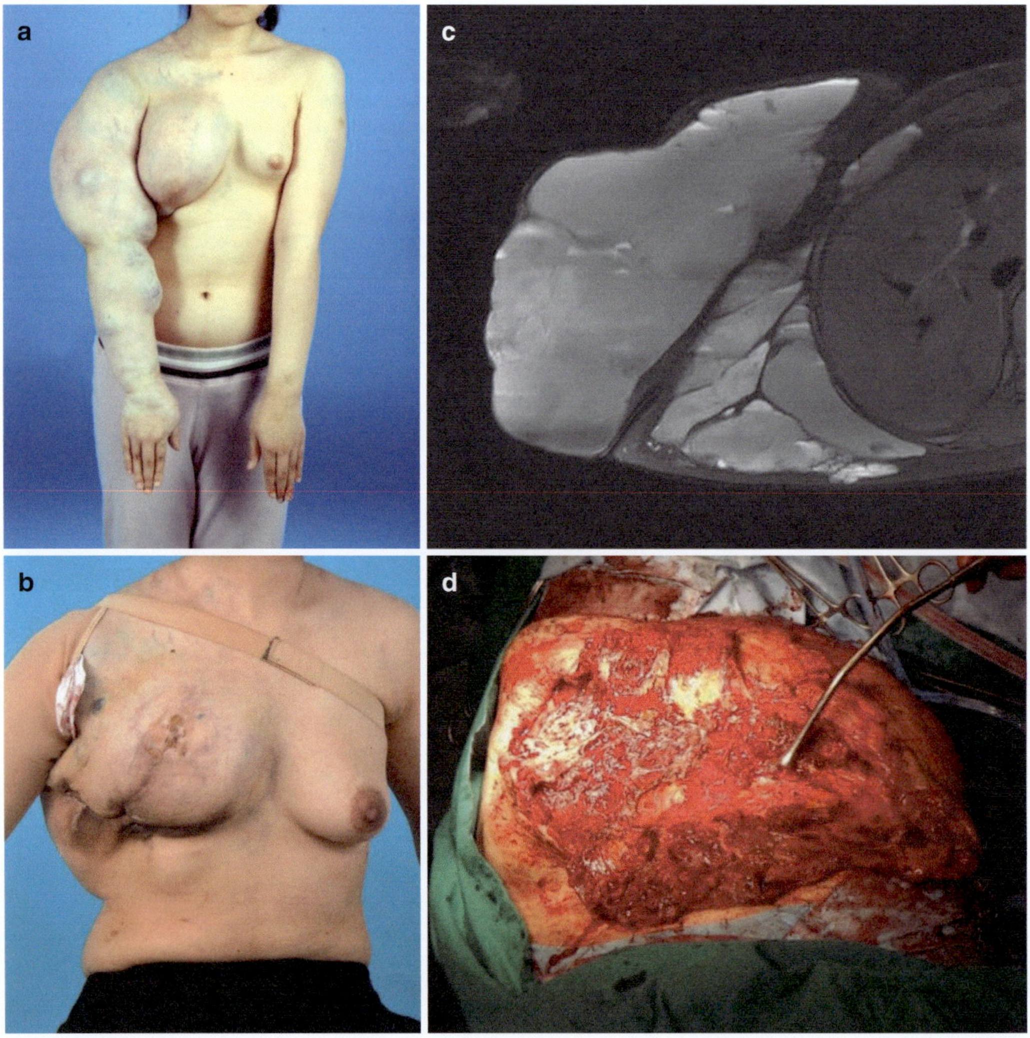

Fig. 13.26 CC: mass on right chest and arm. Dx: Venous malformation. (**a**) preop picture. (**b**) postop picture. (**c**) preop MRI. (**d**) op finding

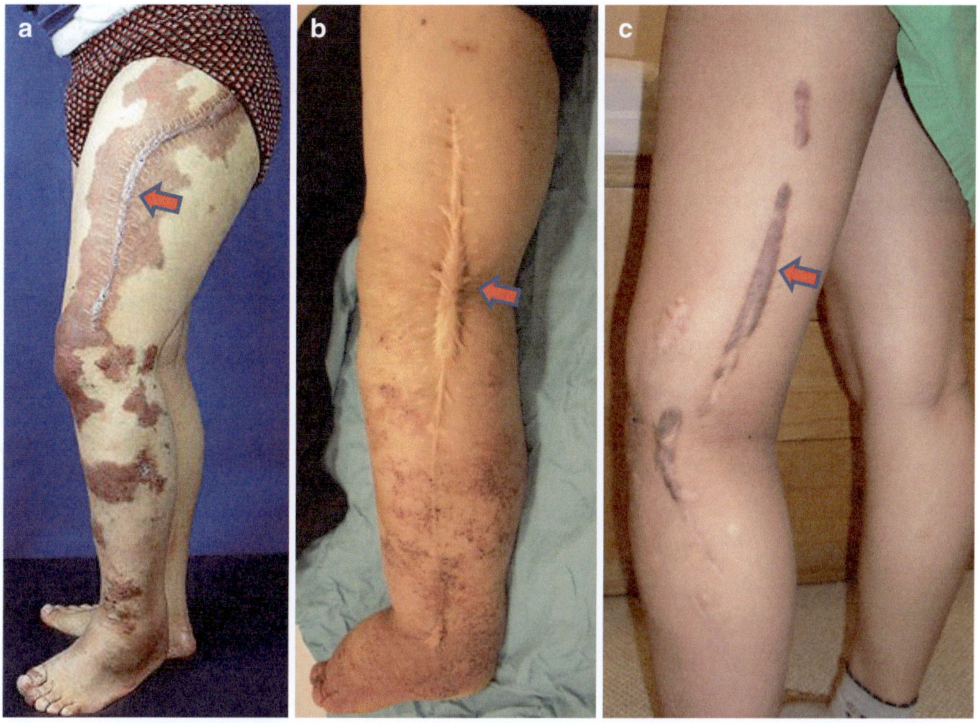

Fig. 13.27 Dx: Klippel–Trenaunay syndrome. (**a**, **b**, **c**) hypertropic scar over marginal vein resection

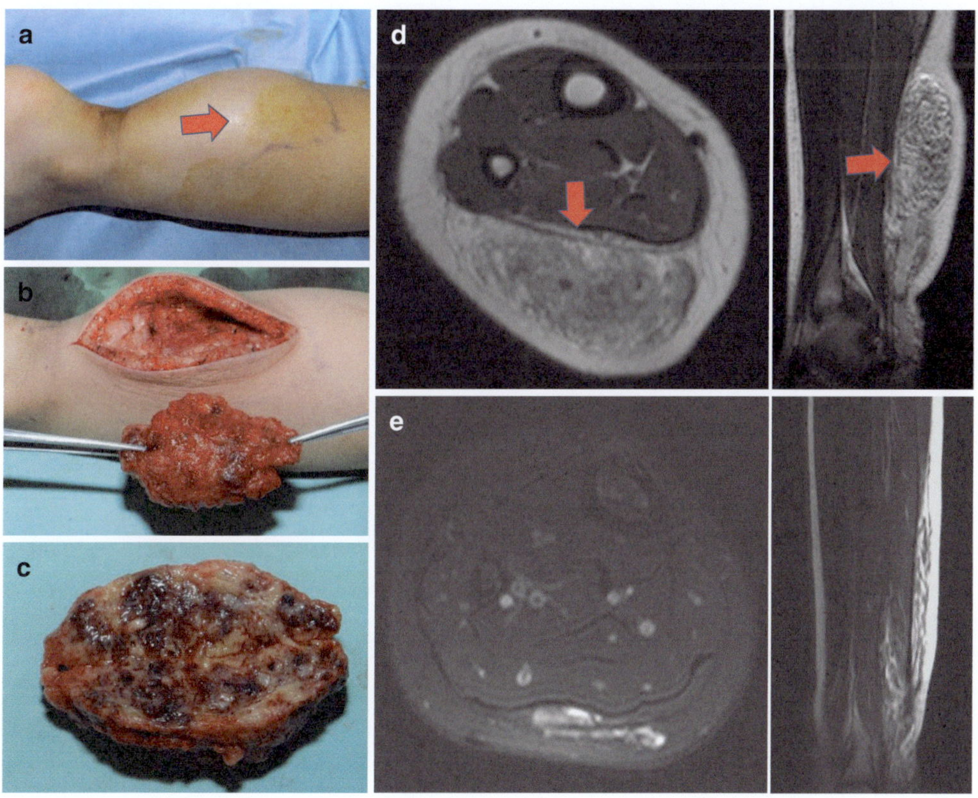

Fig. 13.28 CC: mass on calf. Dx: Venous malformation. (**a**) preop picture. (**b**) op finding: excision of VM mass. (**c**) op specimen. (**d**) preop MRI. (**e**) postop MRI

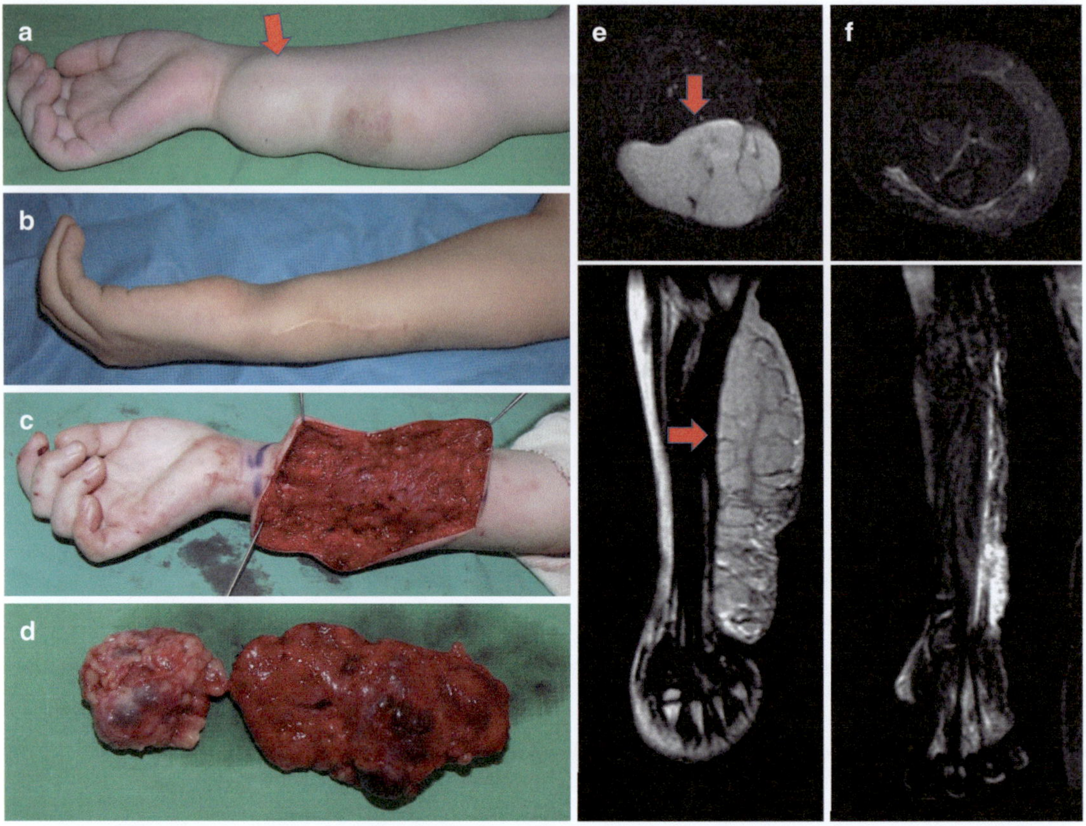

Fig. 13.29 CC: mass on forearm. Dx: Venous malformation. (**a**) preop picture. (**b**) postop picture. (**c**) op finding: excision of VM mass. (**d**) op specimen. (**e**) preop MRI. (**f**) postop MRI

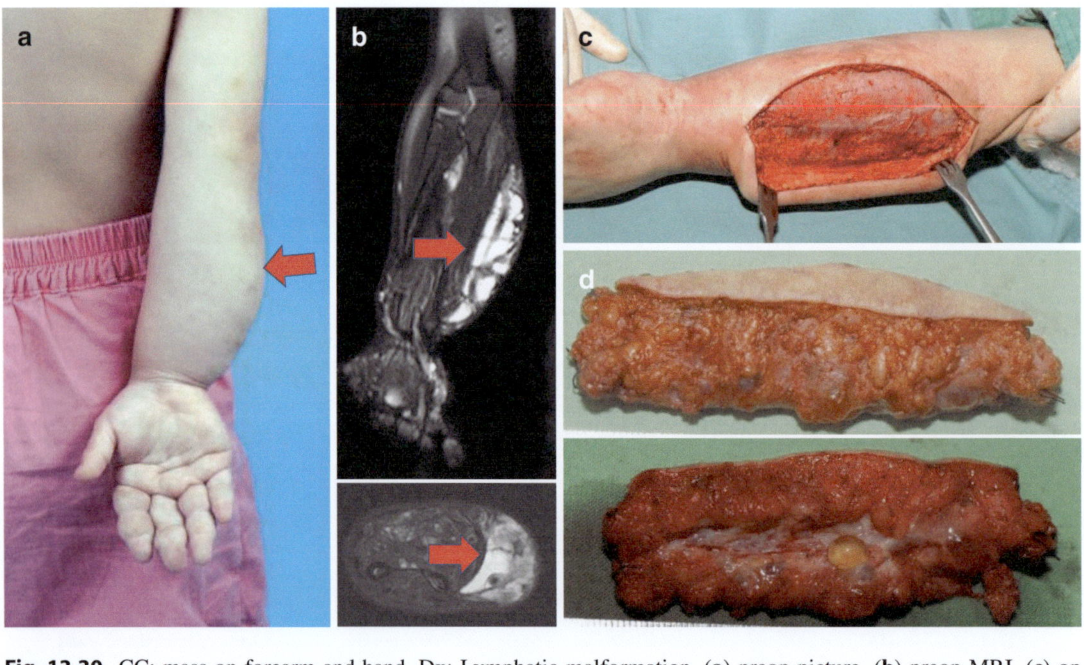

Fig. 13.30 CC: mass on forearm and hand. Dx: Lymphatic malformation. (**a**) preop picture. (**b**) preop MRI. (**c**) op finding: excision of VM mass. (**d**) op specimen

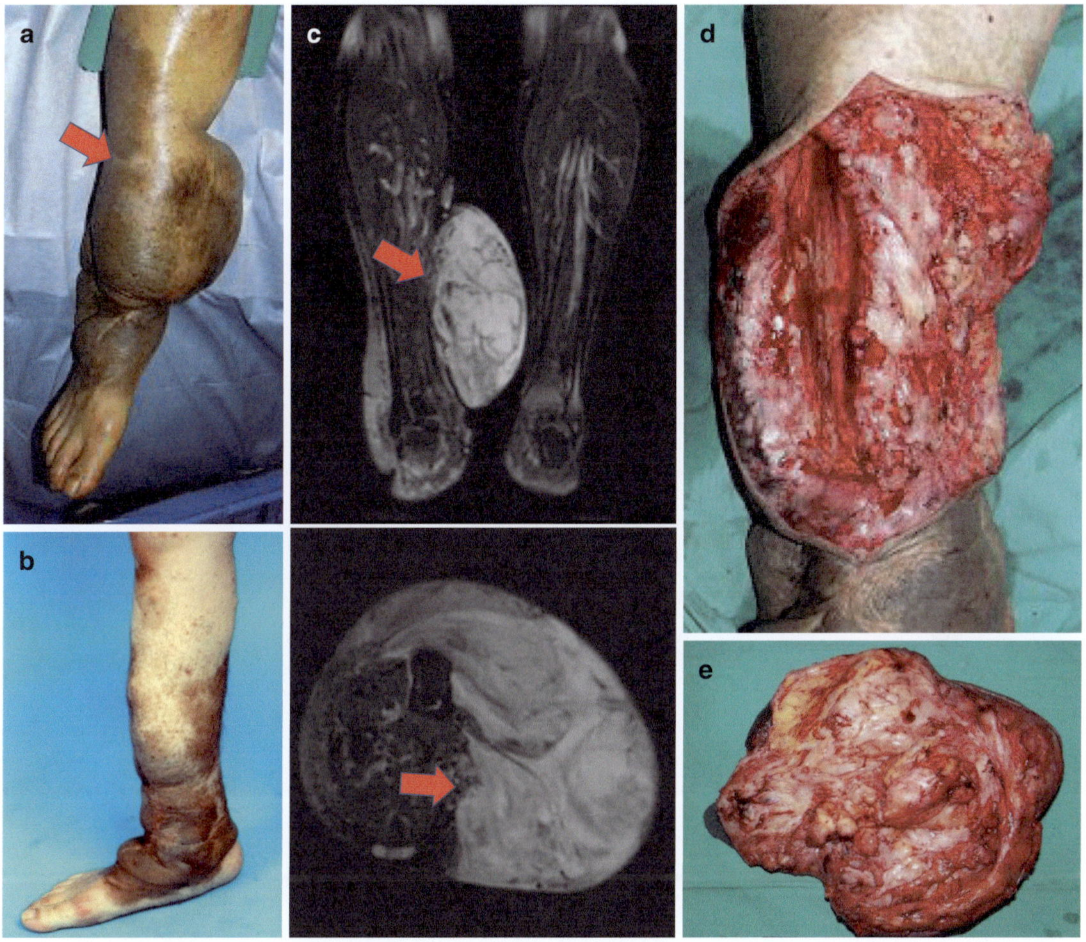

Fig. 13.31 CC: mass on calf. Dx: mixed type of lymphatic malformation and venous malformation. (**a**) preop picture. (**b**) postop picture. (**c**) preop MRI. (**d**) op finding: excision of VM mass. (**e**) op specimen

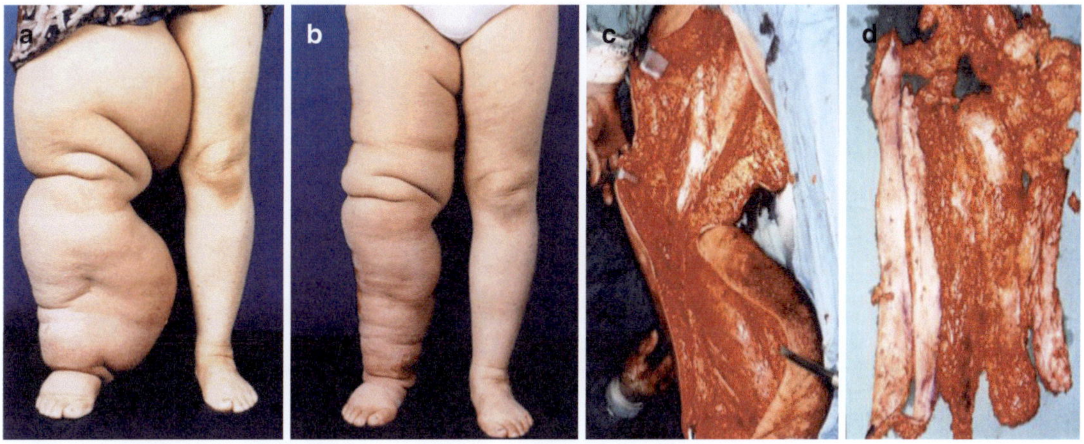

Fig. 13.32 Surgery for lymphedema. (**a**) preop picture. (**b**) postop picture. (**c**) op finding: excision of subcutaneous tissue and superficial fascia. (**d**) op specimen

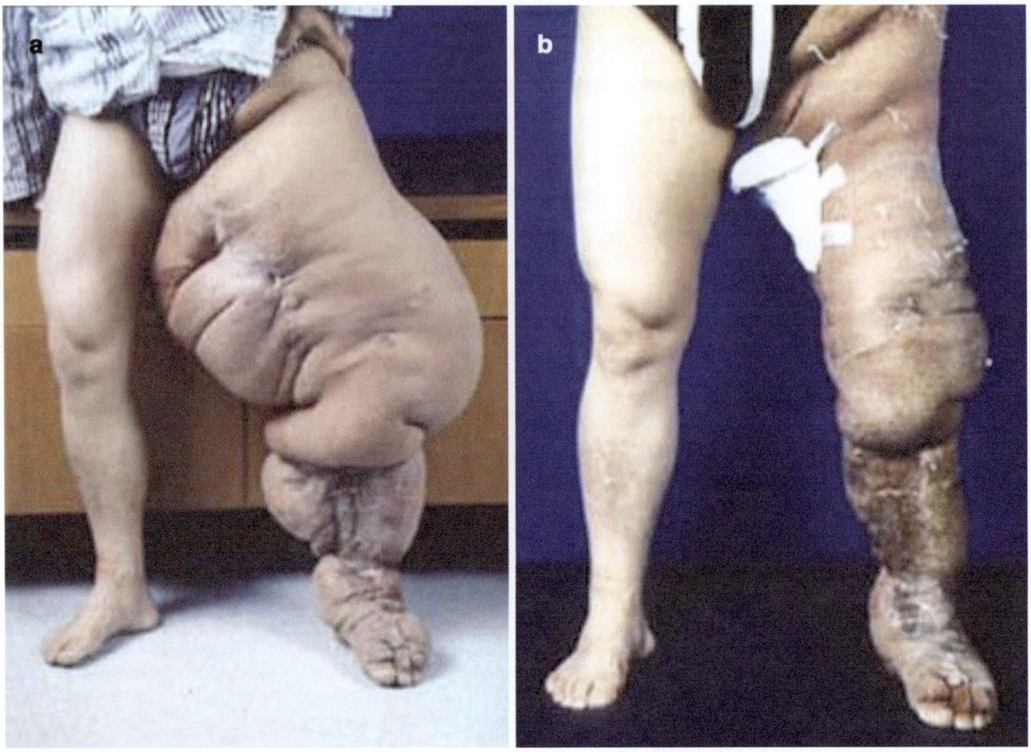

Fig. 13.33 Surgery for lymphedema: Excision of subcutaneous tissue and superficial fascia. (**a**) preop picture. (**b**) postop picture

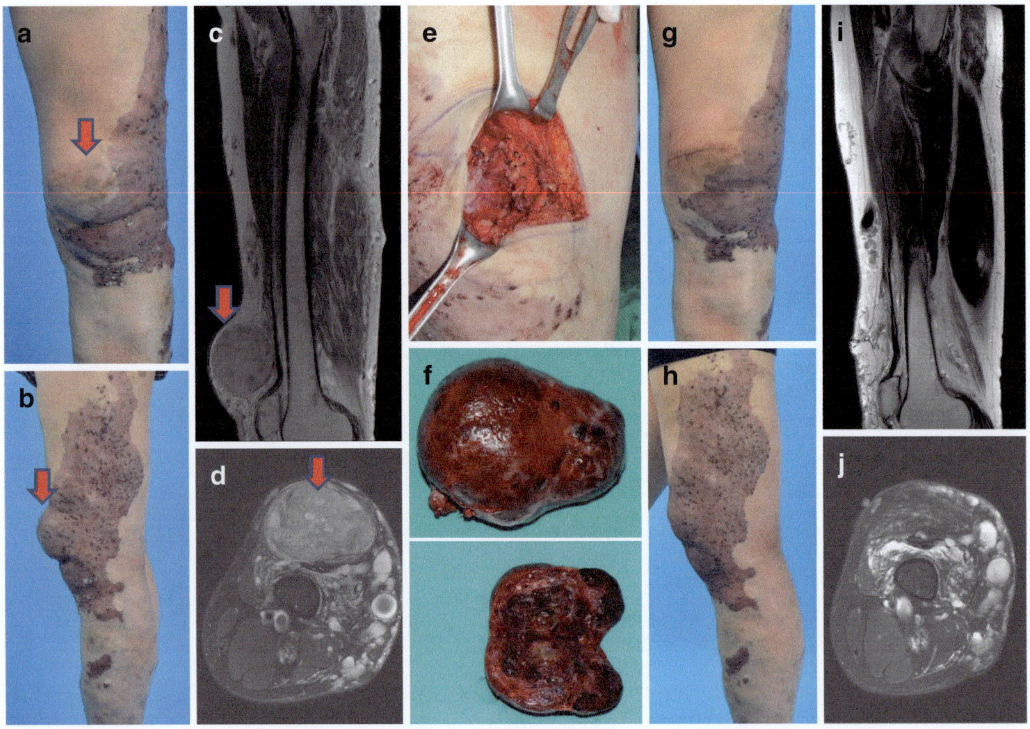

Fig. 13.34 CC: mass on suprapatellar area. Dx: Klippel– Trenaunay syndrome. (**a** and **b**) preop picture. (**c** and **d**) preop MRI. e) op finding: excision of VM mass. (**f**) op specimen. (**g** and **h**) postop picture. (**i** and **j**) postop MRI

References

1. Legiehn GM, Heran MK. Venous malformations: classification, development, diagnosis, and interventional radiologic management. Radiol Clin N Am. 2008;46(3):545–97. vi
2. Yun WS, Kim DI, Rho YN, Do YS, Park KB, Kim KH, et al. Natural course of venous malformation after conservative treatment. Surg Today. 2012;42:950–5.
3. Kim DI, Huh S, Hwang JH, Kim YI, Lee BB. Venous dynamics in leg lymphedema. Lymphology. 1999;32:11–4.
4. Arneja JS, Gosain AK. Vascular malformations. Plast Reconstr Surg. 2008;121(4):195e–206e.
5. Park UJ, Do YS, Park KB, Park HS, Lee BB, Kim DI. Treatment of arteriovenous malformations involving the hand. Ann Vasc Surg. 2012;26(5):643–8.
6. Lee BB, Do YS, Yakes W, Kim DI, Mattassi R, Hyon WS. Management of arteriovenous malformations: a multidisciplinary approach. J Vasc Surg. 2004;39(3):590–600.
7. Visser A, FitzJohn T, Tan ST. Surgical management of arteriovenous malformation. J Plast Reconstr Aesthet Surg. 2011;64(3):283–91.
8. Mattassi, R., 36 surgical treatment of low-flow CVM, in congenital vascular malformations, Y.-W. Kim, et al., Editors. 2017, Springer. p. 269–274.
9. Cox JA, Bartlett E, Lee EI. Vascular malformations: a review. Semin Plast Surg. 2014;28(2):58–63.
10. Roh YN, Do YS, Park KB, Park HS, Lee BB, Kim DI, et al. The results of surgical treatment for patients with venous malformations. Ann Vasc Surg. 2012;26(5):665–73.
11. Kang GB, et al. The usefulness of surgical treatment in slow-flow vascular malformation patients. Arch Plast Surg. 2017;44(4):301–7.
12. Manning SC, Perkins J. Lymphatic malformations. Curr Opin Otolaryngol Head Neck Surg. 2013;21(6):571–5.
13. Parsi K. 34 Management of lymphatic malformations. In: Kim Y-W, et al., editors. Management of congenital vascular malformation: Overview: Springer; 2017. p. 241–56.
14. Zhou Q, et al. Treatment guidelines of lymphatic malformations of the head and neck. Oral Oncol. 2011;47(12):1105–9.
15. Raveh E, et al. Prognostic factors in the treatment of lymphatic malformations. Arch Otolaryngol Head Neck Surg. 1997;123(10):1061–5.
16. Balakrishnan K, et al. Primary surgery vs primary sclerotherapy for head and neck lymphatic malformations. JAMA Otolaryngol Head Neck Surg. 2014;140(1):41–5.
17. Loose DA. Congential vascular malformations. In: Dieter RS, R.A.D. Jr., and R.A.D, editors. Venous and lymphatic diseases: McGraw-Hill; 2011. p. 481–94.
18. Kohout MP, et al. Arteriovenous malformations of the head and neck: natural history and management. Plast Reconstr Surg. 1998;102(3):643–54.
19. Rialon KL, Fishman SJ. 172 Congenital vascular malformations: surgical Management. In: Sidawy AN, Perler BA, editors. Rutherford's vascular surgery and endovascular therapy: Elsevier; 2019. p. 225–1258.
20. Kim JY, Kim DI, Do YS, Lee BB, Kim YW, Shin SW, et al. Surgical treatment for congenital arteriovenous malformation: 10 years' experience. Eur J Vasc Endovasc Surg. 2006;32(1):101–6.
21. Ozcan AV, et al. Surgical treatment for a complex congenital arteriovenous malformation of the lower limb. Tex Heart Inst J. 2013;40(5):612–4.
22. Kapadia SR, Thakore VM, Patel HM. Vascular malformations: an update on classification, clinical features, and management principles. Indian J Vasc Endovasc Surg. 2017;4(4):152–62.
23. Lee BB, Bergan JJ. Advanced management of congenital vascular malformations: a multidisciplinary approach. Cardiovasc Surg. 2002;10(6):523–33.
24. Loose, D.A., 37 Surgical treatment for high-flow CVM, in Congenital vascular malformations, Y.-W. Kim, et al., Editors. 2017, Springer. p. 275–282.
25. Perkins JA, et al. Lymphatic malformations: review of current treatment. Otolaryngol Head Neck Surg. 2010;142(6):795–803, 803 e1.
26. Maftei N, et al. The surgical management of 73 vascular malformations and preoperative predictive factors of major haemorrhage–a single Centre experience. Eur J Vasc Endovasc Surg. 2009;38(4):488–97.
27. Heit JJ, et al. Guidelines and parameters: percutaneous sclerotherapy for the treatment of head and neck venous and lymphatic malformations. J Neurointerv Surg. 2017;9(6):611–7.
28. Loose DA. Surgical management of venous malformations. Phlebology. 2007;22(6):276–82.
29. de Serres LM, Sie KC, Richardson MA. Lymphatic malformations of the head and neck. A proposal for staging. Arch Otolaryngol Head Neck Surg. 1995;121(5):577–82.
30. Hamoir M, et al. Lymphatic malformations of the head and neck: a retrospective review and a support for staging. Head Neck. 2001;23(4):326–37.
31. Ha J, Yu YC, Lannigan F. A review of the management of lymphangiomas. Curr Pediatr Rev. 2014;10(3):238–48.
32. Emery PJ, Bailey CM, Evans JN. Cystic hygroma of the head and neck. A review of 37 cases. J Laryngol Otol. 1984;98(6):613–9.
33. Hancock BJ, et al. Complications of lymphangiomas in children. J Pediatr Surg. 1992;27(2):220–4. discussion 224-6
34. Schneider LF, et al. Surgical management of a dermal lymphatic malformation of the lower extremity. Can J Plast Surg. 2008;16(4):236–8.
35. Mulliken JB, Fishman SJ, Burrows PE. Vascular anomalies. Curr Probl Surg. 2000;37(8):517–84.
36. Peachey RD, Lim CC, Whimster IW. Lymphangioma of skin. A review of 65 cases. Br J Dermatol. 1970;83(5):519–27.
37. Flanagan BP, Helwig EB. Cutaneous lymphangioma. Arch Dermatol. 1977;113(1):24–30.
38. Bauer BS, Kernahan DA, Hugo NE. Lymphangioma circumscriptum--a clinicopathological review. Ann Plast Surg. 1981;7(4):318–26.

14 Lasers in Vascular Anomalies

James D. Phillips and Gresham T. Richter

14.1 Basic Laser Concepts

Lasers, originally an acronym: Light Amplification by Stimulated Emission of Radiation, were developed in the latter half of the twentieth century. Lasers differ from other light sources in their increased *coherence* of the light. This term signifies that, as opposed to a light bulb which produces light energy over a wide range of wavelengths, laser light is composed of a narrow wavelength band. This is accomplished by applying energy (typically electrical input) to a particular population of atoms, the medium of the laser. A medium may be matter in any state such as a gas (e.g., carbon dioxide), a crystal (erbium, ytterbium, or neodymium), or a liquid (e.g., a dye solution). This medium then absorbs and emits photons in a predictable and characteristic manner due to the nature of the elements in the medium. The resulting light is concentrated within a mirrored chamber and then allowed to be released. This produces a narrow beam of light energy which can be used for either its illuminative or heat properties. Pioneers of this technology soon found useful applications within the field of medicine.

In the treatment of vascular anomalies, eradication of pathological tissue while sparing the normal tissue from injury is often difficult. This is due to the diffuse, infiltrative nature that is often characteristic of vascular anomalies; abnormal vessels may be microscopic and widely distributed amongst unaffected structures. Lasers have proved to be very useful in this regard as they may be calibrated to specifically target certain tissues for destruction while sparing the surrounding tissue. This is accomplished through the principle of selective photothermolysis [1]. Based on the wavelength of the laser beam, a target selectively absorbs a disproportionate amount of the laser energy and is thus heated and destroyed while surrounding tissue is relatively unaffected. The target is termed the chromophore and is characterized based on its pigment or color. When treating vascular anomalies, the chromophore is typically hemoglobin. As hemoglobin molecules heat, this leads to swelling and rupture of erythrocytes, leading to aggregation of the cellular debris, a reparative inflammatory response, and ultimately destruction of the endothelium of the vessel [2]. Hemoglobin exists in either oxygenated (red) or deoxygenated (blue/purple) states, and the appropriate laser wavelength for treatment must be selected accordingly based on the nature of the vessels requiring treatment.

J. D. Phillips
Otolaryngology Head and Neck Surgery, Vanderbilt University Medical Center, Nashville, USA
e-mail: james.d.phillips@vumc.org

G. T. Richter (✉)
Otolaryngology Head and Neck Surgery, University of Arkansas for the Medical Sciences, Little Rock, USA
e-mail: GTRichter@uams.edu

A. K. Khanna, S. K. Tiwary (eds.), *Vascular Malformations*,
https://doi.org/10.1007/978-981-15-9762-6_14

Another important consideration in laser selection is that the pulse duration corresponds to the diameter of the vessel being treated. Shorter pulse duration (less laser exposure) is adequate to treat small vessel lesions (< 100 micrometers in diameter). Medium vessel (100–400 micrometers) and large vessel (>400 micrometers) require a progressively longer pulse duration from the laser [3].

The argon laser, with wavelengths from 488–514 nm was one of the first to be applied to vascular and pigmented cutaneous lesions [4]. However, over time the argon laser was noted to have an unacceptably high rate of scarring as well as hyper/hypopigmentation, and so its usage in cutaneous vascular anomalies diminished. Similar issues were found with both copper and krypton lasers. Currently, the more commonly utilized lasers are the pulse dye laser (PDL), the alexandrite, the neodymium-doped yttrium aluminum garnet (Nd:YAG), and the carbon dioxide (CO2) lasers. The following sections will review the particulars of these devices and the clinical scenarios in which they are most useful.

14.2 Capillary Malformation (Port-Wine Stain)

Commonly known as a port-wine stain (PWS), a capillary malformation is a vascular birthmark composed of small, ectatic blood vessels that are near the skin surface. PWS presents as a flat, macular lesion which begins as a reddish color but darkens to more of a purple hue over time. It may be small or widely distributed over the skin's surface, and the majority of PWS have some involvement in the head and neck region. Occurring in over 1 in 1000 births, it is the most common congenital vascular malformation [5]. PWS may occur in isolation or in combination with other vascular malformation or somatic overgrowth.

As capillary malformations darken with time, the involved skin thickens and becomes more raised and nodular. At this point, disfigurement becomes a great concern, compromising a patient's self-image and self-worth [6]. Underlying skeletal overgrowth is another important consideration in terms of the deformity related to PWS. This is postulated to occur from a pathologically increased blood supply leading to a local over-abundance of growth factors [7]. To prevent this eventuality, treatment is recommended as early as infancy. The literature suggests that indeed the earlier that treatment is started, the better the outcome [8, 9].

The mainstay for the treatment of PWS is intermittent pulse dye laser (PDL) therapy. Modern PDL devices produce wavelengths between 595–600 nm, a range that is well absorbed by oxyhemoglobin and to a lesser degree deoxyhemoglobin and melanin. Initial fluence starts between 8–9 J/cm2 and is then increased to obtain the desired clinical response. The skin should have a gray or purpuric change in the treated area (as the target vessels rupture) with the absence of significant blanching which can be an early indicator of blistering possibly leading to a scar. Pulse duration can be varied from 0.45 to 40 ms, and various spot sizes may be selected on the order from 2 to 12 mm. The latest models are equipped with cryogen cooling spray which protects the epidermis from thermal injury, contributing to an excellent safety profile. Alteration in pigmentation has been reported around 1.4%, atrophic scarring at 4.3%, and hypertrophic scarring at 0.7% in appropriately selected candidates [10].

PDL treatment may be performed with or without anesthesia as appropriate according to the age of the patient and subsequently their ability to cooperate. Treatment is often recommended in series with sessions scheduled about every 4–6 weeks. This is to allow for adequate coverage of the entire involved area. A single session may produce a "polka-dotted" appearance, as the overlap of individual laser bursts is spaced to minimize the risk for scarring. Subsequent sessions allow for the treatment of the spaces in between as well as the calibration of the fluence until an ideal setting is reached. If the patient is a child requiring anesthesia, sessions may be spaced out to every 2–3 months to allow for greater intervals between anesthetic exposure. When a plateau is reached in the responsiveness of the color, treatment may be discontinued. However, patients and families should be advised that the rates of recidivism are high. At 5 years after the completion of PDL treatments, 16–50% of patients experience darkening of their lesions [11, 12], thought to be due to vessel regeneration and lesion revascularization [13]. Thus, many individuals will benefit from additional intermittent laser treatment over the course of years.

Results from PDL treatment are typically excellent. As measured by a chromameter, Koster et al. report 50–90% overall clearance with at least 10% improvement with each session [14]. However, certainly there are cases in which lesions are not adequately responsive to PDL. One review cites resistance rates between 20–30% [15]. Risk factors for resistance are felt to include very small vessels as well as vessels that are located deeper in the dermis. Patient age and anatomic location may also play a role. Poor responders may include midfacial lesions in a trigeminal distribution.

In cases of resistance, the use of alternative lasers may be considered. Alexandrite lasers are near-infrared, with wavelengths around 755 nm. This allows for greater penetration in comparison to PDL. Thus, it may be considered for particularly dark or resistant cases. It also has a greater affinity for deoxyhemoglobin, which is present in higher concentrations in large capillary, venular, and venous channels [16]. The Nd:YAG may also be considered for resistant PWS. At a 1064 nm wavelength, it has the greatest depth of penetration. However, since greater fluence settings are often required, the rate of pigmentary change and scarring is higher when compared to PDL [17]. In these cases, cryogen usage for epidermal cooling is paramount.

Another consideration in cases of PDL resistance is the usage of topical rapamycin as a pharmacologic adjunct. An mTOR inhibitor, rapamycin has anti-angiogenesis properties and has been recently been observed to have beneficial effects in a number of applications in the treatment of vascular anomalies. Formulated as a topical cream, the drug has been investigated as a treatment for resistant port-wine stain cases. Early clinical trials of PDL + topical rapamycin have indicated significant improvement in digital photographic image score when compared with PDL + placebo [18]. Usage may increase the overall efficacy and duration of PDL treatment resulting in fewer overall treatments and a longer lasting plateau [13, 19, 20].

Common side effects of PDL treatment are erythema, swelling, and bruising (purpura). This can last from hours to weeks. If a site is overtreated with a high fluence or overlapping spots, blistering can be induced which can lead to scarring. Such wounds are best treated with the liberal application of moisturization ointment and dressing. Hyper/hypopigmentation can occur from direct injury to melanosomes or from postinflammatory reparative changes. This is particularly worrisome with type IV-VI skin patients. Catastrophic events such as ocular injury or fire should be obviated as long as proper eye protection and fire safety precautions are stringently adhered to.

14.3 Infantile Hemangioma

There are multiple possible pharmacologic and surgical treatments for infantile hemangiomas (IHs), and early evaluation by a provider intimately familiar with the pathophysiology of hemangioma is crucial. Previously, a tradition of "benign neglect" was followed by most pediatric providers. However, as more treatment options have been developed over the last decade, a more current approach supports earlier consideration for treatment. One well-designed study demonstrated a long-term benefit in color difference between IH treated with laser versus observation as measured by a colorimeter [21]. Laser therapy is most commonly considered in the following scenarios: early proliferating lesions with skin ulceration or bleeding [22] and involuting hemangiomas with residual telangiectasias [23]. As with port-wine stains, the PDL is the most commonly used in the treatment of hemangiomas because of its excellent uptake by oxyhemoglobin. Families must be advised that the primary outcome expected to be improved with laser treatment is the color of the lesion. Improvement of the growth or bulk of a lesion or cases greater than 3 mm in thickness should not be expected to be significantly affected by PDL, due to limited depth of tissue penetration by this laser [24, 25].

The CO2 laser may be used for skin resurfacing of involuted IHs that have residual atrophic skin or scarring [26]. Particularly protuberant lesions may result in the significant fibrofatty residuum. This bulky, non-pigmented tissue does not respond to laser therapy, and surgical excision is usually necessary to give an acceptable cosmetic outcome.

The CO2 laser is the most commonly used laser in the treatment of subglottic hemangiomas. This laser is effective in reducing the lesion size and thus decreasing symptoms of airway restriction. However, subglottic stenosis may recur if overly aggressive laser treatments are performed [27]. With the broad acceptance of propranolol therapy in the treatment of IHs (including those in the subglottis), CO_2 laser use may not be needed. Instead, combination therapy with oral administration of propranolol and intralesional injection of steroids may often be sufficient.

14.4 Venous Malformation

Venous malformations (VM) are composed of tortuous, thin-walled veins with a single endothelial lining [28]. They are present at birth and typically grow with the patient, though there may be the acceleration of growth in the peri-pubertal years. Venous malformations are slow flow, compressible, and will wax and wane in size. One unique characteristic is swelling induced by dependent positioning due to the gravitational shunting of flow into the vessels. Symptoms arise from the deformity of these lesions as well as space-occupying effects on functions as speech, swallowing, breathing, or musculoskeletal range of motion.

By definition, VMs are filled with post-capillary circulation, deoxygenated hemoglobin. Thus, when selecting a laser to treat these lesions, this is the chromophore that must be targeted. The Nd:YAG laser with a longer wavelength of 1064 nm, and the Alexandrite (755 nm) laser are the most commonly used due to their increased absorption by deoxyhemoglobin when compared to PDL. Similar to PWS, when the hemoglobin is heated, erythrocytes are lysed, and an inflammatory, coagulative response is initiated. Similar to the principles of sclerotherapy, the subsequent inflammatory cascade is destructive to the endothelial lining of the malformation, resulting in the coaptation of the vessel walls to one another, limiting flow through the treated area.

In a recent review, Richter and Braswell summarized the treatment modalities for VMs, which included laser therapy, sclerotherapy, embolization, and surgical excision [29]. The appropriateness of laser therapy is dependent on the site and extent of the venous malformation. Superficial cutaneous and mucosal lesions are the most accessible to laser treatment. However, deeper lesions may be treated via interstitial techniques: direct puncture of the venous malformation with a needle and then introducing a laser fiber into the malformation by passing it through the needle lumen.

The Nd:YAG laser may be used safely on the skin surface, but consideration must be made for the protection of the epidermis as there may be absorption by water leading to thermal damage of the skin surface. This may be achieved by the use of a laser system that has a coordinated emission of a cryogen burst immediately preceding the laser pulse [29, 30]. Alternative techniques may include firing the laser through ice or through chilled sapphire crystals. Smaller, venous telangiectasias may be better treated by the Alexandrite laser, and larger superficial veins will typically respond better to the Nd:YAG [29]. Laser treatment may be combined with sclerotherapy for extensive lesions, and there is evidence to support that pre-treatment with the laser may augment the results of sclerotherapy and decrease the likelihood of ulceration [30]. Similar to PDL therapy, families must be advised that an adequate result may require a series of treatments. Again, providers typically schedule these sessions at least 4–6 weeks apart to allow for the completion of the inflammatory response between treatment. Patients with a low burden of disease may require only 1 to 2 treatments for disease control, but an overall average of 4 treatments is reported [31].

Mucosal VMs respond well to the Nd:YAG laser. Because of the regenerative nature of mucosa and thus lower concern for scarring, concurrent cooling of the mucosal surface is less necessary than when this laser is used on the skin. Lesions of the aerodigestive tract may be accessed via direct visualization with a headlight (in the oral cavity or oropharynx) or with endoscopic techniques (nasopharynx, hypopharynx, larynx, esophagus, or trachea). The laser fiber may be attached directly to a telescope to allow for simultaneous visualization and treatment. Venous malformations of the mucosa of the vulva or anorectal vault also may be safely treated with the Nd:YAG laser [32]. When the laser beam is activated, there is an instant shrinkage of the lesion. Immediately after treatment, ice may be used to cool the area if it is accessible (such as the oral cavity). A short course of postoperative steroids may help alleviate edema and pain. Rare complications include bleeding, scarring, and mucosal sloughing [29, 31, 33].

As mentioned, interstitial techniques may be utilized to introduce the Nd:YAG laser fiber for deeper VMs at any site. Often under ultrasound guidance, a 14-gage needle is inserted directly into the VM, and the fiber is passed through directly into the lumen of the VM. Prior to insertion, one must measure the extent of the exposed fiber such that there is no direct contact with the needle itself. If the exposed fiber is in contact with the needle, the metal may be heated, leading to injury at the insertion site. Direct introduction of the needle in this way permits the ablation of the VM from the inside as the laser is manipulated to different sites [33, 34]. A clear response can be observed in real time via ultrasound imaging as the VM collapses onto itself. Careful consideration must be made that interstitial techniques are not used in close proximity to neural structures as collateral thermal injury may be difficult to anticipate.

14.5 Lymphatic Malformation

Lymphatic malformations, the aberrant development of lymphatic channels, may be classified by their size. Macrocystic disease describes cysts that are 2 cm or greater in diameter whereas microcystic disease is less than 2 cm. Lymphatic malformations are often deep, infiltrative lesions that are not close enough to the skin or mucosa to be amenable to laser treatment. Surgical excision and sclerotherapy represent the mainstays of treatment, with both modalities achieving comparable rates of success [35]. However, some lesions will involve the skin or mucosal surface. These cases present with small vesicular lesions that are deforming and may chronically bleed or weep lymphatic fluid. The area may also be tender. For these, laser therapy has proven to be a useful adjunct to sclerotherapy or surgical excision.

Unlike other vascular anomalies composed of blood-filled channels, lymphatic malformations by definition are filled with lymphatic fluid, with a much lower concentration of hemoglobin. For this reason, the chromophore targeted in lymphatic malformation is water. The CO2 laser, with wavelengths around 10,600 nm, is well absorbed by water and has been used for targeted microablation of tissue and resurfacing [36]. However, because water is ubiquitous throughout the body, it is more difficult to be selective in terms of the ablation of the malformation separate from the surrounding tissue or overlying skin.

The CO2 laser has been effectively applied to lesions of the oral tongue [37], tongue base [38], and larynx [39]. Glade and Buckmiller reported a 10-year experience using CO_2 laser resurfacing of oral LMs, indicating both the efficacy and safety of this technique [37]. In the study, patients underwent an average of 3 laser procedures. Though a small sample size due to the rarity of the disease, all patients reported improvement of symptoms including swelling, bleeding, and pain. Combined with the suspension of the airway and microscopic or endoscopic techniques, serial intervention is often required as lesions wax and wane, and unfortunately, regrowth is common.

14.6 Conclusion

The treatment of vascular anomalies is a diverse and challenging task. As we learn more about these lesions, their genetic causes, and potential therapies, providers must commit to ongoing education in this burgeoning field. The implementation of a multidisciplinary team is an excellent method for providing coordinated, quality care. A program such as this facilitates close communication between colleagues of varied disciplines who share an interest in this area. Examples of specialties that may be involved include interventional radiology, otolaryngology, pediatric surgery, plastic surgery, hematology/oncology, dermatology, and orthopedic surgery. At least one provider on the team who is comfortable with the administration of laser treatments is paramount such that this useful technology can be added to the armamentarium of therapies offered to patients afflicted with vascular anomalies.

References

1. Anderson RR, Parrish JA. Selective photothermolysis: precise microsurgery by selective absorption of pulsed radiation. Science. 1983;220(4596):524–7.
2. Brightman LA, Geronemus RG, Reddy KK. Laser treatment of port-wine stains. Clin Cosmet Investig Dermatol. 2015;8:27–33. https://doi.org/10.2147/CCID.S53118.
3. Keller GS, Toft KM. Lasers in aesthetic surgery. New York: Thieme; 2001.
4. Geronemus RG. Argon laser for the treatment of cutaneous lesions. Clin Dermatol. 1995;13(1):55–8.
5. Frigerio A, Bhama PK, Tan OT. Quantitative three-dimensional assessment of port-wine stain clearance after laser treatments. Lasers Surg Med. 2013;45(10):633–8. https://doi.org/10.1002/lsm.22176.
6. Malm M, Carlberg M. Port-wine stain--a surgical and psychological problem. Ann Plast Surg. 1988;20(6):512–6.
7. Greene AK, Taber SF, Ball KL, Padwa BL, Mulliken JB. Sturge-Weber syndrome: soft-tissue and skeletal overgrowth. J Craniofac Surg. 2009;20(Suppl 1):617–21. https://doi.org/10.1097/SCS.0b013e318192988e.
8. Chen JK, Ghasri P, Aguilar G, van Drooge AM, Wolkerstorfer A, Kelly KM, Heger M. An overview of clinical and experimental treatment modalities for port wine stains. J Am Acad Dermatol. 2012;67(2):289–304. https://doi.org/10.1016/j.jaad.2011.11.938.
9. Ashinoff R, Geronemus RG. Flashlamp-pumped pulsed dye laser for port-wine stains in infancy: earlier versus later treatment. J Am Acad Dermatol. 1991;24(3):467–72.
10. Astner S, Anderson RR. Treating vascular lesions. Dermatol Ther. 2005;18(3):267–81. https://doi.org/10.1111/j.1529-8019.2005.05025.x.
11. Michel S, Landthaler M, Hohenleutner U. Recurrence of port-wine stains after treatment with the flashlamp-pumped pulsed dye laser. Br J Dermatol. 2000;143(6):1230–4.
12. Orten SS, Waner M, Flock S, Roberson PK, Kincannon J. Port-wine stains. An assessment of 5 years of treatment. Archives of otolaryngology–head & neck surgery. 1996;122(11):1174–9.
13. Tan W, Jia W, Sun V, Mihm MC Jr, Nelson JS. Topical rapamycin suppresses the angiogenesis pathways induced by pulsed dye laser: molecular mechanisms of inhibition of regeneration and revascularization of photocoagulated cutaneous blood vessels. Lasers Surg Med. 2012;44(10):796–804. https://doi.org/10.1002/lsm.22101.
14. Koster PH, van der Horst CM, Bossuyt PM, van Gemert MJ. Prediction of portwine stain clearance and required number of flashlamp pumped pulsed dye laser treatments. Lasers Surg Med. 2001;29(2):151–5.
15. Savas JA, Ledon JA, Franca K, Chacon A, Nouri K. Pulsed dye laser-resistant port-wine stains: mechanisms of resistance and implications for treatment. Br J Dermatol. 2013;168(5):941–53. https://doi.org/10.1111/bjd.12204.
16. Izikson L, Anderson RR. Treatment endpoints for resistant port wine stains with a 755 nm laser. Journal of cosmetic and laser therapy: official publication of the European Society for Laser Dermatology. 2009;11(1):52–5. https://doi.org/10.1080/14764170802524452.
17. McGill DJ, MacLaren W, Mackay IR. A direct comparison of pulsed dye, alexandrite, KTP and Nd:YAG lasers and IPL in patients with previously treated capillary malformations. Lasers Surg Med. 2008;40(6):390–8. https://doi.org/10.1002/lsm.20638.
18. Marques L, Nunez-Cordoba JM, Aguado L, Pretel M, Boixeda P, Nagore E, Baselga E, Redondo P. Topical rapamycin combined with pulsed dye laser in the treatment of capillary vascular malformations in Sturge-weber syndrome: phase II, randomized, double-blind, intraindividual placebo-controlled clinical trial. J Am Acad Dermatol. 2015;72(1):151–158 e151. https://doi.org/10.1016/j.jaad.2014.10.011.
19. Jia W, Sun V, Tran N, Choi B, Liu SW, Mihm MC Jr, Phung TL, Nelson JS. Long-term blood vessel removal with combined laser and topical rapamycin antiangiogenic therapy: implications for effective port wine stain treatment. Lasers Surg Med. 2010;42(2):105–12. https://doi.org/10.1002/lsm.20890.

20. Loewe R, Oble DA, Valero T, Zukerberg L, Mihm MC Jr, Nelson JS. Stem cell marker upregulation in normal cutaneous vessels following pulsed-dye laser exposure and its abrogation by concurrent rapamycin administration: implications for treatment of port-wine stain birthmarks. J Cutan Pathol. 2010;37(Suppl 1):76–82. https://doi.org/10.1111/j.1600-0560.2010.01520.x.
21. Kessels JP, Hamers ET, Ostertag JU. Superficial hemangioma: pulsed dye laser versus wait-and-see. Dermatologic surgery: official publication for American Society for Dermatologic Surgery. 2013;39(3 Pt 1):414–21. https://doi.org/10.1111/dsu.12081.
22. Bencini PL, Tourlaki A, De Giorgi V, Galimberti M. Laser use for cutaneous vascular alterations of cosmetic interest. Dermatol Ther. 2012;25(4):340–51. https://doi.org/10.1111/j.1529-8019.2012.01463.x.
23. Franca K, Chacon A, Ledon J, Savas J, Izakovic J, Nouri K. Lasers for cutaneous congenital vascular lesions: a comprehensive overview and update. Lasers Med Sci. 2013;28(4):1197–204. https://doi.org/10.1007/s10103-012-1220-2.
24. Garden JM, Bakus AD, Paller AS. Treatment of cutaneous hemangiomas by the flashlamp-pumped pulsed dye laser: prospective analysis. J Pediatr. 1992;120(4) Pt 1:555–60.
25. Poetke M, Philipp C, Berlien HP. Flashlamp-pumped pulsed dye laser for hemangiomas in infancy: treatment of superficial vs mixed hemangiomas. Arch Dermatol. 2000;136(5):628–32.
26. Brightman LA, Brauer JA, Terushkin V, Hunzeker C, Reddy KK, Weiss ET, Karen JK, Hale EK, Anolik R, Bernstein L, Geronemus RG. Ablative fractional resurfacing for involuted hemangioma residuum. Arch Dermatol. 2012;148(11):1294–8. https://doi.org/10.1001/archdermatol.2012.2346.
27. Bitar MA, Moukarbel RV, Zalzal GH. Management of congenital subglottic hemangioma: trends and success over the past 17 years. Otolaryngology--head and neck surgery: official journal of American Academy of Otolaryngology-Head and Neck Surgery. 2005;132(2):226–31. https://doi.org/10.1016/j.otohns.2004.09.136.
28. North PE, Mihm MC Jr. Histopathological diagnosis of infantile hemangiomas and vascular malformations. Facial Plast Surg Clin North Am. 2001;9(4):505–24.
29. Richter GT, Braswell L. Management of venous malformations. Facial plastic surgery: FPS. 2012;28(6):603–10. https://doi.org/10.1055/s-0032-1329935.
30. Scherer K, Waner M. Nd:YAG lasers (1,064 nm) in the treatment of venous malformations of the face and neck: challenges and benefits. Lasers Med Sci. 2007;22(2):119–26. https://doi.org/10.1007/s10103-007-0443-0.
31. Eivazi B, Wiegand S, Teymoortash A, Neff A, Werner JA. Laser treatment of mucosal venous malformations of the upper aerodigestive tract in 50 patients. Lasers Med Sci. 2010;25(4):571–6. https://doi.org/10.1007/s10103-010-0762-4.
32. Gurien LA, Jackson RJ, Kiser MM, Richter GT. Nd:YAG laser therapy for rectal and vaginal venous malformations. Pediatr Surg Int. 2017;33(8):887–91. https://doi.org/10.1007/s00383-017-4113-4.
33. Glade RS, Richter GT, James CA, Suen JY, Buckmiller LM. Diagnosis and management of pediatric cervicofacial venous malformations: retrospective review from a vascular anomalies center. Laryngoscope. 2010;120(2):229–35. https://doi.org/10.1002/lary.20715.
34. Chang CJ, Fisher DM, Chen YR. Intralesional photocoagulation of vascular anomalies of the tongue. Br J Plast Surg. 1999;52(3):178–81. https://doi.org/10.1054/bjps.1998.3056.
35. Adams MT, Saltzman B, Perkins JA. Head and neck lymphatic malformation treatment: a systematic review. Otolaryngology–head and neck surgery: official journal of American Academy of Otolaryngology-Head and Neck Surgery. 2012;147(4):627–39. https://doi.org/10.1177/0194599812453552.
36. Omi T, Numano K. The role of the CO2 laser and fractional CO2 laser in dermatology. Laser therapy. 2014;23(1):49–60. https://doi.org/10.5978/islsm.14-RE-01.
37. Glade RS, Buckmiller LM. CO2 laser resurfacing of intraoral lymphatic malformations: a 10-year experience. Int J Pediatr Otorhinolaryngol. 2009;73(10):1358–61. https://doi.org/10.1016/j.ijporl.2009.06.013.
38. Edwards PD, Rahbar R, Ferraro NF, Burrows PE, Mulliken JB. Lymphatic malformation of the lingual base and oral floor. Plast Reconstr Surg. 2005;115(7):1906–15.
39. Cohen SR, Thompson JW. Lymphangiomas of the larynx in infants and children. A survey of pediatric lymphangioma. Ann Otol Rhinol Laryngol Suppl. 1986;127:1–20.

15 Endovascular Management of Vascular Malformations

Rashmi Saraf

'Nomenclature has been the major obstacle to our understanding and management of Vascular anomalies'

John Mulliken

15.1 Introduction

Vascular malformations are the result of errors in vascular development. They may cause identifiable birthmarks of the skin and mucosa and a varying degree of underlying soft tissue abnormalities. These lesions predominantly occur in the head and neck and occur in around 0.3% of live births. Detailed analysis and in-depth understanding of the natural history of vascular anomalies is critical for practitioners managing these lesions [1].

Vascular malformations of the head and neck are an important cause of cosmetic and functional disturbances. Depending on the size and locations, significant functional and aesthetic impairment can result from the growth of 'problematic' Hemangiomas or vascular malformations. They present the most formidable challenges to the field of Plastic Surgery and Interventional Radiology. Management of these lesions mandates a comprehensive approach in order to achieve a good cosmetic and functional outcome. Many disciplines are involved in the treatment of these disorders, the majority of which affect the head and neck with frequent involvement of the oral cavity and aerodigestive tract. Apart from capillary malformations, which are usually not treated with interventional therapy, all other types of vascular malformations can be treated with interventional techniques that typically require transarterial, transvenous or direct access.

Interventional therapy is gaining wider acceptance in recent years and is considered the first line of therapy in most of the centres [1].

15.2 Classification

The management of vascular anomalies was plagued by confusion for many years. A lack of understanding of the pathophysiology had resulted in the evolution of bewildering and confusing terminology to describe these lesions. Patients with various kinds of vascular lesions exhibit overlapping clinical signs and symptoms which make the correct diagnosis difficult.

R. Saraf (✉)
Assistant Professor and Incharge, Division of Interventional Neuroradiology, Department of Radiology, Seth G.S. Medical college and KEM hospital, Mumbai, India

A. K. Khanna, S. K. Tiwary (eds.), *Vascular Malformations*,
https://doi.org/10.1007/978-981-15-9762-6_15

A vascular malformation is a generalized term used to describe a group of lesions present at birth, formed by an anomaly of angiovascular or lymphangiovascular structures.

Wegner, in 1880, first separated vascular lesions into angiomas and lymphangiomas. They classified these as simplex, cavernosum or racemosum. This original classification was based on the histological appearance and did not take into account the biological behaviour [1, 2].

The development of the head and neck area involves complex changes (rotations, invaginations, migrations) of the tissues during the first weeks in the uterus. During normal development of the head and neck, the vasculature undergoes series of changes in its branching patterns. Regressions and annexations of arteries account for the unique bidirectional flow in every branch of the head and neck area. The folds between adjacent buds represent critical areas for capillary maturation, primarily on the venous side. After this has occurred, the arterial system can establish the necessary hemodynamic balance. Delay in bud fusion produces specific arterial anatomic variation. If the maturation of the capillary network is simultaneously delayed, vascular lesions may be seen in association with the arterial variations. Even if a malformation is present during the development stages, it will remain as a quiescent defect that will be triggered to produce an irreversible foetal, neonatal, child or adult vascular malformation. Could and colleagues demonstrated that endothelial cells of the cephalic region have a generalized origin from the paraxial mesoderm, which provides blood vessels to specific regions of the face and brain. In general, the neural crest and mesodermal cells originating from a given transverse level occupy the same facial territories and the two cell types cooperate in myogenesis and in vasculogenesis. Related to this contribution, one can recognize some of the clinical syndromes described in the literature and can postulate a link between apparently unrelated territories, like Sturge–Weber syndrome. These disorders are collectively called cerebrofacial arteriovenous metameric syndromes [3].

Before the 1980s, the terminology that was used to describe vascular anomalies was confusing and ambiguous. The descriptive terminology used in the past (port-wine stain, strawberry hemangioma, salmon patch) conjure up a visual approximation to the lesions but have no correlation with the biological behaviour or natural history of these lesions.

In 1982, Mulliken and Glowacki for the first time used clinical behaviour and endothelial cell characteristics to devise a simple biological classification for these lesions. Vascular anomalies were distinctly divided into vascular tumours (Hemangiomas) and vascular malformations. According to this classification, Hemangiomas are vascular tumours that arise from endothelial hyperplasia or excess angiogenesis whereas vascular malformations are congenital lesions resulting from developmental anomalies due to errors in vascular and lymphatic morphogenesis that 'grow' with the patient and have normal endothelial activity. The vascular malformation includes capillary, arterial, lymphatic, venous or a combination of these types. This classification was a breakthrough in the field of vascular malformation as it gave insight into the management of these lesions.

Hamburg Classification was introduced in 1988 after the ISSVA meeting in Hamburg, Germany. It accounts for the underlying anatomical, histological and pathophysiological features of congenital vascular malformations. It also introduces embryological aspects, further subdividing them into either an extratruncular or truncular form, based on the time of developmental arrest during embryonic life. Extratruncular forms of CVMs arise early in embryonic life, while the vascular system is still in the reticular stage. They are in fact mesodermal tissue remnants, that retain the potential of angioblasts to grow and proliferate when stimulated. This is why these lesions may continue to grow and carry a significant risk of a recurrence after therapeutic interventions. Truncular forms arise at a later stage when the developmental arrest occurs during the vascular trunk formation. Truncular lesions have lost the potential to grow and proliferate. Thus, they carry only a minimal risk of recurrence. Truncular lesions are further subdivided into obstructive or dilatative lesions. They present as various degrees of developmental defects of a vascular trunk, which may include agenesis or aplasia on the one hand and aneurysms or persistent embryonic channels on the other [1, 4].

The International Society for the Study of Vascular Anomalies (ISSVA) was formed in 1992 to promote research in the field of vascular anomalies and to create a uniform nomenclature that would facilitate research and clinical practice. It adopted the classifications of vascular anomalies by Mulliken and Glowacki in 1996 and it was further revised in 1997. This is now recognized worldwide as the official system for the classification of congenital disorders of vascular development and also the first biological classification of vascular anomalies. (Table 15.1) [1, 2].

Table 15.1 The first biological classification of Vascular Anomalies (1996)

Vascular Tumours	Vascular Malformations
Infantile Hemangioma	• Slow flow vascular malformation capillary malformation (CM) venous malformation (VM) lymphatic malformation (LM) combined
	High flow vascular malformation • arterial malformation • Arteriovenous fistula • Arteriovenous malformation

This classification is updated regularly, the last being in May 2018. (Table 15.2) [5] The recent update involves more genetic insight into the basic classification. Additional disease entities have since been identified that are complex and less easily classified by generic headings, such as capillary malformation, venous malformation, lymphatic malformation, etc. The general biological scheme of the classification is retained. The section on tumours has been expanded and lists the main recognized vascular tumours, classified as benign, locally aggressive or borderline, and malignant. A list of well-defined diseases is included under each generic heading. Two new sections were created: one dealing with the malformations of individually named vessels (previously referred to as 'truncular' malformations); the second groups lesions of uncertain or debated nature (tumour versus malformation). This classification is meant to be a framework, acknowledging that it will require modification as new scientific information becomes available [5, 6].

For simplification and clear understanding, the Table 15.3 will explain the new terminologies for the older description of vascular anomalies.

Table 15.2 ISSVA Classification—Last Revision May 2018 [5]

Vascular Anomalies				
Vascular Tumours	Vascular malformations			
Benign Infantile hemangioma Congenital hemangioma Tufted Hemangioma Spindle cell Hemangioma Epithelioid Hemangioma Pyogenic granuloma Locally aggressive or borderline Kaposiform Hemangioendothelioma Malignant Angiosarcoma	Simple	Combined	Of major named vessels	Associated with other anomalies
	Slow flow vascular malformation Capillary malformation (CM) Venous malformation (VM) Lymphatic malformation (LM) Combined	Various combination of simple types	Affect Lymphatics Veins Arteries Anomalies of Origin Course Number Length Diameter Valves Communication Persistence	KT syndrome PW syndrome Servelle–Martorell's syndrome Sturge Weber syndrome Maffucci syndrome CLOVES syndrome CLAPO syndrome Proteus syndrome
	High flow vascular malformation Arterial malformation Arteriovenous fistula Arteriovenous malformation			

Table 15.3 Old versus new terminology for common vascular anomalies

Old	New
Capillary Hemangioma	Hemangioma
Port-wine stain Capillary hemangioma Strawberry hemangioma	Capillary malformation
Cavernous hemangioma Ossifying hemangioma	Venous malformation
Lymphangioma Cystic hygroma	Lymphatic malformation

15.3 Diagnosis and Investigation

15.3.1 History and Clinical Examination

Accurate terminology leads to the precise identification of the vascular entity. In most cases, an accurate history and physical examination will help establish the diagnosis.

15.3.2 Investigations

Further investigations are considered for Hemangiomas only if the diagnosis is in doubt. In the case of Vascular malformations, further investigations in the form of MRI is important to assess the size and extent of the lesion, proximity to the airway, multiplicity. It is important in planning the treatment. Imaging is used to confirm the suspected diagnosis, establish the extent of the lesion and document any associated abnormalities.

Magnetic resonance imaging is the investigation of choice as it provides accurate information about the extent of the lesion, better contrast between the lesion and surrounding tissues, and has multiplanar capabilities. It can also help distinguish between the different types of vascular anomalies. It gives a clear idea of the relationship with surrounding important structures such as nerves, orbit and airways. STIR and T2WI with fat suppression in all three planes are important, for defining the complete extent of the lesion. Contrast-enhanced computed tomography has a role in evaluating intraosseous lesions and the bony margins of extensive lesions that are under consideration for resection. Grey-scale ultrasound and Doppler analysis are useful in defining whether the lesion is solid or cystic and to establish the presence or absence of high flow vessels. Angiography, particularly digital subtraction angiography (DSA), has a specific but limited role in the diagnosis of vascular lesions, but should not be used as a first-line investigation. It is, however, useful for mapping out the blood supply of the lesion and in the assessment of the characteristics of the flow of arteriovenous malformations. Direct intralesional injection of contrast medium has a role in the analysis of venous malformation [3, 7].

15.4 Vascular Tumours

15.4.1 Hemangiomas

15.4.1.1 Introduction

Hemangiomas are congenital vascular tumours and considered to be the most common benign tumours of infancy, affecting 5–10% of all infants and up to 30% of premature babies. Vascular tumours are true proliferative neoplasms and demonstrate growth by endothelial hyperplasia with elevated serum markers of proliferation such as VEGF, cell nuclear antigen, GLUT 1. They are comprised of rapidly dividing endothelial cells with a greater incidence in Caucasians, females, premature and low birth weight infants. Hemangiomas proliferate during the first 9–12 months of life and subsequently involute at a variable course over many years (up to 12 years). The head and neck region are the most commonly involved site (60%). Multiple cutaneous lesions are often associated with visceral involvement. Facial Hemangiomas have a predilection for segmental distribution and for regions of embryological fusion. In such cases, workup for potential underlying PHACE syndrome should be undertaken.

Other rare benign vascular tumours include the pyogenic granuloma (also called lobular capillary hemangioma), which is one of the reactive vascular proliferative lesions grouped with vascular tumours. In the borderline category, kaposiform hemangioendothelioma is a childhood tumour that may be associated with thrombocytopenia and consumptive coagulopathy, whereas Kaposi sarcoma is most commonly encountered in the immunocompromised adult. Angiosarcoma is a rare malignant vascular tumour of older adults that most often involves the scalp and skin and is associated with high rates of local recurrence and distant metastases.

15.4.2 Classification

- Based on their clinical behaviour and histology, they have been subdivided into—Infantile Hemangioma and Congenital Hemangioma.

15.4.2.1 Infantile Hemangioma

They are the most common type of vascular tumours and hence most of the Hemangioma description is based on the infantile Hemangioma. They develop shortly after birth and follow the expected course of proliferation with prolonged involution. Positive staining for the histologic marker GLUT1 is highly specific and diagnostic for infantile Hemangioma [4]. At birth, the lesions are often small and inconspicuous, with 60% absent at birth. They are more common in females. Typical Triphasic growth pattern is noted in the Hemangiomas of infancy that is Proliferative, Involuting and Involuted. Shortly after birth, the phase of rapid proliferation occurs, the proliferative phase corresponds to a rapid period of growth of endothelial cells that form syncytial masses with and without vascular lumens. This phase has been defined by the high expression of angiogenic factors such as vascular endothelial growth factor and basic fibroblast growth factor. The typical Hemangioma will begin to involute approximately 10 months after birth and 50% of lesions are completely resolved in 5 years. Involutive phase is hallmarked by diminishing cellularity, interstitial fibrosis and fibrofatty replacement.

Some locations of the Hemangiomas in the Head and Neck regions make them prone to cause functional disturbances and hence they are considered as 'Problematic' Hemangiomas. These regions are lip, orbit, eyelid, nose, ear and airway [3].

15.4.2.2 Congenital Hemangioma

They are rare benign vascular tumours with clinical and histological features that differ from infantile Hemangiomas. They are present at birth, does not follow the natural growth phase of its infantile counterpart and histologically GLUT1 negative [8].

- They are of two types:
  - Rapidly involuting congenital hemangioma
  - Non-involuting congenital hemangioma
- Based on the pattern of involvement of the anatomic region, it may be localized/focal and segmental.

Localized/Focal:

- Arise from a central focus{skin/liver/GIT}.
- Single or multifocal. If lesions are more than five in number, it is advisable to look for liver Hemangiomas.

Segmental:

- They cover an anatomic territory.
- Involves multiple contiguous cervical and facial units with indistinct borders.
- Example:
  - Beard Hemangioma: Lower lip, chin, cheek and preauricular area are strongly associated with subglottic airway involvement [3].
  - *PHACES Syndrome:* Neurocutaneous condition marked by the presence of:

P = Posterior fossa (refers to possible abnormal structures in the brain, particularly the cerebellum)

- Major
- Posterior fossa brain anomalies
- Dandy–Walker complex
- Other hypoplasia/dysplasia of the mid and/or hind brain
- Minor–Midline brain anomalies
- Malformation of cortical development

H = Hemangioma

A = Arterial (refers to possible abnormal arteries in the brain) Anomaly of major cerebral or cervical arteries

- Major
- Dysplasia of the large cerebral arteries
- Arterial stenosis or occlusion with or without moyamoya collaterals
- Absence or moderate-severe hypoplasia of the large cerebral or cervical arteries
- Aberrant origin or course of the large cerebral or cervical arteries, except common arch variants such as the bovine arch
- Persistent carotid-vertebrobasilar anastomosis (proatlantal segmental, hypoglossal, otic, and/or trigeminal • arteries)
- Minor
- Aneurysm of any of the cerebral arteries

C = Cardiac (refers to possible heart abnormalities usually involving the great vessels) Aortic arch anomalies

- Major
- Coarctation of the aorta
- Dysplasia
- Aneurysm
- Aberrant origin of the subclavian artery with or without a vascular ring
- Minor
- Ventricular septal defect
- Right aortic arch/double aortic arch
- Systemic venous anomalies

E = Eyes (refers to possible eye abnormalities)

- Major
- Posterior segment abnormalities
- Persistent foetal vasculature
- Persistent hyperplastic primary vitreous
- Retinal vascular anomalies
- Morning glory disc anomaly
- Optic nerve hypoplasia
- Peripapillary staphyloma
- Minor -
- Anterior segment abnormality
- Sclerocornea
- Cataracts
- Coloboma
- Microphthalmia

Others Ventral/Midline Abnormalities

- Major
- Sternal cleft
- Anomaly of the midline chest and abdomen
- Sternal defect
- Supraumbilical raphe
- Minor hypopituitarism
- Ectopic thyroid
- Midline sternal papule/hamartoma

PHACE syndrome should be considered in infants with large plaque- type facial Hemangiomas. (Figs. 15.1 and 15.2) According to one study in infants with large Hemangiomas, one-third have extracutaneous manifestations consistent with the diagnosis of PHACE syndrome. The most common are cerebrovascular and cardiovascular anomalies. Affected children are classified into two categories, definite PHACE syndrome and possible PHACE syndrome, based on the nature and number of criteria met. *Definite PHACE syndrome* can be diagnosed in one of two different combinations: (1) A characteristic segmental Hemangioma greater than 5 cm in diameter on the face (or scalp) plus one of the major criteria or two minor criteria; (2) Hemangioma of the neck, upper torso or torso and upper arm plus two major criteria. *Possible PHACE syndrome* can be diagnosed in one of three different combinations: (1) Facial Hemangioma greater than 5 cm in diameter plus one minor criterion; (2) Hemangioma of the neck, upper torso, or torso and upper arm plus one major criterion or two minor criteria; or (3) no Hemangioma plus two major criteria. Note that more than one anomaly in one organ system (for example, two heart conditions) only counts for one criterion [9].

- Based on the depth of tissue involved, it may be Superficial, Deep or Compound.

15.4.3 Clinical Features

Most of the description is based on the Infantile Hemangiomas. They are evident shortly after

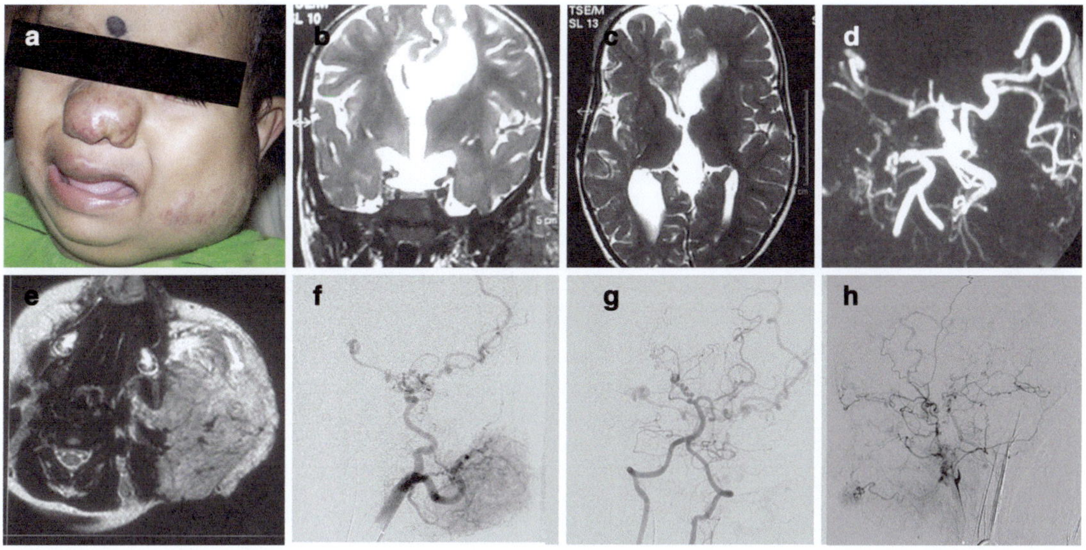

Fig. 15.1 Phace syndrome. 6 month old girl with left cheek swelling present at birth as a mark and gradually increasing in size. 2D Echo showed small ASD. (**a**) Clinical picture at the time of presentation with pinkish discolouration of the overlying skin. (**b, c**) MRI showing cerebral involvement. There is corpus callosal agenesis and pachygyria. (**d**) TOF MRA shows occluded right ICA with reformation of right MCA through unnamed collaterals. (**e**) T2WI showing the hemangioma with multiple signal voids suggestive of high vascularity in the proliferative phase. (**f**) Left CCA angiogram shows hyper vascular left cheek hemangioma and abnormal loopy, cork screw intracranial arteries. There is reformation of left hemispheric arteries through midline collaterals. (**g**) Left Vertebral angiogram shows corkscrew loopy posterior cerebral arteries. (**h**) Right Common carotid angiograms show occluded right ICA and reformation of cortical branches through dural pial collaterals

birth with a well-defined/demarcated, red, expansive lesion. It is firm to soft in consistency. The overlying skin is frequently bright red, cobblestone and elevated during the proliferative phase of growth. Due to rapid growth, soft tissue ischemia, necrosis and ulceration may occur. Sometimes massive growth may cause disfigurement or impact normal function. The lesion is usually pulsatile due to underlying high vascularity in the proliferative phase. At the Onset of involution, there is a change in the colour of the skin to greyish and the course of involution is variable during which they become less tense, flaccid and reduced in size. Residual lesions may appear as telangiectatic tissues (seen as an arborizing network of small, medium and large vessels), fibrofatty lesions, epidermal atrophy [3].

15.4.4 Diagnosis

The lesion is diagnosed clinically in most of the cases and Oral therapy can be initiated on clinical and examination findings alone. MRI is helpful in cases where the diagnosis is in doubt or when further treatment is planned in order to know the nature and extent of the lesion.

15.4.5 Complications

Although Hemangiomas are typically benign, a percentage of them develop life-threatening complications. Potential complications include Kasabach–Merritt Syndrome (consumptive coagulopathy), compression of vital structures (airway), orbital fissure formation, ulceration,

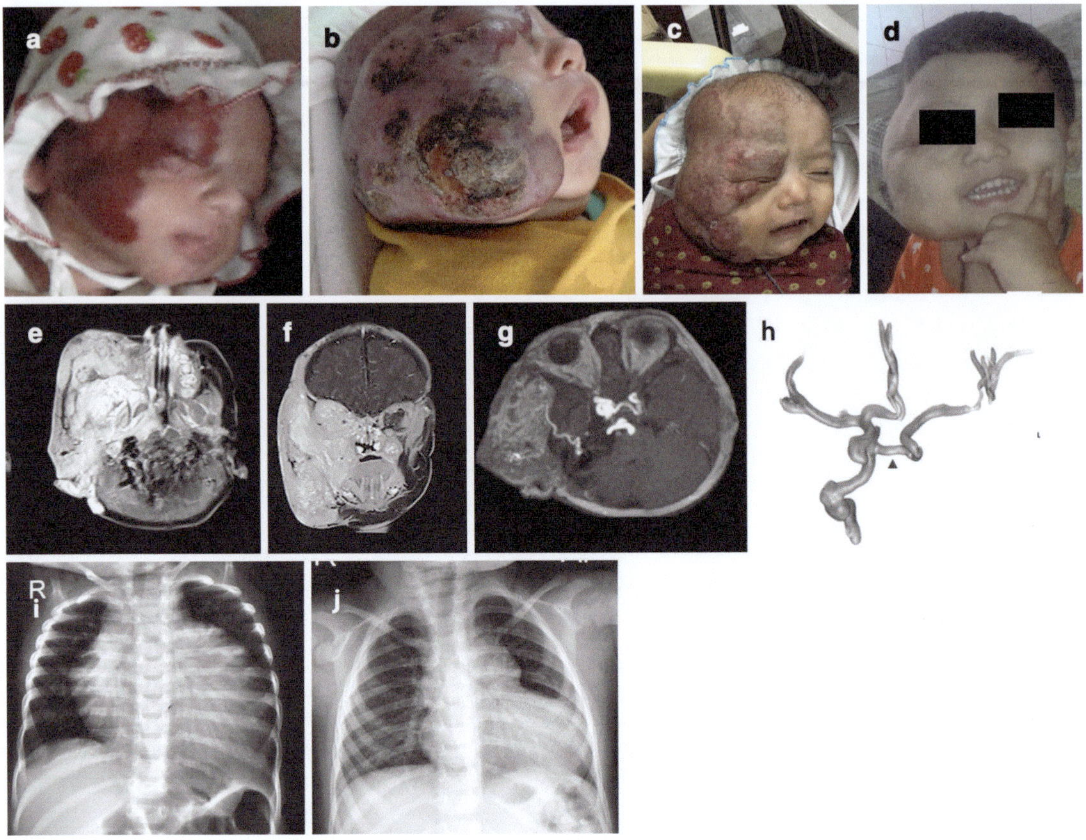

Fig. 15.2 PHACE Syndrome. A 3-day-old patient with right facial reddish discolouration suggestive of hemangioma involving the right cheek, forehead and upper eyelid who presented at 3 months of age when there was a rapid increase in the size of selling with ulceration and necrosis.(**a**) Clinical photograph at presentation. (**b**) Clinical photograph at 3 months of age showing an increase in the size of the lesion with bleeding and ulceration.2D echocardiography showed Right ventricular and right atrial dysfunction with small ASD. After discussion with cardiologist, child was started on propranolol therapy. (**c**) Clinical picture at 8 months of age. There was healing of the lesion with a decrease in ulcerations. She developed otitis media on the right side with episodes of cyanotic spells. MRI was performed at this stage. (**d**) Follow-up at 2 years of age after three sessions of percutaneous bleomycin sclerotherapy showing reduction of the swelling. Complete absence of necrosis and ulcerations on the surface. (**e-g**) Magnetic resonance imaging showing right-sided large segmental hemangioma seen extending up to the middle cranial fossa. (**h**) On angiography, the patient was found to have a persistent primitive maxillary artery which is a rare entity seen in patients with PHACE syndrome. (**i**) Chest radiograph at 6 months of age showing gross cardiomegaly along with features of pulmonary arterial hypertension. 2D Echo at this time showed severe PAH with right-sided heart enlargement, She was started on medical therapy. Primary pulmonary hypertension can sometimes be associated with Large segmental hemangiomas. She was started on intralesional Bleomycin sclerotherapy to accelerate the regression of hemangioma. (**j**) Chest radiograph of the patient 1 year. after Bleomycin treatment showing a reduction in the size of heart as well as pulmonary hypertension which was confirmed with 2D echocardiography

infection and bleeding. These complications usually occur in the rapid proliferative phase and can be associated with a mortality rate as high as 20–30%. Large facial Infantile Hemangioma can be associated with neurological, ophthalmologic and cardiac anomalies (PHACE syndrome).

15.4.6 Management

Reassurance and waiting for spontaneous involution were the mainstay of treatment a decade ago. (Fig. 15.3) The natural history of hemangiomas should influence the timing and type of interven-

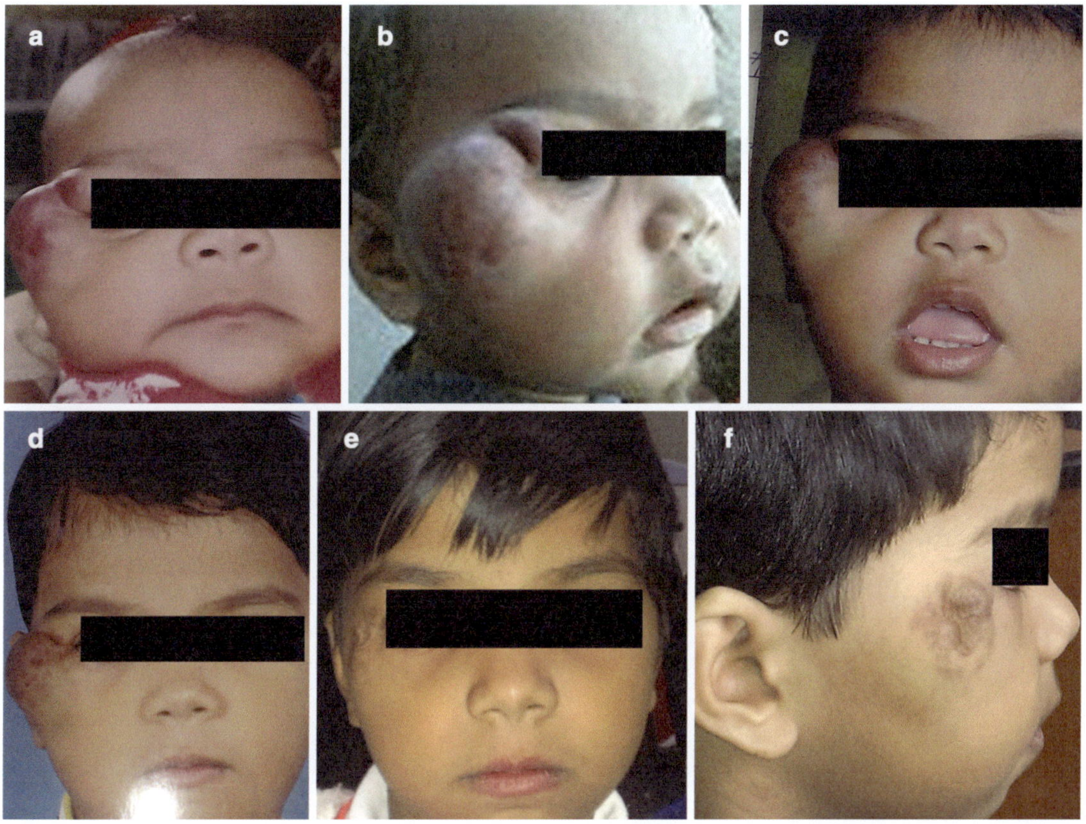

Fig. 15.3 —Infantile hemangioma–Spontaneous regression. (**a**) Clinical picture at one month of age. (**b**) At 5 months of age (**c**) At 2 years of age. (**d**) At 4 years of age. (**e, f**) At 7 years of age

tion. The treatment of choice depends on several factors including the age of the patient and the size and extent of the lesions, as well as their clinical characteristics.

As the understanding of the disease is increasing, more therapeutic options are available and emerging recognition of aesthetic consequences, more and more Hemangiomas are being treated in early phases. It is well recognized that incomplete resolution is common and they may frequently leave fibrofatty residue and scar. In the involution phase, the aim is to improve appearance and function and the treatment should never give a worse result than after natural involution.

Treatment is recommended in the proliferative phase as rapid growth can lead to worsening of function, obstruction/cosmetic issues Various treatments have been used in the management of Hemangiomas, including oral corticosteroids, intralesional injection of fibrosing agents, interferon α2b, radiation, electrocoagulation, cryosurgery, laser therapy, embolization and surgical excision Factors such as patient's age, size and site of lesion and the proximity of the lesion to the vital structure are paramount in the determination of the therapeutic approach and surgical excision. Currently, sclerotherapy is employed largely because of its efficiency and ability to conserve the surrounding tissues [3, 10].

Steroid Therapy: Prednisolone is the first-line drug of choice for the treatment of life- or sight-threatening hemangiomas. The response rate varies from 30 to 90% and depends on the dose, duration and age at the start of treatment. Steroids are useful only in the proliferative phase [10].

Propranolol therapy: It is a non-selective beta-blocker used in 2–3 mg/kg/ day in 3 divided doses. Baseline ECG needs to be done before starting the therapy [11].

It works best in the proliferative phase. Once the Hemangioma is regressed, it needs to be tapered and stopped. (Fig. 15.4) The mechanism of Action is unclear, although the most likely effect is the pharmacological stimulation programmed endothelial cell death (apoptosis). There are no serious adverse effects but some minor effects may be seen like the pharmacologi-

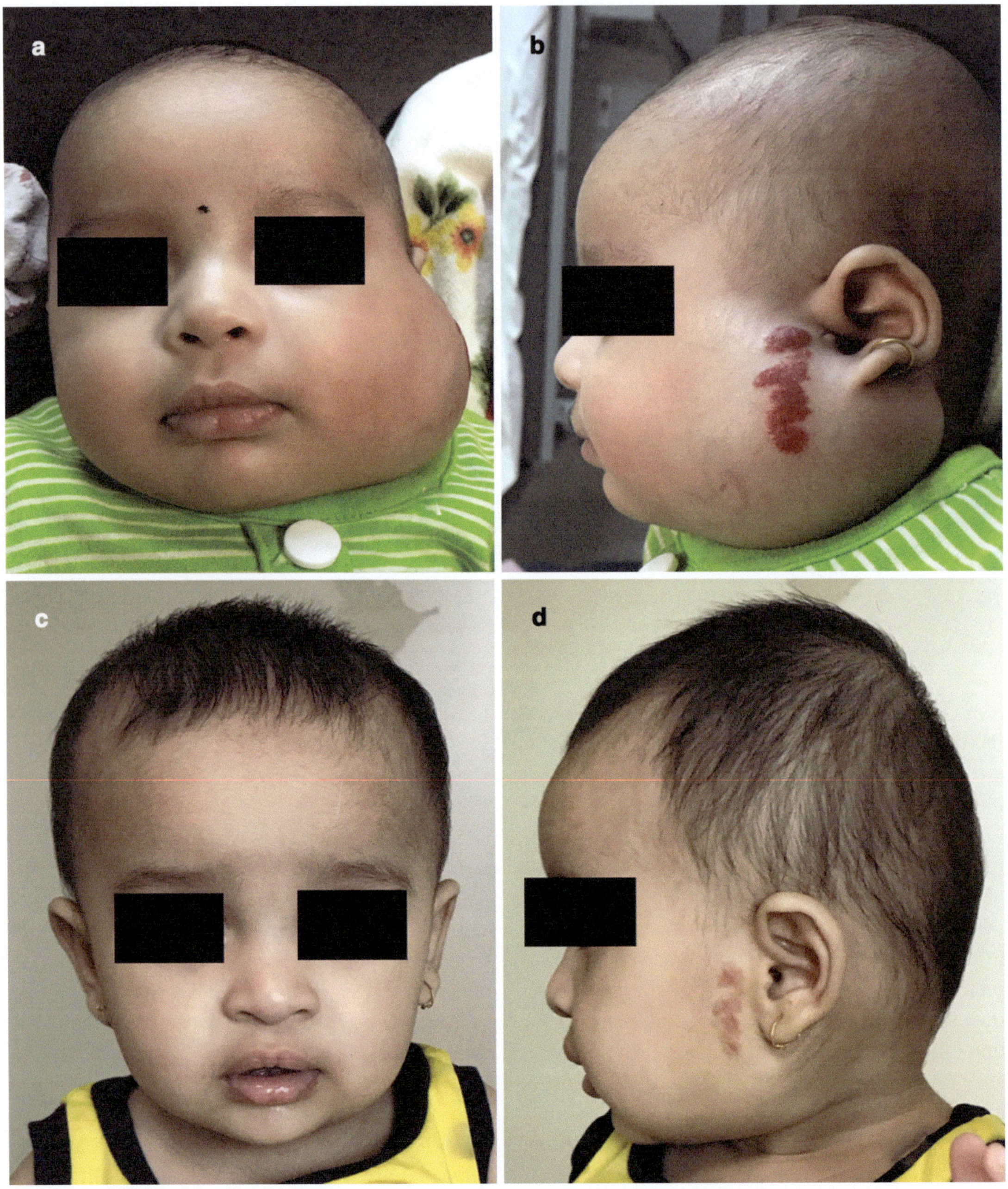

Fig. 15.4 Clinical photographs of a 3-month-old kid who was presented with a left parotid swelling and was managed with Propranolol therapy. (**a**, **b**) Soft, diffuse swelling with overlying skin having reddish discoloration which is pulsatile inferiorly. (**c**, **d**) Patient 6 months after propranolol therapy showing regression of infantile hemangioma with some minor residual tissue

cal stimulation programmed endothelial cell death (apoptosis). There are no serious adverse effects but some minor effects may be seen like hypoglycaemia, somnolence, gastroesophageal reflux, bronchospasm and allergic rash. Propranolol has revolutionized the management of Hemangiomas offers the best medical treatment to date for this purpose. Adverse effects of propranolol are minor like bradycardia, hypotension, hypoglycaemia, bronchospasm, somnolence, gastroesophageal reflux and allergic rash [11, 12]. High-output cardiac failure can occur in infants with very large IH and PHACES syndrome.

Percutaneous Sclerotherapy: Direct puncture of the lesion and sclerotherapy is the mainstay of treatment for lesions not responding to propranolol therapy or for residual lesions. The commonly used sclerosant is Bleomycin. The usual dose is 1 U/kg, with a maximum of 15 units [10, 13]. (Fig. 15.5).

Transarterial Embolization: Endovascular therapy through the feeding arteries can be performed in the proliferative phase. This can lead to rapid regression of the lesion. (Fig. 15.6) This is extremely useful in cases where functional disturbance is a major concern especially in large Hemangiomas and preoperatively if surgical excision is planned [14]. (Fig. 15.7).

Surgical Excision: It is not performed regularly and is usually indicated when there is no response to systemic treatments or for aesthetic reasons, is performed as a simple excision in combination or not with plastic surgery. It is usually preceded by endovascular embolization.

Transarterial onyx may be used for intraosseous hemangiomas which present as firm swellings [15]. (Fig. 15.8).

Laser therapies are done for involuted tissues and mainly for cosmetic reasons.

15.4.7 Tongue/Floor of Mouth Hemangiomas

Although Hemangioma is considered one of the most common soft tissue tumours of the head

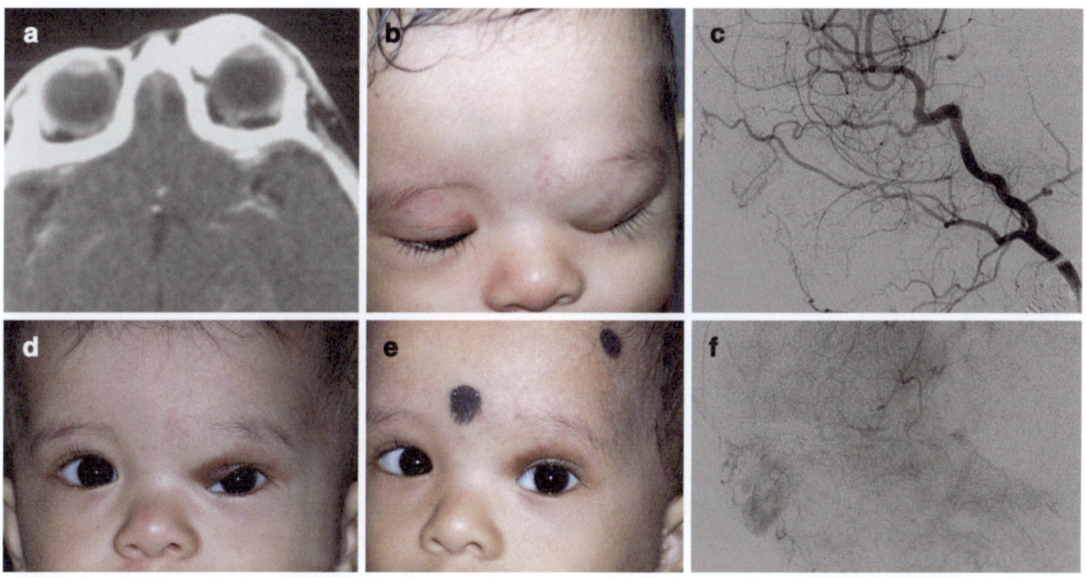

Fig. 15.5 Four-month-old girl with left upper eyelid hemangioma. She was not responding to propranolol therapy. Two sessions of intralesional bleomycin sclerotherapy were performed. Early intervention is advised as there is risk of amblyopia. (**a**) Post-contrast axial CT showing intensely enhancing left upper eyelid lesion suggestive of hemangioma. (**b**) Clinical photograph at the time of presentation shoeing swelling with reddish discolouration. (**d**) After the first session. (**e**) After the final session showing a significant reduction of swelling with normal palpebral fissure. (**c**) & (**f**) Subtraction angiography in Lateral and AP view showing the hypervascular blush of the hemangioma in the proliferative phase

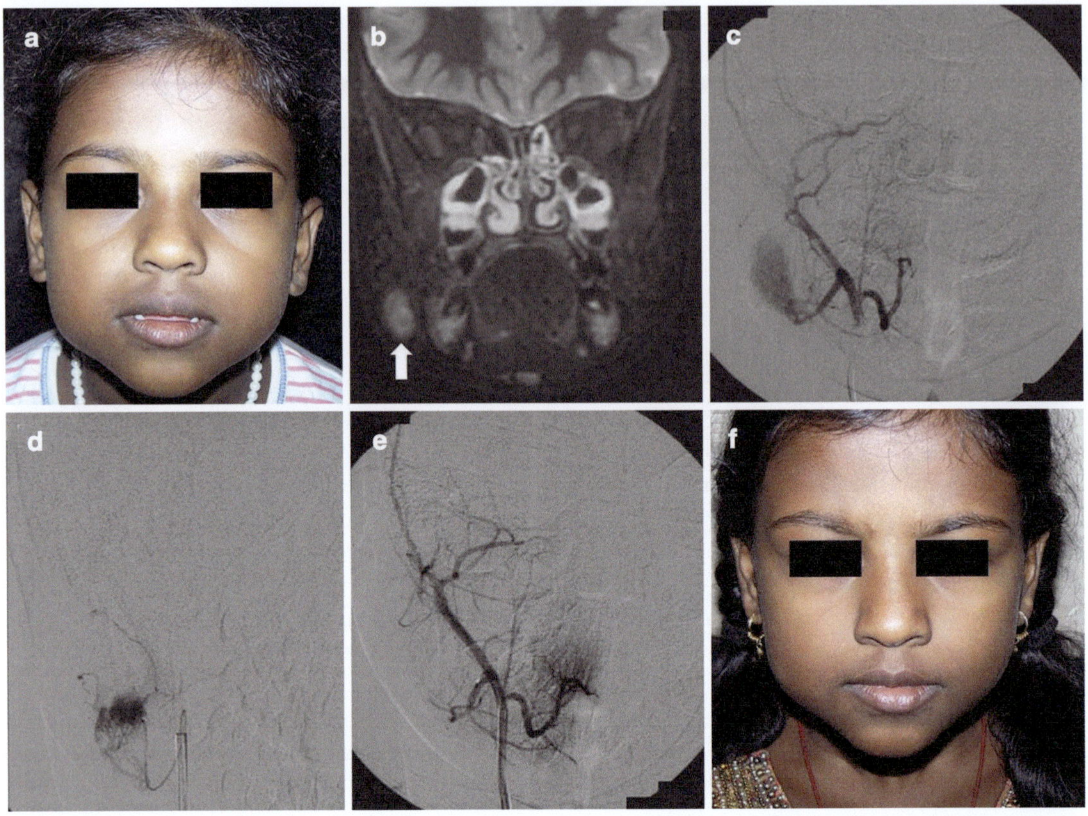

Fig. 15.6 A 7-Year-old girl with right cheek hemangioma treated with transarterial embolization. (**a**) Clinical photograph at presentation showing small right cheek hemangioma. (**b**) Preoperative T2 weight coronal magnetic resonance imaging showing hyperintense soft tissue lesion suggestive of hemangioma. (**c**) right External carotid angiogram showing intense vascular blush. (**d**) Microcatheter navigated into the feeding artery. Transarterial PVA particle embolisation was performed. (**e**) Post-embolisation angiogram showing occlusion of the feeding artery. (**f**) 1 year follow-up clinical photograph showing complete resolution of the right cheek swelling

and neck, it is relatively rare in the oral cavity. Lingual Hemangiomas pose distressing problems to the patients, producing cosmetic deformity, macroglossia, recurrent haemorrhage and functional problems like difficulty in speaking, deglutition and mastication [3].

15.5 Vascular Malformations

15.5.1 Introduction

These are the lesions resulting due to an error in morphogenesis that is populated by stable mature vascular endothelium. No specific sex predominance is noted. They are always present at birth, although may not be noticed and grow commensurate with child's development. (though some may not be apparent until a later stage). They are subclassified based on flow and predominant type of vessel involved. Unlike Hemangiomas, vascular malformations may be associated with skeletal abnormalities. It is believed that the enlargement of these lesions is the result of changes in pressure and flow, ectasia, shunting and collateral proliferation. It may increase in size secondary to various triggering factors such as increased blood flow, arterial occlusion and venous thrombosis. Trauma or hormonal changes can also affect the size of the lesion. The high flow lesion may be stimulated by various factors including endocrine factors (puberty and pregnancy), trauma, iatrogenic insults such as incomplete surgery and proximal embolization and infection [1].

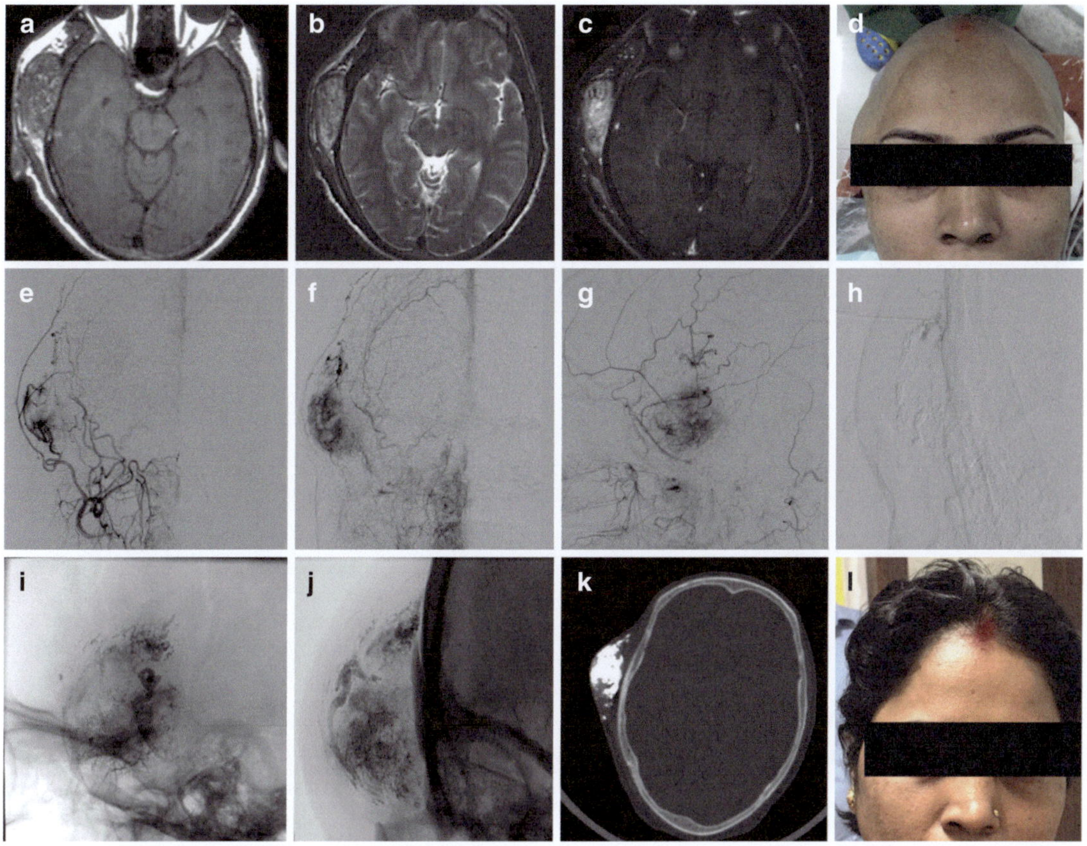

Fig. 15.7 Thirty-two-year-old lady with right temporal scalp swelling since childhood. (**a**, **b** & **c**) MRI T1WI, T2WI, Post-contrast T1WI showing soft tissue lesion in the right temporal scalp region which is intensely enhancing on post-contrast study. (**d**) Clinical picture before embolization. (**e** & **f**) Right ECA angiogram in early arterial and late arterial phase shows intense vascular blush. (**g**) Late arterial phase in lateral view. (**h**) Direct puncture of the lesion done with 24G scalp vein needle. Check angiography to confirm intravascular position of the needle. After confirmation dilute Glue(NBCA) was injected mixed with lipiodol. (**i** & **j**) Plain radiograph in the lateral and AP view respectively showing the Glue cast. The lesion was excised after the embolisation with minimal blood loss. (**k**) Plain CT showing the lipiodol and glue cast within the lesion. (**l**) 4 months Post-surgical excision showing the good clinical and cosmetic result

Progesterone receptors are highly expressed in venous malformation, which might be one of the reasons for the rapid increase in the size of the malformation when hormonal level changes.

Association with Sinus Pericranii: Some Venous malformations are associated with sinus pericranii and intracranial DVAs. Sinus pericranii is particularly suspected when an extracranial venous malformation is found in the presence of calvarial involvement. The sinus pericranii must be occluded before therapeutic injection of the focal lesion [8]. (Fig. 15.23).

15.5.2 Classification

It can be divided into two subtypes based on the flow of the lesion [1].

Low Flow Vascular Malformation: They have no arteriovenous shunts.

- Capillary (Port-wine) malformation
- Venous malformation
- Lymphatic malformation
- Venous lymphatic malformation
- Combination of above

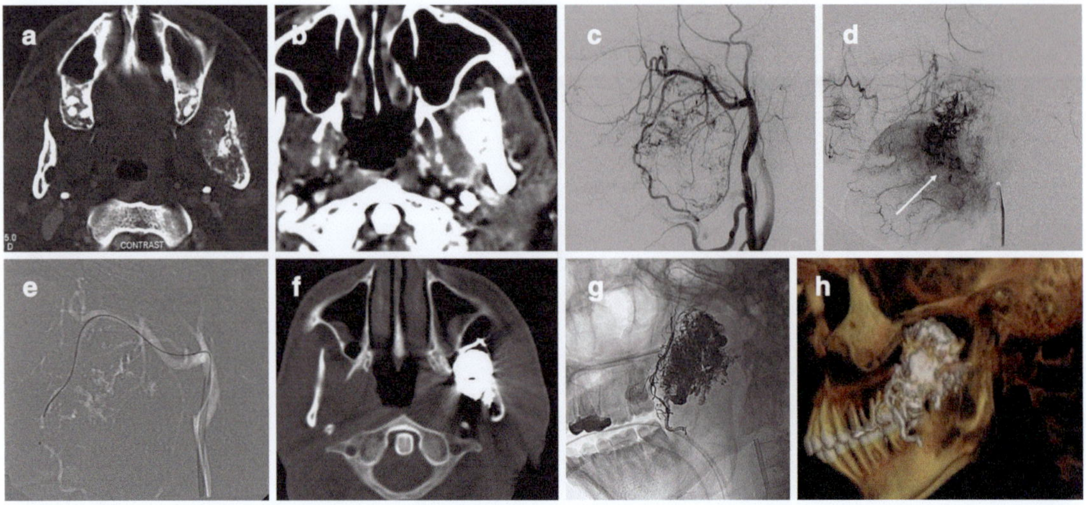

Fig. 15.8 Young boy with firm swelling in the left cheek region. (**a**) CT scan shows an expansile lytic lesion in the rams of the left mandible with soft tissue adjacent to it. (**b**) Post-contrast CT images showing intense contrast enhancement. (**c**, **d**) Catheter angiography shows slow puddling of contrast in the region of the lesion. (**e**) Arterial roadmap showing the catheter position in one of the feeding arteries. Transarterial Onyx injection was done. (**f**, **g**, **h**) Axial CT, Plain radiograph and 3D reconstructed CT image showing the onyx cast within the mandibular lesion

High Flow Vascular Malformation: Associated with Arteriovenous shunting.

- Arteriovenous malformation
- Arteriovenous fistula

15.5.3 Low Flow Vascular Malformation

15.5.3.1 Capillary Malformation (Previously Called Port-Wine Stain/Capillary Hemangioma)

They are made up of postcapillary venules within the papillary and superficial reticular dermis which may dilate with time. They present as flat pink macules but darken and thicken with age resulting in cobblestone appearance. (Figs. 15.9 and 15.10) The capillary malformation is commonly associated with Sturge–Weber Syndrome (Fig. 15.11) and Klippel–Trenaunay Syndrome. They may be associated with enlargement of the affected lip, gingiva, maxilla and mandible. Skeletal overgrowth may not be obvious at birth but progress in childhood. (Fig. 15.12) Pyogenic granuloma frequently develops within port-wine stains, particularly in the oral cavity. (Fig. 15.13) They are extremely difficult to eradicate because of the continual stimulus of local irritation. In patients with dento-alveolar distortions osteotomy can be performed without the fear of bleeding [7, 16].

CVMS (Cerebrofacial Venous Metameric Syndrome)

Encephalotrigeminal angiomatosis or Sturge–Weber syndrome (SWS) is a non-familial disease with a skin discolouration (port-wine stain) in the trigeminal V1 territory, associated with a calcified leptomeningeal venous malformation of the ipsilateral supratentorial hemisphere. Symptoms appear before the second year of age and include problems in cosmesis and neurological problems due to subadjacent cerebral atrophy, leading to epilepsy, deficits and mental retardation. Port-wine stain that represent localized dermal venular malformation are classically present. (Fig. 15.11).

CVMS 1 has involvement of forehead and nose formed from the medial prosencephalic group (olfactory); CVMS 2 arise from the lateral prosencephalic group (optic) with involvement of occipital lobe, eye, cheek and maxilla; CVMS 3

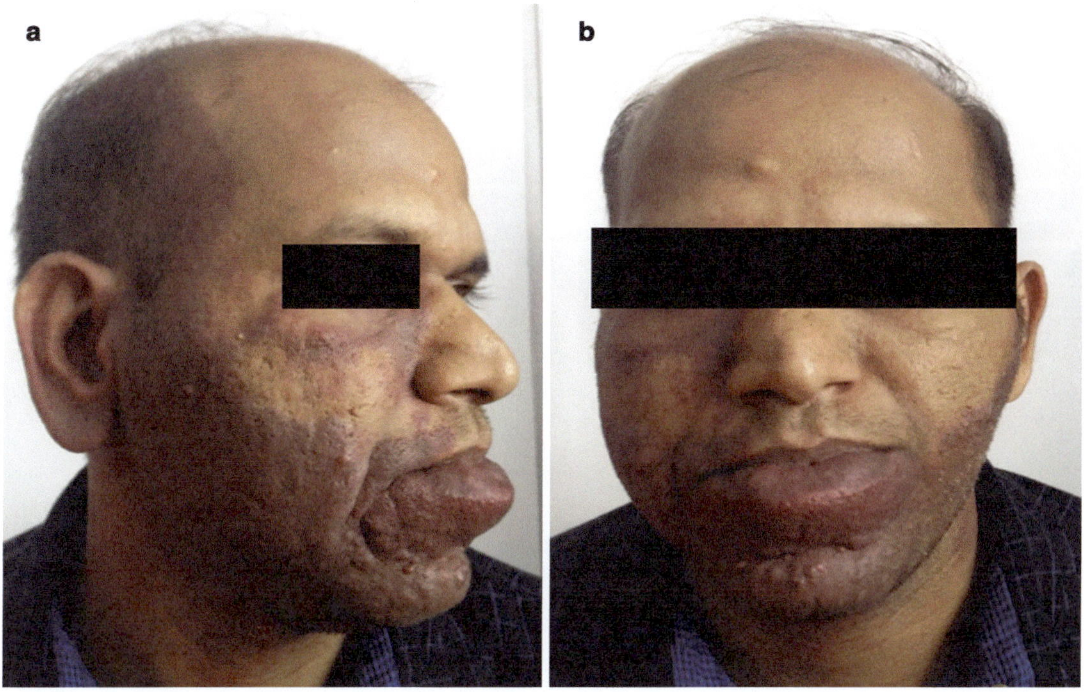

Fig. 15.9 (**a**, **b**) Clinical picture showing port-wine stain

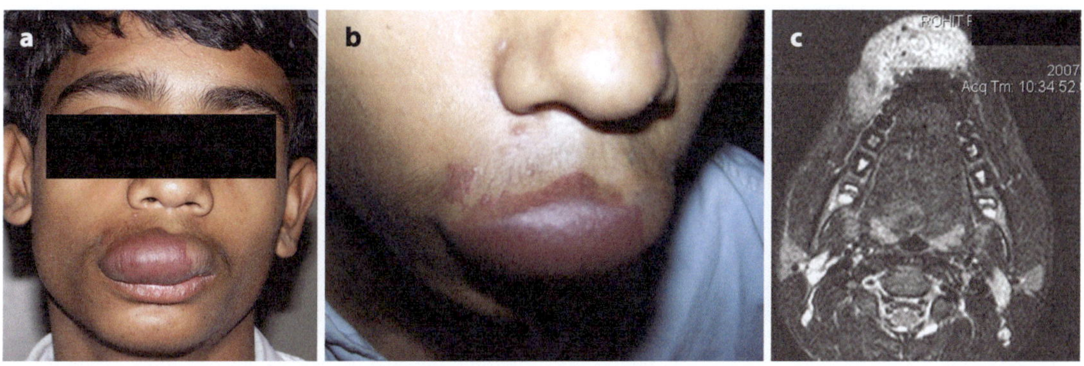

Fig. 15.10 Young boy with upper lip swelling since childhood. (**a**, **b**) Clinical photograph. (**c**) MRI STIR images showing Soft tissue hyperintense lesion flush with the skin that is involving the subcutaneous tissue. This is a diagnostic feature of the capillary malformation. Percutaneous sclerotherapy was attempted with bleomycin however there was no response

arise from the rhombencephalic (otic) group and involve the cerebellum, lower face and mandible [4, 16]. (Fig. 15.12).

15.5.3.2 Venous Malformation

The incidence of venous malformation is 1: 5000–1:10000; approximately 40% of them occur in the head and neck regions. It is the most common vascular malformation present at birth, but they are not always evident. They grow proportionately to the child, expand slowly and often enlarge during puberty. Superficial or deep lesions can be present and they can involve single or multiple anatomical sites. Cheek, neck, eyelids, lips, tongue, soft palate, parapharyngeal space and floor of the mouth are the most com-

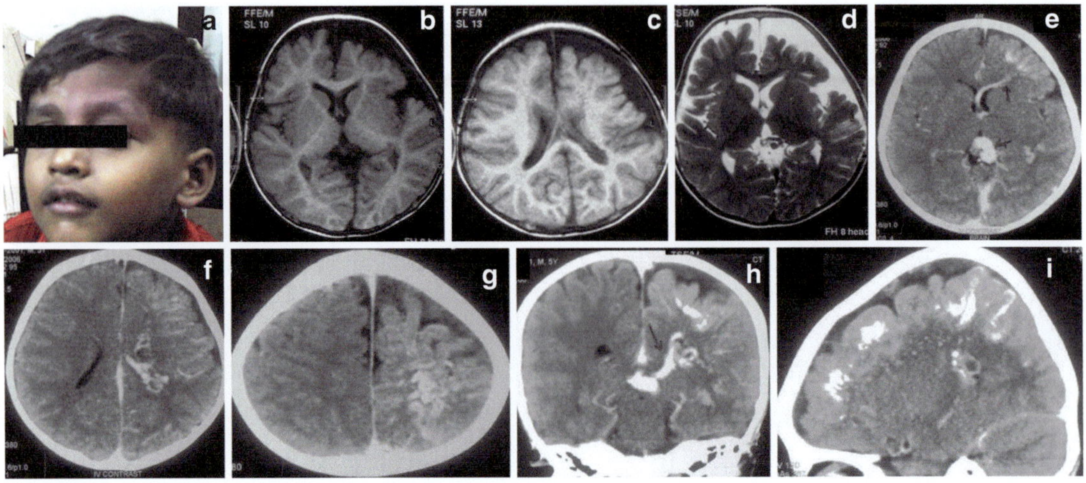

Fig. 15.11 (**a**) Four-year-old boy presenting with left forehead swelling. (**b**, **c**, **d**) MRI and (**e**, **f**, **g**, **h**, **i**) CT scan showing features of venous abnormalities of Sturge–Weber syndrome. (CVMS-1)

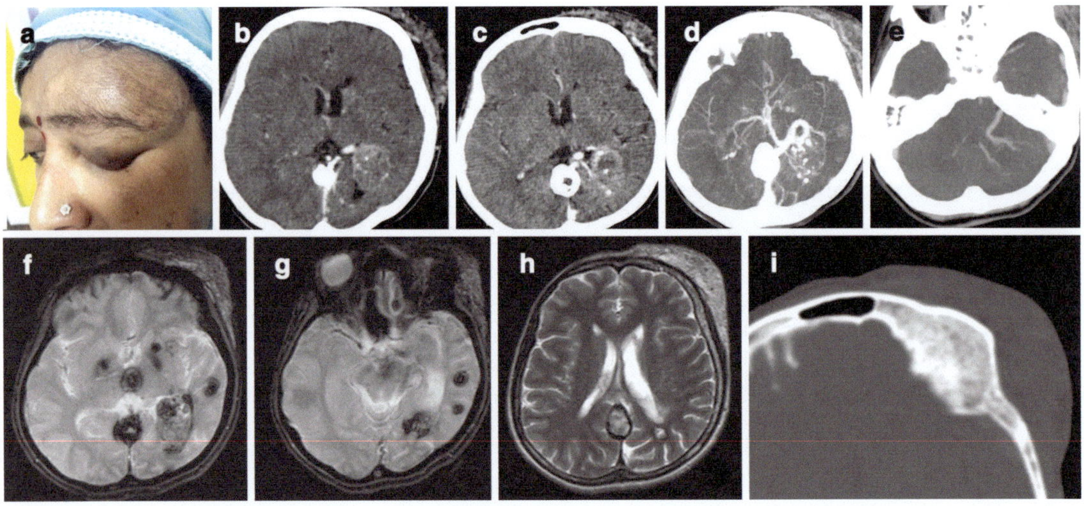

Fig. 15.12 Forty-year-old lady with swelling on the left eyelid. (**a**) Left eye exenteration was done in childhood, the cause of which is unknown. (**b-i**) CT and MRI show the soft tissue swelling suggestive of hemangioma with multiple intracranial venous abnormalities, i.e. developmental venous anomalies with calcifications, cavernomas and bony hypertrophy (CVMS 2 & 3)

mon anatomical sites affected [17]. Head and neck VMs involve both superficial and deep tissues and are often trans-spatial with a predilection for the muscles of mastication [1].

They are caused due to an error in the development within the venous system and are composed of thin-walled, dilated sponge-like channels of variable size and thickness. The typical skeletal changes which can occur are increase in the size of underlying the bone, hypertrophy, distortion of shape. A dramatic increase in size is seen with puberty or other hormonal changes. They can be associated with syndromes like Blue rubber bleb nevus syndrome (TIE2 receptor mutation), Glomuvenous malformation, multiple cutaneomucosal venous malformations, BRBN syndrome and Maffucci syndrome. Blue rubber bleb nevus syndrome comprises of multiple cutane-

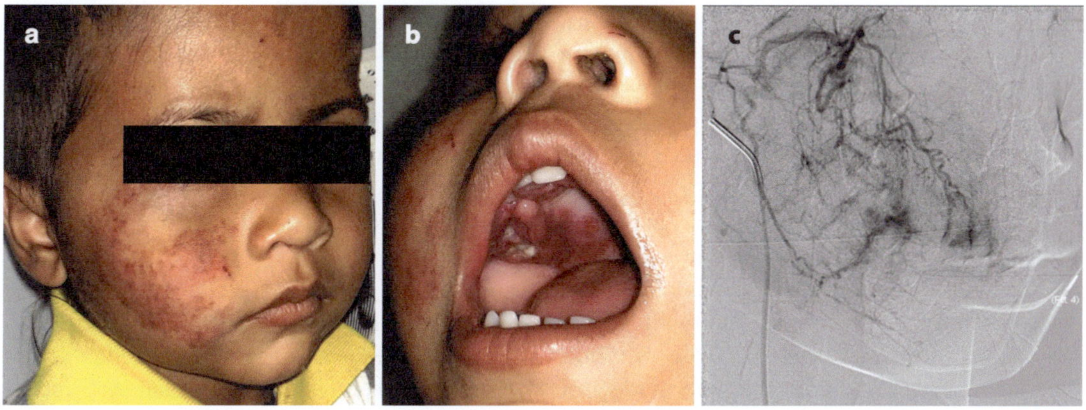

Fig. 15.13 One-year-old boy with pinkish discolouration of the right cheek.(**a**) (**b**) Intraoral view shows mucosal discolouration as well as gum hypertrophy. These findings are suggestive of pyogenic Granuloma. (**c**) Right ECA angiogram in oblique view shows hypervascular blush in the region of upper gums

ous VMS in association with soft tissue and gastrointestinal lesions [16].

15.5.4 Clinical Features

They are frequently obvious at birth and symptoms to depend upon the location of the lesion. Swelling is the most common complaint especially increasing in size on dependency, on waking up in the morning or on Valsalva manoeuvre. Pain or dragging sensation or discomfort is common in venous malformations of head and neck region secondary to pooling of blood in the abnormal venous pools in dependent positions so often in the early morning on awakening or with exertion.

Disfigurement may also be seen with these malformations. Cosmetic issues can lead to psychological stress and feeling of low self-esteem. Venous malformations in the parapharyngeal space, tongue, soft palate may be accompanied by swallowing, speech and airway problems. Compression of adjacent structures leading to an impact on speech, swallowing and respiratory functions. Airway compression is common with extensive lesions [18]. On examination, they are soft, compressible bluish to purplish swelling with ill-defined margins. They increase in size on dependency or Valsalva manoeuvre which is one of the characteristic features of venous malformation. Phleboliths may be palpable. It may be complicated by Trauma or venous stasis can cause clot formation within the lesion leading to pain and sudden increase in swelling. Other cause of a sudden increase in size may be secondary an infection or abrupt intralesional haemorrhage [3, 8].

15.5.5 Investigations

X Rays of the lesion can show Phleboliths. Jaw bone lesions may have honey combed appearance.

USG shows Hypoechoic cystic lesion with a monophasic low-velocity flow or no flow.

CT: Hypoattenuating/heterogenous lesions. Enhances slowly or peripherally. Phleboliths.

MRI: Diagnostic modality of choice. Fat suppressed T2 weighted sequences in all three planes are important. They are classically multilobulated T2 hyperintense multilobulated lesions 'bunch of grapes' hypointense or isointense on T1WI [7, 19].

DSA: No opacification or puddling of contrast in the venous pouches [19].

15.5.6 Management

Cosmetic issues are the most common Indication for the treatment of venous malformations. The aim of therapy is cure for small localized lesions. Control of symptoms or considerable reduction is the aim in multifocal, extensive trans-spatial lesions. Restoring function and improving cosmesis is important while treating these non-lethal lesions [16].

Percutaneous or Permucosal Sclerotherapy:

It involves direct puncture of the lesion and injections of a sclerosant to induce inflammation and thrombosis of the lesion which will lead to long-term fibrosis and hence decrease or eliminate the lesion. This is the first-line therapy of these lesions. Sclerotherapy induces an inflammatory reaction that will worsen the symptoms during the week following intervention. The lesion is punctured directly using a 24-gauge scalp vein needle [20]. Sometimes USG guidance may be necessary. The spinal needle needed for deeper lesions and orbital venous malformations. Multiple sessions are needed based on the site and size of the lesion [3, 21].

15.5.7 Considerations during Sclerotherapy

Under sterile precautions, the lesion is punctured using 24- or 23-gauge scalp vein needle in the softest component. Then aspiration is done to confirm backflow of blood which confirms intralesional positioning of the needle tip. In the presence of good venous backflow, venography is performed with diluted contrast. The Sclerosant mixed with a contrast agent is then injected under the fluoroscopy roadmap guidance. The fluoroscopy helps in looking for spread of the agent, extravasation into surrounding soft tissue and most importantly drainage into adjacent venous system. Simultaneously, it is important to look at the lesion especially in mucosal sites for distension. It is important that during injection, the sclerosant should remain within the lesion and not wash out. To minimize washout, if the vein is superficial, it can be manually compressed while the sclerosant is injected. it should be kept compressed for about 5–10 minutes after that. If the vein is large or deep in location, transvenous occlusion with Coils, glue or balloon can be done before injecting the sclerosant. Post-sclerotherapy, the swelling increase for 48–72 hrs. Symptomatic management is done with analgesics and anti-inflammatory agents (NSAIDs) to minimize the symptoms. Elevation of the head and cold compression are beneficial for a day or two after the sclerotherapy. The usual Interval between sessions should be 4–6 weeks [8, 21, 22, 31].

Follow-up MRI is important to analyse the residual lesion. It can be compared with pre-treatment MRI. A considerable reduction is considered when there is more than 90% reduction of the swelling, especially in larger ones. Sclerotherapy has multiple advantages over Surgery. It is less invasive, good maintenance of cosmesis, reduced hospital stays, outpatient department procedure, no Anaesthesia for Adults, no external scarring [21].

15.5.8 Sclerosants

Ethanol: the volume is assessed based on direct puncture venography. It induces thrombogenesis as a result of chemical damage to the vascular wall and is highly effective but has higher rates of complication. The injection rate and the amount must be carefully controlled under fluoroscopic guidance [23, 24]. The side effect of ethanol use are skin necrosis, neural toxicity, renal toxicity and cardiac arrest [17, 23].

Setrol/STD—Sodium tetradecyl Sulphate is the time-tested agent. It is mixed with non-ionic contrast agent at 66% concentration. It is more efficacious with fewer side effects [25]. Adverse effects are mainly cutaneous necrosis due to extravasation and methemoglobinuria when injected in larger volumes [22, 25]. (Fig. 15.14).

Bleomycin is in the form of powder (15 unit) which is reconstituted with 15 ml of normal saline. Bleomycin has been shown to provide good results and an excellent safety profile. Maximum dose of 1 unit/kg in <1 year of age and in more than >1 year of age, not more than 15 units or mg/session. It has works by multiple mechanisms like cytotoxic, antitumor, antibiotic causing a specific sclerosing effect on vascular malformation [13] (Fig. 15.15).

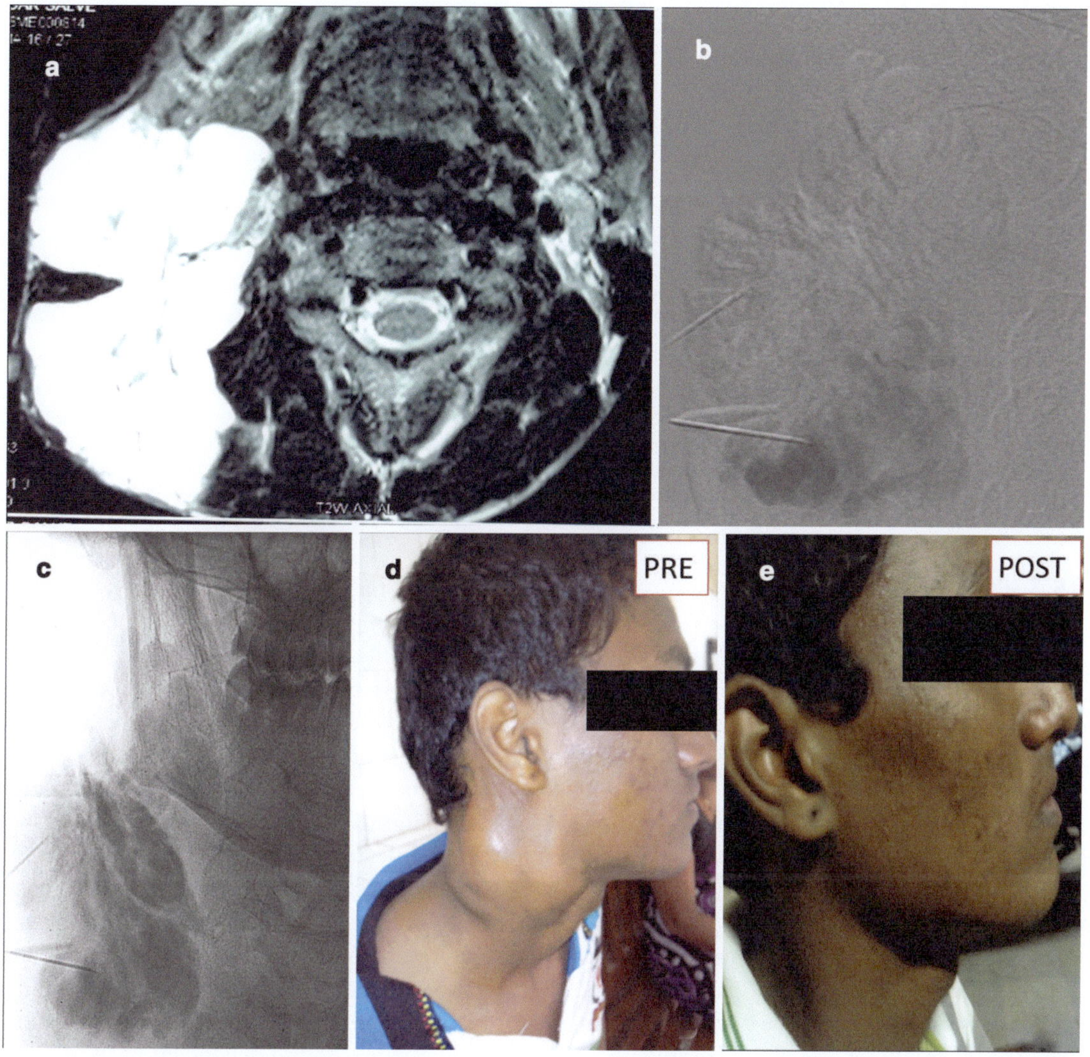

Fig. 15.14 A 16-year-old male presented with a large swelling in the neck. (**a**) Axial magnetic resonance imaging T2WI showing a T2 hyperintense multilobulated in the posterior triangle of the neck suggestive of venous malformation. Percutaneous sclerotherapy was performed with direct puncture sclerosant injection.(sodium tetradecyl sulphate) (**b**) Roadmap showing the spread of the contrast mixed setrol (STD)within the lesion (**c**) Plain radiograph showing the contrast mixed with setrol (STD in the lesion. (**d**) Clinical photograph of the patient at the presentation showing a large soft compressible swelling in the posterolateral aspect of the neck. in the neck region. (**e**) Clinical photograph 6 months post sclerotherapy showing resolution of the malformation

Combination of bleomycin with setrol is more effective with reduced number of sessions and reduced complications. The combination is found to be most effective and associated with the least complications. It is commonly used sclerosant in the author's centre. (Fig. 15.16).

Polidocanol is a mixture of 5% Ethyl alcohol and 95% hydroxyl polyethyldodecane. It works by detergent action which induces rapid overhydration of endothelial cells leading to vascular injury. It is not so commonly used. Direct puncture and NBCA injection with lipiodol may be used for preoperative embolization, if that is bieng considered in a particular case. we recommend the use of glue (NBCA) only for occluding the outflow vein if the VM is draining into an important neck vein. then subsequently sclerose the lesion with sclerosants like STD or bleomycin [30].

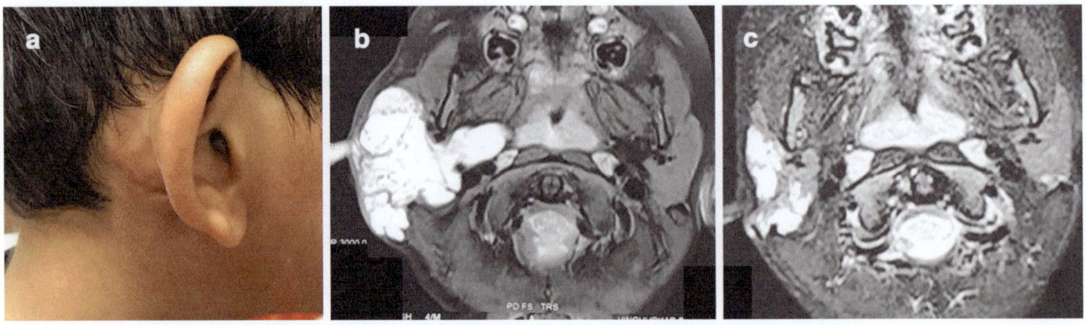

Fig. 15.15 Parotid VM . 7 year old boy with swelling in the posterior and infra auricular region which was increasing in size on dependant position. (**a**) Clinical photograph. (**b**) Presclerotherapy T2WI of MRI showing large Parotid and postauricular Venous malformation. Sclerotherapy was performed using direct puncture intralesional Bleomycin injection. There is a risk of LMN Facial palsy post sclerotherapy hence only bleomycin was used as it is less inflammatory. There were no post-procedural complications. Post-procedure steroid was given for 5 days to control the swelling. (**c**) 6 months post sclerotherapy MRI showing significant resolution of the swelling

15.5.9 Surgical Excision

Indications of excision are *limited in the era of sclerotherapy*. Residual lesions post-sclerotherapy causing cosmetic and functional issues and localized lesions are the only indications for surgery [22].

15.5.10 Specific Locations

The lesions close to the airway need to be managed with airway protection by elective intubation or tracheostomy based on the size, location and extent of the lesion for 2–3 days [18] (Figs. 15.17 and 15.18).

Another important location is orbit. The access is important and General Anaesthesia is needed. Spinal needle is to be used for retroorbital lesions.

Sonographic guidance is of utmost importance for retroorbital lesions. (Fig. 15.19).

Parotid location—Post-sclerotherapy there is an increased risk of lower motor neuron facial nerve paresis. Use of Bleomycin alone as a sclerosant can reduce inflammation and the use of short-term steroids post-sclerotherapy is always suggested [13, 22]. (Fig. 15.15).

Tongue venous malformation needs to be managed carefully as an aggressive approach can lead to necrosis. it requires more number of sessions compared to the other locations. (Fig. 15.20). if the posterior one-third of the tongue is involved with or without parapharyngeal component needs intubation before the sclerosant injection. The intubation is to be continued for 48–72 hours till the edema subsides. Steroid injection helps in the periperiprocedural period. (Fig. 15.21).

Paraspinal venous malformations need special consideration as good imaging is mandatory to look for intracanalicular extension. (Fig. 15.22).

Venous Varix is a separate entity as these distend enormously in dependant position and may drain completely under gravity. The documentation of the communication with draining vein is important. Imaging in the prone position for orbital varies and in dependant position may document the actual size of varix. The treatment considerations are compression of the draining vein during sclerotherapy or actual transvenous blocking of the draining veins is required. in orbital varies, the use of bleomycin alone is important with lateral canthotomy prior to the procedure. This reduces theirs of eyeball compression in the post-procedure period [14, 20]. (Figs. 15.23 and 15.24).

Complications: Infection of the injection site was the commonest complication followed by superficial skin necrosis (2%) due to inadvertent extravascular injection of the sclerosing agent. Most of these are successfully managed with antibiotics and rarely require reconstructive flap surgery. Other minor complications were skin blisters and radiating pain in the neck and

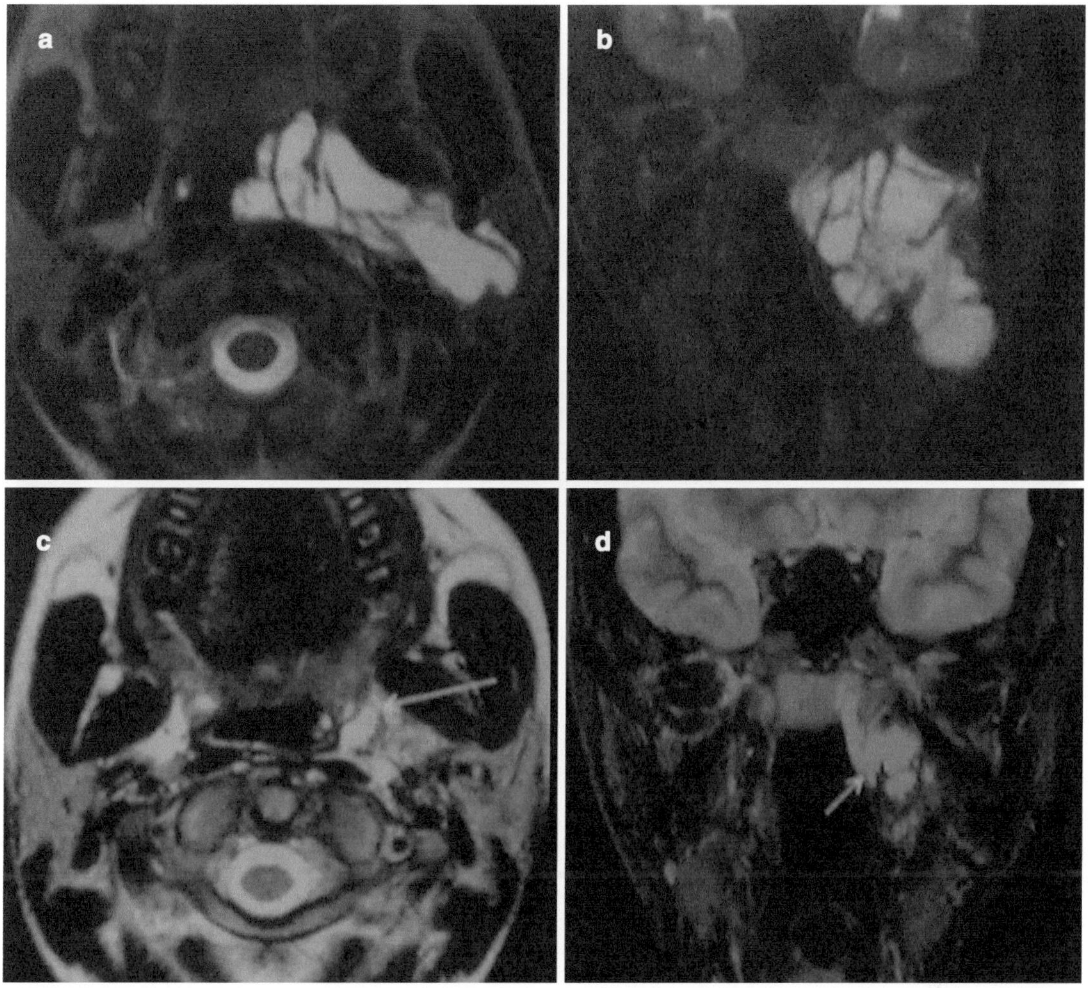

Fig. 15.16 A 16-year-old female present with a left-sided neck swelling extending up to the parapharyngeal space. (**a**) Preoperative Magnetic resonance imaging axial section showing a hyperintense lobulated venolymphatic malformation involving the parotid and the parapharyngeal space. (**b**) Preoperative Magnetic Resonance imaging sagittal section showing hyperintense lobular lymphatic malformation extending from the level of the mandible to the upper border of laryngeal cartilage in the parapharyngeal space. (**c**, **d**) Post bleomycin sclerotherapy magnetic resonance imaging axial and sagittal section showing the considerable reduction in the size and extent of malformation with no clinical evidence of swelling

paraspinal venous malformations. (Fig. 15.25). Bleomycin can sometimes cause flagellate erythema [13, 22]. (Fig. 15.26).

15.5.10.1 Lymphatic Malformation

They are congenital collection of ectatic lymph vessels that form endothelial lined cystic spaces. More than 75% of Lymphatic malformations are found in the neck. They are classified as macrocystic (> = 2 cm), microcystic (<2 cm) or combined. Macrocystic lesions are more easily treated and carry a better prognosis than its microcystic counterpart. The most common location for lymphatic malformations includes the neck (approximately 75%) and Axilla. Cervical lesions are usually of macrocystic type cystic hygroma and those involving the floor of the mouth, cheek, tongue are more likely to be diffuse microcystic type. Cervicofacial malformation leads to the overgrowth and distortion of the underlying maxilla and mandible, as well as adjacent ear cartilage is typical skeletal changes seen with lymphatic malformations. They

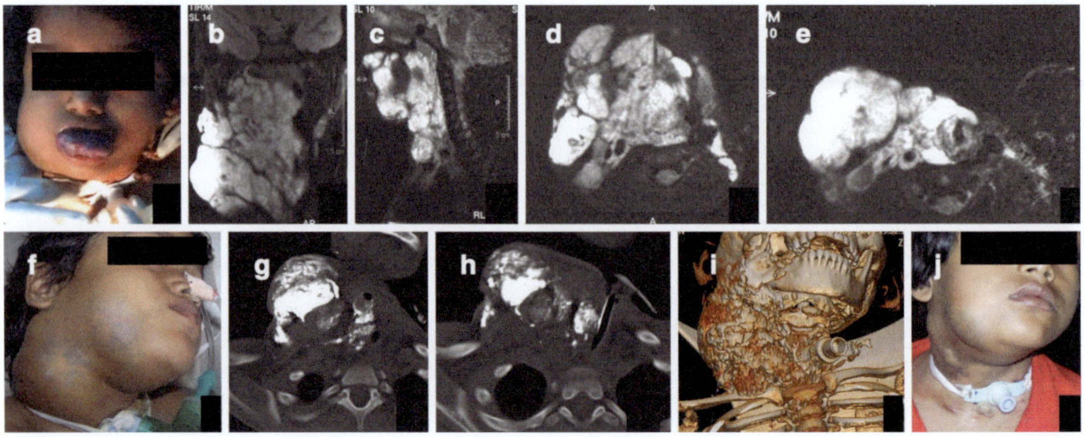

Fig. 15.17 Six- year-old girl presenting with bluish swelling on right side of neck, cheek and tongue noticed since the age of 2 yrs. and is gradually increasing. There was stridor at presentation and a history of snoring. On examination, the swelling was diffuse, large, ill-defined, soft, compressible, non-pulsatile, non-tender along right cheek, tongue and right side of the neck. Swelling is extending into the oropharynx. Swelling increases on valsalva manoeuver and dependent position. Multiple phleboliths were palpable. (**a**) Clinical photograph just before the first session with tracheostomy tube in situ and glossoptosis. (**b**, **c**, **d**, **e**) Coronal, Sagittal and axial MRI images show large transpatial Venous malformation involving the right side of the neck from chin upto anterior chest wall & medially extending up to left pharyngeal tongue, the floor of mouth and laryngeal wall. Elective tracheostomy was performed prior to sclerotherapy. There was difficulty in accessing the trachea due to overlying venous malformation. There was episode of desaturation during the attempt. She was kept on Oxygen support for 2 days and then taken for sclerotherapy. Three sessions of percutaneous sclerotherapy were done in quick succession. The swelling was punctured in the cheek & lateral part of the neck & around the trachea initially to promote the regression of medial dangerous component first. In total 70 cc of 66% STD mixed with Lipiodol was injected at different sites. Post-op. every time, she developed episodes of mild oxygen desaturation (85%) which was managed with nebulization and oxygen support. During the third session when swelling around the trachea was punctured. There was mild extravasation during the injection of Sclerosant following which there was oozing around the tracheostomy tube and from the tube. Managed by compression and surgical and Gelfoam packing. (**f**) Clinical picture before the third session showing a reduction in tongue protrusion. (**g**, **h**, and **i**) CT after the third session shows good Lipiodol cast in the neck region (anterior triangle of the neck) extending into the anterior mediastinum, paratracheal region and in the tracheal wall. Residual swelling was noted in the parapharyngeal region. J. Clinical picture at 4 months follow-up from the last session shows a significant reduction of the swelling. The tracheostomy was closed at this admission

are prone to infection, haemorrhage, pain and mass effect [1] (Fig. 15.27).

15.5.11 Clinical Features

The lesions can be focal, multifocal, diffuse, macrocystic or microcystic. Oral cavity and airway are commonly involved in more diffuse lesions. They usually grow slowly but sometimes may rapidly swell with infections or with hormonal changes such as puberty. The earlier in life they present, the more aggressive it is likely to be and more prone to complications. The lymphatic malformation can cause deformity, pain, airway obstruction, odynophagia, dysphagia, speech difficulty in some patients. Soft, non-compressible lesions and overlying skin normal is observed on physical examination. (Figs. 15.28, 15.29 and 15.30).

15.5.12 Diagnosis

MRI of the lesion appears cystic, septate with fluid-fluid levels. T1WI is hyperintense due to the proteinaceous component of the lymphatic

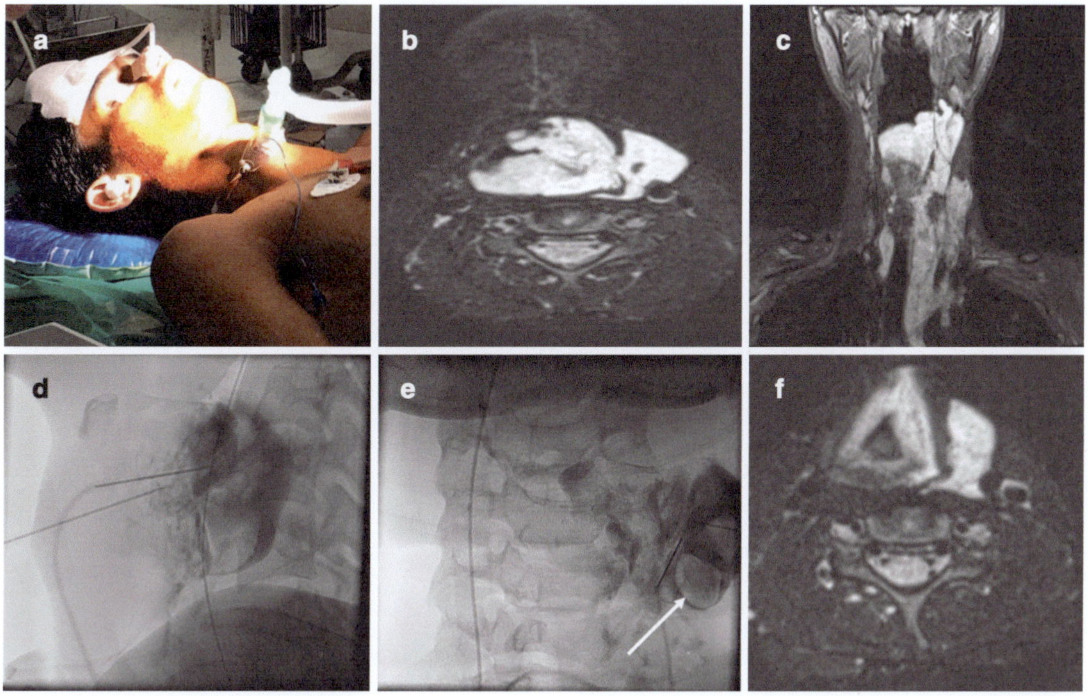

Fig. 15.18 A 19-year-old male presenting with severe dyspnea on lying down and inability to sleep supine. (**a**) Intraoperative clinical photograph showing patient intubate via tracheostomy to provide a patent airway. Difficult tracheostomy as venous malformation is involving larynx and tracheal cartilages and continuing along the anterolateral aspect of the neck down up to the upper mediastinum. (**b**) Preoperative magnetic resonance imaging axial section showing hyperintense malformation involving the laryngeal cartilage and occupying the airway leading to symptoms (**c**) Preoperative magnetic resonance imaging sagittal section showing hyperintense venous malformation extending from the level of laryngeal cartilage to the base of the neck and entering into the mediastinum. (**d**) Intraoperative radiograph showing the direct puncture with the needle to insert sclerosant in the venous malformation. (**e**) Intraoperative plain radiograph showing the filling of venous malformation with the sclerosant mixed with contrast (**f**) Post-operative magnetic resonance imaging axial section showing a decrease in the size of venous malformation and its extension into the laryngeal inlet leading to resolution of symptoms

fluid and rim enhancement may be seen on post-contrast study [19].

15.5.13 Treatment

Sclerotherapy remains the mainstay of treatment for these lesions. Sclerosants used are ethanol, Setrol, Doxycycline, Bleomycin and OK-432. Bleomycin is effective and relatively safer than the rest of the agents. It is the most commonly used sclerosant for microcystic lymphangiomas with minimal adverse effects [13].

In the microcystic variety, the lesion is punctured with 24/23 G scalp vein needle, and sclerosant can be injected intralesional even if there is no backflow of lymphatic fluid or blood. For macrocystic lesions, first, the fluid is aspirated from the large cystic spaces and then Sclerosant is injected. After withdrawing the needle, strapping is advisable in order to oppose the walls of cystic spaces, this prevents refilling of the malformation [1, 13] (Fig. 15.27).

Acevedo et al. performed a literature review of non-surgical treatments for head and neck lymphatic malformations, 66.5% of patients who received OK-432 for lymphatic malformations achieved a complete/excellent or good response, 16.9% achieved a fair/ poor response and 15.4% observed no response. The results of patients

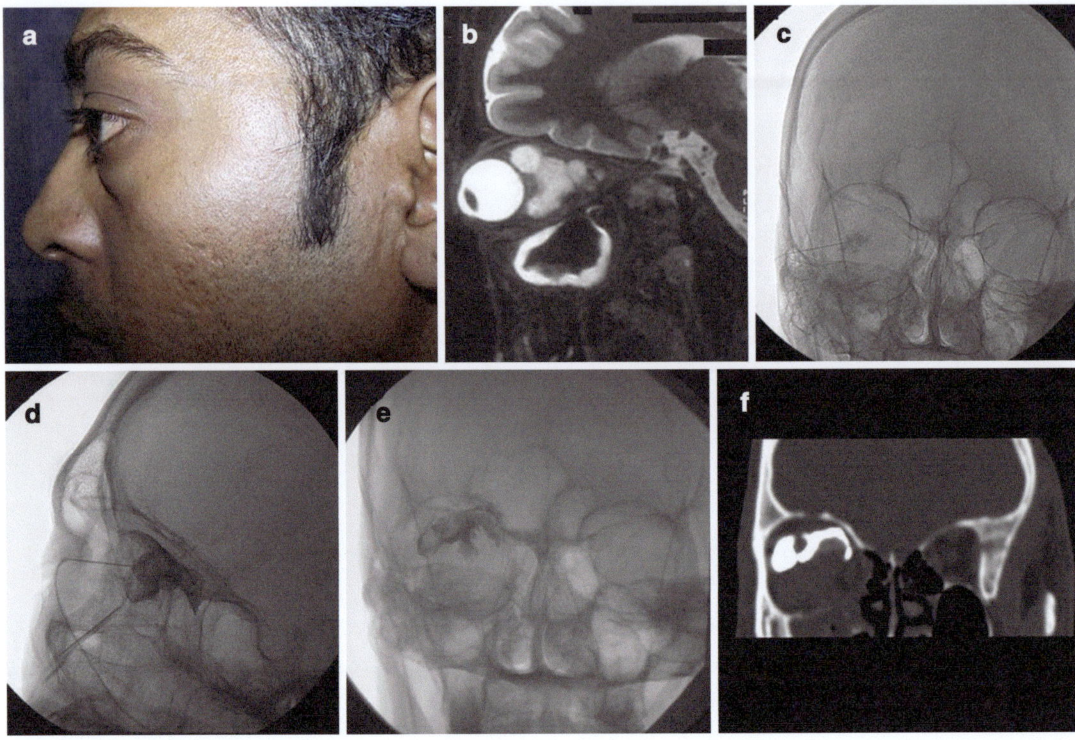

Fig. 15.19 A 22-year-male with right eye proptosis increasing on bending forward. Retrobulbar venous malformation treated with direct puncture sclerotherapy with setrol mixed with contrast (**a**) Clinical photograph at presentation showing right eye proptosis. (**b**) Preoperative T2 weighted sagittal magnetic resonance imaging section showing the T2 hyperintense orbital venous malformation. (**c**, **d**) Plain radiographs during sclerotherapy showing spinal puncture needle positioned in the malformation with contrast within the malformation. USG guidance is helpful in negotiating the needle behind the globe.(**e**) Post-procedure plain radiograph showing the lipiodol cast. (**f**) post-procedure coronal computed tomography reconstruction image showing the lipiodol cast

treated with bleomycin showed 72.3% showing excellent or good response, 18.4% fair/poor response and 11.6% no response [26]. Surgery is also an important consideration in the management of lymphatic malformations especially the microcystic one. During surgical excision, it is important to resect all diseases when possible as failure will result in recurrence.

15.5.14 High Flow Vascular Malformations

15.5.14.1 Arteriovenous Malformations

Arteriovenous malformations (AVMs) are congenital vascular malformations that result from birth defects involving the vessels of both arterial and venous origins, resulting in direct communications between the different size vessels or a meshwork of primitive reticular networks of dysplastic minute vessels which have failed to mature to become 'capillary' vessels termed 'nidus'. (Fig. 15.31 a) These lesions are defined by shunting of high velocity, low resistance flow from the arterial vasculature into the venous system. A systematic classification system developed by various groups of experts (Hamburg classification, ISSVA classification, Schobinger classification, angiographic classification of AVMs,) has resulted in a better understanding of the biology and natural history of these lesions and improved management of AVMs. The Hamburg classification, based on the embryological differentiation between extratruncular and truncular type of lesions, allows the deter-

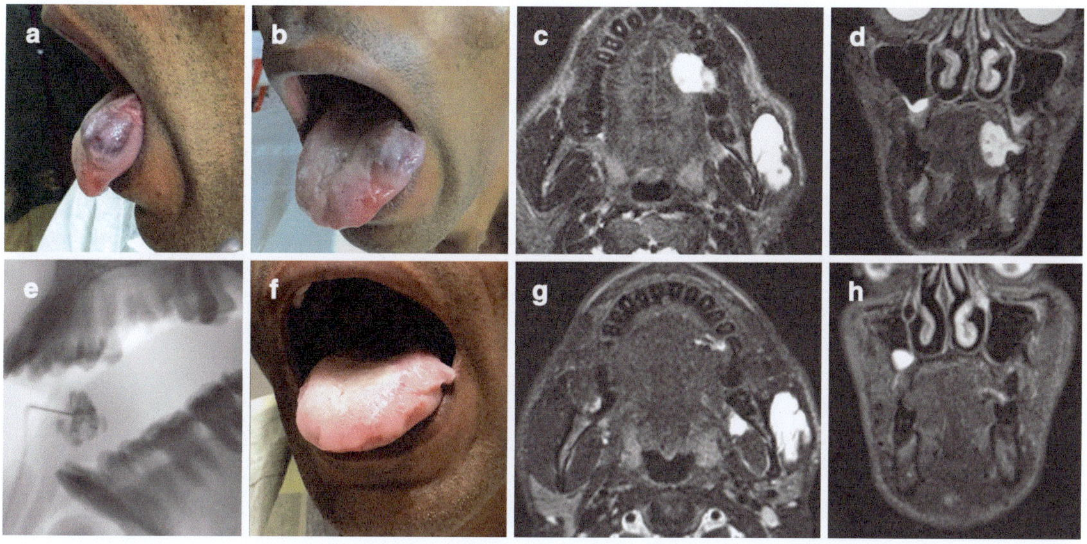

Fig. 15.20 A 30-year-old male presented with swelling in the tongue causing pain. (**a**, **b**) Preoperative clinical photograph showing a purplish bluish soft swelling on the left lateral aspect of the tongue. (**c**, **d**) Preoperative T2 weighted magnetic resonance imaging axial and coronal section showing hyperintense venous malformation in the left lateral side of the tongue and incidentally detected left masseteric Venous malformation. (permucosal sclerotherapy was performed. (**e**) Plain radiograph in lateral view showing needle position within the lesion with contrast and bleomycin cast. Multiple sessions of sclerotherapy were performed for the tongue. The massetric lesion is awaiting treatment.(**f**) Clinical photograph 3 months after the last session for tongue hemangioma shows a considerable reduction of the swelling with normal-appearing tongue mucosa and little redundant mucosa.(**g**, **h**) Control magnetic resonance imaging showing considerable reduction with very small residual tongue and cheek lesion

mination of the potential of progression and recurrence of these lesions. The majority of all AVMs are extratruncular lesions with persistent proliferative potential, whereas truncular AVM lesions are exceedingly rare. Regardless of the type, AV shunting may ultimately result in significant anatomical, pathophysiological and hemodynamic consequences. Therefore, despite their relative rarity, AVMs remain the most challenging and potentially life-threatening form of vascular anomalies [27].

About 50% of the lesions are located in the oral and maxillofacial region, followed by the extremities and trunk. The majority of maxillofacial AVMs are located in the centre of the face—nearly 70% involve the cheek, nose, ears and upper lip. Among vascular anomalies, AVMs are relatively rare accounting for about 1.5% of the lesions. They are believed to be congenital but may not manifest until several years of life. The presentation may vary from completely asymptomatic lesions to significant bleeding, pain, neuropathy or congestive heart failure. They may sometimes be very infiltrative, destructive and may cause life-threatening massive bleeding. Decreased skeletal density may be seen around the lesion. Rapid progressions may occur during periods of hormonal fluctuations such as puberty, pregnancy or hormonal therapy. Arteriovenous fistulas are usually postnatal, it originates from trauma and there is a direct communication between the arteries and the veins. (Fig. 15.31 b) AVMs and AVFs present as soft pulsatile lesions. Soft tissue arteriovenous malformation can involve the soft tissue in various extensions like intramuscular, cutaneous or intraosseous.

Large trans-spatial AVMs pose a therapeutic challenge. There is no single strategy best defining their treatment and despite our best efforts they continue to grow or proliferate like a tumour. These are neither resectable nor curative embolisation is feasible. More studies are needed to understand these lesions and growth

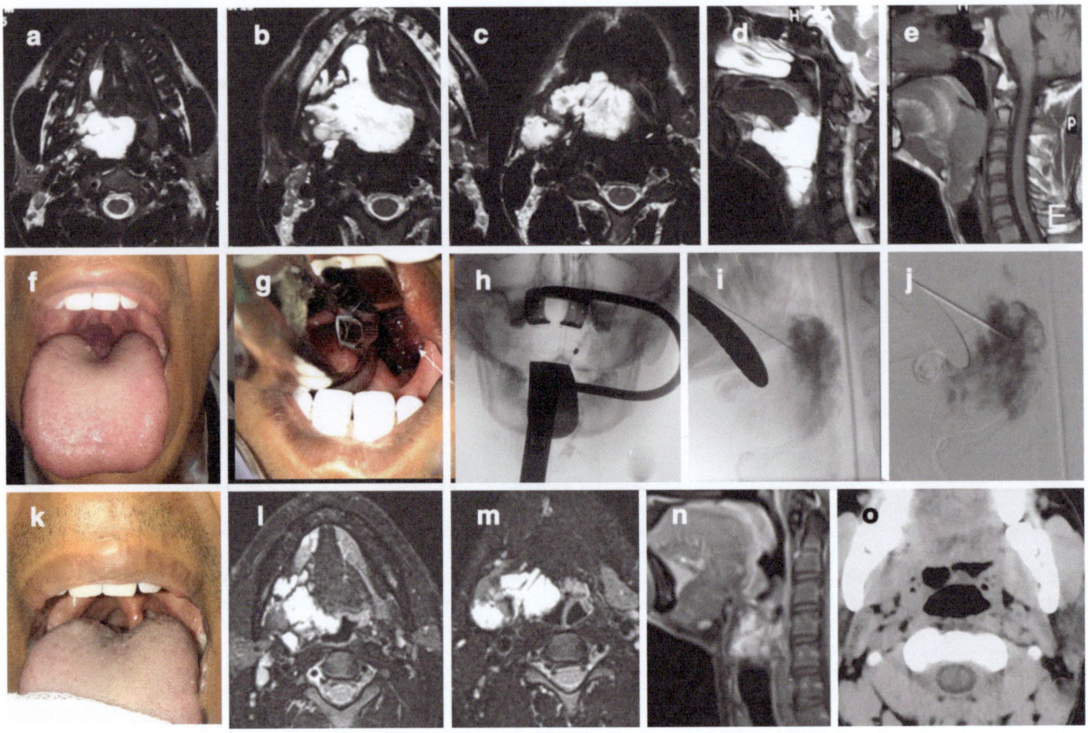

Fig. 15.21 25 year old male presenting with swelling of right submandibular region, dysphagia and hoarseness of voice. On indirect laryngoscopy, purplish mass was seen in the posterior one-third of the tongue and laryngopharynx region. (**a**, **b**, **c**, **d**, **e**) Axial MRI images in STIR sequence show multilobulated trans-spatial venous malformation in the right paraglottic region and extending to the floor of the mouth. There is compression of the airway. Multiple phleboliths are seen as rounded signal voids. (**e**) Sagittal T1WI showing airway compression. (**f**) Clinical photograph showing bulge on the right posterior one-third of the tongue. Percutaneous sclerotherapy through the right submandibular region and permucosal injection was done transorally using spinal needle and mouth retraction by tonsillectomy retractors. (**g**) Transoral view artery retractors showing the lesion. (**h**, **i**) Plain Radiograph and Lat view roadmap (**j**) showing the spread of sclerosant mixed with contrast in the oropharyngeal and laryngopharyngeal region. Tonsillectomy retractor is visible. LP needle is used for the puncture. (**k**) Clinical photograph after 6 months shows a reduction in the swelling. There is a complete resolution of dysphagia and hoarseness of voice. (**l**, **m**, **n**) Post sclerotherapy MRI in axial and sagittal view shows a significant reduction of the swelling and better visualization of the airway (**o**) Plain CT scan after the first session shows the reduction of the swelling in the paraglottic region leading to the opening of the airway

factors if present needs to be identified for better management. Currently, we provide only palliative treatment to these lesions. (Fig. 15.38).

CAMS (Cerebral arteriovenous metameric syndrome) The association of AVMs of the brain, the orbit (retinal or retrobulbar lesions), and the maxillofacial region was named originally after Bonnet–Dechaume–Blanc and Wyburn–Mason. Because of the metameric concept of neural crest development, a rational classification reflecting the putative underlying disorder is proposed and the acronym CAMS was coined. Depending on the involved structures, several CAMS can be differentiated: CAMS 1 as a midline prosencephalic (olfactory) group with the involvement of the hypothalamus, corpus callosum, hypophysis and nose; CAMS 2 as a lateral prosencephalic (optic) group with the involvement of the optic nerve, retina, parieto-temporal-occipital lobes, thalamus and maxilla; and CAMS 3 as a rhombencephalic (otic) group with the involvement of the cerebellum, pons, petrous bone and mandible. CAMS 3 is located in a strategic position on the crossroad between the complex cephalic segmental arrangements and the relatively simplified spinal metamers, and therefore it may bear transitional characteristics. (Figs. 15.37 and 15.40).

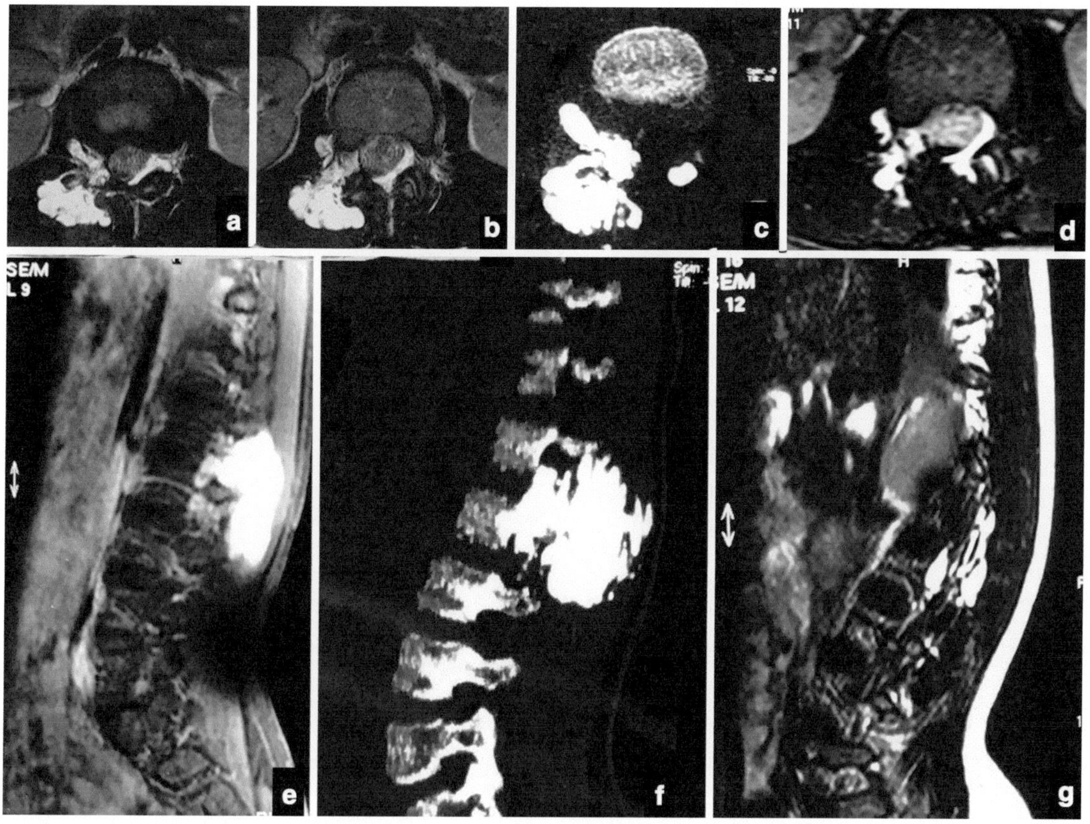

Fig. 15.22 Ten–year-old girl with backache and dragging sensation. No obvious swelling was seen on examination. (**a** and **b**) Spinal MRI axial section at L1–L2 level showed right paraspinal venous malformation. The lesion is extending along the right dorsal nerve root (**e**) Sagittal image showing the longitudinal extent of the lesion. Percutaneous sclerotherapy was done in GA in prone position using 18G spinal needle. USG standby helps in locating the lesion when selling is not obvious. Sclerosant is injected under roadmap guidance. Setrol was mixed with lipiodol for better opacification. (**c**, **f**) Post sclerotherapy CT scan was done to look for the spread of the sclerosant. Intra procedure and Post-procedure period is covered with injectable steroids to prevent nerve root inflammation reconstruction in sagittal view shows good spread of the sclerosant in the entire malformation. (**d**, **g**) Follow-up MRI after 6 months shows a considerable reduction of the swelling and complete symptomatic relief

15.5.15 Investigations

CT—soft tissue lesions that enhance as intense vessels in the arterial phase of CT angiography.

MRI, MRA: Abnormal bunch of serpiginous flow voids with hypertrophied adjacent arteries and veins. in addition, it helps to know the exact location in terms of being intramuscular, cutaneous or intraosseous as it has a lot of implications in surgical planning and outcome [19].

Catheter Angiography: It is the mainstay for diagnosis and planning of treatment. The arterial supply and draining vein depend on the location of the AVM.

Classification: The Schobinger Classification (Table III) was designed to assess AVM lesions in different clinical stages and clinical conditions more accurately based on the patient's clinical status and to select the best suited time for management as a practical guideline.

Schobinger Classification of AVM

- Stage I—Quiescence: Pink-bluish stain, warmth and arteriovenous shunting are revealed by Doppler scanning. The arteriovenous malformation mimics a capillary malformation or involuting hemangioma.

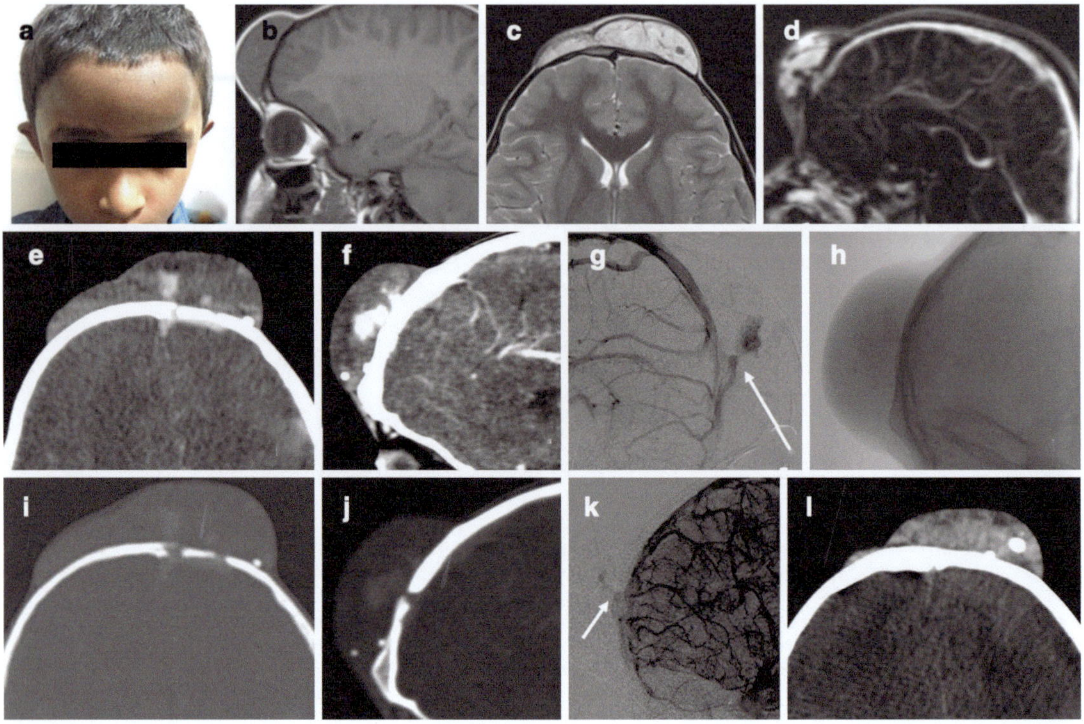

Fig. 15.23 Four-year-old boy with swelling in the forehead noticed since 1 year of age and gradually progressive. (**a**) Clinical photograph showing the forehead swelling. (**b, c**) MRI images in T1WI and T2 WI sequence showing the venous malformation. (**d**) Contrast MR venography showing the sinus pericranii with contrast puddling in the malformation. (**e, f, g, h**) CT venous phase in Brain and bone window and axial and sagittal views respectively showing the bony defect with sinus peicranii. (**i, j, k**) Cerebral angiography in the venous phase documenting the communication. (**l**). CT showing Phlebolith

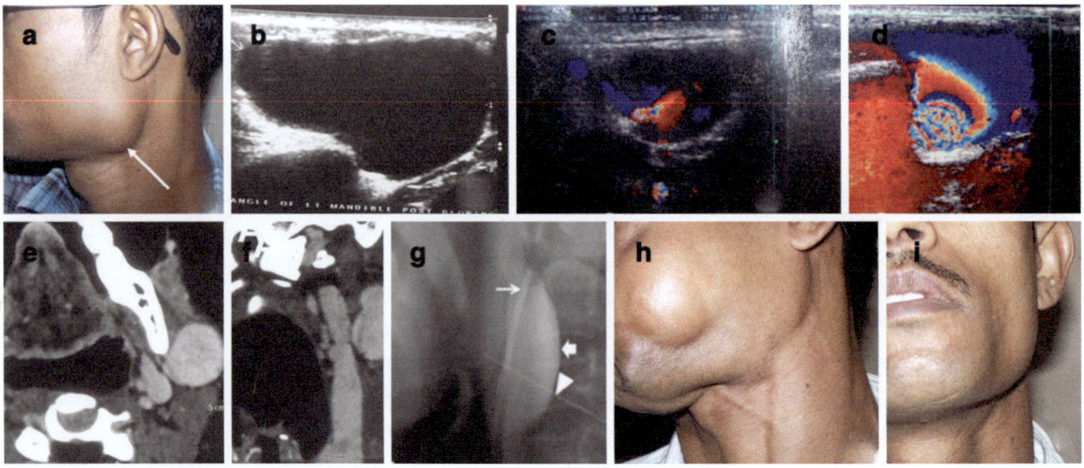

Fig. 15.24 Young male with swelling in the region of angle of the mandible which is increasing on Valsalva manoeuvre. (**a**) Clinical photograph showing the swelling. (**b, c, d**) USG and colour doppler showing the cystic lesion with Ying Yang phenomenon in venous varix. (**e, f**) CT Venography showing communication with the retromandibular vein. (**g**) Direct puncture sclerotherapy was done with compression of the draining vein. (**g**) Plain radiograph showing Contrast stasis and layering within the lesion. (**h, i**) Clinical photograph at follow-up showing cure of the lesion with no visualization of the swelling even on Valsalva

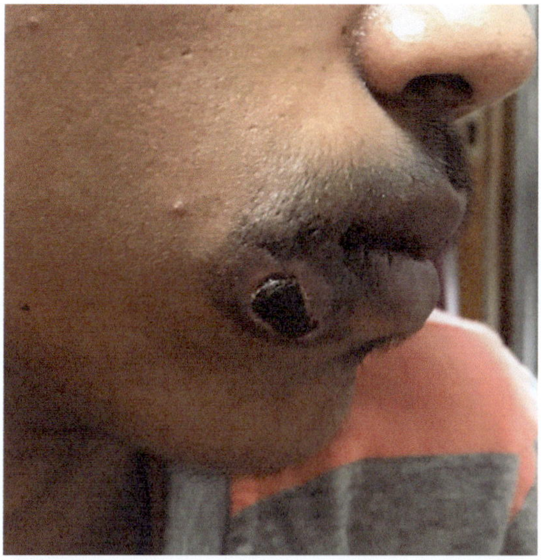

Fig. 15.25 Angle of mouth Venous malformation treated by Percutaneous sclerotherapy. Necrosis post-sclerotherapy

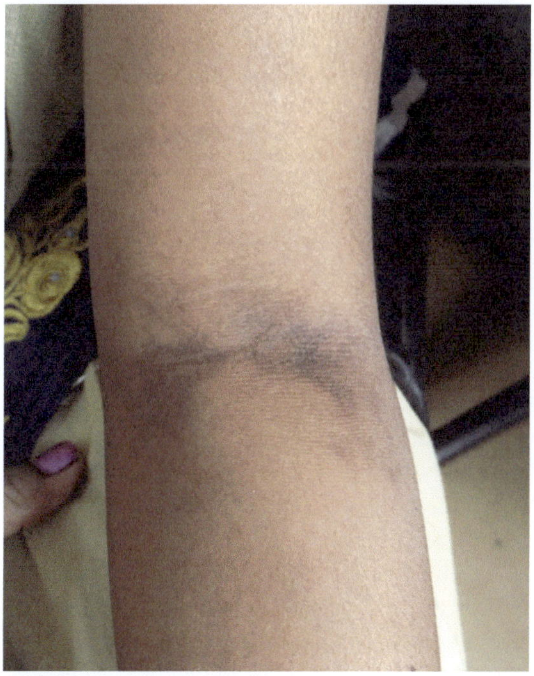

Fig. 15.26 Young girl with neck VM close to the brachial plexus, Bleomycin sclerotherapy was done. There was some drainage of the sclerosant into the systemic circulations there are lot of draining veins in the neck VM. Flagellate discolouration at the elbow. They are seen predominantly at the flexural surface as a side effect of Bleomycin sclerotherapy

- Stage II—Expansion: Stage I plus enlargement, pulsations, thrill, bruit and tortuous/tense veins.
- Stage III—Destruction: Stage II plus dystrophic skin changes, ulceration, bleeding, tissue necrosis. Bony lytic lesions may occur.
- Stage IV—Decompensation: Stage III plus congestive cardiac failure with increased cardiac output and left ventricle hypertrophy.

15.5.16 Treatment

After the diagnosis is established, it's important to determine which therapy is best suited for that location, size and extent of the AVM. A multidisciplinary team approach should be utilized to integrate surgical and non-surgical interventions for optimum care.

The treatment options are Embolization alone or as preoperative step, followed by surgery. Palliative embolization is suggested for large AVMs where surgery is associated with extensive morbidity. Surgical partial treatment often triggers the expansion of the arteriovenous lesions and should be avoided unless life-threatening bleeding cannot be controlled by transarterial or direct percutaneous embolization and rarely transvenous embolization.

Transarterial coil embolization or ligation of feeding arteries where the nidus is left intact, are incorrect approaches and may result in the proliferation of the lesion. Furthermore, such procedures would prevent future endovascular access to the lesions via the arterial route. Surgically inaccessible, infiltrating, extratruncular AVMs are still a therapeutic challenge [27].

Embolization has become an integral part of the treatment of these malformations. Cure of these lesions may be attained by embolization alone or embolization followed by surgical removal. Endovascular therapy includes Transarterial Embolization or Direct Puncture Embolization. Transarterial embolization requires distal navigation and super-selective catheter placement close to the nidus. In small AVMs, the cure can be achieved by this technique alone. (Fig. 15.32) However, if there is residual AVM, direct punc-

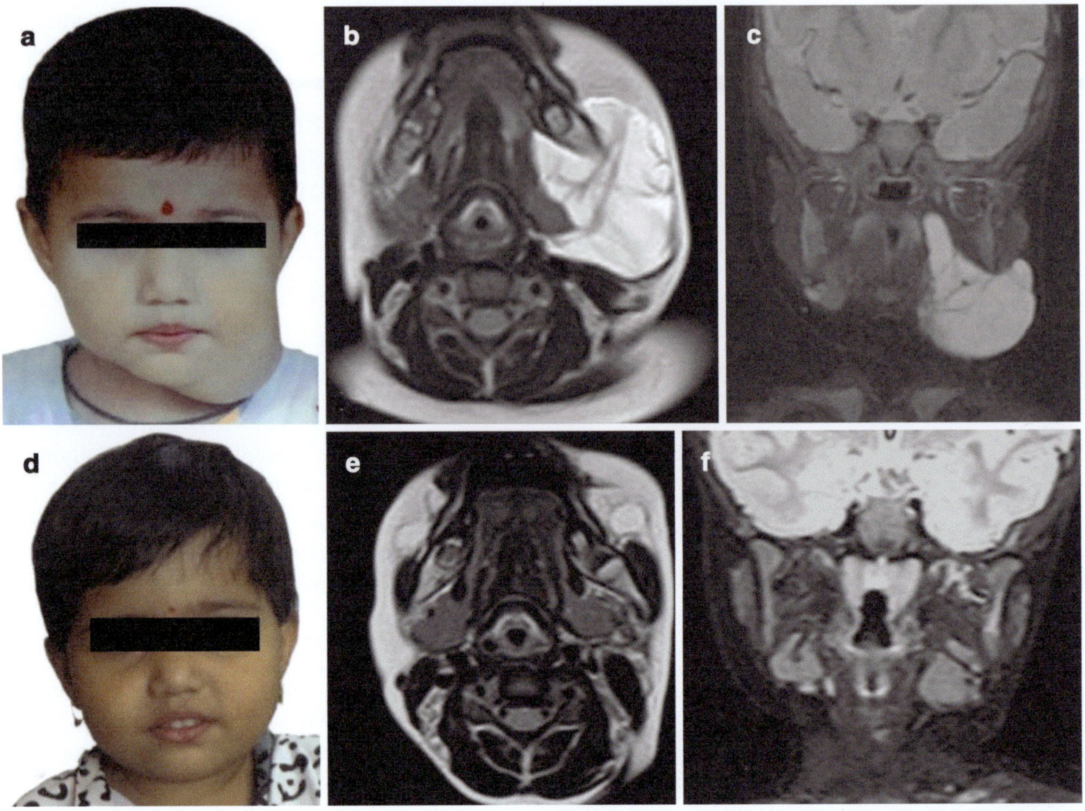

Fig. 15.27 (**a**) Clinical photograph of the patient is showing lower cheek and angle of the mandible swelling (**b**, **c**) Axial (**a**) and Coronal (**b**) T2 weighted Images of MRI show a hyperintense, well-defined mass in left masticator space, mandibular space, para pharyngeal space and is abutting the carotid vessels. Lesion has multiple internal hypointense septae suggestive of Macrocystic Ly9mphangioma or cystic hygroma (**d**, **e**, **f**) Clinical photograph of the patient after 2 years after two sessions of Percutaneous Sclerotherapy shows complete resolution of the swelling which is confirmed on MRI

ture embolization is necessary. (Fig. 15.33) The choice of agent depends upon several factors: the vascular territory to be treated, the type of abnormality being treated, the possibility of superselective delivery of occlusive agents, the goal of the procedure, and the permanence of the occlusion required. The options are Alcohol, NBCA and Onyx. The newer agents are Squid, Phil and Menox, all of them have properties like Onyx. Alcohol is good, effective but has the highest rate of complications. Despite the success that is possible with ethanol, it must be remembered that it is an extremely dangerous intravascular sclerosant that can cause tissue necrosis and cardiopulmonary collapse. Nontarget embolization with ethanol will lead to tissue necrosis as capillary beds are entirely destroyed. Being a fluid agent, ethanol penetrates to the capillary level, devitalising normal tissue. With the advent of Onyx and good embolization and surgical results, the use of alcohol for embolization has come down over the years [15, 27].

The choice of agent currently is between NBCA (Glue) and Onyx, Squid or Menox. The advantages of Onyx seem to hold more for intra-arterial rather than a percutaneous approach. With the currently available limited data, the best strategy may be the individualization of the choice of the liquid embolic agent (*n*BCA versus Onyx) based on the clinical and angiographic

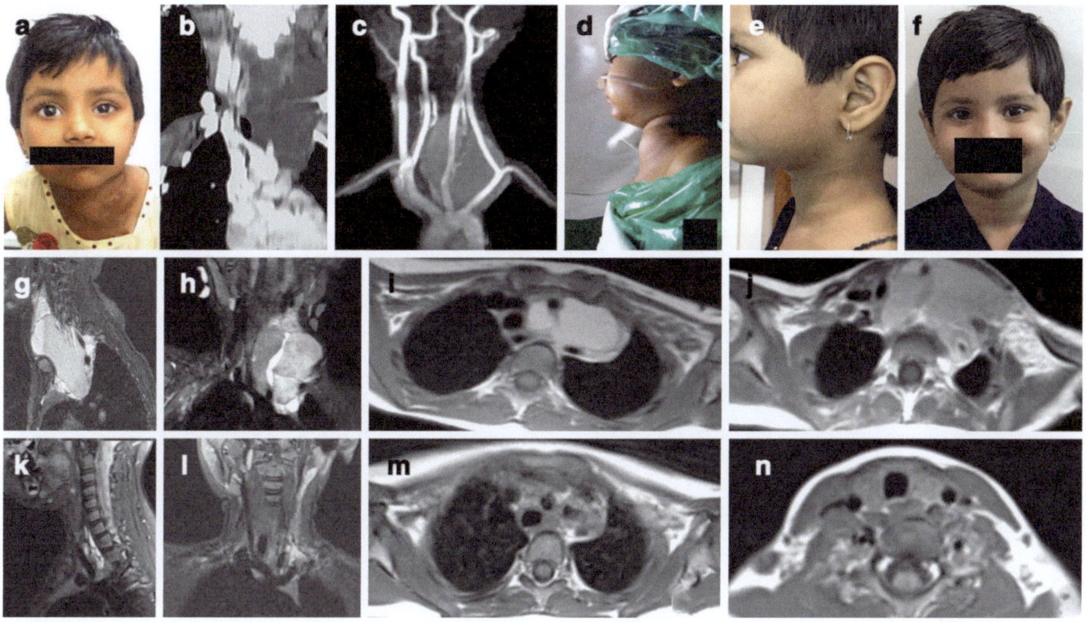

Fig. 15.28 A 5-year-old female presented with a mass on the left side of the neck and supraclavicular region causing left-sided Horner's syndrome. (**a**) Clinical photograph at presentation showing swelling in the left side of the neck as well as miosis and enophthalmos in the left eye and neck swelling. (**b**) Preoperative CT scan in Sagittal reconstruction Preoperative computed tomography of the neck showing a cystic vascular malformation encasing and (**c**) displacing the major great vessels from the root of aorta. (**g**, **h**, **i**, **j**) Preoperative magnetic resonance imaging sagittal, coronal and axial section showing a cystic lesion in the anterior triangle of neck encasing and displacing vital structures of the neck like great vessels—Common carotid, vertebral and left subclavian artery. The trachea is displaced laterally on the right side. The lesion is extending into the upper mediastinum. (**d**) Percutaneous sclerotherapy was performed after puncture and fluid aspiration from the cystic hygroma followed by bleomycin injection (**k**, **l**, **m**, **n**) Magnetic resonance imaging after 6 months of treatment at the same levels as G, H, I and J respectively, showing obliteration of the lymphatic lesion with the restoration of normal neck anatomy. This is the distinct advantage of sclerotherapy over surgery in these lesions. (**e**, **f**) Post-operative clinical photograph showing resolution of the swelling and of Horner's syndrome caused by compression of the superior cervical paravertebral ganglion

characteristics of each patient, as well as the overall estimated cost of the embolization procedure. N-butyl cyanoacrylate (NBCA) belongs to a class of tissue adhesive that is used for Endosurgical vascular ablation. NBCA is used to treat AVMs and AVF. This glue remains in the liquid state until contact occurs with blood, whereby it polymerises from its monomeric form to polymeric form. In this polymerisation process, the cyanoacrylates generate heat, which may contribute to some level of histotoxicity in the adjacent area and angionecrosis [28]. Onyx has good penetration into the AVM nidus and can be injected for a longer duration. The ability to inject slowly during treatment enabled avoidance of the dangerous collaterals of the craniofacial vasculature, which are known to become more prominent in the presence of a vascular malformation. (Fig. 15.34) If the lesion is not easily accessible via an external carotid transarterial approach, percutaneous embolization with *n*BCA is performed. The decision for surgical excision is based on the involvement of muscles and the degree of expected surgical morbidity. Most of the lesions in today's practice are embolized by direct puncture Glue or Onyx injection and subsequent surgical excision [15, 29]. (Figs. 15.35, 15.36, and 15.37).

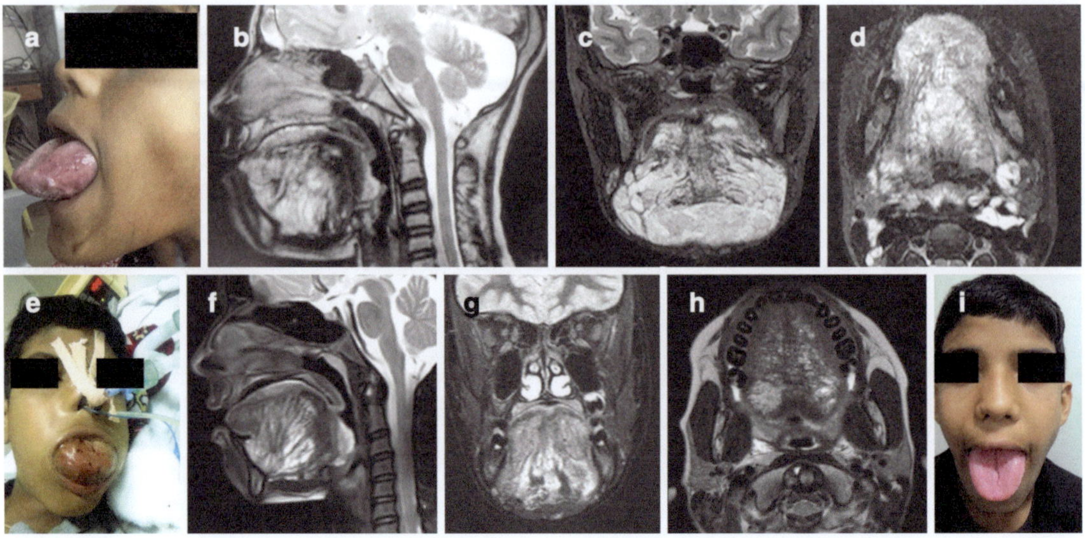

Fig. 15.29 A 10-year-old male presented with swelling in the tongue causing difficulty in eating, breathing. There is macroglossia causing speech difficulty and glossoptosis. (**a**) Clinical photograph on presentation showing macroglossia with prominent reddish papule over the tongue. (**b**, **c**, **d**) Preoperative magnetic resonance imaging sagittal section showing T2 hyperintense lesion with septa involving the tongue in its entirety and the floor of the mouth. The lesion is causing airway compromise. The findings are suggestive of microcystic lymphatic malformation. Bleomycin sclerotherapy was done with prior intubation. 0.5 cc of diluted bleomycin solution was injected in the anterior part of the tongue. The swelling started increasing immediately after injection to the extent that compression was not stopping the bleeding from the puncture site. Local gelfoam and glue injection was done at the puncture site and homeostasis achieved after 3 hrs. (**e**) immediate Post bleomycin sclerotherapy clinical imaging showing a sudden increase in swelling of the tongue for which the patient had to be kept intubated n the ICU for 7 days after which the swelling started to subside. (**f**, **g**, **h**) Post-operative magnetic resonance imaging sagittal, coronal and axial section showing a decrease in the extent, size and intensity of the malformation with normal signal intensity in the majority of the tongue. One more session was done for the floor of the mouth. (**i**) Clinical photograph 8 months post-sclerotherapy showing complete normalization of the tongue mucosa with normal size. There is good speech with no difficulty in swallowing on follow-up

Rarely, in large AVMS, palliative treatment may be done with transarterial particle embolization. Polyvinyl alcohol foam (PVA) is formed by the reaction of polyvinyl alcohol foam with formaldehyde. It is biologically inert and provokes a mild inflammatory reaction. Initially thought to be a permanently occluding agent, PVA is now known to recanalize when used to treat vascular malformations.

Fistulous lesions are more likely to be cured by embolization alone through an intra-arterial and/or direct percutaneous approach.

Intraosseous AVMs: Intraosseous arteriovenous malformations of the maxilla or mandible are rare. They are high flow lesions and they may present with facial swelling, loosening of tooth, gingival bleeding and sometimes with life-threatening haemorrhages, especially after dental extraction. They are characterized by congenital dysmorphogenesis of the arterial and venous structures of the dental arcade. Radiographic findings vary from poorly defined radiolucency to honeycomb, soap-bubble appearance or irregular lacunae. Variable radiographic presentations especially for small lesions delay the diagnosis of this specific rare entity. Computed tomographic angiography (CTA) or magnetic resonance imaging (MRI) may be helpful for diagnosis but DSA is the gold

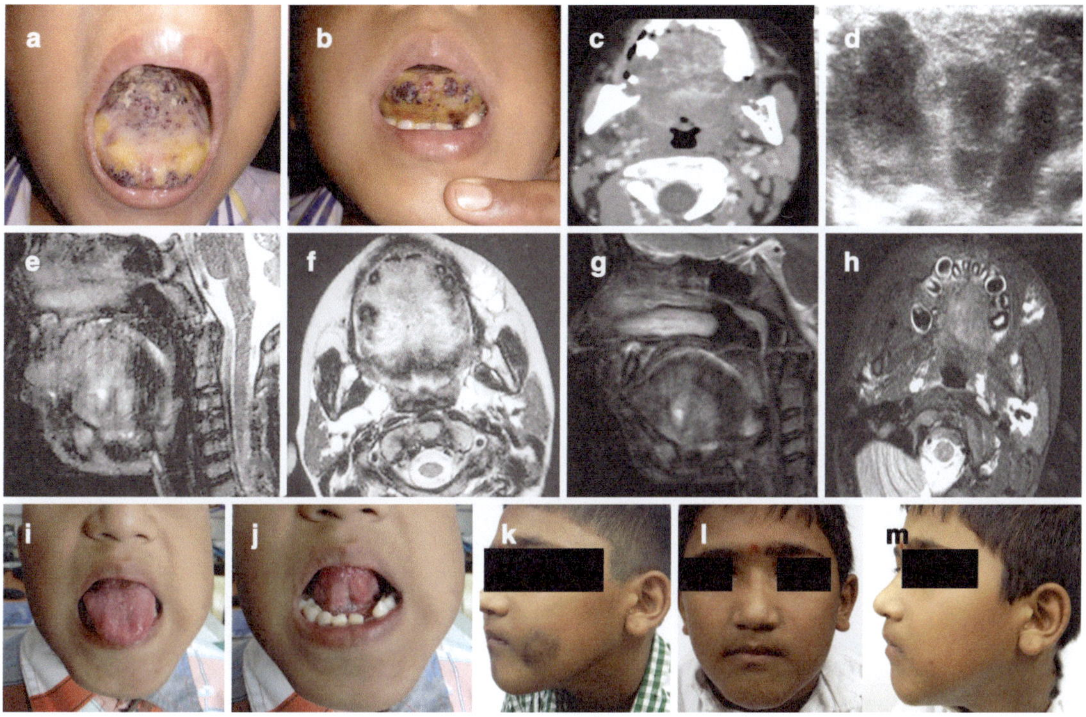

Fig. 15.30 A 4 year-old boy presented with a swelling in the tongue, bleeding intermittently. Speech difficulty with difficulty in swallowing. (**a**, **b**) Clinical photograph at presentation showed swelling in the tongue with punctuate haemorrhage, necrosis, plaques leading to yellowish discolouration of the tongue. (**c**) CT scan showing enhancing lesion of the tongue. (**d**) Ultrasonography of the cheek lesion showed the presence of multiseptate microcystic lesion. (**e**, **f**) Preoperative magnetic resonance imaging axial and sagittal of the tongue showed diffuse slightly hyperintense lymphatic malformation of the tongue and floor of the mouth (**g**, **h**) Post-operative magnetic resonance imaging sagittal and axial section showing considerable reduction of the lymphatic malformation of the tongue after bleomycin sclerotherapy. (**i**, **j**) Post-sclerotherapy clinical photograph showing normalization of the tongue mucosa with the absence of necrosis, haemorrhage and discolouration. (**k**) Left cheek malformation sclerotherapy was done later. Post-sclerotherapy clinical photograph showing hyperpigmentation on the cheek a known side effect associated with bleomycin sclerotherapy. (**l**, **m**) Clinical photograph 6 months after sclerotherapy showing resolution of the cheek hyperpigmentation

standard to define the angioarchitecture and plan the treatment. The management of these high flow complex lesions is challenging due to their intraosseous location, extensive vascularity and maxillo-mandibular involvement. Endovascular embolization is useful and is the standard treatment in the present era with the availability of hardwares and embolic agents. It not only provides a cure or stabilization of symptoms but also preserves the anatomic contiguity and osseous regeneration. Endovascular techniques include Transarterial or Transvenous embolization with particles, liquid embolic agents or coils. Complete devascularization may still be difficult in high flow, complex lesions and direct puncture of the intraosseous pouch can lead to good results in these cases. (Figs. 15.38, 15.39, and 15.40).

The AVM treatment involves great planning and multidisciplinary involvement for achieving the sure and good cosmetic outcome.

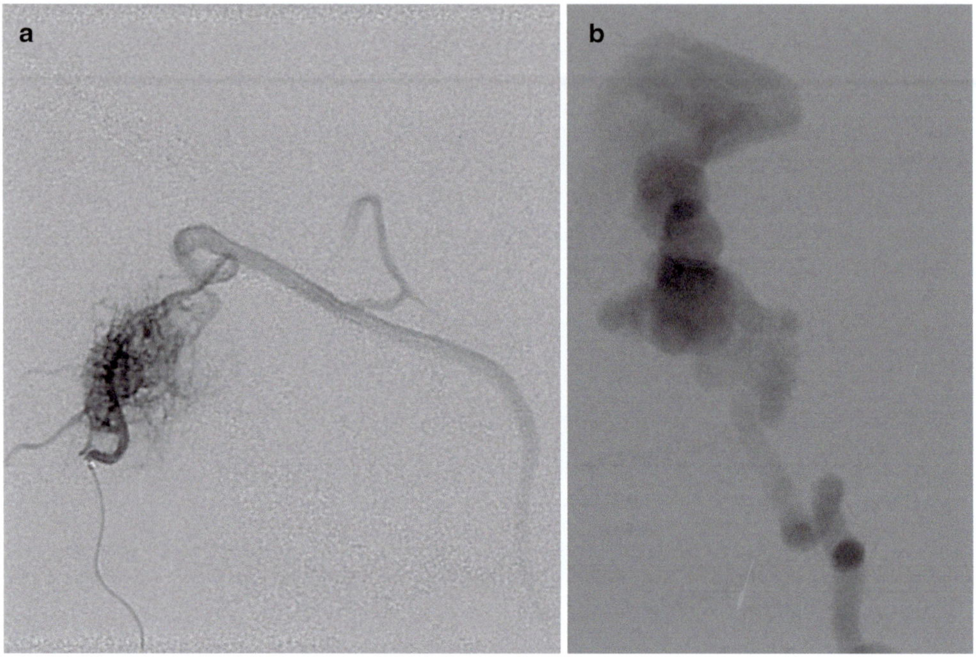

Fig. 15.31 (**a**) Arteriovenous malformation with a nidus (**b**) Arteriovenous Fistula

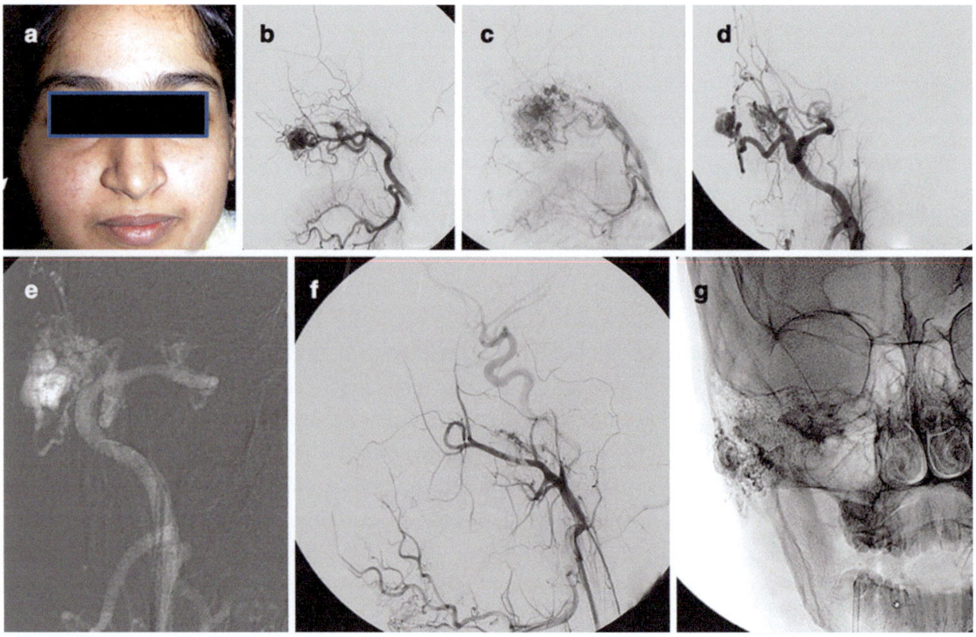

Fig. 15.32 Eighteen Y/F with swelling right cheek which is pulsatile. (**a**) Clinical photograph showing right zygomatic arteriovenous malformation. Transarterial Glue (NBCA) embolisation was performed through two arterial feeders leading to complete cure. (**b**, **c**, **d**) Catheter angiography showing the arterial feeders, the nidus and the draining veins. (**e**) Arterial roadmap showing distal microcatheter position. (**f**) Post Embolization angiogram showing complete obliteration of the AVM nidus. (**g**) Plain radiograph showing glue cast

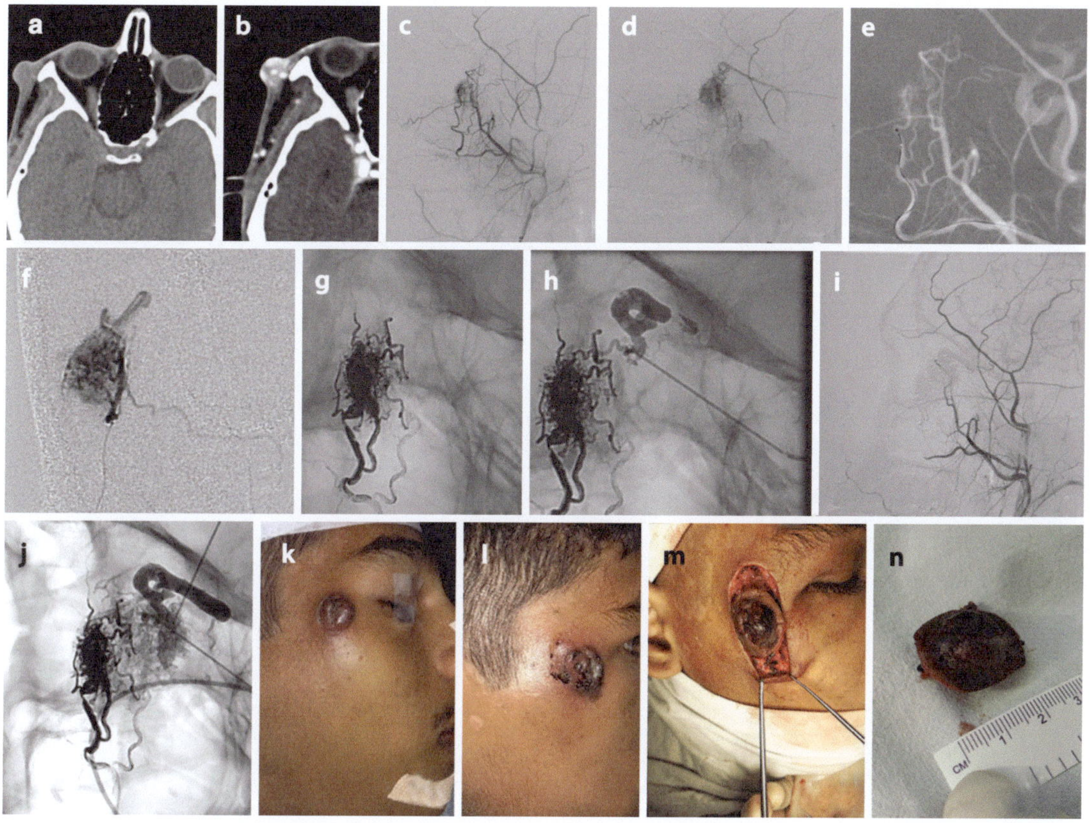

Fig. 15.33 Transarterial ONYX and Direct puncture glue. Young boy with bleeding from the right zygomatic lesion. (**a**, **b**) Ct plain and contrast showing soft tissue lesion with intense enhancement suggestive of high flow vascular malformation. (**c**, **d**) DSA in early and late arterial phase showing the AVM nidus, feeding artery and vein. (**e**) Roadmap showing catheter position (**f**) Microcatheter angiogram demonstrating the AVM nidus and draining vein. Transarterial onyx was injected. However venous penetration could not be achieved. The direct puncture was done and glue was injected to achieve good embolization. (**g**) Needle position. (**h**) post-embolisation angiogram. (**i**) Final cast showing onyx and glue in the nidus and glue in the draining vein. (**j**) Prembolization clinical picture. (**k**, **l**) post-embolisation picture showing blackish staining of the lesion due to ONYX. (**m**, **n**) Introperative photograph and gross specimen showing complete excision with the bloodless field

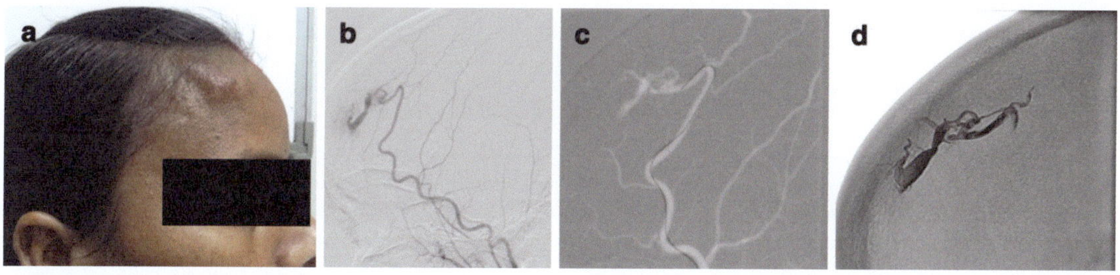

Fig. 15.34 Twenty-five-year-old lady with pulsatile swelling in the forehead. (**a**) Clinical photograph. (**b**) Right External carotid angiogram showing slow flow small forehead AVM. (**c**) Marathon microcatheter was navigated in feeding the frontal branch of the Superficial temporal artery. Menox (Meril Life Sciences, India) was injected under roadmap guidance. (**d**) Menox cast showing good penetration into the nidus and draining vein. (**e**) Post embolization angiogram showing complete obliteration of the AVM nidus. (**f**) on Follow-up, the lesion had regressed in size and firm in consistency. The cast was palpable on examination. (**g**, **h**) Follow-up MRI imaging kenos cast with stable obliteration of the nidus. No abnormal vessel is seen around the cast which is hypo intense in all sequences

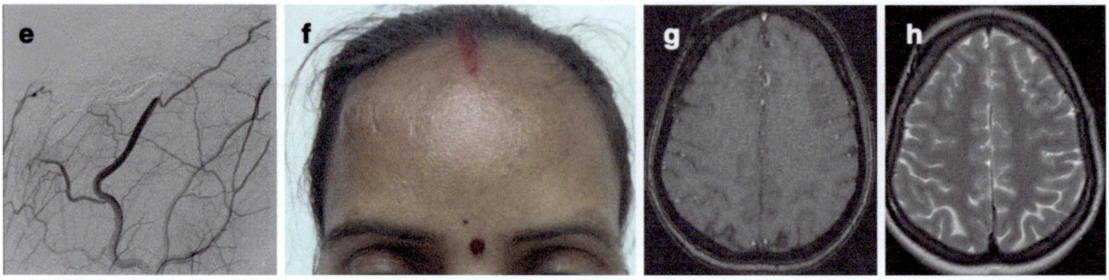

Fig. 15.34 (continued)

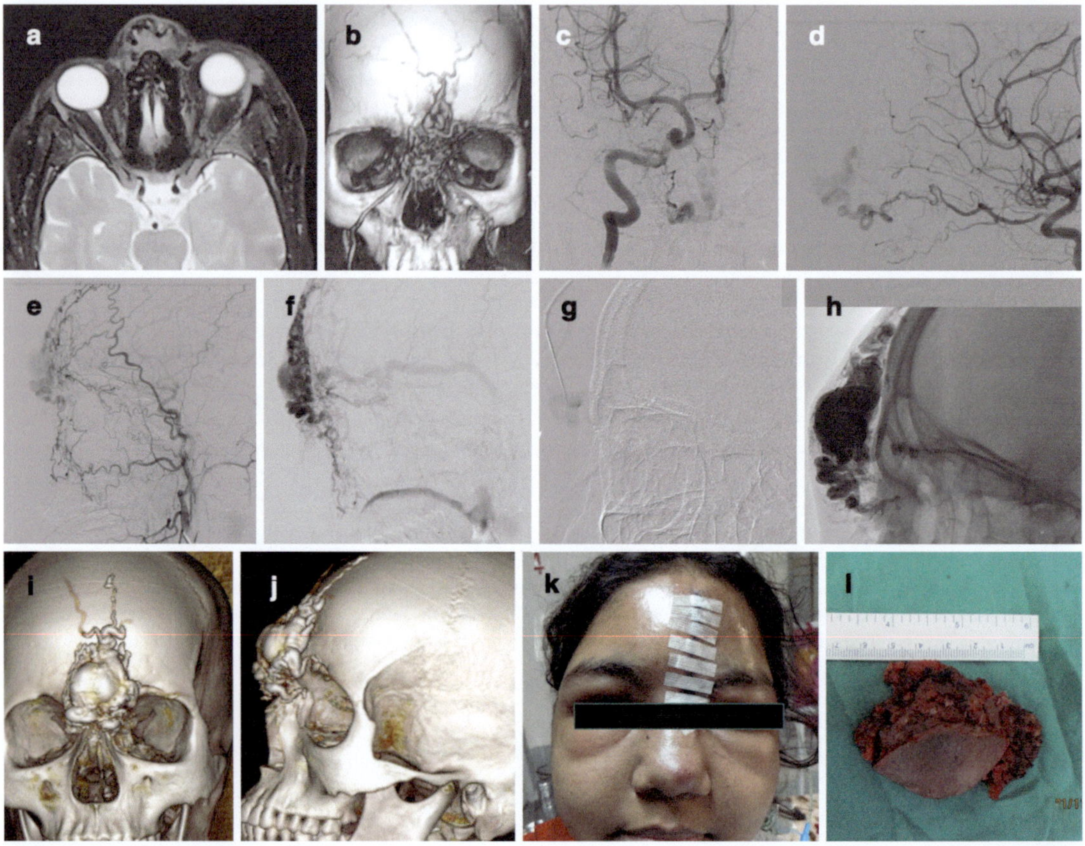

Fig. 15.35 Twenty-two-year-old female with swelling in the forehead noticed at 10 years of age and progressively increasing. (**a**) MRI T2WI showing abnormal signal voids in the glabellar region and forehead in the midline (**b**) 3D reconstructed the image of CT angiography showing the AVM nidus in the midline. (**c**) right ICA angiography (**d**, **e**), Left ICA and Bilateral ECA angiography was performed. The midline forehead AVMs are supplied through bilateral external carotid arteries and also from ophthalmic arteries bilaterally. During Embolization, utmost care needs to be taken to prevent retrograde glue progression into the feeding ophthalmic arteries. (**f**) the entire AVM nidus with the dilated venous pouch in lateral view. (**g**) Direct puncture with 24 G scalp vein needle and angiogram to confirm the intravascular position of the needle. (**h**) Plain radiograph in lateral view showing Final Glue cast. (**i** & **j**) Volume rendered images of CT maxillofacial region showing the entire glue cast. (**k**) Surgical excision of the AVM was done with minimal blood loss. Clinical photograph in the post-operative period. (**l**) Gross specimen of the AVM in entirety

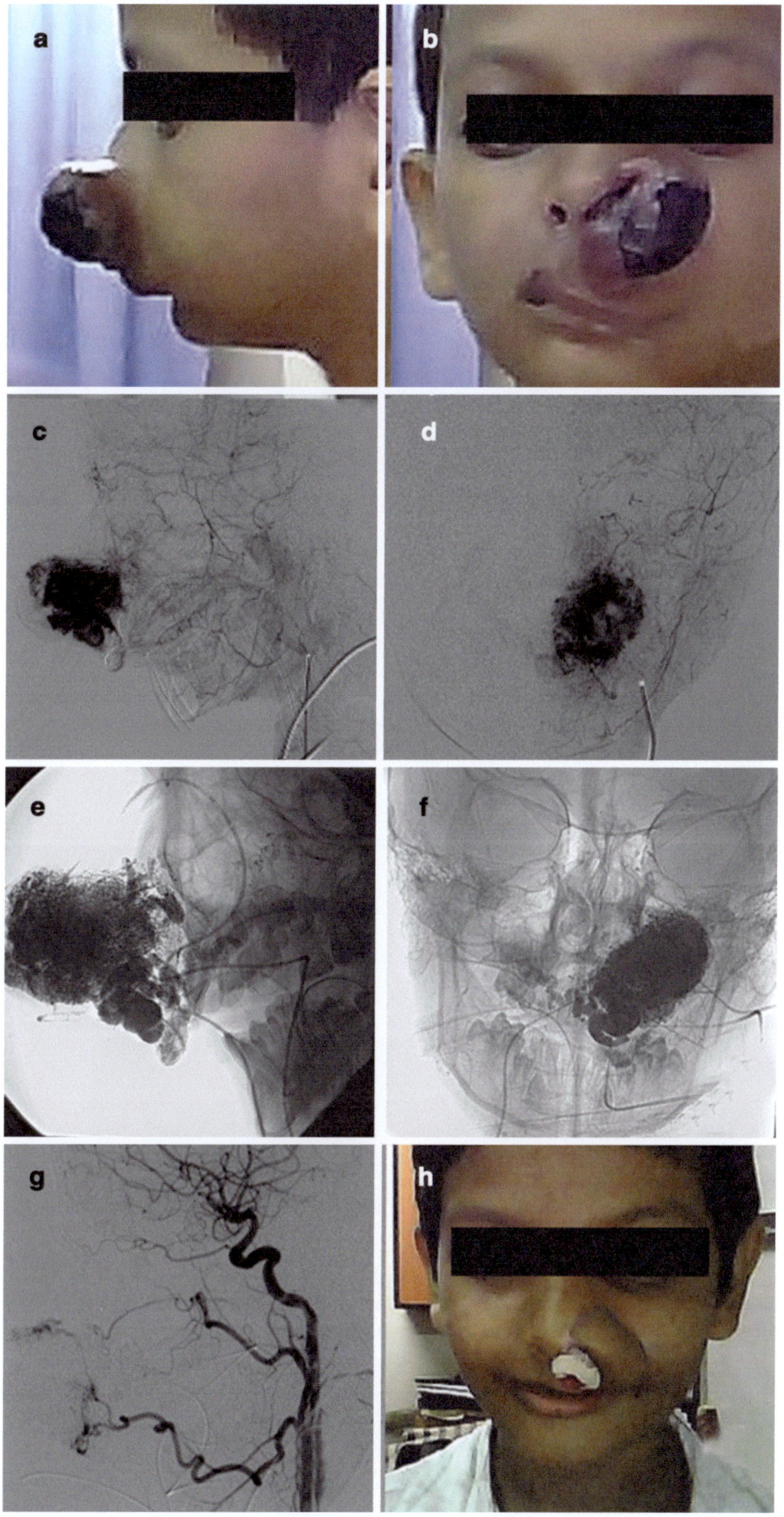

Fig. 15.36 Eight-year-old boy presented with swelling in the left columellar region for 4 years. Presented in the casualty with Sudden massive bleeding from the swelling. Emergency angiography showed high flow fistula from the facial artery to control bleeding. Subsequently, Direct puncture and glue embolization was performed for definitive treatment. (**a**, **b**) Clinical picture preoperatively before direct picture. (**c**, **d**) Catheter angiography in Lateral and AP view showing entire nidus of the Nasal AVM. (**e**, **f**) The Glue cast matching the entire nidus. This produces intraoperative bleeding during surgical excision. (**g**) Post Embolization Common carotid angiogram shows more than 90% obliteration of the AVM nidus. He was operated later. (**h**) Post-op clinical photograph with flap reconstruction

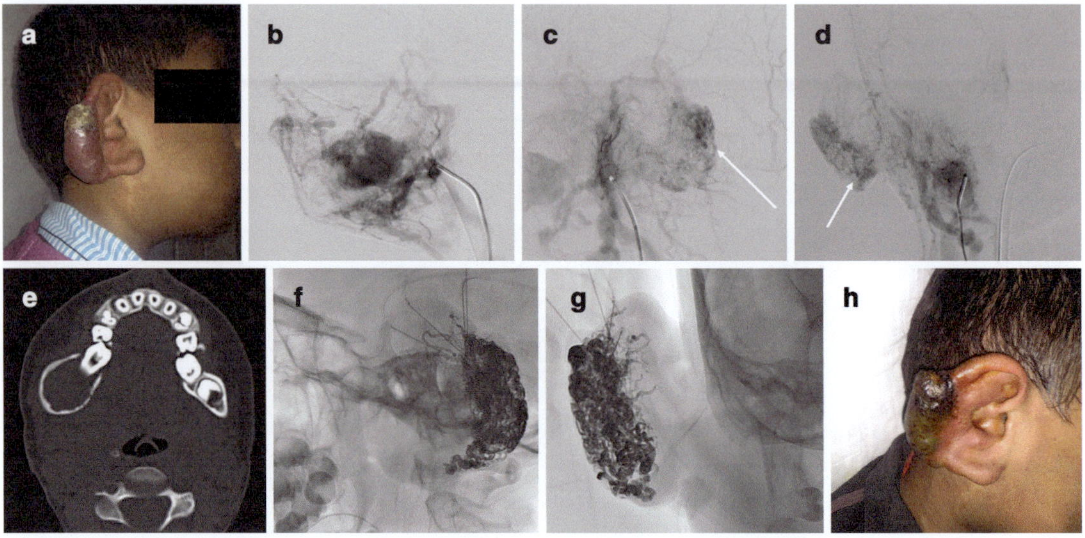

Fig. 15.37 Direct puncture onyx. (**a**) Clinical photograph of a young boy with pinna AVM presented with bleeding from the pinna. (**b**) Catheter angiography in oblique view showing incidentally detected high flow dental arcade intraosseous mandibular AVM . CAMS is a known association with Maxillofacial AVMs. This patient belongs to CAMS 3. (**c**) Lateral and (**d**) AP view showing the Pinna AVM. (**e**). CT Mandible showing lytic lesion. The parents did not want pinna excision hence definitive extensive embolisation for pinna AVM followed by surgical excision of pinna could not be done. Direct puncture ONYX was injected in order to control symptoms and achieve Nidal obliteration at the same time. (**f**, **g**) Onyx cast. (**h**) Clinical photograph post-embolisation showing staining of the malformation causing greyish black discolouration of the lesion. Intraosseous malformation was treated later

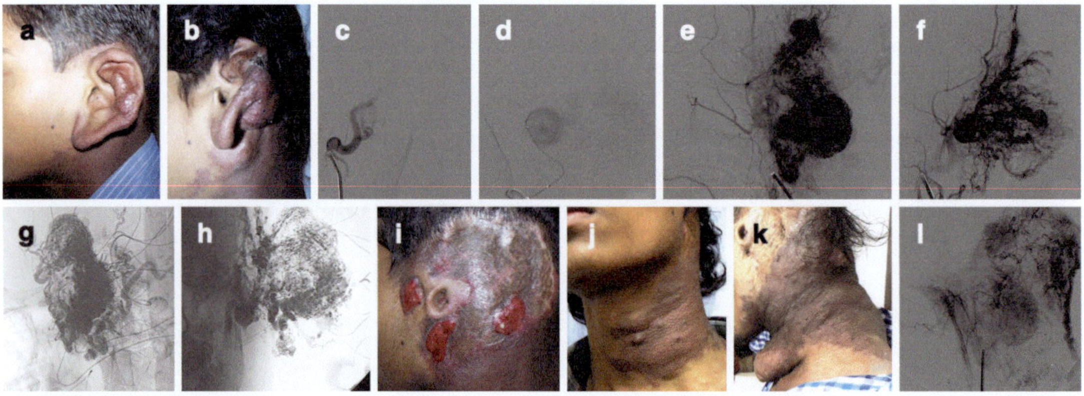

Fig. 15.38 Twelve- year-old boy presented with multiple episodes of bleeding from the pinna. The bleeding used to stop with compression so no treatment was taken. (**a**) Clinical picture at the time of the first presentation. Refused treatment at that time. After 1 year, he came to casualty with massive bleeding. (**b**) Clinical picture 1 year later. Enlarged swelling with ulcerated, necroses area. That was the site of bleeding. (**c**) DSA at the time of emergency embolisation showed high flow fistula which was embolizaed transarterially and bleeding controlled. (**d**) Microcatheter angiogram showing fistula and venous aneurysm. (**e**, **f**) Residual AVM in lateral and AP view. Managed by direct puncture glue embolization. (**g**, **h**) Glue Cast Pinnogram showing adequate embolization. He underwent surgical excision. Since there was a large area of port-wine stain in the post auricular and adjacent neck region. With increased vascularity on DSA (**l**). The placement of the Graft was difficult with long post-operative phase of graft healing. (**i**) (**j**) Follow-up after 2 years from embolisation further increase in neck lesion. (**k**) Ten years follow-up from the first presentation, i.e. at 22 years of age the lesion shows marked increase in the neck and nape lesion suggestive of proliferating AVM. Our current therapeutic approaches are limited in managing these lesions

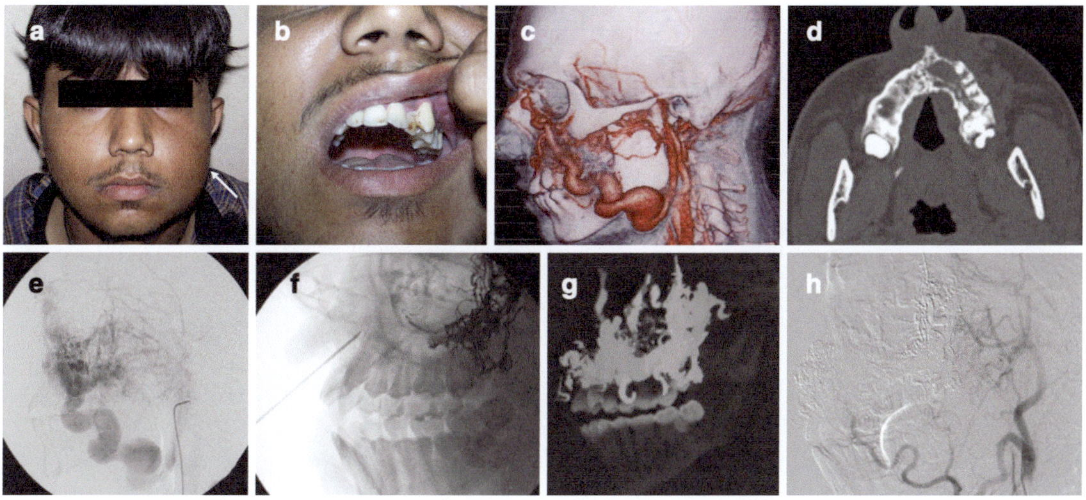

Fig. 15.39 Eighteen- year-old boy with gum bleeds. (**a**, **b**) Clinical photograph showing left cheek swelling. Intramural view shoeing the site of gum bleed adjacent to the left upper incisor. (**c**) CT angiogram reconstructed views show the malformation within the maxilla with large hypertrophied draining vein. (**d**) Axial CT shows a lytic lesion in the left maxilla extending across the midline. (**e**) Left ECA angiogram shows high flow intraosseous AVM in the left maxillary alveolar process supplied by multiple hypertrophied alveolar and nutrient branches from the distal internal maxillary artery and draining through the hypertrophied maxillary vein into the facial vein. (**f**) Transmucosal puncture was done with spinal needle at the site of bony depression and needle positioned within the intraosseous venous pouch and position confirmed by contrast injection. (**g**) Post-treatment CT shows the glue deposition within the intraosseous venous pouch. (**h**) Control angiogram was done after six months. Left ECA angiogram shows stable obliteration of the maxillary intraosseous AVM

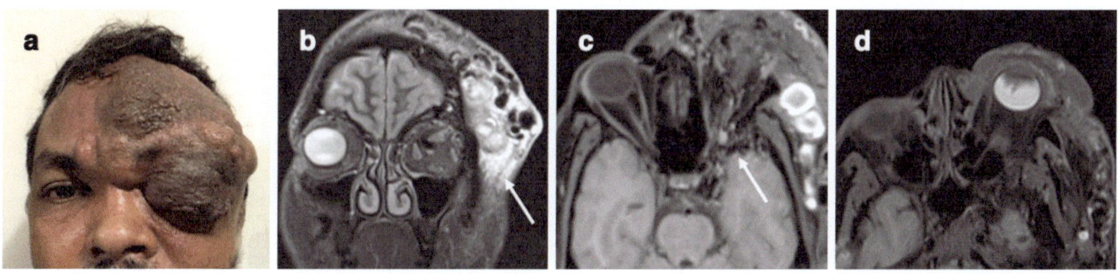

Fig. 15.40 CAMS 2. 35 year old male with large left forehead and eyelid swelling for many years. There is history of episodes of bleeding from the lesion and proptosis and redness of the left eye for 6 months. (**a**) Clinical photograph. (**b**) MRI T2WI showing the superficial scalp and forehead AVM. (**c**) Signal voids are seen within the left greater wing of sphenoid suggestive of intraosseous AVM (Arrow). (**d**) Vitreous haemorrhage. (**e**) Prominent cortical vein in the left frontal region. (**f**) Right ECA angiogram shows frontal cortical direct leptomeningeal Dural arteriovenous fistula on the left side. The supply is through middle meningeal artery crossing the midline and supplying the fistula in the left frontal region (**g**, **h**) Left ECA Angiography showing high flow forehead superficial AVM. (**i**) Axial CT showing left sphenoid wing erosion. (**j**) Left internal maxillary artery angiogram showing the intraosseous Arteriovenous fistula. (**j**, **k**) DYNA CT angiogram showing the contrast within the sphenoid bone suggestive of intraosseous component (**k**) Endovascular embolisation was performed for the intraosseous AVM. Plain radiograph showing the Onyx and Coil cast. (**m**, **n**) The second session was preoperative embolisation of the superficial AVM. Plain radiograph in AP and Lateral view showing the glue cast of the same. (**o**) Clinical picture post Direct puncture Glue embolization. This was followed by Surgical excision

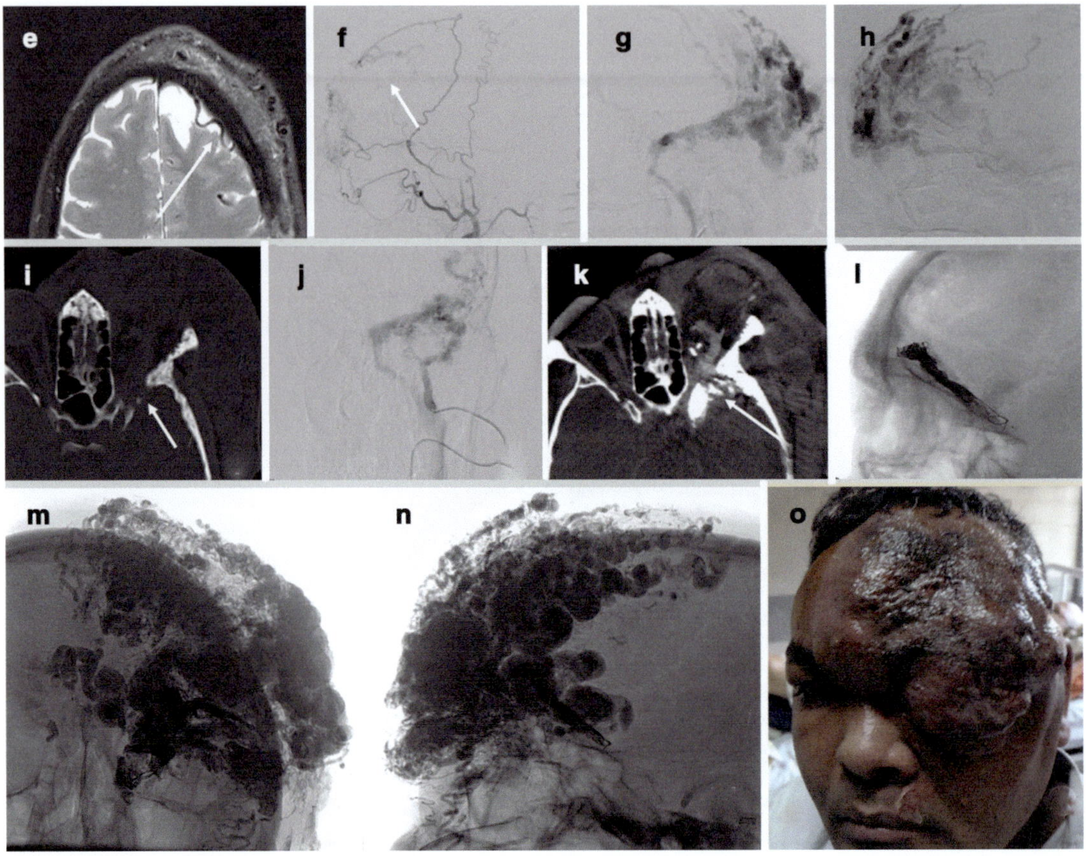

Fig. 15.40 (continued)

15.6 Conclusion

Vascular anomalies represent a wide variety of vessel abnormalities. Correct diagnosis is imperative to accurately ascertain prognosis and plan treatment. Multidisciplinary team approach is mandatory between Interventional radiologists, Plastic Surgeons, Maxillofacial surgeons, ENT surgeons and Paediatricians in the case of children. With the advent of better hardware for interventional procedures and the availability of good embolic agents, a challenging group of vascular malformation can be successfully managed with interventional techniques.

Acknowledgement I would like to sincerely thank the Department of Plastic surgery and the Department of ENT for their constant support in the management of Patients with maxillofacial vascular malformation. I would also extend my heartfelt thanks to Tushar Garg, MBBS Final year student at Seth G.S. Medical College and KEM hospital for support in technical work.

References

1. Legiehn GM, Heran MK. Venous malformations: classification, development, diagnosis, and interventional radiologic management. Radiol Clin N Am. 2008 May;46(3):545–97, vi. https://doi.org/10.1016/j.rcl.2008.02.008.
2. Belov S. Anatomopathological classification of congenital vascular defects. Semin Vasc Surg. 1993;6:219–24.
3. Buckmiller LM, Richter GT, Suen JY. Diagnosis and management of hemangiomas and vascular malformations of the head and neck. Oral Dis. 2010 Jul;16(5):405–18. https://doi.org/10.1111/j.1601-0825.2010.01661.x.

4. Haggstrom AN, Lammer EJ, Schneider RA, Marcucio R, Frieden IJ. Patterns of infantile hemangiomas: new clues to hemangioma pathogenesis and embryonic facial development. Pediatrics. 2006 Mar;117(3):698–703.
5. ISSVA Classification of Vascular Anomalies © 2018 International Society for the Study of Vascular Anomalies Available at "issva.org/classification" Accessed 31 Jan 2019.
6. Wassef M, Blei F, Adams D, Alomari A, Baselga E, Berenstein A, Burrows P, Frieden IJ, Garzon MC, Lopez-Gutierrez JC, Lord DJ, Mitchel S, Powell J, Prendiville J, Vikkula M, ISSVA Board and Scientific Committee. Vascular anomalies classification: recommendations from the International Society for the Study of vascular anomalies. Pediatrics. 2015 Jul;136(1):e203–14. https://doi.org/10.1542/peds.2014-3673.
7. Dubois J, Soulez G, Oliva VL, Berthiaume MJ, Lapierre C, Therasse E. Soft-tissue venous malformations in adult patients: imaging and therapeutic issues. Radiographics. 2001 Nov-Dec;21(6):1519–31.
8. Donnelly LF, Adams DM, Bisset GS. Vascular malformations and hemangiomas: a practical approach in a multidisciplinary clinic. AJR Am J Roentgenol. 2000 Mar;174(3):597–608.
9. Kaban LB, Mulliken JB. Vascular anomalies of the maxillofacial region. J Oral Maxillofac Surg. 1986 Mar;44(3):203–13.
10. Bonet-Coloma C, Mínguez-Martínez I, Palma-Carrió C, Galán-Gil S, Peñarrocha-Diago M, Mínguez-Sanz JM. Clinical characteristics, treatment and outcome of 28 oral hemangiomas in pediatric patients. Med Oral Patol Oral Cir Bucal. 2011 Jan 1;16(1):e19–22.
11. Léauté-Labrèze C. Dumas de la Roque E, Hubiche T, Boralevi F, Thambo JB, Taïeb a. propranolol for severe hemangiomas of infancy. N Engl J Med. 2008 Jun 12;358(24):2649–51. https://doi.org/10.1056/NEJMc0708819.
12. Buckmiller LM, Munson PD, Dyamenahalli U, Dai Y, Richter GT. Propranolol for infantile hemangiomas: early experience at a tertiary vascular anomalies center. Laryngoscope. 2010 Apr;120(4):676–81. https://doi.org/10.1002/lary.20807.
13. Muir T, Kirsten M, Fourie P, Dippenaar N, Ionescu GO. Intralesional bleomycin injection (IBI) treatment for hemangiomas and congenital vascular malformations. Pediatr Surg Int. 2004 Jan;19(12):766–73.
14. Konez O, Burrows PE, Mulliken JB. Cervicofacial venous malformations. MRI features and interventional strategies. Interv Neuroradiol. 2002 Sep 30;8(3):227–34.
15. Arat A, Cil BE, Vargel I, Turkbey B, Canyigit M, Peynircioglu B, Arat YO. Embolization of high-flow craniofacial vascular malformations with onyx. AJNR Am J Neuroradiol. 2007 Aug;28(7):1409–14.
16. Ethunandan M, Mellor TK. Hemangiomas and vascular malformations of the maxillofacial region--a review. Br J Oral Maxillofac Surg. 2006 Aug;44(4):263–72.
17. Chapot R, Laurent A, Enjolras O, Payen D, Houdart E. Fatal cardiovascular collapse during ethanol sclerotherapy of a venous malformation. Interv Neuroradiol. 2002 Sep 30;8(3):321–4.
18. Lungren MP, Patel MN. Endovascular Management of Head and Neck Vascular Malformations. Current Otorhinolaryngology Reports. 2014;2(4):273–84.
19. Flis CM, Connor SE. Imaging of head and neck venous malformations. Eur Radiol. 2005 Oct;15(10):2185–93.
20. Kumar S, Kumar V, Kumar S, Kumar S. Management strategy for facial venous malformations. Natl J Maxillofac Surg. 2014 Jan;5(1):93–6. https://doi.org/10.4103/0975-5950.140188.
21. Zheng JW, Mai HM, Zhang L, Wang YA, Fan XD, Su LX, Qin ZP, Yang YW, Jiang YH, Zhao YF, Suen JY. Guidelines for the treatment of head and neck venous malformations. Int J Clin Exp Med. 2013 May 22;6(5):377–89.
22. Jeyaraj P, Chakranarayan A (2017) Management of vascular malformations of the maxillofacial region using sclerotherapy and sclerothrombotic therapy along with surgery. Int J Dental Res Oral Sci. 2017 Aug; 1(3):20–28.
23. Lee IH, Kim KH, Jeon P, Byun HS, Kim HJ, Kim ST, Kim YW, Kim DI, Choi JY. Ethanol sclerotherapy for the management of craniofacial venous malformations: the interim results. Korean J Radiol. 2009 May-Jun;10(3):269–76. https://doi.org/10.3348/kjr.2009.10.3.269.
24. Spence J, Krings T, TerBrugge KG, Agid R. Percutaneous treatment of facial venous malformations: a matched comparison of alcohol and bleomycin sclerotherapy. Head Neck. 2011 Jan;33(1):125–30. https://doi.org/10.1002/hed.21410.
25. O'Donovan JC, Donaldson JS, Morello FP, Pensler JM, Vogelzang RL, Bauer B. Symptomatic hemangiomas and venous malformations in infants, children, and young adults: treatment with percutaneous injection of sodium tetradecyl sulfate. AJR Am J Roentgenol. 1997 Sep;169(3):723–9.
26. Sannier K, Dompmartin A, Théron J, Labbé D, Barrellier MT, Leroyer R, Touré P, Leroy D. A new sclerosing agent in the treatment of venous malformations. Study on 23 cases. Interv Neuroradiol. 2004 Jun 29;10(2):113–27.
27. Su LX, Fan XD, Zheng JW, Wang YA, Qin ZP, Wang XK, Yang YW, Zhao YF. A practical guide for diagnosis and treatment of arteriovenous malformations in the oral and maxillofacial region. Chin J Dent Res. 2014;17(2):85–9.
28. Han MH, Seong SO, Kim HD, Chang KH, Yeon KM, Han MC. Craniofacial arteriovenous malformation: preoperative embolization with direct puncture and injection of n-butyl cyanoacrylate. Radiology. 1999 Jun;211(3):661–6.
29. Churojana A, Chiewwit P, Chuangsuwanich A, Aojanepong C, Chawalaparit O, Suthipongchai S. Embolization of vascular malformations in

head and neck regions. A single center experience. Interv Neuroradiol. 2004 Mar 14;10(1): 37–46.

30. Cil BE, Vargel I, Geyik S, Peynircioglu B, Cavusoglu T. Venous vascular malformations of the craniofacial region: pre-operative embolisation with direct percutaneous puncture and N-butyl cyanoacrylate. Br J Radiol. 2008 Dec;81(972):935–9. https://doi.org/10.1259/bjr/66893325.

31. Uehara S, Osuga K, Yoneda A, Oue T, Yamanaka H, Fukuzawa M. Intralesional sclerotherapy for subcutaneous venous malformations in children. Pediatr Surg Int. 2009 Aug;25(8):709–13. https://doi.org/10.1007/s00383-009-2414-y.

Radiological Interventions in Vascular Malformations

16

Ajay Savlania and Abhinaya Reddy

16.1 Introduction

Congenital vascular malformations (CVMs) are relatively rare vascular anomalies, resulting from the defect in inborn error of vascular morphogenesis that occurs between fourth and fifth week of the intrauterine period. They remain a difficult diagnostic and pose a therapeutic challenge due to confusing terminology, varied clinical presentations, unpredictable clinical course, inconsistent response to treatment, and high recurrence rates.

To provide a terminology that will serve as a guide for management and results comparison, the International Society for the Study of Vascular Anomalies (ISSVA) has classified these CVMs into four groups: Simple vascular malformations, combined vascular malformations, vascular malformations of major named vessels, and vascular malformations associated with other anomalies. Simple vascular malformations based on arterial component classified into low flow malformation (without arterial component) including venous malformation (VM), lymphatic malformation (LM), capillary malformation (CM), and high flow malformation (with arterial component) including arteriovenous malformation (AVM) and arteriovenous fistula (AVF).

A. Savlania (✉) · A. Reddy
Department of General Surgery, Postgraduate Institute of Medical Education and Research, Chandigarh, India

A multidisciplinary approach is a prerequisite for optimal management of these anomalies with low morbidity. Management of CVMs involves three different approaches, conservative, percutaneous minimally invasive radiological interventions, and open surgery. With recent advances, percutaneous radiological interventional management has replaced traditional surgery as the principal invasive therapy for vascular malformations. In this chapter, we shall outline various malformations with a detailed discussion on percutaneous radiological interventions.

16.2 Venous Malformation

VMs are congenital slow-flow malformations that are morphologically and histologically composed of abnormal, non-proliferating dilated venous channels with mitotically inactive endothelium and scant mural smooth muscle cells [1]. VMs are the most common CVMs accounting for 70–80%, with an estimated incidence of 1-2/10,000 population [2, 3]. They range from simple single-channel vessel dilatation (phlebectasia) to multiple spongiform venous lakes, which usually drain into adjacent normal veins through tributaries. They can involve any part of the body with a predilection to the head and neck (40%), the extremities (40%), and the trunk (20%) [4]. VMs are often asymptomatic, however stiffness, local discomfort, and pain can be the presenting

A. K. Khanna, S. K. Tiwary (eds.), *Vascular Malformations*,
https://doi.org/10.1007/978-981-15-9762-6_16

Table 16.1 Indications for the treatment of venous malformations

S. no.	Indication
1	Disabling pain
2	Bleeding
3	Ulcer
4	Lesion near important structures (synovio-articular)
5	Lesion with functional impairment
6	Cosmetic implications
7	Recurrent thrombosis

complaints due to local compression, congestion, and thrombophlebitis [4]. Localized intravascular coagulation (LIC) is an important phenomenon in this group, resulting from the stasis of blood in the tortuous and slow-flow vessels, increasing the risk of thrombosis as well as severe coagulation disorder such as disseminated intravascular coagulation (DIC) [4, 5].

Indications for Treatment Pain is the primary indication for sclerotherapy in the majority of vascular malformations. VMs in particular location (e.g., synovio-articular), symptomatic gastrointestinal VMs, and disfiguring (e.g., facial, genital) VMs require treatment even in the absence of pain. Other indications are listed in Table 16.1. These lesions have to be treated early in life as these lesions grow with the age. Early intervention results in relatively fewer interventions, smaller volume of sclerosants, and prevents long-term complications [6].

16.3 Pre-Intervention Evaluation

The diagnosis of VMs is based primarily on the clinical features. Investigations are mainly for characterization of the disease, confirmation of the diagnosis and to differentiate from other lesions.

Hematologic Evaluation LIC is an important concern, as it has the potential for more serious thromboembolic events as well as thrombohemorrhagic implications like DIC. Patients with severe LIC would have elevated D-Dimer, low level of fibrinogen, and mildly diminished platelet count (1.0–1.5 Lakhs/ml), in contrast to DIC, which may be having profound thrombocytopenia [1]. Mildly deranged coagulation is not a contraindication for a minimally invasive interventional approach (MIIA).

Ultrasound and Doppler In vascular malformations, ultrasound imaging with gray scale, color mode, and spectral analysis is the first-line imaging modality in the evaluation of VMs. Classic ultrasound findings include compressible tissue, anechoic, ectatic venous spaces separated by echogenic septa, with scant monophasic low-velocity flow [7].

Computed Tomography Secondary signs of osseous involvement such as bony expansion, osteolysis, cortical thinning, and increased trabeculation can be seen on roentgenogram and computed tomogram. Phlebolithiasis are best depicted as small calcification on radiograph and CT [5].

Magnetic Resonance Imaging (MRI) Due to good soft-tissue resolution, best anatomical detail, and the absence of ionizing radiation, MRI is the imaging modality of choice for evaluating VMs. VMs present as lobulated, non-mass like lesions with low to intermediate signal intensity on T1-weighted images and hyperintensity on fluid-sensitive sequences. Fat suppressed T2-weighted and STIR images provide excellent delineation of the extension of the lesions, as VMs may infiltrate multiple tissue planes [8]. Based on MRI, Goyal et al., developed a classification of VMs which correlates with the outcome of the Sclerotherapy Table 16.2 [9].

16.4 Treatment

For the treatment of VMs, a multidisciplinary team approach is recommended, with the aim of proper selection of treatment modality either medical, MIIA, Surgical, or the combination of the above. This should be based on location, extent, and symptoms resulting from VMs. Indications for the intervention are as noted in Table 16.1. The therapeutic strategy should be focused on alleviating the symptoms and improving the patient's quality of life, but should not be focused on complete removal (Fig. 16.1).

Table 16.2 MRI-based classification of venous malformations and their relation to clinical outcome after sclerotherapy

Grade	Definition	Response to Sclerotherapy
Grade 1	Well defined, ≤5 cm in diameter	Most have an excellent response to treatment(clinical obliteration), with no poor results
Grade 2A	Well defined, >5 cm in diameter	Most results in the good or excellent response, though poor outcomes were reported
Grade 2B	Ill defined, ≤5 cm in diameter	Large proportions have poor outcomes. Good and excellent results possible
Grade 3	Ill defined, >5 cm in diameter	No clinical obliteration, the largest number of poor outcomes (little or no improvement).

Medical Management Proper skincare, compression garments, anti-inflammatory are the foremost means of conservative treatment. Anticoagulants (low molecular weight heparin) should be administered to patient with high risk of LIC and elevated D-dimer when going through intervention [1].

16.5 Minimally Invasive Intervention Approach

16.5.1 Sclerotherapy

Percutaneous Sclerotherapy is considered as the first line of treatment when medical treatment fails. It may be combined with additional laser therapy or surgical procedure [10]. Based on pre-intervention diagnostic phlebography, according

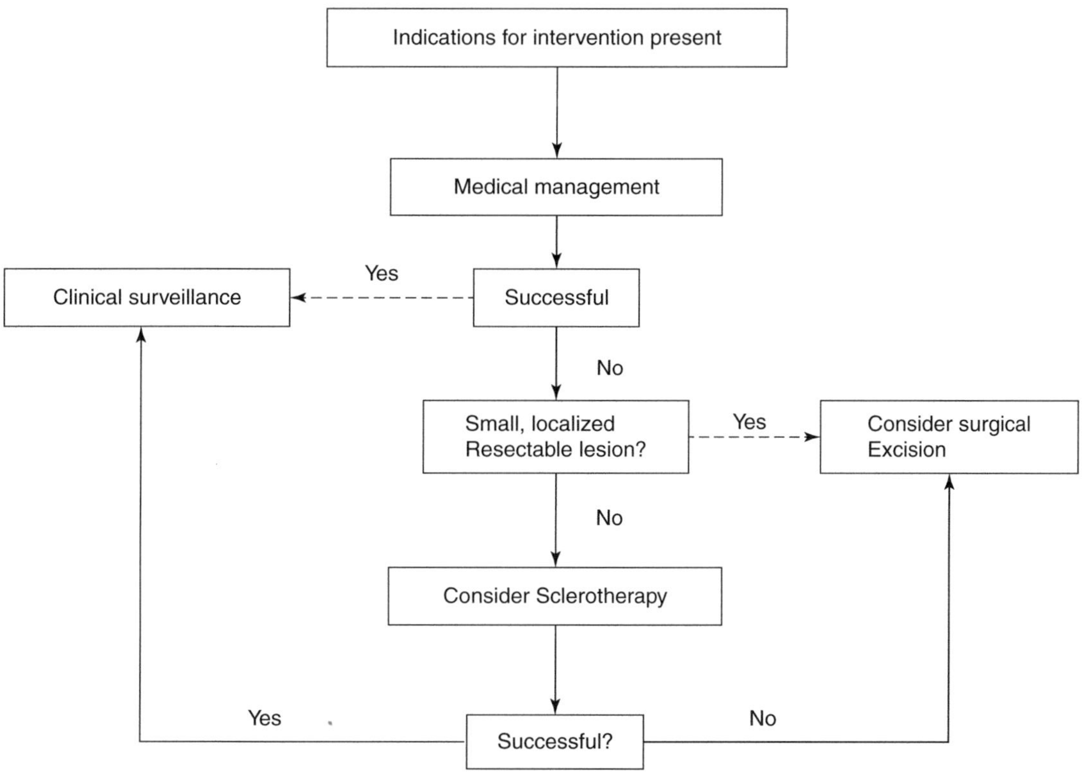

Fig. 16.1 Strategy for selection of the appropriate treatment method for VMs

to patterns of venous drainage VMs are classified into four types with different outcomes after Sclerotherapy as in (Table 16.3, Fig. 16.2). This classification can also predict the risk of complications following sclerotherapy. Sclerotherapy of type I and II VM is uneventful and successful, while in type III and IV VMs sclerotherapy carries a significant risk of complications and may not be possible due to the presence of wide and ectatic veins [11].

Mechanism of Action of Sclerotherapy It disrupts the phospholipids bilayer of the endothelial cells, which leads to a cytotoxic effect on endothelial cells leading to the exposure of subendothelial collagen, activating the coagulation cascade and resulting in thrombosis and fibrosis of the anomalous vessels with reduction of the size [12].

Sclerosing Agents A variety of sclerosants are available which differ in their method of endothelial destruction. Systematic reviews could not identify a significantly superior sclerosing agent in terms of effectiveness. Instead, it is vital to consider the local and systemic side effects of the different sclerosing agents [13, 14]. Frequently used sclerosants in the treatment of VMs are; (a) ethanol, (b) ethanol gel, (c) sodium tetradecyl sulfate, (d) polidocanol, and (e) bleomycin.

Table 16.3 Classification of venous malformations based on phlebography

Type	Description on phlebography
I	Isolated VM with no peripheral drainage
II	VM drain into the normal vein
III	VM drain into dysplastic veins
IV	VM represent dysplastic venous ectasia

VM Venous malformation

(a) **Ethanol:** A very effective sclerosing agent in the treatment of VM. It causes precipitation of endothelial cells and thrombosis of ectatic veins. It should be used with caution as it can result in serious local and systemic side effects like skin hyperpigmentation, necrosis, ulcer, nerve injury, compartment compression, hypoglycemia, deep venous thrombosis, pulmonary embolism, pulmonary vasospasm, cardiac collapse, and death. To minimize these side effects ethanol is injected at a low dose of 0.15 ml/kg over 10 min, in this dose ethanol can be injected without the necessity for pulmonary capillary pressure monitoring [15].

(b) **Ethanol Gel:** Ethanol can be administered as highly viscous gel form to limit diffusion and to keep ethanol in ectatic veins. Compared to ethanol, ethanol gel has a favorable safety profile [1, 16].

(c) **Sodium Tetradecyl Sulfate (STS):** STS has a low complication rate in the treatment of VMs. STS is the active component of the drug Sotradecol [17].

(d) **Polidocanol:** It is a local anesthetic with sclerosants property used in the treatment of VMs. It has fewer side effects compared to ethanol. Polidocanol foam made by using the Tessari technique (1:4 ratio of sclerosant and carbon dioxide) has a higher rate of obliteration compared to liquid Polidocanol [18], Fig. 16.3. Air should not be used to avoid the associated risk of embolism.

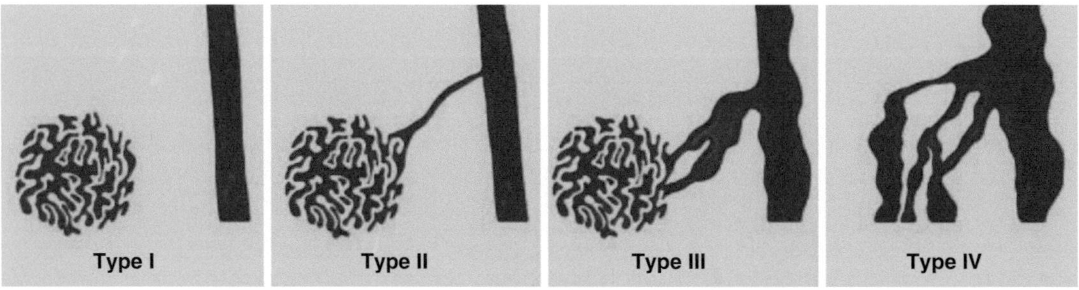

Fig. 16.2 Classification of venous malformation based on diagnostic phlebography

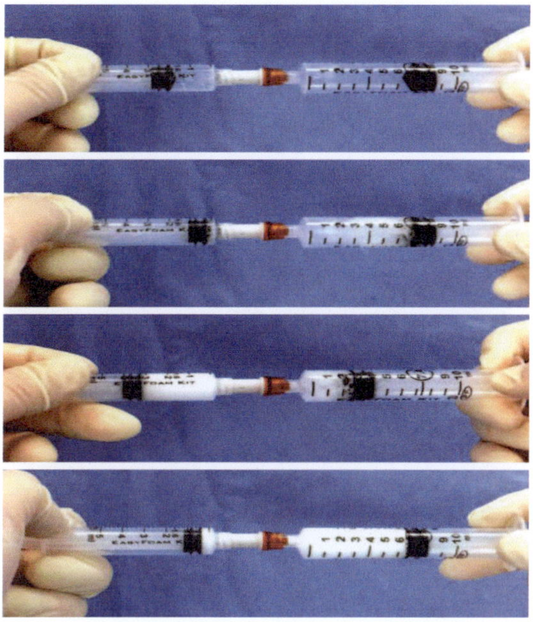

Fig. 16.3 Tessari technique of foam sclerotherapy

(e) **Bleomycin:** Bleomycin is a cytotoxic, antineoplastic antibiotic derived from *Streptomyces verticillus*. Swelling is less intensive after bleomycin compared to ethanol, hence it is a safer agent in patients with VMs causing airway compression. Bleomycin has the potential risk of pulmonary fibrosis and bleomycin-induced neoplasms has been reported in children, thus it should be used with caution [12].

Contraindication Known right-to-left shunts, e.g., patent foramen ovale. (Risk of systemic embolization of the sclerosant).

Anesthesia Sclerotherapy with STS and polidocanol can be performed under analgesia and sedation. General anesthesia is preferred particularly during injection of ethanol and bleomycin.

Application Technique Under real-time ultrasound guidance, direct puncture of the VM is performed with a 20 or 21 gage needle. Once the free flow of blood noted from a needle or a scalp vein puncture, a radio-opaque contrast is injected to obtain a phlebogram of the VM to confirm the position of the needle, estimate the lesion volume and compartmentalization, and to identify draining veins. Four different types of VMs were noted based on phlebograms as in Table 16.3 and Fig. 16.2.

After diagnostic phlebography, a sclerosant is injected slowly under fluoroscopy guidance, which displaces the contrast agent from VM (Fig. 16.4). Local compression of local visible veins or a tourniquet or a pneumatic cuff may be useful to minimize the risk of accidental migration of sclerosant into the deep venous system. The injection should be stopped if there is skin blanching or resistance or extravasation. Depending on the size of the VM, multiple punctures may be required.

16.6 Additional Venous Outflow Occlusion

When a VM is drained by dysplastic, ectatic veins (type III VM) to avoid overflow of contrast into the deep venous system additional occlusion of these ectatic veins is indicated [19]. Through an access needle or a catheter, fibered micro-coils or plug of various types can be placed into the draining veins.

16.7 Endovenous Ablation Techniques

Endovenous laser ablation (EVLA) or Endovenous radiofrequency ablation (ERFA) were successfully used to close ectatic veins (type IV VM), as in lateral marginal vein in patients with Klippel–Trenaunay syndrome and CLOVES syndrome. To reduce the risk of thromboembolism such venous anomalies are ablated endovenously as early as possible [20].

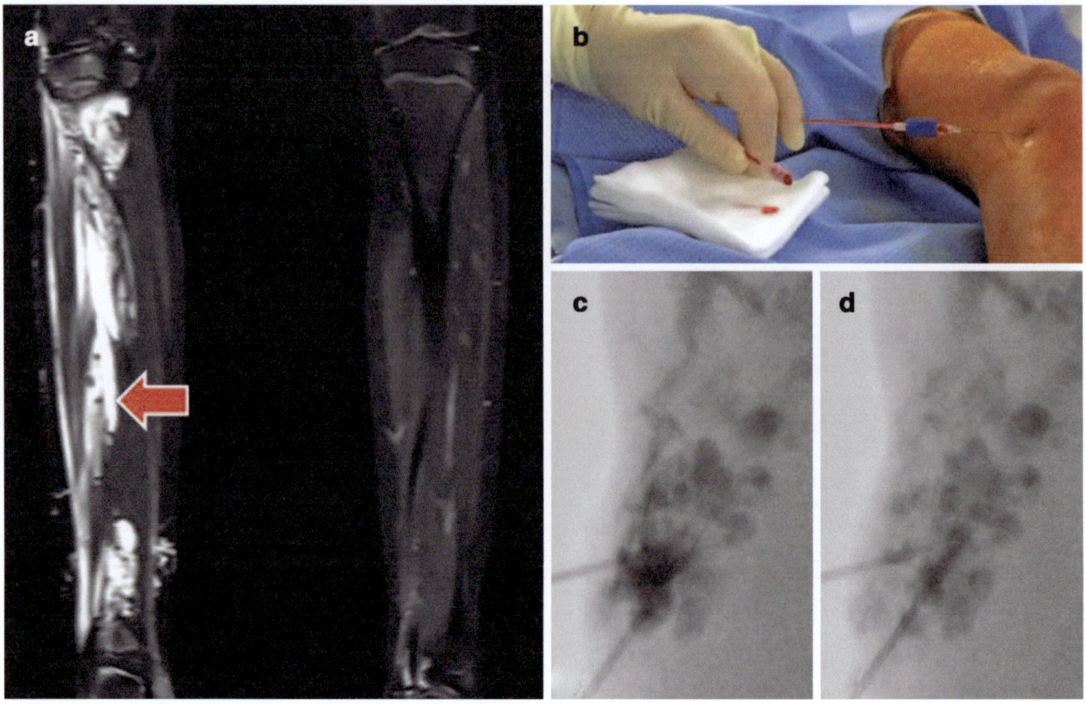

Fig. 16.4 The procedure of sclerotherapy. (**a**) MRI showing hyperintense lesion on T2 weighed image with Phlebolithiasis (arrow), (**b**) Ultrasound-guided percutaneous puncture of the venous malformation, (**c**) Diagnostic phlebogram, (**d**) Injection of sclerosing agent

16.8 Post-Intervention Care

Prophylactic antibiotics are not required. Local compression garments should be worn to help the involution of the lesion. To alleviate pain and edema limb elevation, ice pack, analgesics may be indicated. To prevent deep venous thrombosis prophylactic low molecular vein heparin may be used in large lesions. Particularly where localized intravascular coagulation is detected, prophylactic heparin should be started 5–7 days before and after the treatment session to avoid the risk of DIC. Depending on the size of the lesion and location, multiple treatments are required. Some publications have shown a range of 1–12 sessions to achieve clinical benefits. When re-intervention is necessary, it is done after 6–8 weeks [21].

Outcome In a systematic review by Qiu et al., on the outcomes of sclerotherapy in vascular malformations, 32.5% of the lesions were cured (objective outcomes obtained through measuring the volume of the VM), with up to 30.2% of patients referring total disappearance of symptoms. Improvement in lesion volume was recorded in 58.9% and subjective perception of improvement in symptoms was registered in 60.9% of the treated patients. Little change or failure in reducing the malformation's volume was reported in 8.6% of patients, and 8.9% had no improvement of their symptoms [12].

Surgery It is a good option for small and well localized lesions not compromising vital structures [22].

16.9 Capillary Malformation

CMs are the least common and the most superficial of all the slow-flow VMs. These are classically named as "port-wine stains," composed of dilated and ectatic capillary to venule sized vessels [23].

Clinical Features These are the least common form of VMs seen in 0.3% of children as a macular pink to dark red patch with irregular borders commonly in the trigeminal dermatome distribution [6].

Diagnosis It is diagnosed on the basis of clinical features. Imaging therefore not required, may be useful to evaluate underlying disorders in syndromic patients [24].

16.10 Treatment

Primarily by flash-lamp pulsed-dye laser therapy. Laser, is absorbed by hemoglobin, converted to heat leading to blood vessel wall coagulation, which is achieved by sparing adjacent tissues. This process is known as selective photothermolysis. The results of this therapy are better at younger age, hence should be started as early as possible. Several sessions are usually required for the complete response of the lesion. Some CMs which are resistant to this therapy, other options include photodynamic therapy and intense pulse light therapy [25].

16.11 Lymphatic Malformation (LM)

LMs are traditionally misnamed as "lymphangiomas or cystic hygromas" are the second most common type of vascular malformation [26]. LMs are dilated lymphatic channels or cyst filled with chyle, lined by endothelial cells with lymphatic phenotype. LMs are divided into (a) Macrocystic LMs, (b) Microcystic LMs, and (c) Mixed LMs. (A) Macrocystic LMs are large, intercommunicating cysterns, lined by endothelial cells without an increase in mitotic activity, filled with proteinaceous fluid which contains lymphocytes, macrophages and occasional erythrocytes. (B) Microcystic LMs are composed of small lymphatic channels that may interdigitate with tissue elements. (C) Combined LMs consists of lesions with both macrocystic and microcystic lymphatic channels [22].

Clinical Features LMs usually present within 2 years of life. They are usually present in the neck (70–80%), especially in the posterior triangle and axillary region (20%), less commonly in the mediastinum, retroperitoneum, and extremities [27]. Depending on the location and dimensions LMs can present with various ways. Small superficial lesions may appear as fluid filled vesicles while larger lesions cause swelling and deformity. LMs are non-pulsatile, generally compressible unless very tense and their dimensions are not affected by the change in posture or Valsalva maneuver [28].

LMs are commonly asymptomatic, but may be complicated by the rapid expansion of lesion due to infection, trauma, or bleeding. Large cysts may cause a mass effect on adjoining structures. Superficial lesions are prone to infection, ulceration, bleeding. LMs may be accompanied by tissue overgrowth leading to deformity and functional impairment [29].

Diagnosis LMs diagnosis is based on history, physical examination, and imaging.

Ultrasound On ultrasonography LMs appear as thin wall cystic lesion with posterior acoustic enhancement with thin septa. Doppler signals are absent within cyst except for septa [5]. Microcystic LMs are too small to be noted and present as ill-defined hypoechoic lesion with posterior acoustic enhancement [8].

MRI MRI is the preferred imaging modality for assessment of the lesion. Macrocystic LM appears as well-defined cystic lesion with septae. The cysts have low signal-intensity in T1-weighted images and are hyperintense in T2-weighted images. Microcystic LMs normally appear diffuse areas of low signal-intensity in T1-weighted images and high signal-intensity in T2-weighted images, as the cysts are too small to be identifiable as discrete structures in MRI [12].

Lymphoscintigraphy Using 99mTc labeled human serum albumin or 99mTc-labeled sulfur colloid may be useful for the evaluation of lymphatic function and the characterization of lymphatic anomalies.

Treatment As in all CVMs, a multidisciplinary team management is prerequisite and with an aim of minimizing symptoms and improving quality of life.

Indications for Intervention Symptomatic LMs due to recurrent infection, recurrent bleeding, severe aesthetic deformity, or functional impairment of neighboring structures [19].

Various treatment modalities and strategies in the management of LMs are shown in Fig. 16.5 [29].

16.12 Conservative Management

Physical therapy for the decongestion of LMs is of utmost important in the management of some of the LMs. It include manual lymphatic drainage, movement exercise, and compression therapy with the use of bandages, garments, and pneumatic compression devices. In order to minimize the risk of infection, the patient should be advised on good skincare and prevention of trauma [30].

16.13 Medical Therapy

Recent studies have shown the positive effect of m-Tor inhibitor Sirolimus in extensive lymphatic malformations especially in infants with cervicofacial lesion [31]. However, further studies are necessary to confirm its efficacy and safety.

Sclerotherapy In the recent past surgery was the principal method of management of LMs, with the risk of incomplete resection and functional and cosmetic side effects. But, in recent times sclerotherapy has evolved as the preferred method of management method, especially for macrocystic LMs. In Microcystic LMs sclerotherapy is not possible due to their small size [31]. STS is less effective in LMs [32]. Ethanol carries an increased risk of complications [31]. The most commonly used sclerosants are:

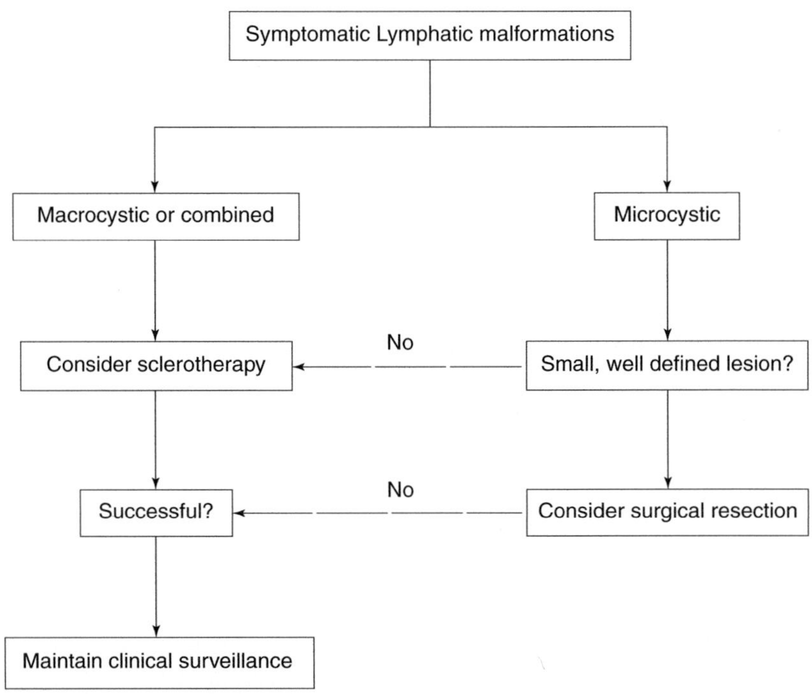

Fig. 16.5 Treatment options and strategy for lymphatic malformations

(a) **Picibanil (OK 432):** It is a lyophilized mixture of group A *Streptococcus pyogenes* with a high capacity to produce fibrosis. It has been shown to be safe and effective in the treatment of LMs in children. To achieve clinical success repeated injections may be necessary. It can induce severe swelling lasting for more than 1 week, hence when airway compromise is suspected, elective intubation and ventilation may be necessary. Another side effect is post-procedural fever, which can be treated with paracetamol for 1–3 days [33].

(b) **Bleomycin:** It is a well-known sclerosant with a low risk of swelling; hence it is the preferred agent for the treatment of macrocystic LMs in the head and neck area. To avoid pulmonary fibrosis bleomycin should be used in small doses [34].

(c) **Doxycycline:** It can be used in both macrocystic and mixed LMs. It is a very effective sclerosant agent that can be used in head and neck LMs with minimal side effects and is widely used [35].

Application Technique Under ultrasound guidance cyst is cannulated with a needle or a 3–5 French pigtail catheter (in larger cyst). Lymphatic fluid is aspirated and contrast is injected to visualize the whole lesion under fluoroscopy. After the aspiration of cyst contents, the LM can be treated with the sclerosant (Fig. 16.6).

16.14 Post-Procedural Care

In patients with cervical LMs treated with a sclerosant, strict observation of the upper airway is recommended. Fever following Picibanil is treated with paracetamol. Positive effects of sclerotherapy are visualized after 4–6 weeks.

Outcome In a study by Alomari et al. reported a complete resolution in 45%, 14%, and 13% of patients with macrocystic, microcystic, and combined lesions respectively [31].

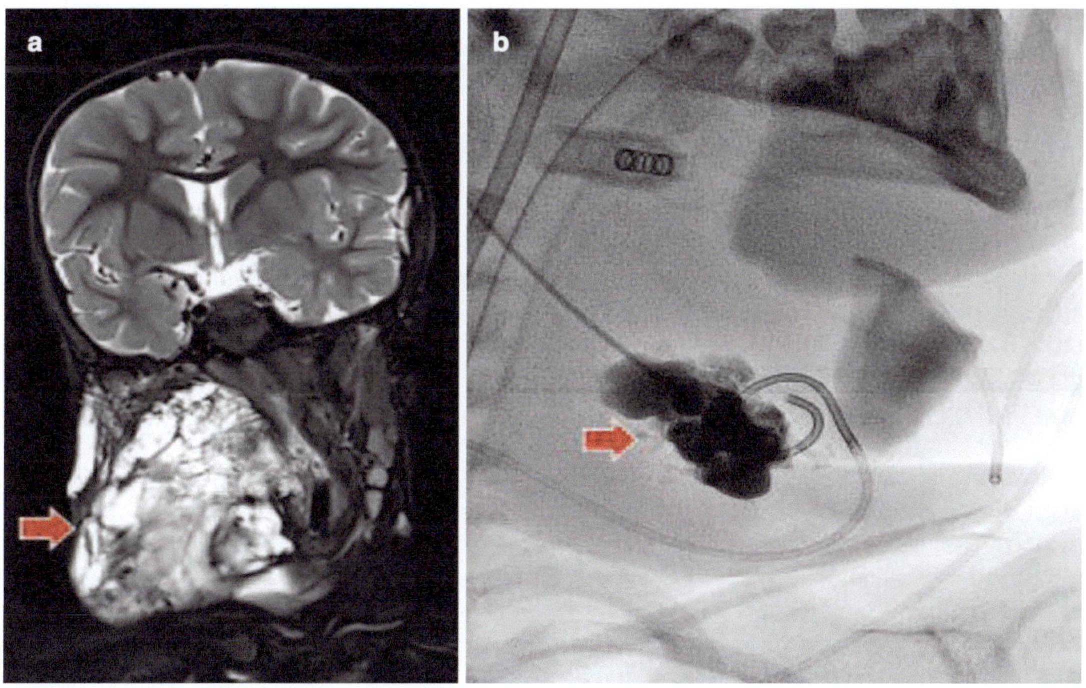

Fig. 16.6 (**a**) Macrocystic lymphatic malformation. Presented as hyperintense macrocystic lymphatic malformation of the neck (arrow). (**b**) Two 3-French pigtail catheters were inserted into the cysts and contrast media was injected before sclerotherapy with OK-432 (arrow)

16.15 Surgical Resection

The majority of LMs can be managed with sclerotherapy. Indications for surgical management include: (a) Small well-localized LMs, (b) Symptomatic microcystic LMs, (c) Macrocystic and combined LMs that can no longer be managed by sclerotherapy, (d) Primary lymphedema. Surgical management of LMs includes resection and reconstruction. Surgical reconstruction is particularly useful in primary lymphedema. Surgical options include lymphatic-venous anastomosis, lympho-venous-lymphatic bypass anastomosis, lympho-lymphatic segmental interposition or lymph nodes transfer from a donor region to an affected area are the most commonly used [36]. Surgical excision in total with reconstruction or staged resection is the surgical options available for LMs other than primary lymphedema. But, these are associated with high risk of local recurrence and with complications like postoperative bleeding and infection [37].

16.16 Arteriovenous Malformations

AVMs are the high flow anomalies resulting from the persistence of primitive blood vessels connecting the feeding arteries and the draining veins, bypassing the capillary bed, which is often partially or completely absent. When there is a single direct connecting channel between an artery and a vein it is called AVF, while in AVM there is a combination of single or multiple feeding arteries and the draining veins separated by a nidus of dysplastic vascular channels [24].

In AVM arteries are larger, tortuous with the destruction of internal elastic lamina in some arteries, and shunting of high-pressure arterial blood directly into the veins, results in fibrosis of intima, hypertrophy of media, and the absence of adventitia in the draining veins [24]. They can occur anywhere in the body, but most commonly intracranial, followed by extracranial head, extremities, trunk, and viscera [38]. Although AVMs occur predominantly sporadically, but genetic predisposition is seen in several clinical syndromes such as Osler–Weber–Rendu syndrome, Parkes Weber syndrome, Congenital Lipomatous Overgrowth, Vascular malformations, Epidermal nevi, and Skeletal deformities (CLOVES) syndrome [39].

Clinical Features Although AVMs are present since birth; their presentation may be delayed till childhood or adulthood. They gradually increase in size with age, rapid growth can be triggered by physical factors such as trauma, thrombosis, infection, or hormonal changes as occur during puberty or pregnancy [40]. AVMs are pink to red cutaneous lesions, warm on touch, with thrill or a bruit. If left untreated the progressive nature of AVMs was best described by the clinical staging of the disease by Schobinger as in Table 16.4 [41].

16.17 Diagnosis

Although in most cases, diagnosis can be made by clinical examination alone, however imaging is necessary for better characterization of the lesion and planning appropriate treatment.

Ultrasonography with Doppler Ultrasonography with different modes, is the first-line investigation in the evaluation of suspicious AVM. It shows a heterogeneously echoic, ill-defined area of hypervascular lesion without any definitive mass, with a dilated network of vessels with multiple arterial feeders and venous drainers,

Table 16.4 Schobinger clinical staging of arteriovenous malformations

Stage	Description	Findings
I	Quiescent	Cutaneous blush or warmth
II	Expansion	Bruit or thrill, increasing size, pulsation, no pain
III	Destruction	Pain, bleeding, infection, skin necrosis, or ulceration
IV	Decompensation	High-output cardiac failure

which are dilated and tortuous due to the arterialization of the veins [39].

MRI: It is required for definitive diagnosis and evaluation of the extent of the lesion. AVM appear ill defined, infiltrating non-mass like lesion with high flow large feeding arteries and draining veins [8, 22].

CTA: Computed tomography angiogram gives less information than MRI, however can be useful when AVMs involving bones, present as a lytic lesion [12].

Conventional Angiography It is an invasive method reserved for the lesions planned for endovascular treatment in the same sitting.

16.18 Treatment

As with intervention in other CVMs, AVMs involve a multidisciplinary system with individualization of the treatment. The indications for the treatment of AVMs are as summarized in Table 16.5.

For proper treatment planning, a detailed local anatomy, shunt type, clinical and hemodynamic consequence of and risk of recurrence are to be assessed properly. For the selection of appropriate treatment option Cho et al. developed an angiography based classification system, dividing AVMs into four types, as in Table 16.6 and Fig. 16.7 [42]. He also noted that type II was the most curable lesions while type IIIa and IIIb were more difficult to cure, with higher failure and recurrence rates [42].

The main therapeutic options in the management of AVMs are sclerotherapy, embolization, and surgical resection (Fig. 16.8).

Table 16.5 Indications for the treatment of arteriovenous malformation

Absolute	Relative
Hemorrhage	Progressive pain/discomfort
Increasing risk of high-output heart failure	Functional impairment or severe cosmetic deformity with an impact on daily life and quality of life
Complications of chronic venous hypertension	Vascular-bone syndrome with progressive skeletal deformities
Lesions which are life and/or limb threatening	Lesions located in regions with a high risk of complication
Lesions threatening vital functions	Lesions with recurrent infection and sepsis

16.19 Conservative Therapy

Compression garments improve the symptoms of AVMs and quality of life. Analgesics may be required to control pain.

16.20 Embolotherapy

Consists of intravascular injection of inert agents. It is the first choice in the management of AVMs, as it has low morbidity with acceptable results, but with the high risk of local recurrence. Embolotherapy is also used preoperatively in some cases where surgical resection of the nidus has been planned [10]. Interventionist's should be aware of various properties of differet materials and their delivery mechanisms. The goal of the endovascular embolotheray is to occlude nidus/fistula as well as early draining veins while sparing the normal arterial branches supplying adjacent areas [12]. Embolization or ligation of proximal arteries may lead to the development of collaterals from branches and the obliteration of the best arteries, which further lead to management difficulties [31].

Commonly used agents in embolotherapy are ethanol, N-butyl cyanoacrylate (NBCA), ethylene-vinyl-alcohol-copolymer (EVOH), in some cases to optimize the hemodynamics additionally coils or vascular plugs for further treatment. But they occlude only feeding vessels never reach the nidus. Hence they are used as an adjuvant, never mere coiling. They are used in combination in the management of AVMs.

Ethanol It is a very potent embolic agent in the management of symptomatic AVMs. However it is associated with a high risk of tissue necrosis, nerve injury, and systemic effects, as ethanol is a low vis-

Table 16.6 Angiographic classification of arteriovenous malformations and their preferential treatment approach

Type	Morphology	Description	Treatment approach
I	Arteriovenous fistulae	≤ 3 arteries to one drainage vein	DP/ TV
II	Arteriovenous fistulae	Multiple arteries draining into one draining vein	DP/ TV
III	Arteriolo-venulous fistulae without dilatation	Multiple arteries shunting into multiple venules	
IIIa	Arteriolo-venulous fistulae without dilatation	Multiple arteries shunting into multiple venules with non-dilated fistulae (appear as blush or fine striations)	TA
IIIb	Arteriolo-venulous fistulae with dilatation	Multiple arteries shunting into multiple venules with dilated fistulae (appear as a complex vascular network)	TA also amenable to DP

DP Direct Puncture, *TV* trans venous access, *TA* Trans arterial approach

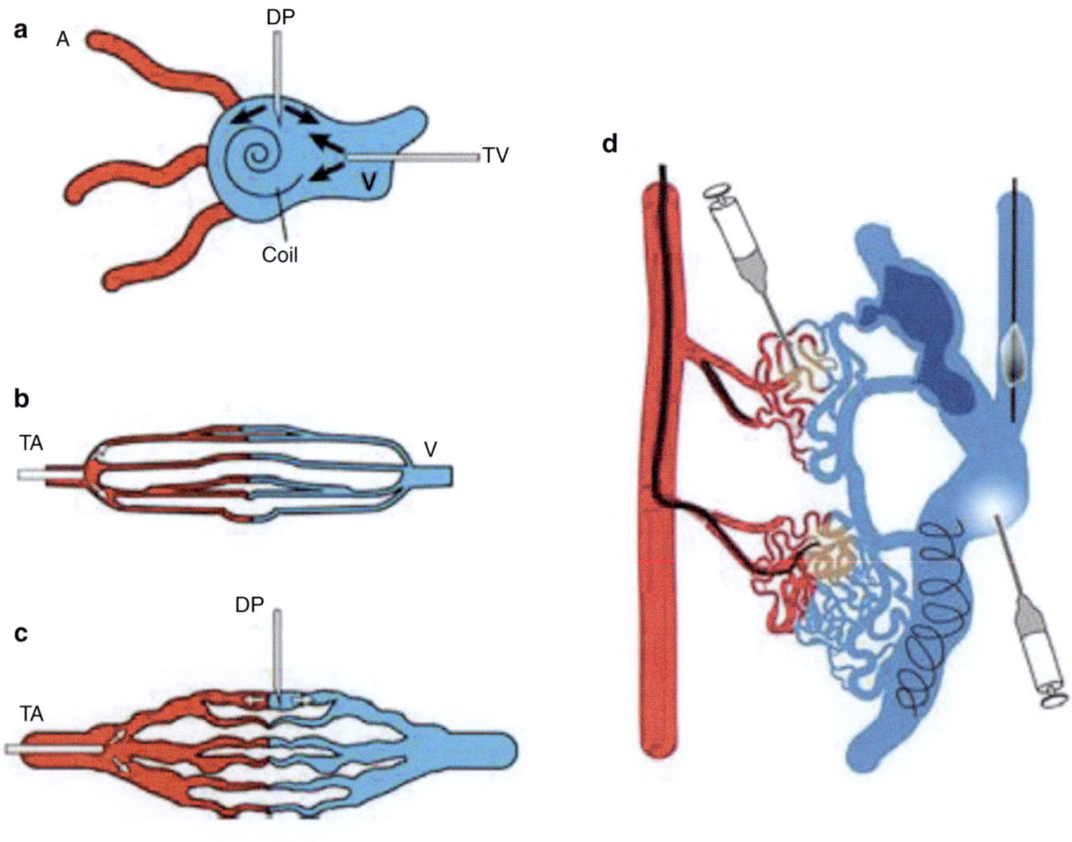

Fig. 16.7 Schematic representation of angiographic classification and access route adapted from Cho et al. (**a**) Transvenous approach and direct puncture of the nidus for type I and II, (**b**) Transarterial approach for type IIIa, (**c**) Transarterial approach and direct puncture for type IIIb. (**d**) Mixed lesions may require a combined approach. *A* artery, *V* vein, *TV* Trans Venous, *DP* Direct Puncture, *TA* Trans arterial

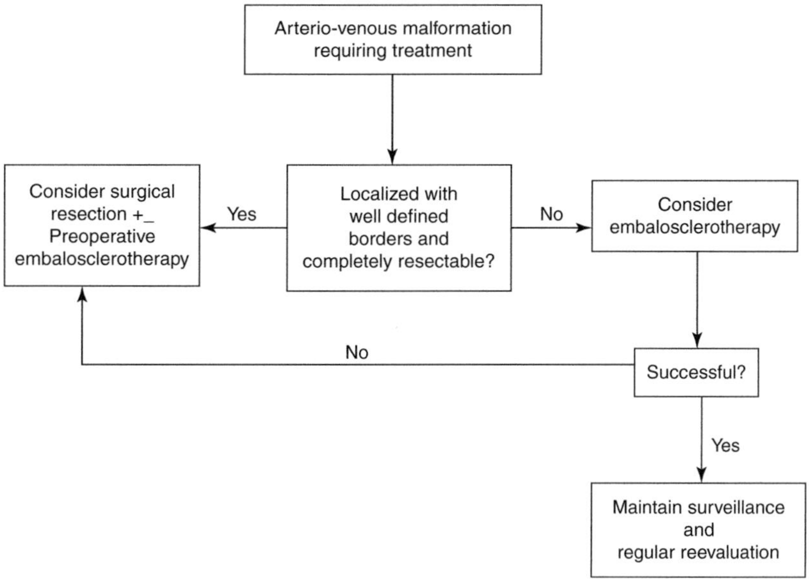

Fig. 16.8 Treatment options in arteriovenous malformations

cous substance it passes through the nidus very quickly into lung circulation. Hence pulmonary arterial pressure (PAP) monitoring is done continuously during ethanol embolization of AVMs. PAP above 25 mm of Hg after 10–15 min of ethanol embolization indicates the systemic spread of ethanol [42]. Most intervention radiologists use low dose ethanol at 0.5 ml per Kg body weight in small aliquots.

N-butyl Cyanoacrylate It is a liquid agent, polymerizes irreversibly on the exposure of the anions in the blood. To enable fluoroscopic visibility and adjust polymerization time, NBCA is mixed with lipiodol at the ratio of 1:1 to 1:5 and the catheters are flushed with 5% glucose solution. Another drawback of NBCA is the potential risk of catheter tip adhesion.

Ethylene-Vinyl-Alcohol-Copolymer (EVOH) It is a non-adhesive liquid embolic agent mixed with dimethyl sulfoxide (DMSO) and radiopaque tantalum powder. EVOH has a longer casting time compared to NBCA, which allows penetration into the nidus (Fig. 16.9). As it is radio-opaque agent with a longer casting time, it can be slowly administered under fluoroscopy guidance using road map techniques (Fig. 16.10). Using EVOH refluxed around the catheter tip as a plug, the active forward push of EVOH into the whole nidus is possible even against the blood flow (Plug and push technique (Fig. 16.11). The important side effect of EVOH is, injection is very painful and to be performed under general anesthesia.

Plug and Coils Can be used in simple AVMs like type I. They are also used in outflow occlusion in type II lesions [43].

Technique Baseline diagnostic catheter angiography is performed to determine the flow characters and morphology of malformation and classified into four types as in Table 16.6 [42]. In most cases embolization can be done transarterial approach, often requiring direct puncture sclerotherapy of the nidus after embolizing feeding arteries. Retrograde transvenous embolization of the nidus can be performed in dominant venous outflow as in type I and II AVMs [43].

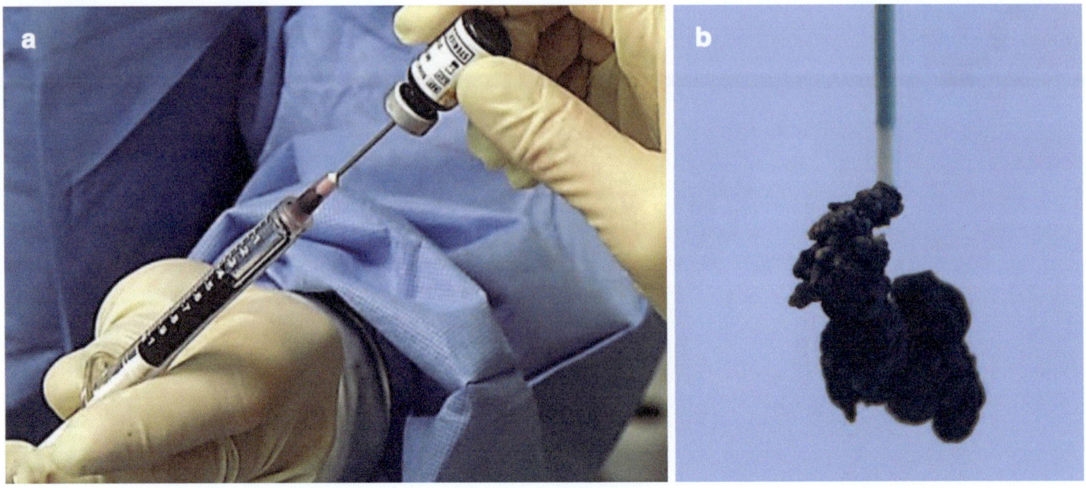

Fig. 16.9 Ethylene-vinyl-alcohol-copolymer (EVOH). EVOH is a non-adhesive liquid embolic agent mixed with dimethyl sulfoxide (DMSO) and radio-opaque tantalum powder (**a**, **b**)

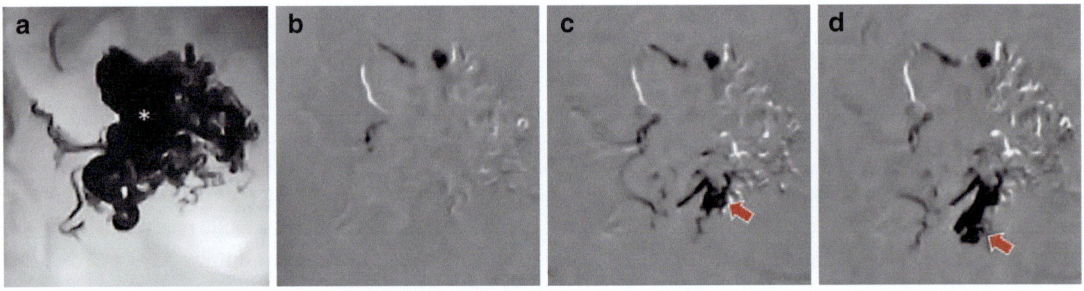

Fig. 16.10 Controlled administration of EVOH in a controlled manner under fluoroscopy guidance (**a**, **b**). The distribution of EVOH can be followed easily using the "roadmap" technique (arrow in **c**, **d**)

16.21 Post-Procedure Care

Good analgesic coverage to control pain with opioids, to avoid stressful post-intervention period. Pain may prevent the patient to complete treatment series with multiple sessions. It is mandatory to closely monitor skin and neurovascular assessment during the immediate post-intervention period. Long-term surveillance with intermittent imaging should be performed to rule out recurrence.

Sclerotherapy Various sclerosants and their mechanism of action are explained in detail in venous malformation. High flow and collateral flow of AVMs, may dilute the sclerosant agent or redirect it away from the targeted area. Hence a combination of embolization and sclerotherapy known as embolosclerotherapy is used which makes sclerosant safe and effective in previously embolized AVMs.

Outcome of Embolosclerotherapy Because of the variability in the method of evaluation of the results of sclerotherapy, limited studies in evaluating sclerotherapy are available. In a retrospective analysis of Do et al. ethanol embolization had a cure and partial response rate of 40% and 28% respectively, with a complication rate of 52% [44].

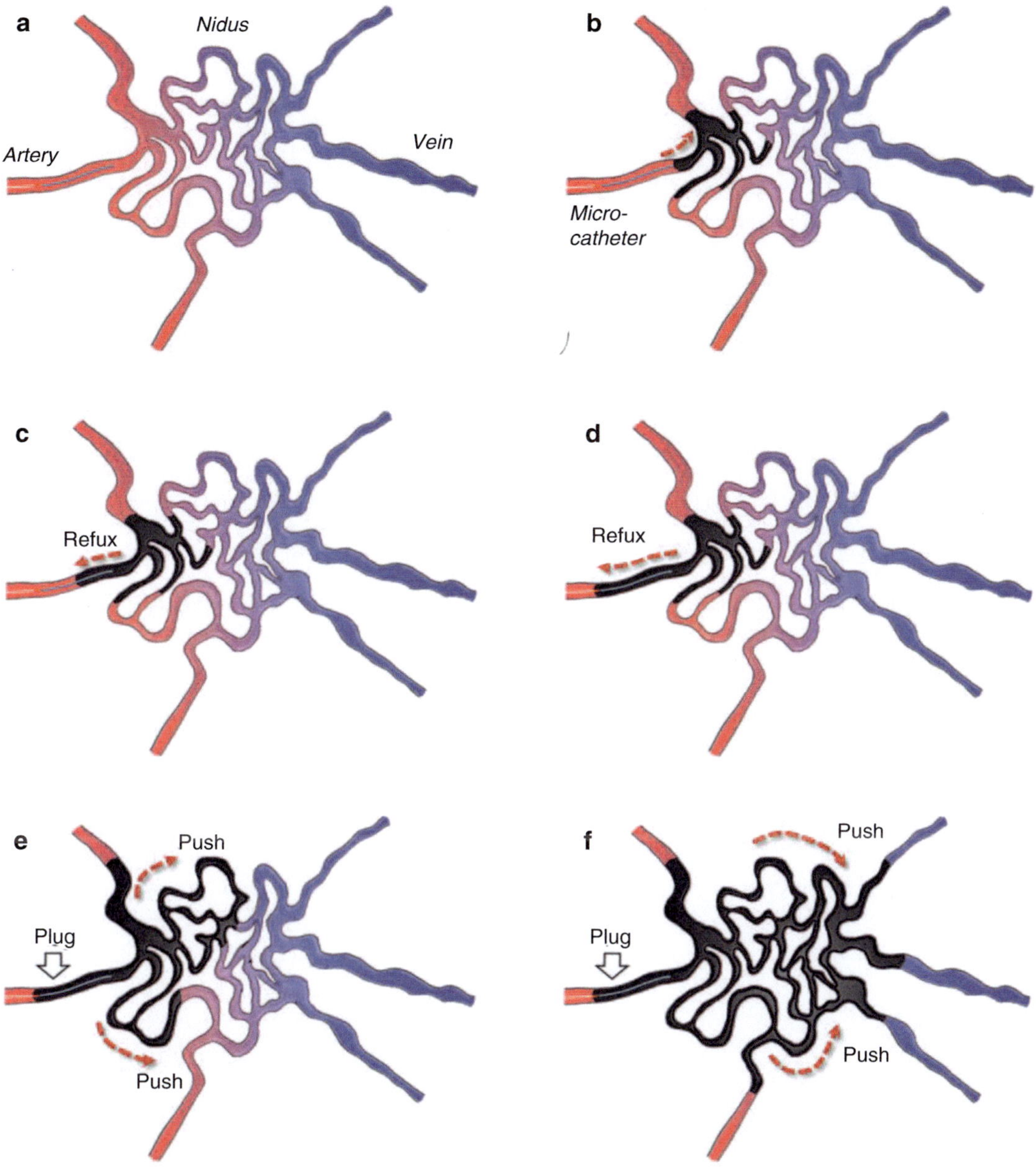

Fig. 16.11 Plug and push technique. Using the reflux of EVOH as a plug around the detachable tip of the microcatheter, an active forward flow of EVOH into the whole nidus is possible regardless of the flow direction (**a–f**)

Surgical Resection It is another method in the management of AVMs, it is used alone or in the combination of embolosclerotherapy. Surgery is indicated in lesions, which are localized, well-defined borders that can be resected with minimal bleeding with a low chance of recurrence, increasing the chance of cure. In the case of diffuse AVMs surgical resection is challenging and may lead to extensive bleeding, which may require reconstruction after large resections. To minimize the risk of recurrence complete resection should be aimed [45]. Hence surgical resection for diffuse AVMs is indicated only in life-threatening bleeding, progressive growth of

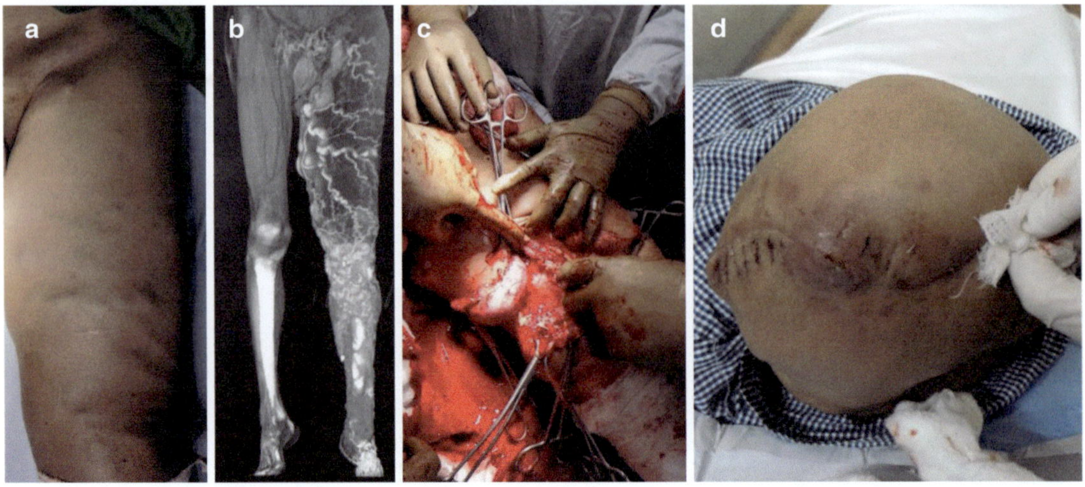

Fig. 16.12 (**a**) Clinical image of high flow arteriovenous malformation with recurrent episodes of bleeding and patient had gangrene of foot and leg due to AVM shunting and ischemia to leg (not shown in picture) (**b**) CT angiography showing diffuse arteriovenous malformation (**c**) Intraoperative image, performing above knee amputation with ligation of femoral artery for gangrene of leg (**d**) Above knee amputated stump

AVMs with a cosmetic deformity or functional impairment which are persistent despite the use of other treatment modalities. Preoperative embolization is frequently beneficial and should be performed before 24–48 h before the planned surgical procedure (Fig. 16.12).

16.22 Conclusion

A good understanding of the classification of the CVMs, extent, and the hemodynamic consequence of such lesion is necessary for selecting the appropriate treatment option or selecting the sequence of treatment options for optimal management of these lesions with low recurrence rates. In recent times, with the advances in minimally invasive interventional radiological techniques, this challenging group of diseases can be managed better with acceptable morbidity and outcome and has replaced traditional open surgery as the preferred treatment modality.

References

1. Dompmartin A, Vikkula M, Boon LM. Venous malformation: update on aetiopathogenesis, diagnosis and management. Phlebology. 2010;25(5):224–35.
2. Wassef M, Blei F, Adams D, Alomari A, Baselga E, Berenstein A, Burrows P, Frieden IJ, Garzon MC, Lopez-Gutierrez JC, Lord DJ. Vascular anomalies classification: recommendations from the international society for the study of vascular anomalies. Pediatrics. 2015;136(1):e203–14.
3. McRae MY, Adams S, Pereira J, Parsi K, Wargon O. Venous malformations: clinical course and management of vascular birthmark clinic cases. Australas J Dermatol. 2013;54(1):22–30.
4. Flors L, Hagspiel KD, Park AW, Norton PT, Leiva-Salinas C. Vascular malformations and tumors. Part 2: low-flow lesions. Radiología (English Edition). 2019;61(2):124–33.
5. Behr GG, Johnson CM. Vascular anomalies: hemangiomas and beyond—part 2, slow-flow lesions. Am J Roentgenol. 2013;200(2):423–36.
6. Kapadia SR, Thakore VM, Patel HM. Vascular malformations: an update on classification, clinical features, and management principles. Indian J Vasc Endovasc Surg. 2017;4(4):152.
7. Johnson CM, Navarro OM. Clinical and sonographic features of pediatric soft-tissue vascular anoma-

lies part 2: vascular malformations. Pediatr Radiol. 2017;47(9):1196–208.
8. Flors L, Leiva-Salinas C, Maged IM, Norton PT, Matsumoto AH, Angle JF, Hugo Bonatti MD, Park AW, Ahmad EA, Bozlar U, Housseini AM. MR imaging of soft-tissue vascular malformations: diagnosis, classification, and therapy follow-up. Radiographics. 2011;31(5):1321–40.
9. Goyal M, Causer PA, Armstrong D. Venous vascular malformations in pediatric patients: comparison of results of alcohol sclerotherapy with proposed MR imaging classification. Radiology. 2002;223(3):639–44.
10. Ranieri M, Wohlgemuth W, Müller-Wille R, Prantl L, Kehrer A, Geis S, Klein S, Lamby P, Schiltz D, Uller W, Aung T. Vascular malformations of upper and lower extremity–from radiological interventional therapy to surgical soft tissue reconstruction–an interdisciplinary treatment. Clin Hemorheol Microcirc. 2017;67(3–4):355–72.
11. Puig S, Aref H, Chigot V, Bonin B, Brunelle F. Classification of venous malformations in children and implications for sclerotherapy. Pediatr Radiol. 2003;33(2):99–103.
12. Legiehn GM, Heran MK. A step-by-step practical approach to imaging diagnosis and interventional radiologic therapy in vascular malformations. In: Seminars in interventional radiology. New York: © Thieme Medical Publishers; 2010, June. Vol. 27, No. 02, p. 209–231.
13. Qiu Y, Chen H, Lin X, Hu X, Jin Y, Ma G. Outcomes and complications of sclerotherapy for venous malformations. Vasc Endovasc Surg. 2013;47(6):454–61.
14. Ali S, Mitchell SE, Outcomes of venous malformation sclerotherapy: a review of study methodology and long-term results. In: Seminars in interventional radiology. New York: Thieme Medical Publishers; 2017, September. Vol. 34, No. 03, p. 288–293.
15. Orlando JL, Caldas JGMP, Campos HGDA, Nishinari K, Wolosker N. Outpatient percutaneous treatment of deep venous malformations using pure ethanol at low doses under local anesthesia. Clinics. 2010;65(9):837–40.
16. Teusch VI, Wohlgemuth WA, Hammer S, Piehler AP, Müller-Wille R, Goessmann H, Uller W. Ethanol-gel sclerotherapy of venous malformations: effectiveness and safety. Am J Roentgenol. 2017;209(6):1390–5.
17. Park HS, Do YS, Park KB, Kim KH, Woo SY, Jung SH, Kim DI, Kim YW, Hyun D, Cho SK, Choo IW. Clinical outcome and predictors of treatment response in foam sodium tetradecyl sulfate sclerotherapy of venous malformations. Eur Radiol. 2016;26(5):1301–10.
18. Yamaki T, Nozaki M, Sakurai H, Takeuchi M, Soejima K, Kono T. Prospective randomized efficacy of ultrasound-guided foam sclerotherapy compared with ultrasound-guided liquid sclerotherapy in the treatment of symptomatic venous malformations. J Vasc Surg. 2008;47(3):578–84.
19. Burrows PE, Mason KP. Percutaneous treatment of low flow vascular malformations. J Vasc Interv Radiol. 2004;15(5):431–45.
20. Berber O, Holt P, Hinchliffe R, Thompson M, Loftus I. Endovenous therapy for the treatment of congenital venous malformations. Ann Vasc Surg. 2010;24(3):415–e13.
21. Veräjänkorva E, Rautio R, Giordano S, Koskivuo I, Savolainen O. The efficiency of sclerotherapy in the treatment of vascular malformations: a retrospective study of 63 patients. Plast Surg Int. 2016;2016:*1*.
22. Roh YN, Do YS, Park KB, Park HS, Kim YW, Lee BB, Pyon JK, Lim SY, Mun GH, Kim DI. The results of surgical treatment for patients with venous malformations. Ann Vasc Surg. 2012;26(5):665–73.
23. Aboutalebi A, Jessup CJ, North PE, MihmJr MC. Histopathology of vascular anomalies. Facial Plast Surg. 2012;28(06):545–53.
24. Restrepo R. Multimodality imaging of vascular anomalies. Pediatr Radiol. 2013;43(1):141–54.
25. Mulligan PR, Prajapati HJS, Martin LG, Patel TH. Vascular anomalies: classification, imaging characteristics and implications for interventional radiology treatment approaches. Br J Radiol. 2014;87(1035):20130392.
26. Marler JJ, Mulliken JB. Current management of hemangiomas and vascular malformations. Clin Plast Surg. 2005;32(1):99–116.
27. El-Merhi F, Garg D, Cura M, Ghaith O. Peripheral vascular tumors and vascular malformations: imaging (magnetic resonance imaging and conventional angiography), pathologic correlation and treatment options. Int J Cardiovasc Imaging. 2013;29(2):379–93.
28. Colletti G, Valassina D, Bertossi D, Melchiorre F, Vercellio G, Brusati R. Contemporary management of vascular malformations. J Oral Maxillofac Surg. 2014;72(3):510–28.
29. Carqueja IM, Sousa J, Mansilha A. Vascular malformations: classification, diagnosis and treatment. Int angiol: A Journal of the International Union of Angiology. 2018;37(2):127–42.
30. Lee B, Andrade M, Bergan J, Boccardo F, Campisi C, Damstra R, Flour M, Gloviczki P, Laredo J, Piller N, Michelini S. Diagnosis and treatment of primary lymphedema. Consensus document of the International Union of Phlebology (IUP)-2009. Int Angiol. 2010;29(5):454–70.

31. Alomari AI, Karian VE, Lord DJ, Padua HM, Burrows PE. Percutaneous sclerotherapy for lymphatic malformations: a retrospective analysis of patient-evaluated improvement. J Vasc Interv Radiol. 2006;17(10):1639–48.
32. Thomas DM, Wieck MM, Grant CN, Dossa A, Nowicki D, Stanley P, Zeinati C, Howell LK, Anselmo DM. Doxycycline sclerotherapy is superior in the treatment of pediatric lymphatic malformations. J Vasc Interv Radiol. 2016;27(12):1846–56.
33. Müller-Wille R, Wildgruber M, Sadick M, Wohlgemuth WA. Vascular anomalies (part II): interventional therapy of peripheral vascular malformations. In: RöFo-Fortschritte auf dem Gebiet der Röntgenstrahlen und der bildgebenden Verfahren. Stuttgart: © Georg Thieme Verlag KG; 2018, October. Vol. 190, No. 10, p. 927–937.
34. Yang Y, Sun M, Ma Q, Cheng X, Ao J, Tian L, Wang L, Lei D. Bleomycin A5 sclerotherapy for cervicofacial lymphatic malformations. J Vasc Surg. 2011;53(1):150–5.
35. Cheng J. Doxycycline sclerotherapy in children with head and neck lymphatic malformations. J Pediatr Surg. 2015;50(12):2143–6.
36. Elluru RG, Balakrishnan K, Padua HM. Lymphatic malformations: diagnosis and management. In Seminars in pediatric surgery. Philadelphia: WB Saunders; 2014, August. Vol. 23, No. 4, p. 178–185.
37. Greene AK, Perlyn CA, Alomari AI. Management of lymphatic malformations. Clin Plast Surg. 2011;38(1):75–82.
38. Mulliken JB, Fishman SJ, Burrows PE. Vascular anomalies. Curr Probl Surg. 2000;37(8):517–84.
39. Nassiri N, Cirillo-Penn NC, Thomas J. Evaluation and management of congenital peripheral arteriovenous malformations. J Vasc Surg. 2015;62(6):1667–76.
40. Donnelly LF, Adams DM, Bisset GS III. Vascular malformations and hemangiomas: a practical approach in a multidisciplinary clinic. Am J Roentgenol. 2000;174(3):597–608.
41. Grigg C, Anderson D, Earnshaw J. Diagnosis and treatment of hereditary hemorrhagic telangiectasia. Ochsner J. 2017;17(2):157–61.
42. Cho SK, Do YS, Shin SW, Kim DI, Kim YW, Park KB, Kim EJ, Ahn HJ, Choo SW, Choo IW. Arteriovenous malformations of the body and extremities: analysis of therapeutic outcomes and approaches according to a modified angiographic classification. J Endovasc Ther. 2006;13(4):527–38.
43. Wohlgemuth WA, Müller-Wille R, Teusch VI, Dudeck O, Cahill AM, Alomari AI, Uller W. The retrograde transvenous push-through method: a novel treatment of peripheral arteriovenous malformations with dominant venous outflow. Cardiovasc Intervent Radiol. 2015;38(3):623–31.
44. Do YS, Yakes WF, Shin SW, Lee BB, Kim DI, Liu WC, Shin BS, Kim DK, Choo SW, Choo IW. Ethanol embolization of arteriovenous malformations: interim results. Radiology. 2005;235(2):674–82.
45. Uller W, Alomari AI, Richter GT. Arteriovenous malformations. In: Seminars in pediatric surgery. Philadelphia: WB Saunders; 2014, August. Vol. 23, No. 4, p. 203–207.

17 Low-Flow Venous and Lymphatic Malformations: Permanent Ablations with Ethanol Sclerotherapy

Alexis M. Yakes, Alexander J. Continenza, and Wayne F. Yakes

17.1 Terminology of Hemangiomas and Vascular Malformations

Pediatric deep and cutaneous vascular lesions (hemangiomas) and vascular malformations, having been confused by many clinicians for decades, have been finally classified accurately by Mulliken, Glowacki, and coworkers, after denovo research into endothelial cell characteristics, numbers of mast cells present, and endothelial cell in vitro characteristics [1–6]. Most pediatric hemangiomas are not present at birth, clinically manifest within the first month of life, and exhibit a rapid growth phase in the first year of life. More than 90% of pediatric hemangiomas spontaneously regress to near-complete resolution by 5–7 years of age. Hemangiomas occur with a reported incidence of 1–2.6% [1, 6, 7]. Hemangiomas in the proliferative phase are characterized by rapid growth, significant endothelial cell hyperplasia forming syncytial masses, thickened endothelial basement membrane, ready incorporation of tritiated thymidine into the endothelial cells, and the presence of large numbers of mast cells [1–3].

After this period of rapid expansion in the proliferative phase, hemangiomas can stabilize and grow commensurately with the child. Because of the complex nature of hemangiomas, the proliferative phase may continue as the involutive phase slowly begins to dominate. Involuting hemangiomas show diminished endothelial cellularity and replacement with fibrofatty deposits, exhibit a unilamellar basement membrane, demonstrate no uptake of tritiated thymidine into endothelial cells, and have normal mast cell counts. [1–3]

Vascular malformations are vascular lesions that are present at birth and grow commensurately with the child. Trauma, surgery, hormonal influences caused by birth control pills, and the hormonal swings during puberty and pregnancy may cause a vascular malformation to expand and grow hemodynamically, thus increasing symptoms. Vascular malformations demonstrate no endothelial cell proliferation, contain large vascular channels lined by flat endothelium, have a unilamellar basement membrane, do not incorporate tritiated thymidine into endothelial cells, and have normal mast cell counts. They may be formed from any combination of primitive arterial, capillary, venous, or lymphatic elements

A. M. Yakes
University of Kansas Medical Center, The School of Medicine, Kansas City, KS, USA
e-mail: ayakes@kumc.edu

A. J. Continenza
The University of Minnesota Medical Center, Minneapolis, MN, USA

W. F. Yakes (✉)
The Yakes Vascular Malformation Center, Englewood, Colorado, USA
e-mail: Wayne.yakes@yakesvascularmalformationcenter.com

A. K. Khanna, S. K. Tiwary (eds.), *Vascular Malformations*,
https://doi.org/10.1007/978-981-15-9762-6_17

with or without direct arteriovenous (AV) shunts. Vascular malformations are true structural vascular anomalies resulting from inborn errors of vascular morphogenesis and the incomplete resorption of the early developmental primitive vascular structures. Current research is attempting to link genetic markers and somatic mutations to vascular malformation occurrences.

Eponyms have further clouded and confused the nomenclature of hemangiomas and vascular malformations in the literature. Maffucci's syndrome (or Kast's syndrome) has been defined as a condition whereby the patient has multiple exophytic enchondromas of bone and coexistent hemangiomatosis [8–11]. In the current corrected classification system, hemangiomatosis should be termed venous malformations. Ollier's disease is Maffucci's Syndrome without venous malformations. Despite the fact that Ollier's Disease, Maffucci's Syndrome, and Kast's syndrome are non-familial, somatic mutations of IDH1 and IDH2 are determined as causative for these lesions [11].

The Riley-Smith syndrome, a rare autosomal dominant disorder, has been previously characterized by macrocephaly, pseudopapilladema, intestinal polyposis, pigmentation of the penis, and multiple hemangiomas [12]. The term "hemangioma" should be replaced with "venous malformation". Capillary malformations and lymphatic malformations may also be present with the Riley-Smith syndrome. The Riley-Smith syndrome, Bannayan's syndrome, Bannayan–Zonana syndrome, Bannayan–Riley–Ruvalcaba syndrome, and Ruvalcaba-Myhre-Smith syndrome are a spectrum of similar autosomal dominant heritable congenital vascular anomalies [12–15]. These syndromes belong to a family of hamartomatous polyposis syndromes, which also includes Peutz-Jeghers syndrome, Juvenile Polyposis, Cowden Syndrome, Proteus syndrome, and Proteus-like syndrome due to a mutation of the PTEN gene. They are also known as PTEN Hamartoma Tumor Syndromes (PHTS) [16]. Proteus syndrome, also known as Wiedemann syndrome, is a rare congenital disorder causing skin overgrowth, atypical bone development, and abnormal blood and lymphatic vessels [13, 17].

Gorham syndrome, Gorham-Stout syndrome, and Trinquoste syndrome are similar entities described as osteolysis (disappearing bone disease) caused by an underlying hemangiomatosis [18]. The term "hemangiomatosis" should be replaced by "intraosseous vascular malformation", usually a venous malformation. AVMs also may stimulate bone resorption, but also may cause bone overgrowth, particularly if the AVM is involving an epiphysis.

The Blue Rubber Bleb Nevus syndrome (or Bean's syndrome) are other confusing eponyms, but are also unusual in that they are an autosomal dominant heritable condition associated TEK tyrosine kinase. It is characterized by subcutaneous (rubbery) venous malformations that spontaneously grow and occur in the skin, extremities, trunk, and then enlarge. More severe forms can have venous malformations involving the intestines and in the CNS that can hemorrhage. This can cause neurological deficits or significant GI blood loss. Surgery may be required [19].

Another confusing group of clinical eponyms (Klippel–Trenaunay syndrome, naevus vasculosus osteohypertrophic, verrucous hypertrophycans, osteohypertrophic naevus flammeus, angioosteohypertrophy syndrome) all describe a congenital entity characterized by unilateral lower limb (usually) hypertrophy, cutaneous skin capillary malformations with pigmentations and port-wine stains, lymphatic malformations, a normal, hypoplastic, or atretic deep venous system, occasional extension of the vascular malformation into the pelvis and trunk, a lower extremity retained embryonic lateral venous anomaly (Servelle's vein), and increased subcutaneous fat in the affected limb [20–22]. A similar group of eponyms Parkes–Weber syndrome, Klippel–Trenaunay–Weber syndrome, Klippel–Trenaunay–Weber–Rubashov syndrome, Giant Limb of Robertson represent similar clinical entities, that the same features of the Klippel–Trenaunay syndrome with the coexistence of multiple arteriovenous fistulae [23–25]. The Klippel–Trenaunay syndrome and Parkes–Weber syndrome usually occur in the lower extremity, but occasionally can affect the upper extremity [25]. In the upper extremity, the Parkes–Weber syndrome is more commonly seen, although in the Klippel–Trenaunay syndrome it is much more common overall. Servelle-Martorell syndrome is characterized by limb VMs, rarely AVMs, with lower extremity bone hypoplasia [24, 25].

PHACE syndrome refers to a neurocutaneous syndrome associated with facial hemangiomas, cardiac defects, eye abnormalities, coarctation of the aorta, posterior fossa brain abnormalities, and arterial malformations; P = Posterior Fossa; H = Hemangioma; A = Arterial lesions in the head and neck; C = Cardiac abnormalities and Coarctation of the Aorta; E = Eye abnormalities, eye maldevelopment, hemorrhages, seizures, developmental delays, brain strokes, and skin ulcers [26].

CLOVES syndrome eponym is defined as: C = Congenital; L = Lipomatous tissue; O = Overgrowth; V = Vascular Malformations; E = Epidermal nevi; S = Spinal and skeletal anomalies with scoliosis. CLOVES syndrome is characterized by lipomatous overgrowth with concurrent LM, VM, CM, AVMs, epidermal nevus, and spinal/skeletal anomalies/scoliosis [27].

Sturge–Weber syndrome is characterized by ipsilateral facial and leptomeningeal CM, eye anomalies, glaucoma, seizures, mental retardation, and also referred to as encephalotrigeminal angiomatosis. It is caused by a somatic activating mutation occurring in the GNAQ gene [28–30]. Plain x-ray intracranial "trans-track" calcifications are diagnostic of this syndrome on skull x-rays due to calcifications in the second and third cerebral cortex layers thought related to the anoxic injury.

Rendu–Osler–Weber syndrome is identical to Hereditary Hemorrhagic Telangiectasia (HHT). It is characterized as an autosomal dominant heritance with the formation of abnormal malformations in the skin, mucus membranes, brain, lungs, liver, intestines, nasal, and oral cavity. Pulmonary AVF occurs in around 50% of patients requiring closure to prevent stroke and paradoxical emboli to the brain and body. Pulmonary AVF may indeed be multiple in this condition. Brain AVMs (10% of patients) may also require treatment. Liver AVMs (30–70%) may require treatment. Repeated epistaxis requiring treatment is a common problem and often leads to anemia [31–36]. Patients often undergo multiple bilateral Internal Maxillary artery particle embolizations resulting ultimately in arterial occlusions of this artery. When transarterial embolization is no longer possible due to chronic Internal Maxillary artery occlusions, I have proven that direct puncture with 23 g needles into the nasal mucosal in the bleeding nasal turbinates and injecting a 50% mixture of ethanol and non-ionic contrast is extremely effective in controlling epistaxis by directly accessing the CVMs and treating them.

The overabundant capillary malformations that surround one or all three branches of the Trigeminal nerve causing the characteristic port-wine stain (or nevus flammeus) along the distributions Ophthalmic, Maxillary, and/or Mandibular braches of the Trigeminal nerve which arises from the Trigeminal Ganglion (or also termed Gasserian Ganglion; also termed the Semilunar Ganglion) in Meckel's Cave containing the cell bodies of incoming sensory nerve fibers. The overabundant capillary malformations engulf the sensory nerve fibers in the dermis along one, two, or all three of the major branches of the Trigeminal nerve; the Ophthalmic nerve (V1), the Maxillary nerve (V2), and the Mandibular nerve (V3). Intracranially there is leptomeningeal angiomatosis (capillary-venous malformations) on the brain ipsilateral to the port-wine stains. The ocular choroid is another common site involved with capillary-venous malformations resulting in glaucoma and buphthalmos. These phenomena result in 70–80% of patients having seizures. In Tuberous Sclerosis, another form of these phakomatoses along with Sturge–Weber Syndrome, also results in the patient suffering from seizure activity.

Venous malformations with glomus cells (glomangioma, glomovenous malformation) are usually hereditary (64%), like Blue Rubber Bleb Nevus Syndrome, and account for 5% of venous anomalies. Histologically, glomovenous malformations consist of distended venous cannels (venous malformations) with flattened endothelium surrounded by a variable number of maldifferentiaed smooth muscle-like "glomus cells" in the wall. It is an autosomal dominant with variable penetrance and affects any body part. Unlike venous malformations, however, compressive garments cause pain and should be avoided. Sclerotherapy and surgery are the primary forms of treatment, just like venous malformations [37, 38].

The Kasabach–Merritt phenomenon is an unusual condition that can be missed clinically until it becomes severe enough to cause symptoms to warrant clinical investigations as to why a pediatric, or even adult patient suffers from a severe coagulopathy. It was first reported by two pediatricians in 1940: Haig Haigouni Kasabach and Katherine Krom Merritt [39]. They associated, as have many physicians through the years, this coagulopathic condition with pediatric hemangioma as it occurred in neonatal infants. The landmark publications of Mulliken et al [1–6] are now known to occur with Kaposiform Hemangioendothelioma (KHE) and Tufted Angiomas [39, 40]. In children and adults, this Kasabach–Merritt phenomenon can also occur with extensive involvement of the body with venous malformations [41]. Symptoms include low platelet counts, low fibrinogen levels, D-dimers positive, and disseminated intravascular coagulopathy (DIC). This DIC state can vary from mild to a severe lethal form in KHE. In extensive VMs it is a milder non-lethal form of DIC.

KHE occurs in neonates in the liver or the soft tissues of the body (trunk, extremities, head and neck, etc.). In the liver, it causes a high-flow shunting condition with resultant cardiac failure and even death. Transarterial large particle embolization is usually curative to occlude the innumerable intra-hepatic shunts. There is a report of Kasabach–Merritt Phenomenon in hepatic KHE whereby despite embolization the neonate died secondary to coagulopathy, liver failure, and sepsis [42]. Unless embolized, over 2/3 of patients with heart failure complications will die [42, 43]. Larger particle size must be used to prevent shunting to the lungs and death in these compromised patients. Extra-hepatic KHE trunk and extremities do cause the Kasabach–Merritt Syndrome. Treatment to reverse the DIC coagulopathy can be done medically with various Vincristine regimens [44] and also by embolization [45]. However, this is the illogical thinking of “either this or that” being done regarding treatment. The mentality of “both and” should be employed to double the therapeutic effects of Vincristine coupled with emergent embolization in this disease with high mortality to allow two synergistic procedures to more quickly potentiate each other’s efficacy to save the life of these severely compromised children [46].

The Kasabach–Merritt phenomenon can also exist silently in an asymptomatic state in the patients with extensive venous malformations involving a large area of their body mass. They frequently do not exhibit any signs of symptoms of DIC coagulopathy and only have symptoms referable to the venous malformation [41]. Patients present for endovascular treatment and undergo sclerotherapy treatment over a large part of their venous malformations. This sclerotherapy procedure then consumes further the patient’s already lowered platelets and fibrinogen, dropping these levels precipitously, then sending the patient into a clinical DIC state. Thus, in any patient with an extensive body involvement of venous malformations, a hematologic work-up should be performed to prevent sending a patient into a DIC crisis acutely post-treatment. The hematologist clinically manages these issues with pre-operative administration of platelets, blood transfusions, fresh frozen plasma, aminocaproic acid (Amicar), and the like. The hematologist then manages the patient post-embolization obtaining blood studies to determine what treatments may or may not be required to replace the blood elements consumed by the sclerotherapy treatment. Knowledge of their hematologic condition prior to treatment is essential to proper management of this unusual patient population.

These are the more significant of the confusing terms and syndromes published in the world’s literature and in clinical practice involving various vascular malformations. The ISSVA modern classification system can eliminate all current confusion, and all clinicians can finally speak the same language. Accurate terminology will lead to the precise identification of clinical entities and ultimately to enhanced patient care. The remainder of this chapter will use this modem classification system originated by Mulliken, Glowacki, and coworkers, now adopted by ISSVA.

MR has replaced CT in most cases for evaluating vascular malformations. CTA still has an important role in AVM evaluations. MR has proven to be a mainstay in the initial diagnostic evaluation as well as in assessing endovascular therapy at follow- up. MR can determine and distinguish between high-flow and low-flow malformations. Further, various imaging sequences make it possible to determine relationships to adjacent anatomic structures such as organs, bone, muscles, nerves, and so on. High-flow malformations typically demonstrate signal voids on most sequences. These flow voids are felt to be predominantly due to time-of-flight phenomenon with turbulence-related dephasing also contributing to signal loss. Gradient Echo (GE) sequences image AVMs as vascular structures with significant increased signal. An additional feature to differentiate high-flow lesions from low- flow lesions is the presence of enlarged feeding arteries and dilated draining veins. Several characteristics of low-flow malformations have been described in the literature, including a serpentine pattern with internal striations or septations associated with focal muscle atrophy [47]. Low-flow malformations, which include venous malformations, glomovenous malformations, and lymphatic malformations, demonstrate a characteristic higher signal intensity that is greater than skeletal muscle in both Tl-and T2-weighted images with fat suppression. However, it is less than subcutaneous fat on Tl-weighted images and greater than fat on T2-weighted images. The high-intensity MR signal seen on fast spin-echo sequences with long TR-TE has been attributed to stagnant flow in these abnormal vascular spaces. STIR sequences show VMs and LMs to advantage. MR characteristics of low-flow malformations that we were the first to publish include a propensity for multifocal discontinuous involvement, a tendency for orientation along the long axis of an affected extremity, a tendency to follow neurovascular distributions suggesting a developmental origin, occasional extension into tendon sheaths, and associated enlargement of subcutaneous fat. These additional characteristics have proven very helpful in the differential diagnosis of problematic cases, particularly mixed malformation lesions [47]. MR commonly demonstrates the full extent of a low-flow lesion to a more accurate degree than arteriography and closed-system or direct puncture venography. Furthermore, given the propensity of low-flow malformations to be multifocal, MR can be used to guide a direct puncture evaluation of unsuspected areas of adjacent involvement. In anatomic regions such as the head and neck, in which closed-system venography is impossible to perform, MR can be very informative and completely delineate the extent of a VM, LM, or glomovenous malformation lesion (Figs. 17.1, 17.2 and 17.3).

Post-procedure, patients are then revived from general anesthesia and sent to the recovery room for observation. After patients are deemed stable in the recovery room, they are usually sent to the routine hospital ward to be observed for 2–4 h. Medical management on the ward consists of Decadron therapy intravenously according to body weight, intravenous fluids, droperidol injection (Inapsine, Janssen Pharmaceuticals, Inc., Titusville, NJ) given intravenously as needed to control postoperative nausea, oral or intramuscular Ketorolac Tromethamine (Toradol, Syntex Laboratories, Inc., Palo Alto, CA) therapy according to body weight in adult patients is very helpful to control pain and diminish swelling. Various oral and intravenous pain medications are usually ordered on an as needed basis. Discharge medications usually include methylprednisolone tablets (Medrol Dose Pack, Upjohn Co., Kalamazoo, MI) after discharge to aid in the resolution of swelling. Patients usually exhibit focal swelling in the area of malformation that was treated post-procedure. Most patients will resolve the majority of the swelling by 2 weeks. In those patients with lower extremity and foot malformations, swelling may last longer because the leg and foot are not only dependent but are

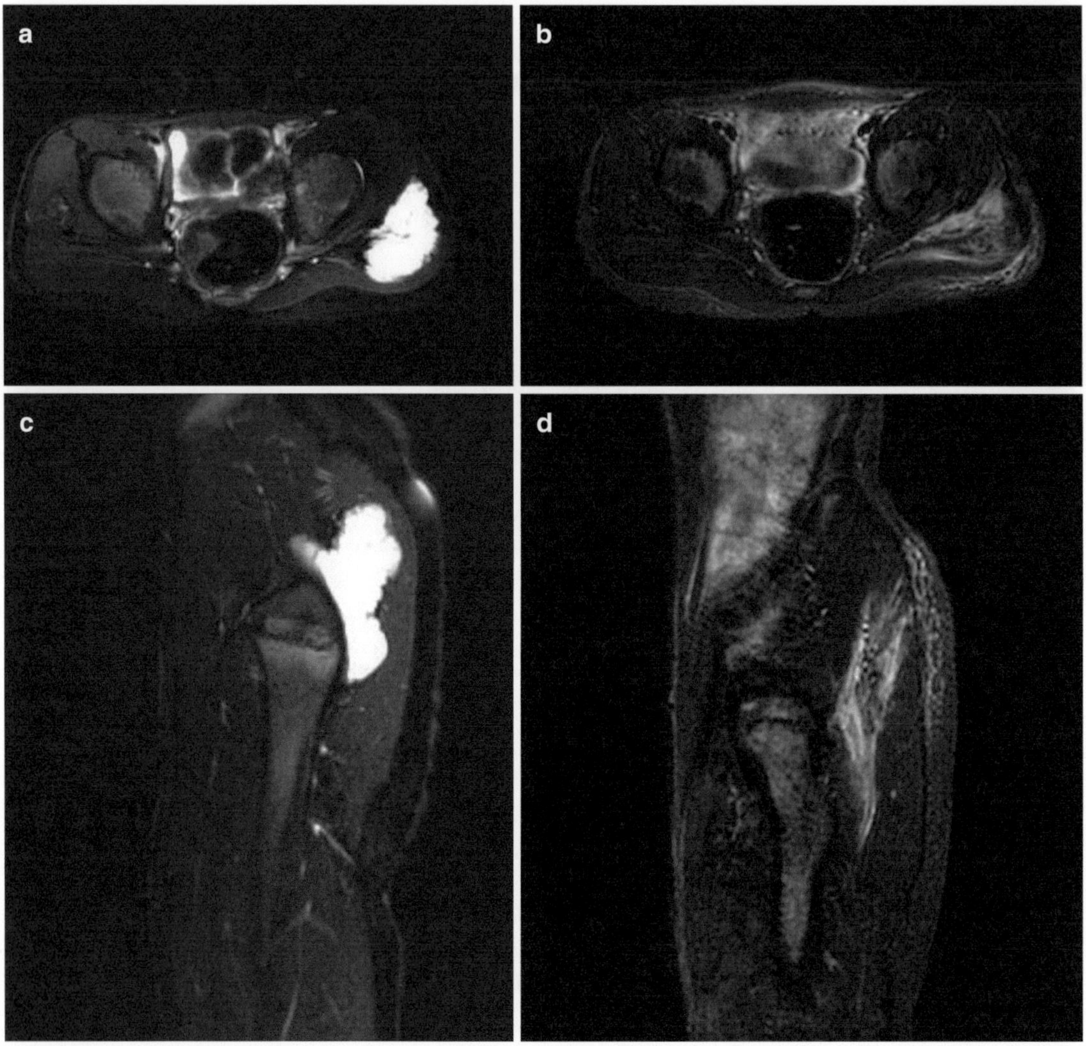

Fig. 17.1 (**a**) Right buttock growing painful mass. Axial MR with STIR imaging sequences consistent with venous or mixed Venous-Lymphatic malformations. (**b**) Follow-up MR showing significant treatment. (**c**) Sagittal MR with STIR imaging sequences again demonstrate a venous or mixed Venous-Lymphatic malformations. (**d**) MR 2 months later with MR showed signal decrease indicative of malformation treatment

also weight-bearing structures. Usually, after 4 weeks, all swelling is resolved, and the patient, being at a new baseline, is ready for follow-up endovascular ethanol therapy as necessary.

After serial therapy, MR and CDI can be used to document the efficacy of therapy. Pain can be a frequent cause for seeking treatment. In those patients who do present with a pain syndrome, serial devascularization of the malformation will usually remove or at least dramatically reduce the amount of pain the patient suffers.

17.1.1 Endovascular Occlusive Agents

Endosurgical vascular ablation (embolotherapy) has evolved as one of the cornerstones of modern Interventional Radiology. The extensive array of catheters, guide wires, endovascular ablative agents (embolic materials), and imaging systems are a tribute to the hard work, insight, and imagination of the many dedicated investigators in this area. Because of significant laboratory research,

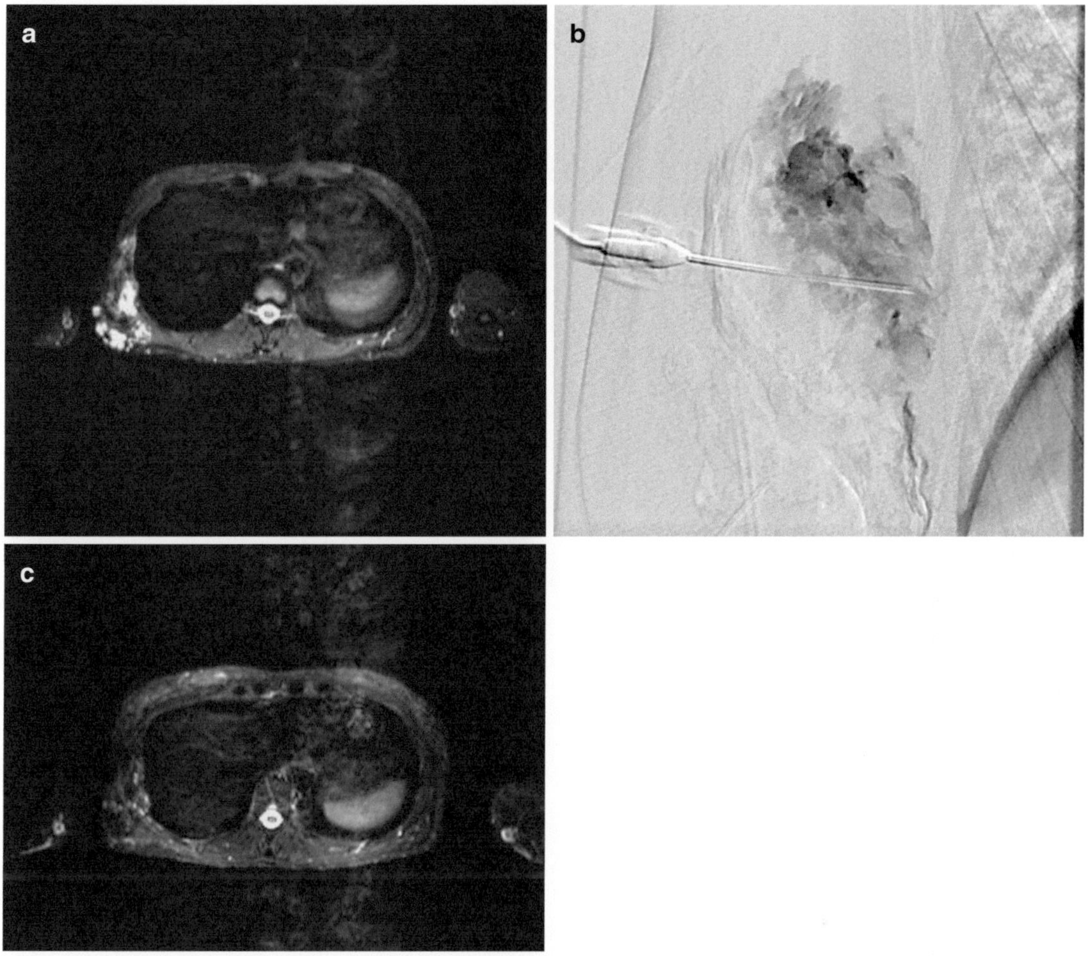

Fig. 17.2 (**a**) Right lateral chest wall venous malformation. (**b**) Direct puncture ethanol injection. (**c**) Dramatic loss of signal in the right chest wall venous malformations indicative of fibrosis within the lesion

clinical research, and extensive clinical experience, the judicious use of endosurgical vascular ablative therapy is common in modern clinical practice. Now that it is firmly established as an essential therapeutic tool, its role will only continue to grow.

There are now many endovascular ablative agents that are used in various clinical scenarios. The choice of agent depends upon several factors: the vascular territory to be treated, the type of abnormality being treated, the possibility of superselective delivery of an occlusive agent, the goal of the procedure, and the permanence of the occlusion required. The following are some occlusive agents that have been used to treat vascular anomalies.

17.1.2 Venous and Lymphatic Malformations

Venous malformations (VMs) may be asymptomatic, cosmetically deforming, cause pain, induce neuropathy, ulcerate, hemorrhage, induce changes of abnormal bone growth, bone osteolysis, and resorption, cause pathologic fractures, induce a thrombocytopenia, and cause the Kasabach–Merritt syndrome. Once it is decided that therapy is warranted, then arteriography and venography should be performed. Venography best identifies the extent of abnormal vascular mass. Arteriography usually shows no arterial abnormality; however, occult AVF may be pres-

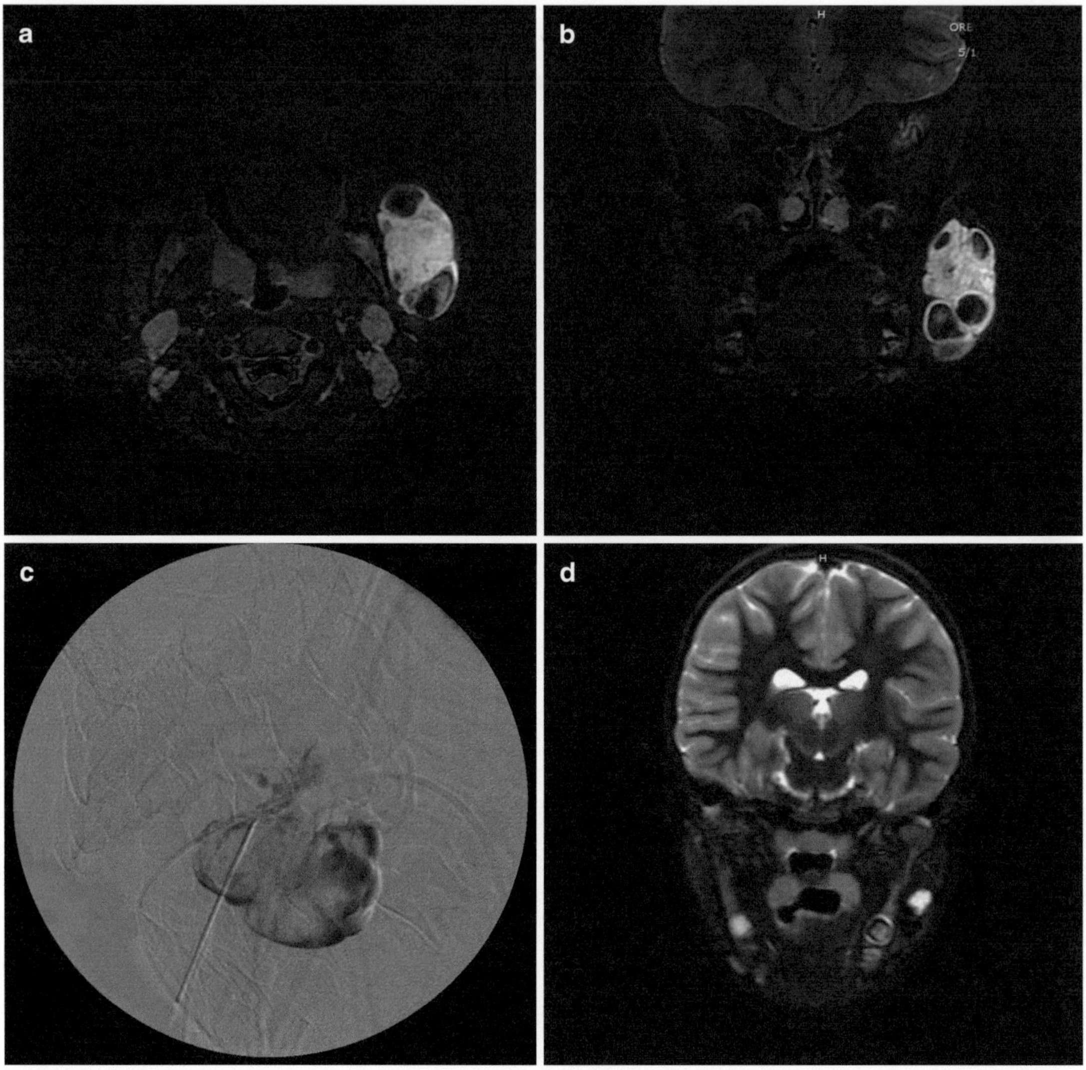

Fig. 17.3 (**a**) Giant left face venous malformation with large calcified phleboliths. (**b**) Left face venous malformation with bright signal and calcified phleboliths. (**c**) Direct puncture DSA into left venous malformation. (**d**) 2-year MR follow-up study shows dramatic reduction of the bright signal within venous malformation

ent in mixed lesions and must be documented by arteriography prior to therapy. After scrutinizing all baseline studies, an appropriate treatment plan can be presented to the patient and the referring clinician [48–90].

Many authors have treated patients with venous malformations in all anatomic locations. All patients were treated by direct percutaneous puncture with 18–23 g needles to directly access the abnormal venous vascular elements. Transarterial ablation with ethanol is never performed in venous and lymphatic malformations unless a concurrent congenital AVF is present. Ethanol will thrombose from the capillary bed backward into the arterial system, thus sparing the venous malformation and resulting in tissue devitalization. Direct puncture techniques into the lesion directly attack the venous malformation itself. Thus, the inflow arterial system and capillary bed are not affected and any tissue loss will be minimized. If the venous malformation has transdermal involvement, then skin injury will always occur with eschar formation and ultimate healing by scar formation despite the type of sclerosant embolic agent being injected. Several sclerosant embolic agents are used to treat venous malformations; Bleomycin, foam sclerotherapy, Polidocanol, Sodium Tetradecyl Sulfate (STS), and Doxycycline [64, 65, 69, 70]. Ethanol is universally successful for treatment VMs and LMs in the 90%–100% malformation ablation range and the other sclerosants that have shown less efficacy in the 60% to 80% malformation ablation range [63–70].

Lymphatic malformations (LMs) arise from vein buds in their abnormal morphogenesis. Lymphatic malformations are similar histologically to venous malformations except that, instead of red blood cells being present within the vascular spaces, lymph fluid is present. Lymphatic malformations can have large saccular spaces (macrocystic) or very small luminal spaces (microcystic). Lymphatic malformations have the same imaging characteristics on MR as do vein malformations in that they demonstrate increased signal on STIR and T-2 sequences with fat suppression. As in MR for venous malformations, lymphatic malformations are also best imaged using STIR or T-2 sequences with fat suppression [91]. The old inaccurate term "cystic hygroma" should be replaced by the more appropriate term "lymphatic malformation". Lymphatic malformations respond to percutaneous ethanol therapy in similar fashion to venous malformations [67–69]. Some success in shrinkage of LMs has also been noted with Bleomycin and Doxycycline [64–66, 69, 70]. Serial ethanol injection into cystic and microcystic LMs is universally successful [50, 66–69, 71, 73, 78]. In essence, in the world's published literature, Bleomycin, foam, sclerotherapy, Polidocanol, Sodium Tetradecyl Sulfate, and Doxycycline have a published success of 60–80% efficacy. Absolute ethanol has a published success rate of 90–100% efficacy [64].

17.2 Summary

Vascular anomalies (hemangiomas and vascular malformations) pose some of the most significant challenges in the practice of medicine today. Chest, abdomen, and pelvis vascular anomalies cause unique clinical problems with regard to their anatomic locations. Clinical manifestations of these lesions are extremely protean. Because of the rarity of these lesions, the experience of most clinicians in their diagnosis and management is limited, augmenting the enormity of the problem and leading to misdiagnoses and poor patient treatment outcomes. Vascular anomalies are best treated in medical centers where patients with these maladies are seen regularly and the team approach is used. The occasional embolizer will never gain enough experience to adequately treat these problematic lesions, and these patients should be referred to centers that routinely deal with vascular anomalies and the complicated issues with which they present. Only in this fashion can significant experience be gained, improved judgment in managing these lesions, and definitive statements develop in the treatment of vascular anomalies. Ethanol directed by direct puncture techniques allow access to the vascular malformation requiring treatment and is the best possibility of effecting a permanent ablation of the vascular lesion itself [50–54, 58, 59, 62–68, 71–90].

References

1. Mulliken JB, Glowacki J. Hemangiomas and vascular malformations in infants and children: a classification based on endothelial characteristics. Plast Reconstr Surg. 1982;69:412–22. 1982/03/01
2. Mulliken JB, Zetter BR, Folkman J. In vitro characteristics of endothelium from hemangiomas and vascular malformations. Surgery. 1982;92:348–53. 1982/08/01
3. Glowacki J, Mulliken JB. Mast cells in hemangiomas and vascular malformations. Pediatrics. 1982;70:48–51. 1982/07/01
4. Finn MC, Glowacki J, Mulliken JB. Congenital vascular lesions: clinical application of a new classification. J Pediatr Surg. 1983;18:894–900. 1983/12/01

5. Upton J, Mulliken JB, Murray JE. Classification and rationale for management of vascular anomalies in the upper extremity. J Hand Surg Am. 1985;10:970–5. 1985/11/01
6. Young A. Pathogenesis of vascular malformations. Vascular birthmarks: hemangiomas and malformations. Philadelphia: Saunders; 1988. p. 107–13.
7. Jacobs AH, Walton RG. The incidence of birthmarks in the neonate. Pediatrics. 1976;58:218–22. 1976/08/01
8. Lowell SH, Mathog RH. Head and neck manifestations of Maffucci's syndrome. Arch Otolaryngol. 1979;105:427–30. 1979/07/01
9. Carleton A, Robb-Smith AH. Kast's syndrome (multiple haemangiomata associated with chondromata or ollier's dyschondroplasia). Proc R Soc Med. 1939;32:266. 1939/02/01
10. Silve C, Juppner H. Ollier disease. Orphanet J Rare Dis. 2006;1:37. 2006/09/26. https://doi.org/10.1186/1750-1172-1-37.
11. Amary MF, Damato S, Halai D, et al. Ollier disease and Maffucci syndrome are caused by somatic mosaic mutations of IDH1 and IDH2. Nat Genet. 2011;43:1262–5. 2011/11/08. https://doi.org/10.1038/ng.994.
12. Riley HD, Smith WR. Macrocephaly, pseudopapilladema, and multiple hemangiomata: a previously undescribed heredofamilial syndrome. Pediatrics. 1960;26:293–300.
13. Wiedemann HR, Burgio GR, Aldenhoff P, et al. The proteus syndrome. Partial gigantism of the hands and/or feet, nevi, hemihypertrophy, subcutaneous tumors, macrocephaly or other skull anomalies and possible accelerated growth and visceral affections. Eur J Pediatr. 1983;140:5–12. 1983/03/01
14. Bannayan GA. Lipomatosis, angiomatosis, and macrencephalia. A previously undescribed congenital syndrome. Arch Pathol. 1971;92:1–5. 1971/07/01
15. Higginbottom MC, Schultz P. The Bannayan syndrome: an autosomal dominant disorder consisting of macrocephaly, lipomas, hemangiomas, and risk for intracranial tumors. Pediatrics. 1982;69:632–4. 1982/05/01
16. Hobert JA, Eng C. PTEN hamartoma tumor syndrome: an overview. Genet Med. 2009;11:687–94. 2009/08/12. https://doi.org/10.1097/GIM.0b013e3181ac9aea.
17. Biesecker LG, Happle R, Mulliken JB, et al. Proteus syndrome: diagnostic criteria, differential diagnosis, and patient evaluation. Am J Med Genet. 1999;84:389–95. 1999/06/09
18. Gorham LW, Stout AP. Massive osteolysis (acute spontaneous absorption of bone, phantom bone, disappearing bone); its relation to hemangiomatosis. J Bone Joint Surg Am. 1955;37-A:985–1004. 1955/10/01
19. Bean WB. Blue Rubber-Bleb nevi of the skin and gastrointestinal tract. In: Vascular spidders and related lesions of the skin. Springfield, IL: Charles C Thomas; 1958. p. 178–85.
20. Baskerville PA, Ackroyd JS, Browse NL. The etiology of the Klippel- Trenaunay syndrome. Ann Surg. 1985;202:624–7. 1985/11/01. https://doi.org/10.1097/00000658-198511000-00015.
21. Gloviczki P, Hollier LH, Telander RL, et al. Surgical implications of Klippel- Trenaunay syndrome. Ann Surg. 1983;197:353–62. 1983/03/01. https://doi.org/10.1097/00000658-198303000-00017.
22. Phillips GN, Gordon DH, Martin EC, et al. The Klippel-Trenaunay syndrome: clinical and radiological aspects. Radiology. 1978;128:429–34. 1978/08/01. https://doi.org/10.1148/128.2.429.
23. Weber PF. Hemangiectatic hypertrophy of limbs-congenital phlebarteriectasis and so-called congenital varicose veins. Br J Child Dis. 1918;15:13–7.
24. Langer M, Langer R, Friedrich JM. Congenital angiodysplasias of types F.P. Weber, Klippel-Trenaunay and Servelle-Martorell. J Mal Vasc. 1982;7:317–24. 1982/01/01
25. Karuppal R, Raman RV, Valsalan BP, et al. Servelle-Martorell syndrome with extensive upper limb involvement: a case report. J Med Case Rep. 2008;2:142. 2008/05/06. https://doi.org/10.1186/1752-1947-2-142.
26. Metry D, Heyer G, Hess C, et al. Consensus statement on diagnostic criteria for PHACE syndrome. Pediatrics. 2009;124:1447–56. 2009/10/28. https://doi.org/10.1542/peds.2009-0082.
27. Alomari AI. Characterization of a distinct syndrome that associates complex truncal overgrowth, vascular, and acral anomalies: a descriptive study of 18 cases of CLOVES syndrome. Clin Dysmorphol. 2009;18:1–7. 2008/11/18. https://doi.org/10.1097/MCD.0b013e328317a716.
28. Shirley MD, Tang H, Gallione CJ, et al. Sturge-Weber syndrome and port-wine stains caused by somatic mutation in GNAQ. N Engl J Med. 2013;368:1971–9. 2013/05/10. https://doi.org/10.1056/NEJMoa1213507.
29. Weber FP. Right-Sided hemi-hypotrophy resulting from right-sided congenital spastic hemiplegia, with a morbid condition of the left side of the brain, revealed by radiograms. J Neurol Psychopathol. 1922;3:134–9. 1922/08/01. https://doi.org/10.1136/jnnp.s1-3.10.134.
30. Sturge WA. A case of partial epilepsy, apparently due to a lesion of one of the vasomotor centers of the brain. Trans Clin Soc Lond. 1879;12:162.
31. Rendu HJ. Epistaxis repetees chez un sujet porteur de petits angiomes cutanes et muqueux. Gaz Hop. 1896;135:1322–3.
32. Osler W. On a family form of recurring epistaxis, associated with multiple telangiectasia's of the skin and mucus membranes. Bull Johns Hosp. 1901;12:3333–7.
33. Babington BG. Hereditary epistaxis. Lancet. 1865;2:362–3.
34. Weber FP. Multiple hereditary developmental angiomata (telangiectasia) of the skin and mucus membranes associated with recurring hemorrhages. Lancet. 1907;2:160–2.

35. Hanes FM. Multiple hereditary telangiectasia is causing hemorrhage (hereditary hemorrhagic Telangiectasia). Bull Johns Hopkins Hosp. 1909;20:63–73.
36. Abdalla SA, Letarte M. Hereditary haemorrhagic telangiectasia: current views on genetics and mechanisms of disease. J Med Genet. 2006;43:97–110. 2005/05/10. https://doi.org/10.1136/jmg.2005.030833.
37. Boon LM, Mulliken JB, Enjolras O, et al. Glomuvenous malformation (glomangioma) and venous malformation: distinct clinicopathologic and genetic entities. Arch Dermatol. 2004;140:971–6. 2004/08/18. https://doi.org/10.1001/archderm.140.8.971.
38. Boon LM, Vanwijck R. Medical and surgical treatment of venous malformations. Ann Chir Plast Esthet. 2006;51:403–11. 2006/09/29. https://doi.org/10.1016/j.anplas.2006.07.023.
39. HH Kasabach KM. Capillary hemangioma with extensive Purpura: report of a case. Am J Dis Child. 1940;59:1063–70. https://doi.org/10.1001/archpedi.1940.01990160135009.
40. Enjolras O, Wassef M, Mazoyer E, et al. Infants with Kasabach-Merritt syndrome do not have "true" hemangiomas. J Pediatr. 1997;130:631–40. 1997/04/01
41. Dompmartin A, Acher A, Thibon P, et al. Association of localized intravascular coagulopathy with venous malformations. Arch Dermatol. 2008;144:873–7. 2008/07/23. https://doi.org/10.1001/archderm.144.7.873.
42. Kim EH, Koh KN, Park M, et al. Clinical features of infantile hepatic hemangioendothelioma. Korean J Pediatr. 2011;54:260–6. 2011/09/29. https://doi.org/10.3345/kjp.2011.54.6.260.
43. Daller JA, Bueno J, Gutierrez J, et al. Hepatic hemangioendothelioma: clinical experience and management strategy. J Pediatr Surg. 1999;34:98–105. discussion 105–106. 1999/02/18
44. Fernandez-Pineda I, Lopez-Gutierrez JC, Chocarro G, et al. Long-term outcome of vincristine-aspirin-ticlopidine (VAT) therapy for vascular tumors associated with Kasabach-Merritt phenomenon. Pediatr Blood Cancer. 2013;60:1478–81. 2013/04/24. https://doi.org/10.1002/pbc.24543.
45. Enomoto Y, Yoshimura S, Egashira Y, et al. Transarterial embolization for cervical hemangioma associated with Kasabach-merritt syndrome. Neurol Med Chir (Tokyo). 2011;51:375–8. 2011/05/27. https://doi.org/10.2176/nmc.51.375.
46. Garcia-Monaco R, Giachetti A, Peralta O, et al. Kaposiform hemangioendothelioma with Kasabach-Merritt phenomenon: successful treatment with embolization and vincristine in two newborns. J Vasc Interv Radiol. 2012;23:417–22. 2012/03/01. https://doi.org/10.1016/j.jvir.2011.12.007.
47. Rak KM, Yakes WF, Ray RL, et al. MR imaging of symptomatic peripheral vascular malformations. AJR Am J Roentgenol. 1992;159:107–12. 1992/07/01. https://doi.org/10.2214/ajr.159.1.1609682.
48. Shin BS, Do YS, Lee BB, et al. Multistage ethanol sclerotherapy of soft-tissue arteriovenous malformations: effect on pulmonary arterial pressure. Radiology. 2005;235:1072–7. 2005/04/19. https://doi.org/10.1148/radiol.2353040903.
49. Bisdorff A, Mazighi M, Saint-Maurice JP, et al. Ethanol threshold doses for systemic complications during sclerotherapy of superficial venous malformations: a retrospective study. Neuroradiology. 2011;53:891–4. 2010/11/30. https://doi.org/10.1007/s00234-010-0803-5.
50. Yakes WFPS. Diagnosis and management of vascular anomalies. Interv Radiol. 1992;1:152–89.
51. Yakes WF, Pevsner P, Reed M, et al. Serial embolizations of an extremity arteriovenous malformation with alcohol via direct percutaneous puncture. AJR Am J Roentgenol. 1986;146:1038–40. 1986/05/01. https://doi.org/10.2214/ajr.146.5.1038.
52. Yakes WFPS, Gibson MD, Haas DK, Pevsner PH, Carter TE. Alcohol Embolotherapy of vascular malformations. Semin Interv Radiol. 1989;6:146–61.
53. Yakes WF. Extremity venous malformations: diagnosis and management. Semin Interv Radiol. 1994;11:332–9.
54. Yakes WF, Luethke JM, Merland JJ, et al. Ethanol embolization of arteriovenous fistulas: a primary mode of therapy. J Vasc Interv Radiol. 1990;1:89–96. 1990/11/01
55. Jo JY, Chin JH, Park PH, et al. Cardiovascular collapse due to right heart failure following ethanol sclerotherapy: a case report. Korean J Anesthesiol. 2014;66:388–91. 2014/06/10. https://doi.org/10.4097/kjae.2014.66.5.388.
56. Ko JS, Kim JA, Do YS, et al. Prediction of the effect of injected ethanol on pulmonary arterial pressure during sclerotherapy of arteriovenous malformations: relationship with dose of ethanol. J Vasc Interv Radiol. 2009;20:39–45.; quiz 45. 2008/11/26. https://doi.org/10.1016/j.jvir.2008.10.012.
57. Shin BS, Do YS, Cho HS, et al. Effects of repeat bolus ethanol injections on cardiopulmonary hemodynamic changes during embolotherapy of arteriovenous malformations of the extremities. J Vasc Interv Radiol. 2010;21:81–9. 2010/02/04. https://doi.org/10.1016/j.jvir.2009.09.026.
58. Yakes WFYA. Arteriovenous malformations: the Yakes classification system and its therapeutic implications. Egyptian J of Vasc Endovasc Surg. 2014;10:9–23.
59. Yakes WFBI. Interventional treatment of arterio-venous malformations. Gefasschirurgie. 2014;19:325–30.
60. Puig S, Aref H, Chigot V, et al. Classification of venous malformations in children and implications for sclerotherapy. Pediatr Radiol. 2003;33:99–103. 2003/01/31. https://doi.org/10.1007/s00247-002-0838-9.
61. Doppman JL, Pevsner P. Embolization of arteriovenous malformations by direct percutaneous puncture. AJR Am J Roentgenol. 1983;140:773–8. 1983/04/01. https://doi.org/10.2214/ajr.140.4.773.
62. Yakes WF. Endovascular management of high-flow arteriovenous malformations. Semin Intervent Radiol. 2004;21:49–58. 2004/03/01. https://doi.org/10.1055/s-2004-831405.

63. Yakes WF. Invited discussion: sclerotherapy of craniofacial venous malformations: complications and results. Plast Reconstr Surg. 1999;104:12–5.
64. Yakes WF. Use of multiple sclerosant agents in vascular malformation management: a world in endovascular confusion and chaos. J Vasc Interv Radiol. 2015;26:1494–6. 2015/09/27. https://doi.org/10.1016/j.jvir.2015.06.002.
65. Zhang J, Li HB, Zhou SY, et al. Comparison between absolute ethanol and bleomycin for the treatment of venous malformation in children. Exp Ther Med. 2013;6:305–9. 2013/10/19. https://doi.org/10.3892/etm.2013.1144.
66. Burrows PE. Endovascular treatment of slow-flow vascular malformations. Tech Vasc Interv Radiol. 2013;16:12–21. 2013/03/19. https://doi.org/10.1053/j.tvir.2013.01.003.
67. Furukawa H, Sasaki S, Oyama A, et al. Ethanol sclerotherapy with 'injection and aspiration technique' for giant lymphatic malformation in adult cases. J Plast Reconstr Aesthet Surg. 2011;64:809–11. 2010/10/16. https://doi.org/10.1016/j.bjps.2010.09.003.
68. Impellizzeri P, Romeo C, Borruto FA, et al. Sclerotherapy for cervical cystic lymphatic malformations in children. Our experience with computed tomography-guided 98% sterile ethanol insertion and a review of the literature. J Pediatr Surg. 2010;45:2473–8. 2010/12/07. https://doi.org/10.1016/j.jpedsurg.2010.07.023.
69. Shiels WE 2nd, Kang DR, Murakami JW, et al. Percutaneous treatment of lymphatic malformations. Otolaryngol Head Neck Surg. 2009;141:219–24. 2009/08/01. https://doi.org/10.1016/j.otohns.2009.04.001.
70. Mathur NN, Rana I, Bothra R, et al. Bleomycin sclerotherapy in congenital lymphatic and vascular malformations of head and neck. Int J Pediatr Otorhinolaryngol. 2005;69:75–80. 2005/01/04. https://doi.org/10.1016/j.ijporl.2004.08.008.
71. Vogelzang RL, Yakes WF. Vascular malformations: effective treatment with absolute ethanol. In: Pearce WH, JST Y, editors. Arterial surgery management challenging problems. Stamford, CT: Appleton and Lange Publishers; 1997. p. 553–60.
72. Yakes WF, Krauth L, Ecklund J, et al. Ethanol endovascular management of brain arteriovenous malformations: initial results. Neurosurgery. 1997;40:1145–52.; discussion 1152–1144. 1997/06/01. https://doi.org/10.1097/00006123-199706000-00005.
73. Yakes WF, Luethke JM, Parker SH, et al. Ethanol embolization of vascular malformations. Radiographics. 1990;10:787–96. 1990/09/01. https://doi.org/10.1148/radiographics.10.5.2217971.
74. Yakes WF. AVMs – how I treat them: alcohol. Ces Radiol. 2008;62:146–52.
75. Yakes WF. Endovascular management of high-flow arteriovenous malformations. Zhonghua Kou Qiang Yi Xue Za Zhi. 2008;43:327–32. 2008/11/27
76. Yakes WF, Yakes AM. Auricular AVMs: diagnosis and treatment. Egyptian J Vasc Endovasc Surg. 2014;10:31–16.
77. Do YS, Yakes WF, Shin SW, et al. Ethanol embolization of arteriovenous malformations: interim results. Radiology. 2005;235:674–82. 2005/04/29. https://doi.org/10.1148/radiol.2352040449.
78. Yakes WF. Current Endosurgical vascular ablative management strategies for vascular malformations. Progress in Angiology. 1991;1:387–90.
79. Vinson AM, Rohrer DG, Willcox CW, et al. Absolute ethanol embolization for peripheral arteriovenous malformation: report of two cures. South Med J. 1988;81:1052–5. 1988/08/01
80. Mourao GS, Hodes JE, Gobin YP, et al. Curative treatment of scalp arteriovenous fistulas by direct puncture and embolization with absolute alcohol. Report of three cases. J Neurosurg. 1991;75:634–7. 1991/10/01. https://doi.org/10.3171/jns.1991.75.4.0634.
81. Yakes WF, Rossi P, Odink H. How I do it. Arteriovenous malformation management. Cardiovasc Intervent Radiol. 1996;19:65–71. 1996/03/01
82. Yakes WF. Management of Bone and Soft Tissue Vascular Malformations of the spine. JVIR. 2002;13:294–8.
83. Cho SK, Do YS, Kim DI, et al. Peripheral arteriovenous malformations with a dominant outflow vein: results of ethanol embolization. Korean J Radiol. 2008;9:258–67. 2008/06/06. https://doi.org/10.3348/kjr.2008.9.3.258.
84. Lee BB, Baumgartner I, Berlien HP, et al. Consensus document of the international union of angiology (IUA)-2013. Current concept on the management of arterio-venous management. Int Angiol. 2013;32:9–36. 2013/02/26
85. Rabe E, Pannier F. Sclerotherapy in venous malformation. Phlebology. 2013;28(Suppl 1):188–91. 2013/03/27. https://doi.org/10.1177/0268355513477282.
86. Ierardi AM, Mangini M, Vaghi M, et al. Sclerotherapy of peripheral venous malformations: a new technique to prevent serious complications. Vasc Endovascular Surg. 2010;44:282–8. 2010/04/21. https://doi.org/10.1177/1538574410362117.
87. Keljo DJ, Yakes WF, Andersen JM, et al. Recognition and treatment of venous malformations of the rectum. J Pediatr Gastroenterol Nutr. 1996;23:442–6. 1996/11/01
88. Settecase F, Hetts SW, Nicholson AD, et al. Superselective intra-arterial ethanol sclerotherapy of feeding artery and nidal aneurysms in ruptured cerebral arteriovenous malformations. AJNR Am J Neuroradiol. 2016;37:692–7. 2015/11/14. https://doi.org/10.3174/ajnr.A4584.

89. Vogelzang RL, Atassi R, Vouche M, et al. Ethanol embolotherapy of vascular malformations: clinical outcomes at a single center. J Vasc Interv Radiol. 2014;25:206–13.; quiz 214. 2014/01/28. https://doi.org/10.1016/j.jvir.2013.10.055.
90. Yakes W, Huguenot M, Yakes A, et al. Percutaneous embolization of arteriovenous malformations at the plantar aspect of the foot. J Vasc Surg. 2016;64:1478–82. 2016/10/26. https://doi.org/10.1016/j.jvs.2015.10.092.
91. Reinhoff WF. Congenital arteriovenous fistula: an embryological study with the report of a case. Johns Hopkins Hosp Bull. 1924;35:271–84.

18 Emergencies in Vascular Malformations

Sumit Kapadia

18.1 Introduction

The aim of this chapter is to present an overview of the different emergency presentations of various vascular malformations including identification, clinical features, diagnostic criteria as well as management principles.

Venous malformation (VM) is one of the most common vascular malformations and is a low flow variety. It grows in proportion with the body, exhibiting lifelong growth, and does not regress spontaneously [1]. Other low flow malformations include lymphatic malformations (LM) and capillary malformations (CM). The high-flow ones are termed as Arteriovenous malformations (AVM) which consist of multiple arteriovenous shunting within a nidus which consists of a capillary network [2].

Clinical presentation of vascular malformations is extremely variable and ranges from asymptomatic spots of simple visual concern to lesions with high blood flow or located in critical sites that may be life-threatening [3]. In this chapter, we shall focus on the emergency or critical clinical presentations of various vascular malformations.

S. Kapadia (✉)
Vascular and Endovascular Surgeon, Venus Hospital, Baroda, Gujarat, India

18.2 Capillary Malformations

Although these are commonly recognized as port-wine stains, they are sometimes a part of syndromes like Sturge–Weber syndrome and can affect the eyes as well as the brain. The most significant clinical ophthalmic manifestation is glaucoma, which should be recognized and treated early. However, the most common manifestation is increased choroidal vascularization which is recognized by a characteristic image at the back of the eye known as "tomato ketchup." This lesion is usually asymptomatic in childhood but can lead to retinal detachment in adult life [4].

Brain involvement or leptomeningeal angiomatosis usually occurs on the same side as the capillary malformation and is evident clinically as epileptic symptoms with focal tonic-clonic seizures on the contralateral side of the body, with onset during the first year of life. Response to treatment is variable and most seizures usually become resistant to antiepileptic drugs, leading to slow progressive hemiparesis [5].

18.3 Lymphatic Malformations

Traditionally described as lymphangioma or cystic hygroma, these lymphatic malformations (LM) most frequently involve the head and neck region and present as soft, easily compressible masses

A. K. Khanna, S. K. Tiwary (eds.), *Vascular Malformations*,
https://doi.org/10.1007/978-981-15-9762-6_18

(Figure) with thin overlying skin that may swell in dependent positions or when venous pressures increase (crying or Valsalva) [6]. Bleeding within the cyst or a mixed veno-lymphatic malformation may result in blue discoloration of the overlying skin. When they spread, cervical lesions may compress the pharynx or trachea when the mediastinum is involved and sudden growth of a cervical lymphatic malformation may be an emergency because the airways can be compromised, sometimes leading to respiratory distress. Such sudden growth can be triggered by accidental injury, sclerotherapy, bleeding, or infection [6].

The most common treatment option for LM is the use of sclerosants using various agents like absolute ethanol, Sodium Tetradecyl Sulfate (STS), or bleomycin These agents cause irreversible damage to the endothelium, inducing local inflammation and ultimately leading to fibrosis.

Multiple sessions are often required to achieve regression of the lesion. Swelling, a consistent consequence of sclerotherapy, can cause upper airway obstruction requiring observation in the intensive care unit, intubation, and sometimes even a tracheostomy [7].

The only potentially curative modality for LM is surgical resection. The goals of resection focus on gross debulking of defined anatomic field, limiting blood loss, and minimizing damage to surrounding structures. It is vital to remember that complete or radical resection is typically not without damage to surrounding normal structures especially nerves [8]. Hence, over time relapse may occur, which can be dealt with by sclerotherapy.

18.4 Venous Malformations

Venous malformations (VM) have low blood flow and are categorized as either superficial or deep, and as localized, multicentric, or diffuse [9]. The appearance of most superficial ones is purple color; the subcutaneously located or mucosal ones appear more bluish or greenish whereas the deeper intramuscular ones may appear as ill-defined swelling with normal overlying skin. Mucosal VM especially present with bleeding on minor trauma (Fig. 18.1).

Within the digestive tract, the most common site of the VM is in the small intestine which occasionally may be asymptomatic. Intestinal location of VMs can be associated with severe complications ranging from chronic anemia to acute abdominal conditions due to massive gastrointestinal bleeding (hematemesis or melena), intussusception, or volvulus that ultimately require an emergency surgery [10]. Such gastrointestinal VM may be a part of the Blue Rubber Bleb Naevus Syndrome in which there are associated multiple cutaneous VM which are blue in color and rubbery in consistency.

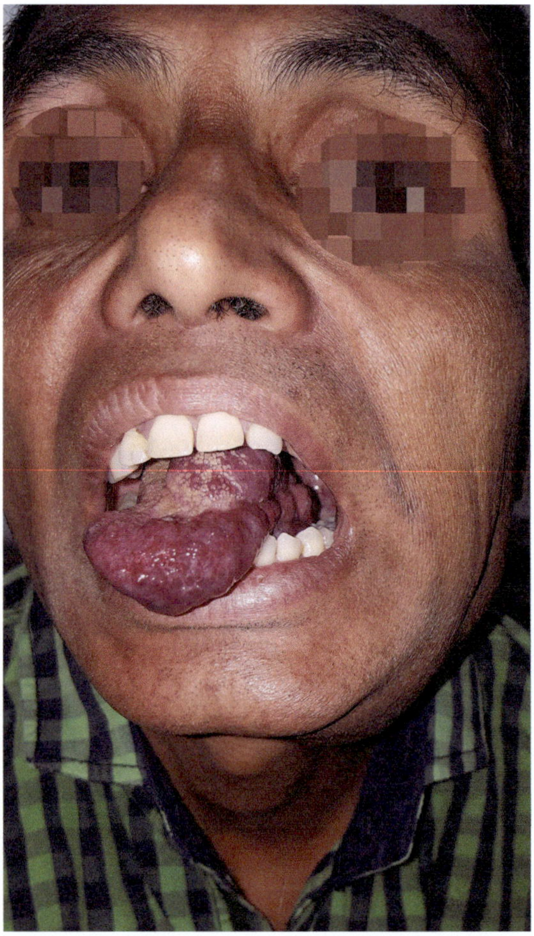

Fig. 18.1 Vascular malformation of tongue causing bleeding

Sudden increase in the size of VM is typical of bleeding within the VM. Trauma or accidental injury to subcutaneous or intramuscular VM can lead to hematoma or neurologic symptoms due to adjacent nerve injury or compression.

Apart from bleeding, the other major complication associated with VM, especially extensive VM or syndromes like Klippel–Trenaunay Syndrome (KTS in Fig. 18.2) is a coagulation disorder called Localized Intravascular Coagulation (LIC) [11]. Localized intravascular coagulopathy occurs due to stasis within the dilated and distorted low flow vessels with the formation of thrombin and subsequent conversion of fibrinogen to fibrin, which is followed by fibrinolysis and evidence of fibrin degradation products like d-dimer.

Newly formed microthrombi in LIC bind to intravascular elementary calcium deposits and form pathognomonic stone-like structures called "phleboliths." These phleboliths can often be palpated in patients with superficial VM, whereas in deep VM, they can be visualized on plain radiography or T-2 weighted MRI. The presence of phleboliths may represent indication for anticoagulation especially when the accompanying lesion is large and extensive [12].

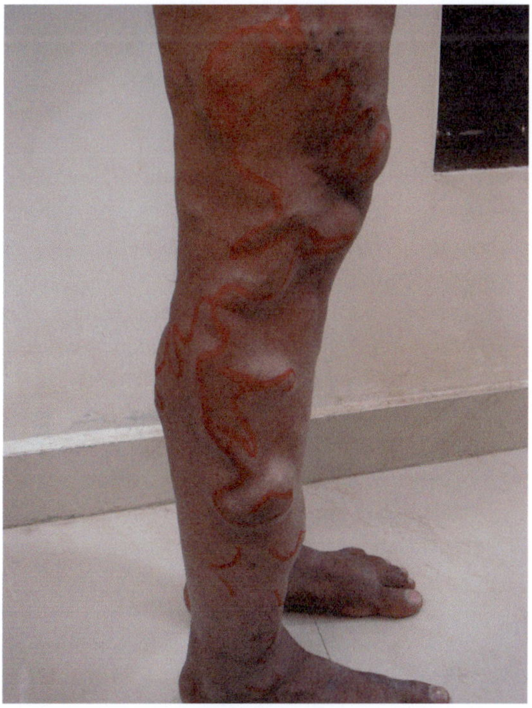

Fig. 18.2 Klippel–Trenaunay syndrome

LIC is of important clinical concern due to the potential for more serious thrombo-embolic events, including superficial thrombosis, deep venous thrombosis or pulmonary embolism as well as thrombo-hemorrhagic Disseminated Intravascular Coagulation (DIC) with life-threatening hemorrhage.

The conversion of LIC to DIC is marked by the consumption of platelets and factors of coagulation. Increase in prothrombin time and decrease in coagulation factor V are the earliest blood test findings. A number of events such as sclerotherapy, surgical resection, bone fracture, prolonged immobilization, and pregnancy or menstruation are known to trigger the conversion of the LIC to DIC, with hemorrhage related to consumption of coagulation factors and multiorgan failure related to disseminated microvascular thrombosis [13].

Additionally, low fibrinogen level and high d-Dimer reflects high consumption due to clotting associated with high fibrinolysis and increased risk for bleeding and requires preventive management by low molecular weight heparin (LMWH) which also helps to treat the pain caused by LIC and to prevent decompensation of severe LIC to DIC. Traditionally pain associated with VMs was considered as an inevitable consequence of the pathogenesis and progression of VM. However, recently the pain in the VM has been found to have a close relationship with underlying coagulopathy to cause LIC in many VM patients [14].

A hypercoagulable status is commonly associated with VMs and may present with chronic intermittent superficial thrombosis, Deep vein Thrombosis (DVT), or Pulmonary Embolism. Therefore, a thrombotic risk profile to evaluate a hypercoagulable state should be performed in all VM patients as a routine part of diagnostic evaluation prior to surgery or sclerotherapy, a detailed coagulation profile is critical in order to identify those patients at increased risk of hemorrhage due to an impaired primary hemostasis.

18.5 AV Malformations

AVM is a high-flow malformation with multiple arteriovenous shunting within a nidus which consists of a capillary network. The commonest sites are intracranial followed by extracranial head and neck, extremity, trunk, and visceral [14]. The clinical presentation ranges from an asymptomatic mass to cardiac failure. Bleeding occurs more frequently with AVM than with other vascular malformations, while other presenting symptoms include pain, ulcer, ischemic steal, or skin changes of venous hypertension (Figs. 18.3, 18.4, 18.5 and 18.6).

The four stages of AVM as proposed by Schobinger are as under [1]:

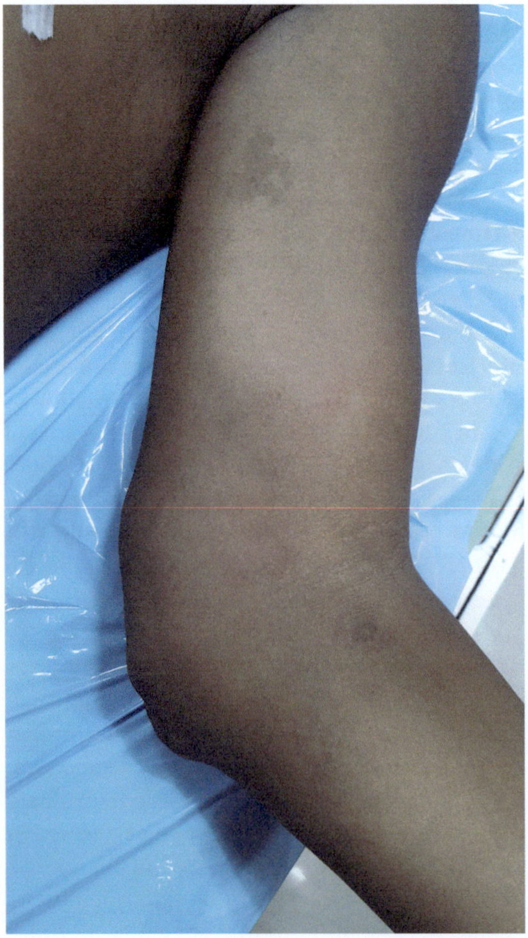

Fig. 18.3 Elbow AVM causing pain

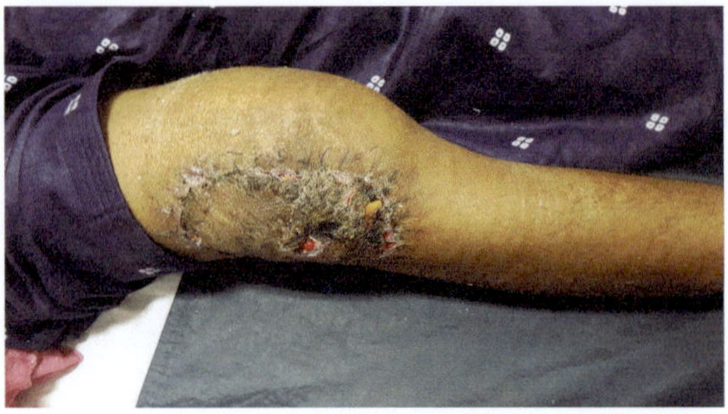

Fig. 18.4 AVM over knee with bleeding. Note incision for attempted but failed surgical treatment

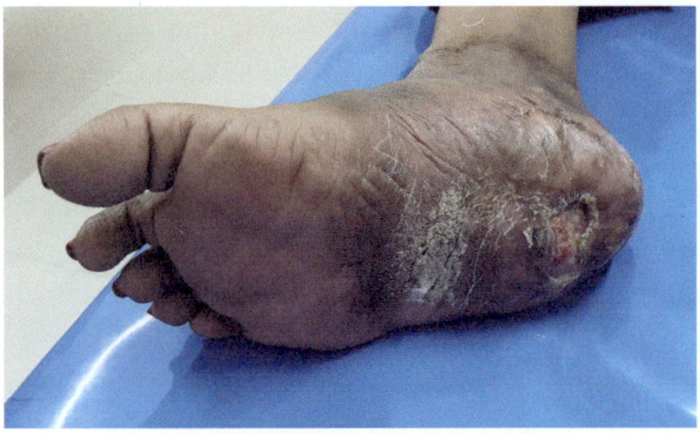

Fig. 18.5 Foot AVM causing ulcer

- Stage 1: *Quiescent*. The malformation is apparently stable and does not grow. This phase is transient in almost all cases, but it can last for decades.
- Stage 2: *Growing*. Spontaneously, or after physical or hormonal changes, the AVM becomes larger and the growth rate is unpredictable.
- Stage 3: *Symptomatic*. Growth brings the AVM close to the skin or mucosa, nerves, and major vessels. This can cause ulceration, bleeding due to rupture, or lead to pain due to irritation of nerves.
- Stage 4: *Decompensating*. High-flow diversion of blood through the AVM can which can lead to the development of dilated cardiomyopathy and, ultimately, heart failure.

Specific emergencies related to the location of AVM include the following:

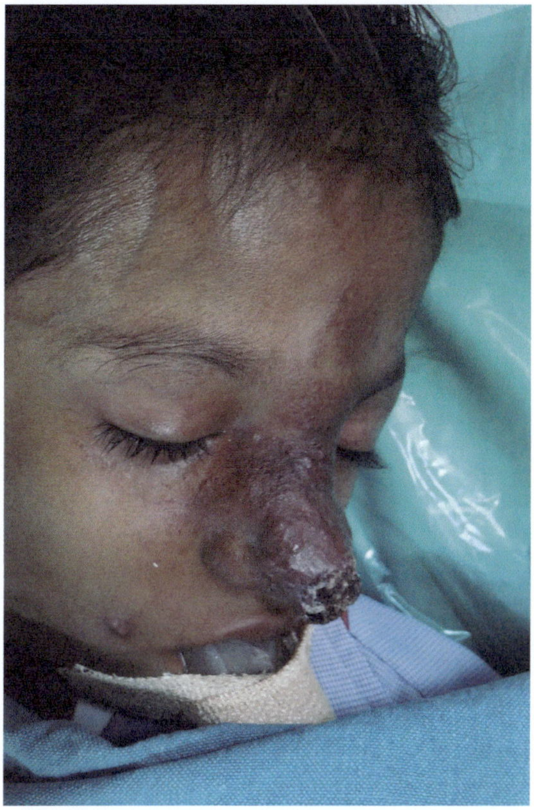

Fig. 18.6 Nose AVM presented with massive bleeding

1. *Brain and Spinal AVM*: Hemorrhage is the commonest presentation of brain AVM, followed by seizures and headaches. The overall risk of hemorrhage for brain AVM is 2–4% per year. Larger nidus, deep infratentorial location, and deep vein drainage are independent predictors of increased risk of hemorrhage. Also, ruptured brain AVMs have higher rates of rebleeding within the first year of presentation [15].

   The current treatment options include conservative management, surgical resection, stereotactic radiosurgery, endovascular embolization, or combinations of these treatments (multimodal therapy) [16].

   Spinal AVMs most frequently occur in the thoracolumbar region and progressive congestive myelopathy is the predominant clinical presentation. However, cervical lesions may present with subarachnoid hemorrhage [17].

2. *Pulmonary AVM*: Pulmonary arteriovenous malformations are abnormal direct communications between pulmonary arteries and pulmonary veins without the interposition of a capillary bed. Approximately 80–90% of patients presenting with PAVMs eventually present as Hereditary Hemorrhagic Telangiectasia (HHT) or Rendu–Osler–Weber Syndrome, whereas the remaining are sporadic cases [18].

   HHT may be clinically diagnosed on the basis of the Curacao criteria [19]. Three criteria are thus needed among the following:

   - Multiple mucocutaneous telangiectases
   - Spontaneous and recurrent epistaxis
   - Visceral involvement
   - A family first-degree history of HHT

   Often, thrombosis develops within the dilated venous sacs. In addition, there is a proliferation of anaerobic bacteria due to the right to left extracardiac shunt. This leads to paradoxical embolism and often leads to thromboembolic stroke or cerebral abscess events. Adams et al. reported that transient ischemic attacks and lacunar brain strokes are usually the first clinical manifestation of pulmonary embolism resulting from PAVM [20]. Yet a brain abscess is the most serious neurological complication of PAVM and occurs in 5–10% of patients with PAVM [21]. The reason is that right to left shunting in the lungs enables bacteria to avoid the filtering effect of pulmonary capillaries and consequently, the brain becomes the first and the most frequently affected target for bacterial emboli [22].

   Hemoptysis or hemothorax due to spontaneous rupture of a fistula sac is rare and usually occurs in pregnancy. This can often lead to a life-threatening situation with hypotension and shock and is diagnosed by X-ray or CT scan chest. Immediate therapeutic options include angiographic embolization. However, in presence of multiple AVMs, a posterolateral thoracotomy with wedge resection or lobectomy is the preferential choice because of low mortality and minimal recurrence rate [23].

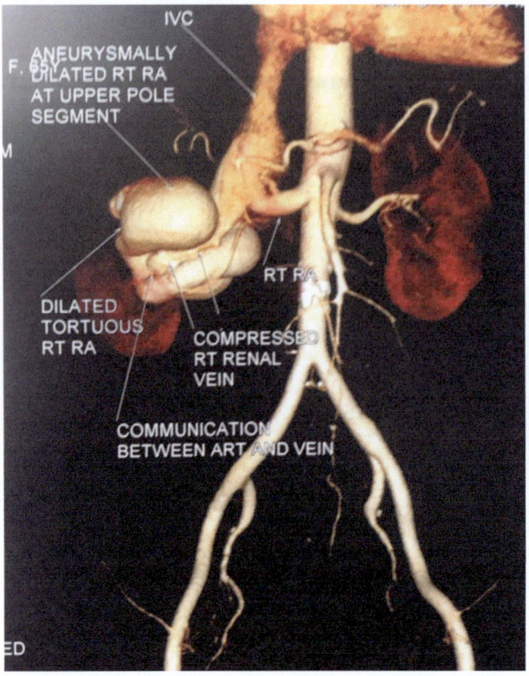

Fig. 18.7 CT angiography shows right Renal AVM with aneurysm

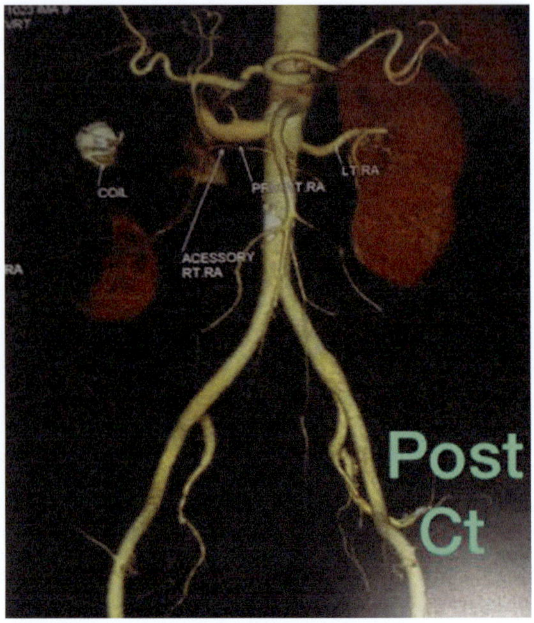

Fig. 18.8 Post-AVM embolisation CT angiography confirms total occlusion of renal AVM

The aim of transcatheter embolization is to occlude all the PAVM feeding arteries by a selective catheterization of pulmonary arteries by using a coaxial system, via a percutaneous femoral approach. Embolization materials used for this purpose include fibered coils, detachable coils, or the Amplatzer plug device. The anchor technique consists of coil blockage within a small collateral branch of the main feeding artery immediately upstream of the PAVM. This allows anchoring of the coil and thus creates a scaffold of the first coil, which permits the blockage of other subsequent devices and also prevents further accidental device mobilization and distal migration to the left circulation [24].

3. *Renal AVM*: Congenital renal AVM are uncommon and sometimes associated with HHT; Some of them present as congenital AV fistula which are high-flow shunts associated with venous aneurysm (Figs. 18.7 and 18.8). The majority of patients present with hematuria, flank pain, or perinephric hematoma. If asymptomatic, they may present later with arterial hypertension and the occurrence of high-output cardiac failure ranges from 5 to 30% in these patients [25].
4. *Pelvic AVMs* may produce severe pain, pelvic congestion, sexual dysfunction, and occasionally, high-output cardiac failure and hemorrhage. Although the primary blood supply of pelvic AVMs is from hypogastric arteries, there may be multiple feeding branches from the inferior mesenteric artery, middle sacral artery, lumbar artery, and femoral arteries. Because of the complexity of feeding branches, complete surgical treatment is often not possible, and recurrences after successful surgical intervention are common. Hence, endovascular embolization is the accepted therapeutic option for these patients [26].
5. *Uterine AVM*: Congenital AVM is rare, although acquired AVM is more commonly encountered due to uterine surgery, curetting, or infection (Fig. 18.9). Uterine AVMs frequently cause sudden massive bleeding in

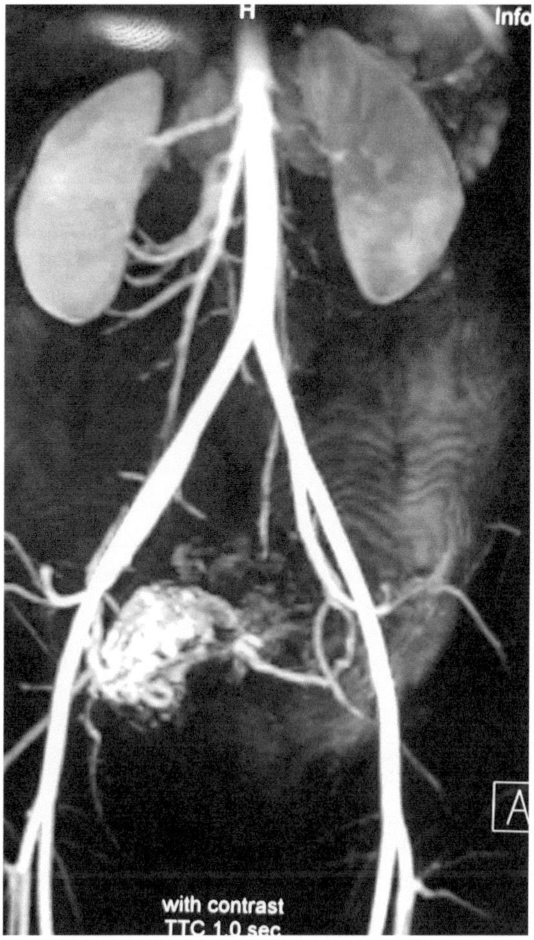

Fig. 18.9 MRI angiography shows uterine AVM

young patients, and in an unstable patient, appropriate diagnosis is important because emergent treatment with D&C can worsen the underlying condition, leading to profuse uterine hemorrhage, shock, and potentially hysterectomy [27]. Emergency angioembolization is the preferred treatment of choice and has excellent results, often avoiding the need for hysterectomy (Figs. 18.10 and 18.11).

6. *Gastrointestinal AVM*: AVM of the pancreas or common bile duct (CBD) is a vascular anomaly in which blood flows from the arterial system directly into the portal venous system without passing through the capillaries. This can lead to hemobilia or massive upper

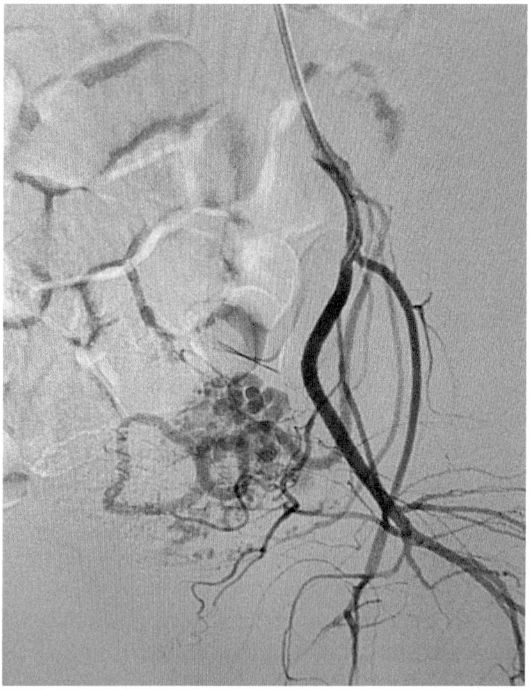

Fig. 18.10 Uterine AVM (before embolisation)

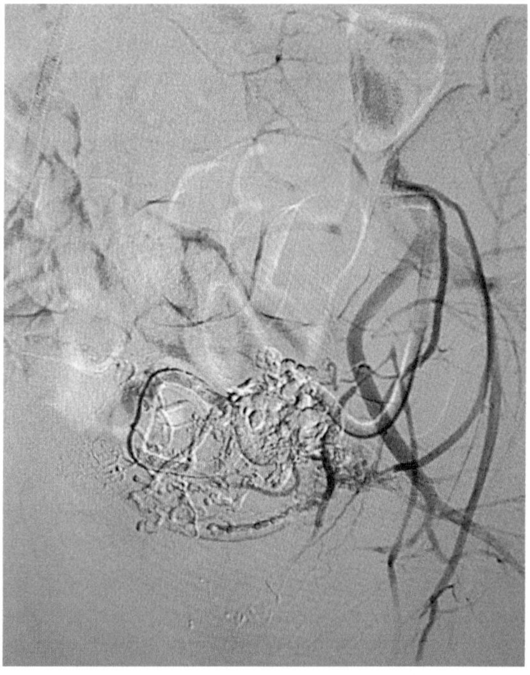

Fig. 18.11 Uterine AVM (after embolisation)

gastrointestinal (GI) bleeding and may be fatal. The treatment can be angioembolization or emergency laparotomy and pancreatoduodenectomy [28].

18.6 Treatment Principles of AV Malformations

These high-flow AV malformations are relatively rare and are far more difficult to treat. Surgical ligation of the feeding arteries of a high-flow AVM is ineffective and can be counterproductive as it often results in rapid recruitment of collaterals, which may render subsequent interventions ineffective.

Complete elimination of the nidus of an AVM is the only possibility for a total cure. However, this is often difficult to accomplish surgically. Debulking, incomplete resection, or ligation of arterial branches lead to recurrence of the malformation. Additionally, difficult surgical exposure and extensive blood loss are common during surgical resection of deep AVMs.

Successful endovascular embolization (embolotherapy) of the nidus of an AVM often requires super-selective catheterization of numerous arterial feeding branches. This is facilitated by using coaxial microcatheter systems. A 2-F to 3-F microcatheter is coaxially introduced through a 4-F to 5-F selective catheter and can be manipulated into the terminal feeding artery. Embolic agents are then delivered via the microcatheter, which is ideal for delivering liquid agents, particles, and small coils. The aim of embolization is to obliterate the nidus while simultaneously minimizing non-target embolization. For adequate embolization, it is recommended to use a combination of any of the three delivery routes: transarterial, transvenous, and direct puncture of the skin [29].

Selection of the appropriate agent for embolotherapy is as essential as correct patient selection. Various embolic materials available include: ethanol, N-butyl cyanoacrylate (NBCA), polyvinyl-alcohol (PVA) particles, ethylene vinyl alcohol copolymer (Onyx), and endovascular coils and vascular plugs [30]. Figures 18.12 and 18.13 show the use of glue or NBCA in an AVM of the lip, with complete obliteration of nidus. For another complex lesion in post-auricular region, embolisation using Onyx is demonstrated in Figs. 18.14 and 18.15.

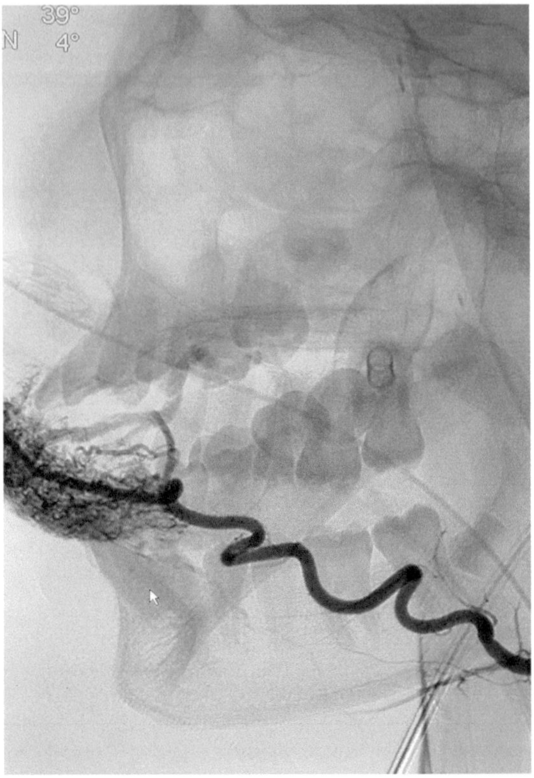

Fig. 18.12 Angiography shows nidus of lip AVM (before embolization)

Gorham-Stout syndrome (disappearing bone disease, phantom bone disease, diffuse skeletal hemangiomatosis) is a very rare syndrome characterized by multiple intraosseous vascular malformations inducing massive osteolysis. The truncal bones and upper extremities are most commonly affected. The vascular malformation may be localized or diffuse, and the degree of bone resorption is variable. Patients with this disorder often present during childhood with an antecedent history of minor trauma resulting in a pathologic fracture.

Localized intravascular coagulopathy (LIC) occurs due to stasis within these vessels with the formation of thrombin and subsequent conversion of fibrinogen to fibrin, which is followed by

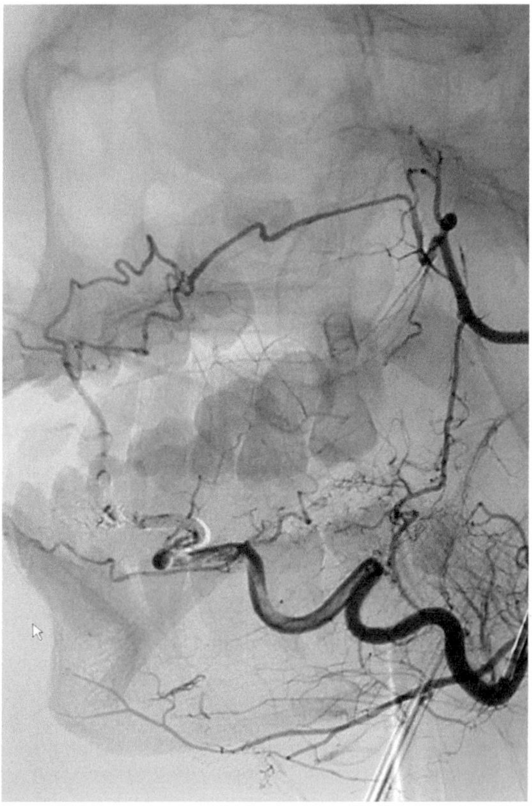

Fig. 18.13 Completion angiography shows obliteration of nidus of lip AVM (after glue embolisation)

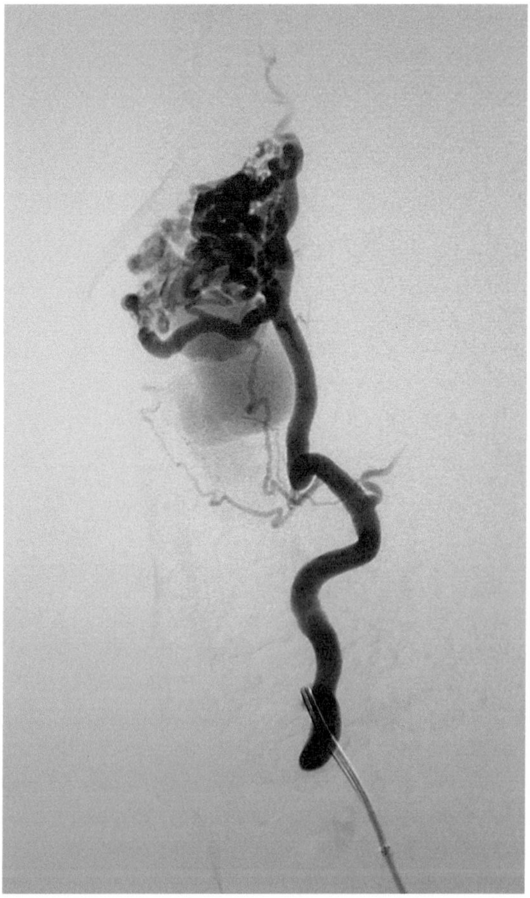

Fig. 18.14 Digital Subtraction Angiography shows nidus of ear AVM

fibrinolysis and evidence of fibrin degradation products like d-dimer LIC is of important clinical concern due to the potential for leading to more serious thrombo-embolic events, including STP, DVT, PE and the associated pulmonary hypertension, and thrombo-hemorrhagic DIC with life-threatening hemorrhage which can occur during or following surgical resection or sclerotherapy. Extensive CVM with large surface area, muscle involvement, and/or palpable phleboliths are strong predicting criteria for coagulation disorders associated with CVM. Assessment of the coagulation profile and D-dimer levels is indicated in patients with extensive CVMs. Coagulation profile and D-dimer levels are indicated in patients with extensive CVMs.

LIC as characterized by elevated D-dimer levels has been observed in approximately 40% of patients with CVMs. Patients with severe LIC would present with highly elevated D-dimer levels associated with low fibrinogen levels. Anticoagulation with LMWH can be used to treat the pain caused by LIC and to prevent decompensation of severe LIC to DIC.

AVM patients can present with pain, functional impairment, concerns about cosmetics, cutaneous and/or muscular ischemia, infection, and even ulceration(s) due to "steal phenomena" and subsequent diminished distal arterial blood flow.

If extensive, AVMs can lead to severe episodes of life-threatening hemorrhage, limb-threatening ischemia, and high-output cardiac failure due to large volume arteriovenous shunting. It may occasionally involve vital or critical structures like airways, eyes, or manifest by extension into the brain, perineum, genitals or intra-articular location (Hauert disease).

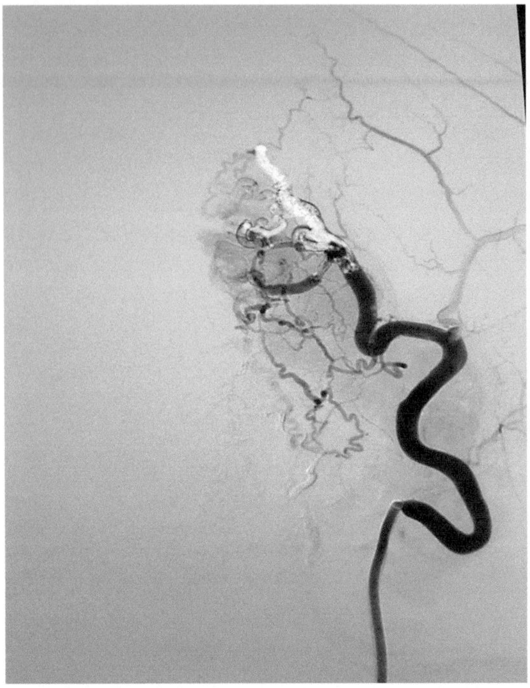

Fig. 18.15 Post-onyx embolization of ear AVM

In cases of trauma, secondary infection, abrupt hemorrhage of the lesions, or changes in hormonal levels can lead to pain, swelling, and even bleeding [13]. Venous malformations in parapharyngeal space, tongue, and soft palate may be accompanied by swallowing, speech, and airway problems.

18.7 Conclusion

Vascular malformations remain one of the most complex and ill understood diseases treated by vascular surgeons and interventionalists. A proper knowledge of emergency presentations of these infrequent disorders helps in deciding and delivering appropriate treatment.

Treatment of these vascular anomalies is challenging and often involves various therapeutic options. Multidisciplinary approach with full integration of open surgical and endovascular therapy has become the mainstay of treatment in the contemporary management of VMs.

References

1. Collcti G, Valassina D, Bcrtossi D, Mclciorrc F, Vercellio G, Brusati R. Contemporary management of vascular malformations. J Oral Maxillofac Surg. 2014;72:510–28.
2. Lee BB, Baumgartner I, Berlien P, Bianchini G, Burrows P, Glovicki P, et al. Diagnosis and treatment of venous malformations consensus document of the International Union of Phlebology (IUP): updated 2013. Int Angiol. 2015;34(2):97–144.
3. Redondo P. Vascular malformations: concept, classification, pathogenesis and clinical features. Actas Dermosifiliogr. 2007;98:141–58.
4. Tallman B, Tan OT, Morelli JG, Piepenbrink J, Stafford TJ, Trainor S, et al. location of port-wine stains and thelikelihood of ophthalmic and/or central nervous systemcomplications. Pediatrics. 1991;87:323–7.
5. Kramer U, Kahana E, Shorer Z, Ben-Zeev B. Outcome ofinfants with unilateral Sturge-weber syndrome and earlyonset seizures. Dev Med Child Neurol. 2000;42:756–9.
6. Wittekindt C, Michel O, Streppel M, Roth B, Quante G, Beutner D, Guntinas-Lichius O. Lymphatic malformations of the head and neck: introduction of a disease score for children, Cologne disease score (CDS). Int J Pediatr Otorhinolaryngol. 2006 Jul;70(7):1205–12.
7. Adams MT, Saltzman B, Perkins JA. Head and neck lymphaticmalformation treatment: a systematic review. Otolaryngol Head Neck Surg. 2012;147(4):627–39.
8. Cox JA, Bartlett E, Lee EI. Vascular malformations: a review. Semin Plast Surg. 2014;28:58–63.
9. Wassef M, Blei F, Adams D, Alomari A, Baselga E, Berenstein A, et al. Vascular anomalies classification: recommendations from the International Society for the Study of vascular anomalies. Pediatrics. 2015;136:e203–14.
10. Muñoz MR, Bueno A, La Torre CD, Cerezo VN, Rebolledo BN, Cervantes GC, et al. Surgical emergencies in intestinal venous malformations. Eur J Pediatr Surg. 2018;28(01):101–4.
11. Dompmartin A, Acher A, Thibon P, et al. Association of localized intravascularcoagulopathy with venous malformations. Arch Dermatol. 2008;144:873–7.
12. Mazoyer E, Enjolras O, Bisdorff A, Perdu J, Wassef M, Drouet L. Coagulation disorders in patients with venous malformation of limbs and trunk: a study in 118 patients. Arch Dermatol. 2008;144:861–7.
13. Levi M. Current understanding of disseminated intravascular coagulation. Br J Haematol. 2004;124:567–76.
14. Mattassi R, Loose DA, Vaghi M. Hemangiomas and vascular malformations: an atlas of diagnosis and treatment. Milan: Springer Verlag Italia; 2003.
15. Abecassis IJ, Xu DS, Batjer HH, Bendok BR. Natural history of brain arteriovenous malformations: a systemic review. Neurosurg Focus. 2014;37(3):1–11.

16. Derdeyn CP, Zipfel GJ, Albuquerque FC, Cooke DL, Feldman E, Sheehan JP, et al. Management of brain arteriovenous malformations: a scientific statement for healthcare professionals from the American Heart Association/American Stroke Association. Stroke. 2017;48:e200–24.
17. Kim LJ, Spetzler RF. Classification and surgical management of spinal arteriovenous malformations. Neurosurgery. 2006;70(S3):195–201.
18. Cottin V, Plauchu H, Bayle JY, Barthelet M, Revel D, Cordier JF. Pulmonary arteriovenous malformations in patients withhereditary hemorrhagic telangiectasia. Am J Respir Crit Care Med. 2004;169:994–1000.
19. Shovlin CL, Guttmacher AE, Buscarini E, Faughnan ME, Hyland RH, Westermann CJ, et al. Diagnostic criteria for hereditaryhemorrhagic telangiectasia (Rendu-Osler-Weber syndrome). Am J Med Genet. 2000;91:66–7.
20. Adams HP, Subbiah B, Bosch E. Neurologic aspects of hereditaryhemorrhagic telangiectasia. Arch Neurol. 1977;34:101–4.
21. Hall WA. Hereditary hemorrhagic telangiectasia (Rendu-Osler-weber disease) presenting with polymicrobial brain abscess. J Neurosurg. 1994;81:294–6.
22. Press OW, Ramsey PG. Central nervous system infectionsassociated with hereditary hemorrhagic telangiectasia. Am J Med. 1984;77:86–92.
23. Lacombe P, Lacout A, Marcy PY, Binsse S, Sellier J, Bensalah M, et al. Diagnosis and treatment of pulmonary arteriovenousmalformations in hereditary hemorrhagictelangiectasia: an overview. Diagn Interv Imaging. 2013;94:835–48.
24. Mager JJ, Overtoom TT, Blauw H, Lammers JW, Westermann CJ. Embolotherapy of pulmonary arteriovenous malformations: long-term results in 112 patients. J Vasc Interv Radiol. 2004;15:451–6.
25. Cura M, Elmerhi F, Suri R, Bugnone A, Dalsaso T. Vascular malformations and arteriovenous fistulas of the kidney. Acta Radiol. 2010;51(2):144–9.
26. Christenson BM, Gipson MG, Smith MT. Pelvic vascular malformations. Semin Intervent Radiol. 2013;30:364–71.
27. Grivell M, Reid M, Mellor A. Uterine arteriovenous malformations: a review of current literature. Obstet Gynecol Surg. 2005;60(11):761–7.
28. Song KB, Kim SC, Park JB, et al. Surgical outcomes of pancreatic arteriovenous malformation in a single center and review of literature. Pancreas. 2012;41:388–96.
29. Lee BB, Do YS, Yakes W, Kim DI, Mattassi R, Hyon WS. Management of arteriovenous malformations: a multidisciplinary approach. J Vasc Surg. 2004 Mar;39(3):590–600.
30. Lam K, Pillai A, Reddick M. Peripheral arteriovenous malformations: classification and endovascular treatment. Appl Radiol. 2017;46(5):15–21.

19 Quality of Life in Vascular Malformations

Seema Khanna and Rahul Khanna

19.1 Introduction

Vascular malformations are congenital lesions, which may present at birth or later in life and may cause significant morbidity and even mortality in children and adults. The nomenclature of these vascular lesions has been a source of confusion among physicians for various reasons. The terms vascular lesions, vascular malformations, and hemangiomas have often been used interchangeably and inappropriately. Vascular lesions can be subclassified biologically into vascular tumors or vascular malformations based on their endothelial characteristics or radiologically into hemangiomata, vascular and lymphatic malformations based on their vascular dynamics [1].

The classification given by Mulliken and Glowacki in 1982 [2] segregates the endothelial malformations into two main groups, hemangiomas, and vascular malformations on the basis of their natural history, cellular turnover, and histology. Hemangiomas exhibit cellular proliferation, are small or absent at birth, rapidly grow during infancy but involute during childhood. On the other hand, vascular malformations are composed of dysplastic vessels, are present at birth, grow proportionate to the child's growth, and do not regress [3].

S. Khanna (✉) · R. Khanna
Department of General Surgery, Institute of Medical Sciences, BHU, Varanasi, Uttar Pradesh, India

A. K. Khanna, S. K. Tiwary (eds.), *Vascular Malformations*,
https://doi.org/10.1007/978-981-15-9762-6_19

From a clinician viewpoint, these lesions have to be diagnosed correctly so as to initiate the appropriate treatment. A team approach comprising of various subspecialties like surgeons, radiologists, pediatric oncologist, intervention radiologists, and orthopedic surgeons may be required for optimum treatment. They will provide medical therapy, imaging, image guided interventions, surgery, laser therapy, and follow up for short- and long-term complications. Optimum treatment of such patients is usually lacking because the uncommonality of lesions leads to inexperience on part of clinicians and a paucity of randomized controlled trials, which would provide Level I evidence for adequate management of vascular malformations.

19.2 Factors Affecting Quality of Life in Vascular Malformations Patients

As vascular malformations present in myriad presentations and are chronic in nature because of the long time interval needed to cure or treat these patients, the quality of life (QOL) would presumably be negatively affected.

The factors affecting the quality of life can be numerous. Vascular malformations on the face and head and neck regions causing cosmetic disfigurement would lead to social embarrassment and social isolation. The most important concern of these patients is camouflage of the lesion, not complete cure (Fig. 19.1). Extensive lesions as in Klippel Trenaunay syndrome lead to limb hypertrophy and limb disproportion. This may interfere with the occupation and day-to-day working of these otherwise healthy young adults leading to dissatisfaction at workplace and anxiety about progress in life. Lesions involving chest wall and breasts in females (Fig. 19.2) are usually wide-

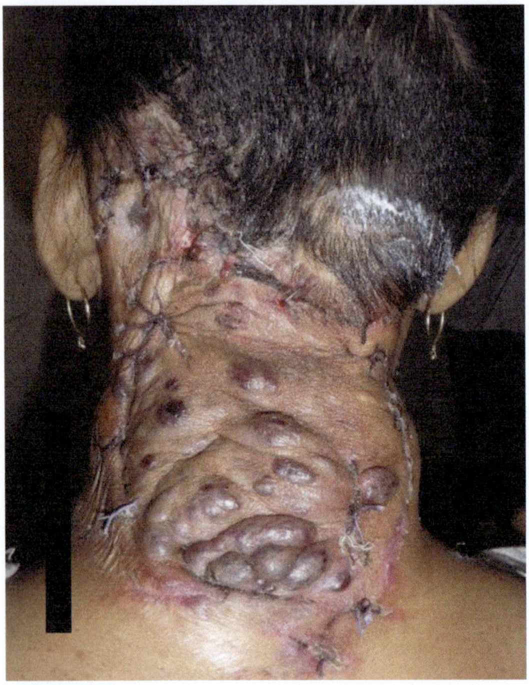

Fig. 19.1 Photograph showing extensive vascular malformation in head and neck region

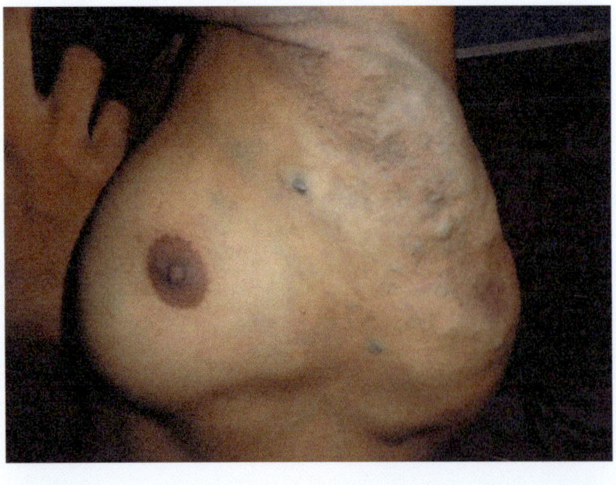

Fig. 19.2 Vascular malformation of chest wall extending into breast with lymphatic component

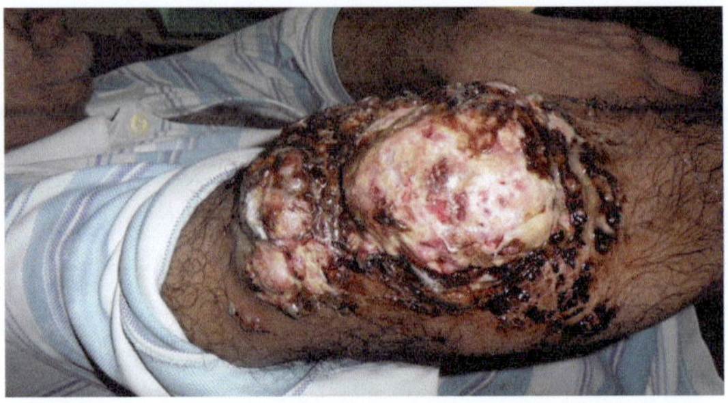

Fig. 19.3 Vascular malformation on elbow joint prone to recurrent bleeding

spread, may extend into the neck and therefore be not amenable to complete extirpation. This may cause emotional problems, affect family life and mental health. Surface vascular malformations on upper limbs (Fig. 19.3) may be a cause of pain and bleeding off and on leading to substantial morbidity. Counselling regarding avoidance of trauma may do little to alleviate the fear and anxiety of patients. Patients with vascular malformations not only suffer from cosmetic disfigurement but may have various degrees of functional impairment, recurrent infections, bleeding episodes, and sometimes life-threatening complications like heart failure. Social stigmatization, negative reaction from strangers, stress, sadness, and low self-esteem has been reported with such lesions.

Assessment of QOL in such patients may guide the clinician toward better management of the vascular malformation lesions.

19.3 Impact of Treatment on Quality of Life in Vascular Malformation

The investigations needed are actually few, especially in a resource-starved country like India and unnecessary investigations should be avoided. The noninvasive tests like duplex scan, standard T_1 and T_2 weighted MRI should form the mainstay of diagnostic strategy. Duplex ultrasonography provides important information regarding constituents, blood flow, velocity, and main feeding artery of the lesion [4]. Standard T_1 and T_2 weighted Magnetic Resonance Imaging (MRI) helps differentiate between high flow and low flow lesions. Bone X-rays may be needed for limb length discrepancies.

Venous photoplethysmography determines the functional status of venous system. Infrared limb volumetry is useful for extremity VM. TC-99 m RBC whole-body blood pool scintigraphy (WBBPS) known as "trans venous angioscan" is able to detect abnormal blood pooling throughout the body [5]. Invasive studies like venography, arteriography, or lymphangiography remain the reference standard for management of all congenital vascular malformations as they form the "road maps" of the treatment plan.

In vascular malformations, treatment is recommended when it causes cosmetic disfigurement, pain, or functional restrictions [6]. Superficial localized malformations are best treated by surgical excision. However, clinical and radiological evaluations may be misleading and the malformation could be found to be considerably more extensive during surgery (Fig. 19.4). Malformations that are deeply situated or extensive require combination therapy with sclerotherapy, image-guided embolization, and single staged surgical excision (Fig. 19.5). The physicians should bear in mind that the post-surgery cosmetic result could be less than satisfactory and on occasion even worse than the preoperative presentation.

Evidently, quality of life in all aspects would be negatively affected when treatment is multistaged and protracted. Malformations with a significant intramuscular component could require excision of significant muscle mass and thus could lead to functional disability. Considering that vascular malformations are essentially benign lesions with a projected normal life expectancy, such functional disability could adversely impact the quality of life. Focused physiotherapy to overcome such disability and counselling can have a positive effect.

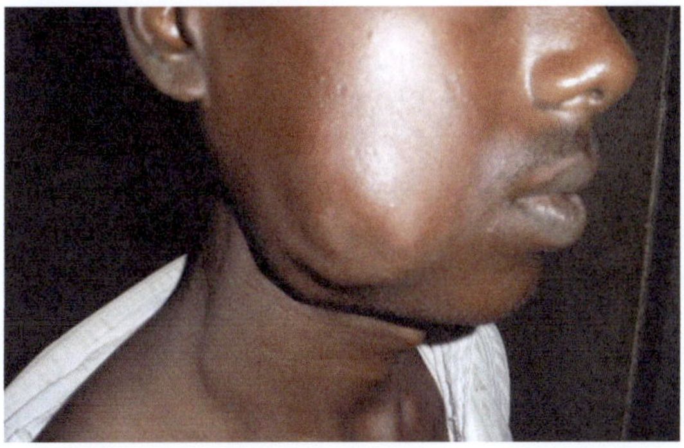

Fig. 19.4 Vascular malformation of cheek. Complete extirpation may lead to disfigurement

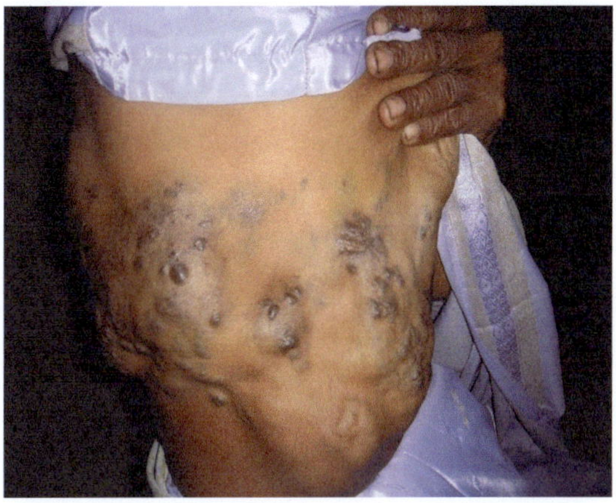

Fig. 19.5 Vascular malformation involving muscles of abdomen

Vascular malformations of the head and neck region can be extremely vascular and lead to local tissue gigantism. Complete extirpation of such lesions is difficult (Fig. 19.1) and in the absence of very high-quality reconstructive surgery the postoperative cosmetic results can sometimes be disastrous. Such patients though with little functional impairment can be severely affected emotionally and psychologically. They may become reclusive, reticent, and chronically depressed. Such patients have difficulty in finding a life partner or a satisfactory occupation and may be reluctant to venture out in public without a concealing outfit.

19.4 Impact of Treatment Failure on Quality of Life

Treatment failure is a fairly common occurrence in patients with vascular malformations. This is primarily because of underestimating the extent of the lesion on clinical evaluation and imaging studies leading to incomplete surgical excision. Unanticipated extension into adjacent muscles can lead to intraoperative dilemmas and the surgeon is more likely to err on the side of a more conservative than desired excision. Also, the vascularity of the lesion may be underestimated and if the patient is being operated in a center where surgical expertise is lacking or modern vessel sealing devices are not available then a failure of the adequate excision or even midway abandonment of the procedure is a strong possibility. A surface vascular malformation may be innocuous in appearance and a surgeon unaccustomed to such cases may grossly underrate the potential intraoperative difficulties (Fig. 19.4). Such patients who have incomplete surgery in the first instance are destined for multiple and prolonged further interventions. This can very adversely affect the patient's morale, his emotional status, physical well-being, and daily routine.

19.5 Quality of Life

The World Health Organization (WHO) conceptualizes positive health encompassing not only physical well-being but also psychological and social well-being. Psychologists assess the state of "well being" with a certain objective and subjective parameters. The objective parameter is the standard of living of an individual and the subjective component of well-being as expressed by each individual is referred to as the "quality of life."

Quality of life (QOL) is defined by WHO [7] as "the condition of life resulting from the combination of the effects of the complete range of factors such as those determining health, happiness and including comfort in the physical environment and a satisfying occupation, education, social and intellectual attainments, freedom of action, justice and freedom of expression [8]."

Various instruments have been developed over time and the exact scale that can measure QOL best is still evolving. American psychologist John Flanagan in 1970s designed the quality of life scale (QOLS), which has been adapted for use in chronic illness groups. QOLS in its present format contains 16 items that measures six conceptual domains of quality of life, namely, material and physical well-being, relationships with other people, social, community and civic activities, personal development, and fulfillment and satisfaction and the last domain which was added after interaction with patients having chronic illnesses was independence, i.e., the ability to do for yourself [9]. Another instrument that is used commonly now to measure QOL is 36 item Short Form Health Survey. SF-36 is designed for self-administration, telephonic administration, or a personal interview [10].

The SF-36 includes one multiple-item scale that assesses eight health concepts.

These include:

1. Limitations in physical activities because of health problems.
2. Limitations in social activities because of physical or emotional problems.
3. Limitations in usual role activities because of physical health problems.
4. Bodily pain.
5. General mental health (psychological distress as well-being).
6. Limitations in usual role activities because of emotional problems.
7. Vitality (energy and fatigue).
8. General health perceptions.

This tool is popular with researchers because of its brevity and comprehensiveness.

19.6 Scales Used for Assessment

Various questionnaires used in assessing QOL in vascular malformations are:

	Questionnaire	Factors assessed
I	SF-36	1. Limitation in physical activities: of health problem 2. Limitation in social activities: of physical or emotional problem 3. Limitation in usual role activities because of physical health problem 4. Bodily pain 5. General mental health 6. Limitation in usual role activities because of emotional problems 7. Vitality 8. General health perceptions
II	Dermatology specific QOL questionnaire (DLQI) (Over last/week) [11]	1. How itchy, sore, painful skin is 2. How embarrassed you were 3. How much did it affect shopping, looking after home garden 4. Affecting wearing of clothes 5. Affecting social or leisure activities 6. Affecting sport 7. Affecting working or studying 8. Problems with partner, friends, or relatives 9. Any sexual difficulties 10. How much problem treatment is causing
III	Skindex 29 (over last 4 weeks)	1. Symptoms Domain—7 items, e.g., pain, irritation, and bleeding 2. Emotions Domain—10 items, e.g., affecting relationships and stay at home
IV	Pain Disability Index	1. Family/home responsibility 2. Recreation 3. Social activities 4. Occupation 5. Sexual behavior 6. Self-care 7. Life support activity
V	Patient Health Questionnaire (PHQ-15) (for last 7 days)	1. Stomach pain 2. Back pain 3. Pain in arms and legs 4. Menstrual cramps 5. Headache 6. Chest pain 7. Dizziness 8. Fainting spells 9. Feeling your heart pound 10. Shortness of breath 11. Problem during sexual behavior 12. Constipation/stools/diarrhea 13. Nausea, gas, and indigestion 14. Low energy 15. Trouble sleeping
VI	HADS Hospital Anxiety And Depression Scale	1. I feel tense 2. I still enjoy the things I used to enjoy 3. I get a frightening feeling that something awful will happen 4. I can laugh and see the funny side of things 5. Worrying thoughts 6. I feel cheerful 7. I can sit at ease and feel relaxed 8. I feel as if I am slowed again 9. I get "butterflies" 10. I have lost interest in my appearance 11. I feel restless 12. I look forward to things 13. I panic 14. I can enjoy a good look/TV

19.7 Various Parameters of Quality of Life to Be Assessed

Various studies have been carried out on different aspects like preoperative, postoperative, or psychological assessment. Ilias Karapantozos et al. [12] assessed QOL in patients of hereditary hemorrhagic telangiectasia (HHT) after the management of epistaxis by Nd:YAG laser by using SF-36 and a short 5-item questionnaire. It was found that diseases like HHT are not the cause of mortality but epistaxis causes loss of work hours, anxiety, and discomfort, which is the cause of reduced scores in both physical and mental dimensions. Even a single laser treatment caused an increase in the QOL scores thereby emphasizing the fact that morbidity due to various reasons directly or indirectly diminishes the QOL.

Proper counseling in the initial visits could do much to alleviate the fear of family members, especially in case of infantile hemangiomas (IH). Moyakine et al. [13] have used a Dutch version (D-IH-QOL) of a validated infantile hemangioma-specific QOL questionnaire to focus on the impact of infantile hemangioma on QOL in young children with an IH in the growth phase, when its impact is maximal on parents psychosocial well-being. Their study revealed that the impact was relatively mild on patients and their parents at the age of 4.4 months. The authors were of the opinion that it could be because the parents were already reassured during their initial consultation. Also because infantile hemangiomas do not cause pain or systemic illness, the impact on QOL may be relatively low. The four main domains assessed in the above questionnaire were PEF (Parent Emotional functioning), PPF (Parent psychosocial functioning), CPS (Child physical Symptoms), and CSI (Child Social Interacting). This is a robust tool as it incorporates both parent and child assessments, which depict the overall QOL in a patient's family.

Oduber Charlene et al. [14] have used a dermatology-specific QOL questionnaire that contains 29 items divided amongst three subscales, namely, (A) Symptoms (B) Emotions (C) Functioning. Questions refer to the previous 4 weeks. High Skinden—29 scores correlate with a lower QOL. According to the authors, they found that a total score lower than 40 indicates a negligible negative impact on QOL, suggesting that Klippel-Trenaunay patients score higher than the rest on mental health, role emotional, and vitality. A possible explanation may be that since KTS patients have congenital malformations since birth, they have been coping with emotional problems since birth and are better able to put things into perspective. It was also concluded that in the various QOL questionnaires available, along with a generic questionnaire, dermatology-specific questionnaire is useful as a generic questionnaire can be used to compare different types of diseases while a dermatology-specific questionnaire will be useful for comparing diseases involving the skin (Fig. 19.2). Screening of patients can be done for psychological distress with short questionnaires (e.g., HADS, PHQ-15) during the history taking. But whether this will result in better patient care needs to be evaluated. Fahrni et al. drive home an important perspective. That QOL in vascular malformations is matchable in certain spheres, probably because of the younger age of these patients. They also found that increased number of interventions does not lower the QOL, contrary to expectations. Also, there was no significant difference in QOL scores between patients of arterial vascular malformations and capillary vascular malformations [15].

Assessment of pain and somatic symptoms, anxiety, and depression is also desirable for a complete analysis of these patients. A Pain Disability Index (PDI) has been devised which measures the magnitude of the self-reported disability in seven areas of daily living. The questionnaire comprises 11 items to be rated on a numeric scale ranging from "0" for "no disability" to 10 for maximum disability yielding a score between 0 and 110.

Somatic symptoms can be assessed using the patient Health Questionnaire (PHQ). The PHQ-15 is a self-administered subscale derived from a full PHQ. Patients are asked to rate the severity of symptoms experienced in last 4 weeks as "0" (not bothered at all), "1" (bothered a little), "2" (bothered a lot). Thus, the total PHQ-15 score ranges from 0 to 30. Scores ≥10 represent moderate levels of somatic distress [16].

Assessment of symptoms of anxiety and depression can be done used HADS (Hospital Anxiety and Depression Scale). The depression and anxiety subscales comprise seven items each to be rated on a four-point Likert Scale [15] which ranges from 0 to 3 where "0" is "not at all" and "3" is "mostly," sum score ranging from 0 to 21. HADS-D subscale for depression and HADS-A subscale for anxiety of ≥8 points is defined as elevated, i.e., clinically relevant levels of depressive and anxiety symptoms. A threshold of ≥17 points from a total of HAD-S and HADS-A subscales means clinically relevant levels of psychological distress [17].

Thus, each patient has to be assessed and evaluated as an individual and management has to be tailor-made for every patient depending on the site of lesion, extent of lesion, the circumstances, and the availability of the resources [18].

19.8 Conclusion

The aim of treatment of any illness is complete cure but vascular malformations are entities that are difficult to treat because of their varied presentation, unpredictable course of illness, and often unsatisfactory response to the treatment strategies. A correct diagnosis of the lesion is important. The classification given by Mulliken and Glowacki, which is also accepted by the International Society for the Study of Vascular Anomalies, should be followed in all cases.

A comprehensive, multidisciplinary approach is essential while treating such patients and management strategy be planned assiduously. Unnecessary investigations should be avoided. This will help in improving the quality of life of these patients. Formation of support groups, helping patients by interacting with each other, educating about the disease process, proper pretreatment counseling, and psychological intervention may improve QOL in vascular malformation patients.

References

1. Bailey and Love: Short practice of surgery. 27th edn, Vol 1. p. 612–5.
2. Mulliken JB, Glowacki J. Hemangiomas and vascular malformations in infants and children : a classification based on endothelial characteristics. Plast Reconstr Surg. 1982;69:412–23.
3. Donnely LF, Adams DM, Bisset III GS. Vascular malformations and hemangiomas : a practical approach in a multidisciplinary clinic. AJR. 2000;174:597–607.
4. Lee BB. New approaches to the treatment of congenital vascular malformations—a single centre experience. Eur J Vasc Endovase Surg. 2005;30:184–96.
5. Lee BB, Kim DI, Hun S, Kiim HH, Choo IW, Byum HS, et al. New experiences with absolute ethanol Sclerotherapy in management of a complex form of congenital venous malformation. J Vasc Surg. 2001;33:764–72.
6. Rautio R, Saarinen J, Laranne J, Salenius JP, Keski-Nisula L. Endovascular treatment of venous malformations in extremities: Results of sclerotherapy and the quality of life after treatment. Acta Radiol. 2004:397–402.
7. WHO. WHO chr. 1976;30(8):312.
8. Nagpal R, Sell H. Subjective wellbeing. Reg. Health papers No. 7, SEARD, WHO, New Delhi; 1985.
9. Burckhardt, CS, Anderson KL. The Quality of life Scale (QOLS): Reliability, validity and utilization. Health and Quality of life outcomes; 2003.
10. Ware Jr JE, Sherbourne CD. The MOS 36-item short-form health survey (SF-36) conceptual framework and item selection. Med Care. 1992;30(6):473–83.
11. Mishra N, Rastogi MK, Agrawal S. Dermatology specific quality of life in vitiligo patients and its relation with various variables: A Hospital based cross-sectional study. J Clin Diagn Res. 2014;8(6):YCOI–YCO3.
12. Karapantzos I, Tsempiris N, Goulis DG, Hoecke HV, Cauwenberge PV, Danielides V. Management of epistaxis in hereditary hemorrhagic telangiectasia by Nd: YAG laser and quality of life assessment using the HR-QOL questionnaire. Eur Arch Otorhinolaryngol. 2005;262:830–3.
13. Moyakine AV, Spillekom-van Koulel S, Kupers EM, Vander Vleuten CJM. Influence of infantile hemangioma severity and activity on QOL of patients and their parents: A cross-sectional a study. Pediatr Dermatol. 2018;35:628–34.
14. Oduber Charlene EU, Khemlani K, Smett JHS, Hennekam RCM, Vander Horst CMAM. Base line

quality of life in patients with Klipple-Trenaunay syndrome. JPRAS. 2010;63:603–9.
15. Fahrni JO, ChoEn Young N, Engelberger RP, et al. Quality of life in patients with congenital vascular malformations. J Vasc Surg Venous Lymphat Disord. 2014;2(1):46–51.
16. Chron MM. Dermatol Clin. 2013;30(2):231–236.
17. Nguyen HL, Donadurer GF 3rd, Tollefson MN. Quality of life; a systematic review and meta-analysis. JAMA Dermatol. 2018;154(6):661–9.
18. Dubois J, Soulez G, Olivia VL, et al. Soft tissue venous malformations in adult patients: imaging and therapeutic issues. Radiographics. 2001;21:1519–31.

Genetics of Vascular Malformations

20

Shashi Prakash Mishra and Ajay K. Khanna

20.1 Definition and Introduction

The term "vascular anomaly" refers to a wide spectrum of congenital malformations and tumors of vascular origin ranging from inconsequential birthmarks to life-threatening and severely disfiguring conditions. Throughout most of the recorded history, they have been believed to result from the emotions, thoughts, or desires of the expectant mother. In the mid-19th century, Scottish anatomist William Hunter questioned this theory of "maternal impression" and introduced the concept of vascular anomaly [1, 2]. However, lack of systematic categorization of these diverse lesions held back medical progress for over a century. While mothers were no longer blamed, the limited diagnostic knowledge often led to inappropriate management and unnecessary anxiety.

In 1982, Mulliken and Glowacki studied the cellular characteristics of vascular anomalies and consequently divided them into vascular tumors and vascular malformations [3, 4]. This division is still the basis for the International Society for the Study of Vascular Anomalies [5] classification [6] comprising a detailed taxonomy for dozens of different vascular entities. This classification was later on revised in May 2018 with an intent to evolve as our understanding of the biology and genetics of vascular malformations and tumors continues to grow [5]. Paolacci et al. worked [7] on vascular anomalies with highlighting molecular bases, genetic testing, and therapeutic approaches.

20.2 The Structure of Blood Vessels

The fundamental structure of a blood vessel is that of a tube formed by a single layer of endothelial cells (ECs). The mature vasculature consists of specialized vessels such as arteries, arterioles, veins, venules, and capillaries that differ in diameter, location in the body, and the composition of supporting layers surrounding the EC tube [8]. These vessels are also arranged in a hierarchical order—large arteries carry blood from the heart to small capillaries via intermediate arterioles. The blood is returned to the heart by veins and via intermediate venules [8].

Capillaries are the smallest branches of mature vessels localized throughout the body. They are the most abundant vessel type and facilitate direct exchange of molecules with the tissues they vascularize [9]. They consist of the EC tube surrounded by a supporting layer of pericytes embedded within a basement membrane (BM).

S. P. Mishra
Department of General Surgery, Institute of Medical Sciences, Banaras Hindu University, Varanasi, Uttar Pradesh, India
e-mail: spmishra.gs@bhu.ac.in

A. K. Khanna (✉)
Department of Surgery, Institute of Medical Science, Banaras Hindu University, Varanasi, India

A. K. Khanna, S. K. Tiwary (eds.), *Vascular Malformations*, https://doi.org/10.1007/978-981-15-9762-6_20

Capillaries are the main sites of nutrient exchange between blood and tissue, given their simple wall structure and large surface-area-to-volume ratio. They also adapt their EC layer structure according to different organ needs. For example, in muscle, the capillary endothelial layer is continuous; in endocrine glands it is fenestrated, while in liver sinusoids it is discontinuous. Further specialized regions such as the blood–brain barrier and the blood–retina barrier include tight junctions in their endothelia. These structures ensure the maintenance of impermeability to various molecules [9].

Arterioles and venules have a thicker outer supporting layer compared to that of capillaries. This supporting layer consists of an internal elastic lamina (IEL), a layer of vascular smooth muscle cells (vSMCs) tightly associated around the EC tube, a basement membrane and an external elastic lamina (EEL).

Arteries and similar large vessels are composed of three layers: the tunica intima, the tunica media, and the tunica adventitia. The intimal layer is composed of the EC tube supported by the IEL; the medial layer consists of multiple concentric layers of vSMCs supported by the EEL; the adventitial layer is composed of fibroblasts embedded in extracellular matrix (ECM) and also supported by an EEL. The adventitial layer also has its own blood supply, called the vasa vasorum (Latin, "the vessels of the vessels"). The layers of vSMCs and elastic laminae contribute to vessel tone and control vessel diameter which in turn regulates blood flow and blood pressure [9].

Apart from the vascular system, the lymphatic system has its own unique network of lymphatic vessels. Lymphatic capillaries consist of a single layer of lymphatic endothelial cells with microvalves in their walls. The lymphatic ECs are embedded in ECM and are connected to the surrounding tissue via anchoring filaments. Lymphatic capillaries join to larger lymphatic vessels that contain valves to direct lymph flow in one direction. They are supported by pericytes and a basement membrane.

The combination of vSMCs and pericytes is collectively known as mural cells as they both form a supporting layer around the EC tube. Although both cell types are believed to originate from a common mesenchymal progenitor, the prototypical vSMC and pericyte are distinct from one another in terms of localization, morphology, and function in the vascular bed [10]. While vSMCs generally adopt a spindle-shaped morphology [11], pericytes may appear as either elongated stellate-shaped cells with multiple cytoplasmic extensions wrapped around the endothelium or rounded compact shapes, depending on the organ in which the pericyte resides [10]. vSMCs are highly abundant around vessels that require regulation of vascular tone and contractility, whereas pericytes are generally localized around smaller vessels such as capillaries, precapillary arterioles, and postcapillary venules. Since a single pericyte can make contacts with several ECs, they are thought to mediate cell communication between neighboring ECs [10]. Despite these differences between vSMCs and pericytes, there exists a vSMC-pericyte phenotypic spectrum where some mural cells have mixed characteristics [10].

20.3 Embryonic Development of Blood Vessels

Blood vessel development in the early embryo occurs by two sequential processes: vasculogenesis and angiogenesis. Vasculogenesis refers to the de novo formation of a primitive vascular network from the differentiation, migration, and coalescence of mesoderm-derived angioblasts into aggregations known as blood islands [12]. The generation of these angioblasts from the mesoderm is mediated by basic fibroblast growth factor (FGF2) signalling to its receptor FGFR [8]. The angioblasts proliferate and differentiate into endothelial cells, which then begin to form the tube of the vessel. These processes are dependent on VEGF signalling [8]. VEGF-A is secreted by mesenchymal cells near the blood islands and is received by VEGFR receptors expressed on the angioblasts in the blood islands [13, 14]. EC tubes then connect to form the primary capillary plexus in vascular islets. Subsequently, ECs are specified to either an arterial or an venous fate, in response to both hemodynamic stimuli and molecular signalling. Arterial specification is mediated by Notch-induced expression of the HEY1 and HEY2 transcription factors [15], whereas venous specification is mediated by the COUP transcription factor 2 that downregulates Notch signalling [16, 17].

Angiogenesis is the sprouting of new vessels and branches from preexisting vessels. It involves complex multistep processes and requires intricate coordination of ECs. Normally the ECs in stable vessels are in a quiescent state until pro-angiogenic signals are detected. In response, ECs dismantle their cell–cell junctional contacts, activate matrix metalloproteases that degrade the surrounding basement membrane and start to migrate to form the new vessel branch. These sprouting ECs are subdivided into two groups—tip cells and stalk cells. Tip cells "lead" the sprouting branch by invading into the future vessel region guided by gradients of angiogenic signals, while stalk cells "follow" behind to support the tip cells and maintain contact with the parental vessel [18]. EC sprouting continues till the tip cells connect and fuse to an adjacent vessel via anastomosis. New cell–cell junctions are established and a continuous lumen is formed. At the same time, supporting mural cells (vSMCs and pericytes) are recruited to the sprouting vasculature by PDGFB and TGF-beta1 signalling, to stabilize the growing vessels [19, 20].TGF-beta1 promotes vSMC differentiation and maturation [17]. Complete absence of pericytes in mice results in EC hyperplasia, suggesting that pericytes help to regulate and silence EC growth during vascular sprouting [21]. Finally, the deposition of a new basement membrane encourages re-establishment of a quiescent EC phenotype. Since angiogenic sprouting involves mature vessels to first undergo destabilization before allowing new vessel branches to form, this destabilization may also lead to vascular regression [22].

Following vasculogenesis and angiogenesis, the vasculature must mature to become fully functional. This involves vascular pruning, which is the selective branch regression of the initial primitive plexus. Pericytes expressing the type I transmembrane glycoprotein Endosialin play an important role in vascular pruning, by promoting timely selective vessel regression in the immature vascular plexus, via endothelial cell apoptosis [23]. Maturation of the vasculature also involves vascular remodelling and adaptation to suit local tissue needs. To do so requires the recruitment and differentiation of supporting mural cells, deposition of an extracellular matrix, and further differentiation of ECs to acquire tissue-adapted phenotypes [24]. Vascular remodelling is highly sensitive to environmental cues and can actively change in response to different local demands, such as oxygen levels and changes in blood pressure. As mentioned previously, PDGFB and TGF-Beta1 signaling are important for vessel maturation due to their roles in stimulating mural cell differentiation, proliferation, migration, and production of ECM [24]. In addition, the Angiopoietins and Ephrins are also important secretory factors required for remodelling and maturation of the nascent vasculature. In particular, ANG1 plays a major role in stabilizing and protecting what is otherwise a leaky immature vasculature by promoting pericyte adhesion and tightening endothelial junctions [25].

Interestingly, the ANG1 antagonist ANG2 is exclusively expressed in adult tissues such as the ovary, placenta, and uterus that undergo vascular remodelling [26]. Ephrin-B2 functions to distinguish developing arterial and venous vessels and also facilitates the association of mural cells to the endothelium [24, 27]. Eventually, once the developing vasculature is stabilized, it enters into a quiescent state characterized by resting ECs forming a tight barrier between blood and surrounding tissue [24]. ECs have a long half-life and remain as such till stimulated by a new angiogenic signal.

In the mature adult vasculature, exogenous application of the molecular players described above, such as the VEGFs, Angiopoietins, and Ephrins, have been shown to be able to recapitulate their function as they would in the embryonic vasculature. For example, administration of VEGF alone can trigger the formation of new vessels, but these are immature and leaky.

Subsequent administration of ANG1 can stabilize and protect vessels from VEGF-induced leakiness [22].

20.4 Vascular Malformations Are Errors of Angiogenesis

Errors in molecular control of angiogenesis and vascular remodeling cause vascular anomalies which are localized lesions of arteriovenous, capillary, or lymphatic origin, and can occur in several distinct tissues including skin, mucosa, visceral organs, and bone. They can be congenital, or appear in adult life [28].

Developmental vascular anomalies are divided into two classes: hemangiomas and vascular malformations, based on endothelial cell properties and clinical course. Both hemangiomas and vascular malformations look similar to histology, therefore clinical history and EC behavior are key diagnostic criteria. Hemangiomas are characterized by actively proliferating neoplastic ECs, while vascular malformations are nonneoplastic abnormal expansile lesions of vascular tissue in which ECs have a normal cell cycle. A hemangioma grows rapidly in the form of a tumor and typically undergoes regression within the first decade of life. On the other hand, vascular malformations never regress and grow proportionally with the child [3, 4, 6]. While hemangiomas are basically tumors of the endothelium, vascular malformations are defects in morphogenesis of the vascular tree and can affect any segment of the system—arterial, venous, or capillary. Most characterized human vascular malformations have intact primary vasculatures, but harbor varying degrees of defects in angiogenesis and maintaining vessel stability [28].

The International Society for the Study of Vascular Anomalies (ISSVA) classifies all vascular anomalies into the two major aforementioned categories—hemangiomas and malformations, and further subdivides each category according to more specific clinical behavior and endothelial properties [6]. Hemangiomas are subdivided into benign, malignant, locally aggressive, or borderline. Vascular malformations are further categorized according to the type and number of vessels affected, be it simple, combined, of a major named vessel or in association with other vascular anomalies. Simple malformations refer to lesions that are localized to one type of vessel, such as capillary, lymphatic, or venous malformations. Combined vascular malformations can refer to mixed-vessel lesions such as capillary-venous, capillary-arteriovenous, or capillary-venous-arteriovenous malformations. Malformations in combination with other syndromic diseases include Klippel–Trenaunay and Parkes-Weber syndromes which are characterized by limb overgrowth, and Sturge–Weber syndrome which involves eye, bone, and soft tissue defects [6].

20.5 The Genetics of Vascular Malformations

Both sporadic and inherited forms of vascular malformations have been described in the literature. Inherited forms of distinct vascular malformations have been found to be caused by mutations in several genes, whose protein products are known modulators of angiogenesis, regulate ECvSMC communication as well as recruitment and migration of vSMCs. These genetic findings, along with studies in animal models, have paved the way to understanding the molecular pathogenesis of these diseases as well as uncover crucial pathways that regulate vessel development and homeostasis.

Angiopoietins and its TIE tyrosine kinase receptors are a class of ligand-receptor families that are crucial for vessel remodelling. Dominant activating mutations in *TIE2* cause Multiple Cutaneous and Mucosal Venous Malformations (VMCM; MIM 600195), which is characterized by a bluish hue lesion on skin and mucosa [29]. On histology, abnormally dilated vessels were coated by an irregular and patchy layer of smooth muscle cells [29]. The causative heterozygous missense mutations in *TIE2* resulted in a dominant ligand-independent hyperphosphorylation of the encoded receptor, which when expressed in endothelial cells increased the survival of ECs [30]. This pro-survival effect of the constitutively active receptor was found to be mediated by the recruitment and phosphorylation of the adaptor protein ShcA [31]. It is hypothesized that the survival of ECs may contribute to lesion formation seen in VMCMs [30]]. These findings in human genetic studies have also been partly corroborated in mouse studies. Deletion of Tie1 in mouse led to immediate postnatal death, partly due to system-wide hemorrhage and edema as a result of poor structural integrity of vascular ECs [32]. Tie2-null mutations in mice, on the other hand, were embryonic lethal, due to a malformation of the vascular network. Vessels were dilated and failed to sprout proper branches [32]. These findings implicate both Tie1 and Tie2 receptors in proper endothelial cell function and angiogenesis. Combined with the reported human data, both loss and over-activation of TIE receptors cause vascular defects in vivo. In addition, mice depleted of Angiopoietin-1, a ligand for TIE2, exhibited similar angiogenic defects similar to its *Tie2-/-* counterpart [25], while transgenic overexpression of the antagonist ligand Angiopoietin-2 also caused severe widespread vessel discontinuities [26]. Taken together, these data highlight the Angiopoietins and TIE receptors as critical regulators of vessel development.

TGFβ and its receptors have also been shown to be necessary for the establishment and maintenance of vessel wall integrity. In human, Hereditary Hemorrhagic Telangiectasia type 1 (HHT1, MIM 187300) and type 2 (HHT2, MIM 600376) are caused by heterozygous mutations in the genes endoglin (ENG) and activin receptor-like kinase 1 (ALK1), respectively [33, 34]. Telangiectasias are focal dilations of postcapillary venules appearing as red or purple clusters in the skin, lung, liver, and brain. HHTs are characterized by multisystemic vascular dysplasia and recurrent hemorrhage [34]. Both ENG and ALK1 are transmembrane co-receptors of the TGFβ receptor family, and are expressed in endothelial cells. Manifestation of disease is attributed to haploinsufficiency of either one of the co-receptors causing reduced TGFβ signalling—a key activator in EC migration and proliferation [35]. TGFβ1 knockout mice die mid-gestation due to defects in yolk sac vasculature and hematopoiesis [36]. In these mice, differentiation of mesodermal precursors to endothelial cells appears to be normal, however, the tubes that are formed from these endothelial cells were weak with reduced cell adhesiveness.

Integrins are another important class of cell surface receptors that mediate adhesion between the endothelium and ECM. Targeted deletion of β1 integrin in either mural cells or vascular smooth muscle cells in mice caused aneurysms and hemorrhaging [37]. In these mice, mural cells showed reduced cell adhesion and spreading which compromised vessel wall integrity [37], while the vascular smooth muscle cells could not maintain their differentiated state and transformed into a "synthetic" phenotype which is associated with injury. Mutations in β1 integrin have not yet been found in human vascular anomalies, however, one of the causative genes for Cerebral Cavernous Malformation (CCM, MIM 116860) is KRIT1, which regulates β1-integrin-dependent angiogenesis by competing with β1-integrin for binding to the integrin cytoplasmic domain associated protein 1α (ICAP1α) [38]. CCMs are malformations in the brain characterized by dilated vascular lesions that lack smooth muscle and elastic tissue. Clinically, CCMs can cause seizures, headaches, and strokes [39]. Mutations in KRIT1, CCM2, and PDCD10 cause cerebral cavernous malformations type 1 (MIM 116860), type 2 (MIM603284), and type 3 (MIM 603285), respectively.

Other genetically defined vascular malformations include Glomuvenous Malformation (GVM, MIM 138000), which is caused by autosomal dominant mutations in GLMN. GVMs are purple-bluish nodules mainly localized in the skin, and characterized by abnormally differentiated vSMCs in the form of "glomus cells" within dilated venous lesions [40]. It is not completely clear how loss of a single GLMN allele results in this phenotype, however, it is speculated that TGFβ signaling is downregulated which then affects EC-vSMC cross-talk and subsequent differentiation of vSMCs [28]. Sometimes mutations in a single gene can cause two clinically distinct vascular malformation syndromes. Mutations in RASA1 cause both capillary malformation—arteriovenous malformation (CM-AVM, MIM608354) and Parkes-Weber Syndrome (PKWS, MIM 608355). CM-AVMs are capillary malformations with an additional fast-flow arteriovenous lesion. They appear as pink, red, or brown small multifocal lesions in the skin. PKWS is similar but also includes overgrowth of limbs where the vascular malformation is localized and may cause congestive heart failure with age [28]. RASA1 encodes the p120RasGAP protein, which inactivates Ras, controls cell motility, and interacts with AKT to inhibit apoptosis. The exact mechanism controlling the formation of CM-AVMs by RASA1 is not completely known.

20.6 Classification of Vascular Anomalies

The classification of vascular anomalies aims to unify and clarify the complex terminology used by multidisciplinary professionals. Accurate terminology is crucial for achieving the right diagnosis, and thereby, proper management [41, 42]. The first classification based on endothelial characteristics of the vascular anomalies was introduced by Mulliken and Glowacki in 1982. It has since been revised and expanded by the International Society for the Study of Vascular Anomalies (ISSVA) to include the latest knowledge about genetics and clinical associations [43]. The essential framework of the ISSVA classification is the division of vascular anomalies into congenital malformations and proliferative tumors [44] (Fig. 20.1).

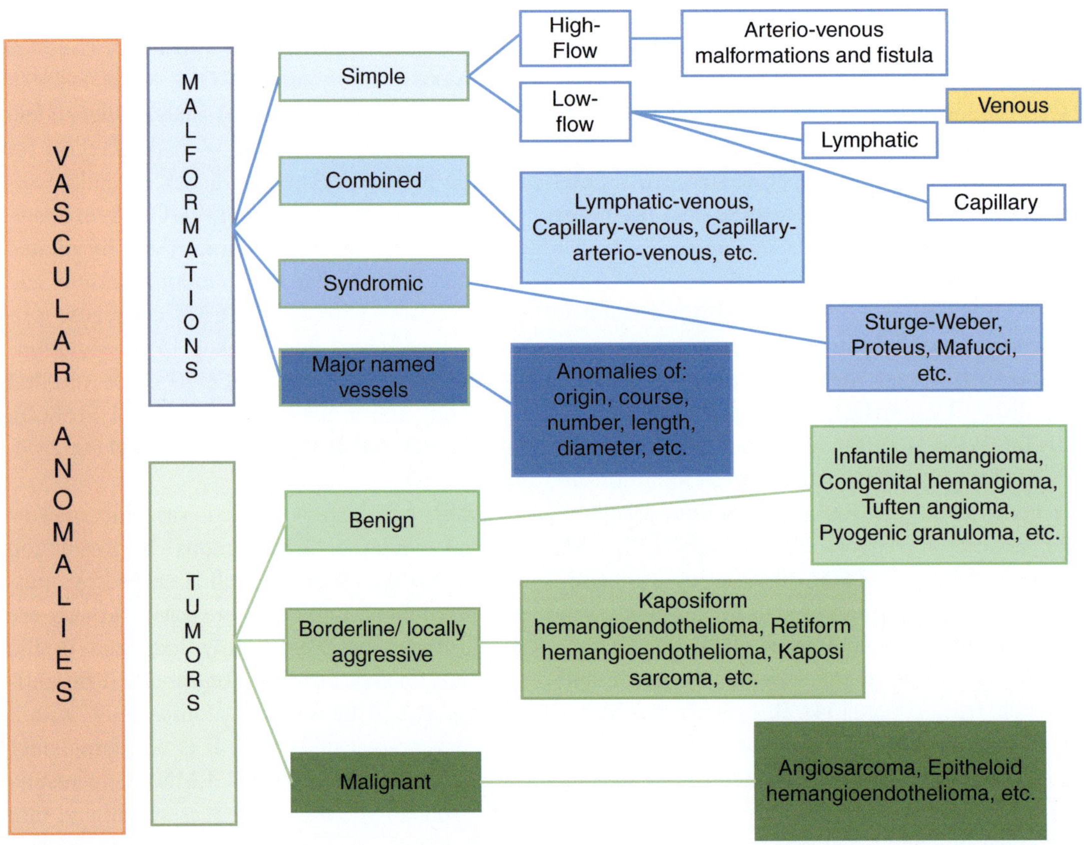

Fig. 20.1 Outline of the current ISSVA classification of vascular anomalies [6]

Vascular malformations are structural defects resulting from local disturbances in the fetal vascular morphogenesis. Their further categorization is based on their predominant vessel type or combinations of different vessel types, as well as associations with other anomalies [45]. Moreover, vascular malformations are often divided into low- and high-flow lesions for the clinical relevance of their pressure conditions [46, 47]. Vascular tumors, in turn, are proliferative lesions with mitotic activity. They are divided into benign, borderline, or locally aggressive, and malignant tumors according to their clinical behavior. Infantile hemangioma is the most common vascular tumor and also the most common pediatric tumor, affecting 4–10% of all children [48]. It has a unique clinical course of early proliferation and spontaneous involution. Congenital hemangioma, tufted angioma, and kaposiform hemangioendothelioma are examples of rare vascular tumors with clinical courses different from infantile hemangioma [49].

20.7 Vascular Tumors (Hemangiomas)

Although hemangiomas have historically been considered vascular malformation, it is important to note that they are histologically distinct based on cellular composition as well as clinical behavior. Hemangiomas are neoplastic lesions with endothelial hyperplasia whereas vascular malformations are congenital lesions with normal epithelial turnover [3, 4]. This distinction is of particular importance as it leads to diverging diagnosis as well as treatment of these conditions [50]. In terms of clinical presentation, hemangiomas are not typically present at birth, but instead appear shortly after and demonstrate rapid postnatal growth followed by slow involution. In contrast, vascular malformations are always present at birth.

Histologically, cells of hemangiomas demonstrate rapid endothelial hyperplasia as compared with the flat endothelium of a vascular malformation. This appears to be significant in that expression of various vascular endothelial growth factor receptors (VEGFR) are affected in hemangiomas, with one study demonstrating that VEGFR1 was markedly reduced whereas VEGFR2 activity was increased [51]. In another study, VEGFR mutations were found to be polymorphic, particularly those associated with infantile hemangiomas [52].

Syndromes associated with hemangiomas include Von Hippel–Lindau and Maffucci syndromes.

20.7.1 Von Hippel–Lindau Syndrome

Von Hippel–Lindau (VHL) syndrome is an autosomal dominant condition that causes a predisposition to both benign and malignant neoplasms, including retinal, cerebellar, spinal hemangioblastoma, renal cell carcinoma, pheochromocytoma, and pancreatic tumors [53]. In particular, the clinical hallmark of VHL is considered angiomata of the retina and hemangioblastoma of the cerebellum. Genetically, there have been several mutations of the VHL tumor suppressor gene, found on chromosome 3, which have been associated with the syndrome [54]. Notably, VHL can be subdivided into two clinical phenotypes, which have also demonstrated specific genetic associations. Type 1, which presents with retinal and central nervous system (CNS) hemangioblastoma, renal cell carcinoma, but not pheochromocytoma, is generally associated with large deletion or truncation mutations of the VHL gene, thus resulting in little or no function of the transcribed protein. In contrast, type 2, which is characterized by the presence of pheochromocytoma, is usually associated with missense mutation of the VHL gene that results in functional but limited protein [54]. Further evidence of a genotype–phenotype association has also been demonstrated by the lower prevalence of renal cell carcinoma in patients with complete VHL gene deletions [55, 56].

20.7.2 Maffucci Syndrome

Maffucci syndrome is characterized by spindle cell hemangiomas in addition to enchondromatosis. Notably, the enchondromas associated with Maffucci syndrome have been shown to have malignant potential, with one study demonstrating progression to chondrosarcoma in 30% of the patients [57]. The hemangiomas in this syndrome are generally cutaneous and subcutaneous, rarely causing acute bleeding [58]. The inheritance of Maffucci syndrome has mostly been reported as sporadic, with several mutations associated with the development of enchondromas [59]. In one study, 77% of patients with Maffucci syndrome carried isocitrate dehydrogenase mutations in their tumors, specifically IDH1 (98%) or IDH2 (2%) [60]. These mutations in cartilage tumors were associated with hypermethylation and downregulated expression of several genes. Notably, even tumors positive for these mutations demonstrated "intraneoplastic mosaicism," a condition in which there exists a mixture of cells that did and did not express the mutant protein.

20.8 Capillary Malformations

The majority of capillary malformations are considered sporadic and not linked to any genetic mutations. A subset of patients will have associated arteriovenous malformations (CM-AVM) [61]. These are described as multifocal capillary lesions surrounded by a pale halo and most commonly located on the head and neck. CM-AVM has been linked to an autosomal dominant, loss-of-function mutation in the RASA1 gene, located on 5q11-q23 and encodes p120 RASGAP. 3. Loss-of-function mutations lead to dysregulation in cell growth and proliferation. Notably, some patients with CM-AVM will have Parkes-Weber syndrome [61].

20.8.1 Sturge–Weber Syndrome

Sturge–Weber syndrome is classically characterized by facial cutaneous capillary malformations (port-wine stains) in association with intracranial vascular anomalies that can cause seizures and mental retardation. There is no clear hereditary pattern in this syndrome, but there is evidence for somatic mosaicism, which occurs in the somatic cells of the body and is the expression of multiple genotypes due to mitotic errors [62]. Although this is a highly variable syndrome, there is some evidence that the syndrome may be caused by a somatic mosaic mutation in the GNAQ gene on chromosome 9q21 [63], which encodes for guanine nucleotide-binding protein G(q) subunit α. Guanine nucleotide-binding proteins are a family of heterotrimeric proteins that couple transmembrane receptors to intracellular pathways and are activated by a GTPase. Interestingly, the single-nucleotide mutation of GNAQ in vascular endothelial cells seems to occur earlier in development than the mutations that occur in nonsyndromic port-wine stains. Although the exact involvement of this protein in phenotypic expression of Sturge–Weber syndrome is unknown, one hypothesis suggests involvement in vasculogenesis via endothelin, which is a G-protein coupled receptor [64, 65].

20.9 Venous Malformations

Venous malformations are the most common vascular malformation evaluated in referral centers. Vikkula et al estimate the incidence to range from 1 in 5000–10,000 live births [66]. These slow-flow lesions are classically blue-violet in color, but can vary widely in clinical presentation. It is crucial to properly identify these anomalies as they can be associated with coagulopathies. A small subset of cutaneomucosal venous malformations is inherited in an autosomal dominant manner. Two large families with known inherited venous malformations have demonstrated single amino acid substitution (R849W) in the gene encoding a tyrosine kinase receptor (TIE2) exclusive to endothelial cells [66]. Although the effects of the substitution are not yet known, it is proposed that mutant TIE2 receptors disrupt the cell cycle of endothelium, ultimately leading to an absence of smooth muscle cells within the malformation, a histological feature unique to cutaneomucosal venous malformations [66].

Another subset of venous malformation is the glomuvenous malformation (GVM), which is a blue-violet raised lesion with a distinct cobblestone surface that is very painful. Lesions contain "glomus cells," which are modified smooth muscle cells that resemble glomus bodies, the arteriovenous complexes involved in temperature regulation [66]. The gene instigated in GVM development is glomulin, which maps to 1p21-p22.3

20.9.1 Blue Rubber Bleb Nevus Syndrome

Blue rubber bleb nevus syndrome (BRBNS), also known as bean syndrome, is a syndrome of generalized small venous malformation found mostly on the trunk and upper arms. These malformations are typically bluish, soft, and easily compressible, and histologically are cavernous spaces lined by a single layer of endothelial cells separated by varying amounts of collagenous and fibrous tissues [67]. Although its lesions have often mistakenly been termed as "angiomas" or "hemangiomas," it is important to note that they are histologically venous malformations. Genetically, most cases of BRBNS are sporadic, although some familial cases have been linked to chromosome 9p, which encodes for the receptor tyrosine kinase TIE2, believed to be involved in vascular morphogenesis [29]. In addition to the skin manifestation of BRBNS, there is also occasional involvement of the gastrointestinal system [68]. Unlike the cutaneous lesions of BRBNS, intestinal lesions can bleed resulting in anemia as well as cause systemic complications such as disseminated intravascular coagulation [69]. A few cases of CNS involvement have also been described, in which patients present with focal seizures or other neurologic symptoms as a result of compression from the lesions. The lesions of BRBNS usually present at birth or in early childhood and tend to increase in size and frequency with age [68].

20.10 Arteriovenous Malformations

Cutaneous arteriovenous malformations (AVMs) are not believed to be heritable with the exception of hereditary hemorrhagic telangiectasia (HHT), an autosomal dominant disorder characterized by AVMs mostly of the mucosa and viscera, but can also involve the skin [66]. There are four subtypes of HHT, but only HHT1 and HHT2 will be discussed as they comprise ~85% of the cases [70]. HHT1 has been linked to a heterozygous mutation on chromosome 9q34, which contains the gene that encodes endoglin. HHT2 is caused by a mutation in ACVRL1 gene on chromosome 12q, which contains the ALK1 gene that codes for activin receptor-like kinase I, ACVRLK1 [71]. Comparisons of HHT1 and HHT2 suggest that HHT1 has a higher incidence of pulmonary lesions; however, it should be noted that there is a great deal of phenotypic variability within each syndrome and clinically the forms are treated in the same manner [72].

A penetrance of 97–100% has been reported [73, 74]. Epistaxis is primarily the presenting symptom and 62% will manifest the disease by age of 16 years and 90% before age of 21 years [75]. Telangiectasias of the mucosa are most commonly located on the face, including the tongue, lips, conjunctiva, and nasopharynx.

In the viscera, various vascular malformations can occur, including arterial aneurysms, arteriovenous fistulas, and poorly formed masses of angiectasia, phlebectasia, and angioma [76]. Pulmonary AVMs have been reported in 4.6–20% of cases and are associated with significant morbidity [77]. These lesions can lead to massive hemorrhage, heart failure, and paradoxical emboli. Lesions within the liver are associated with pronounced fibrosis, which can progress to cirrhosis. One study found that 17 of 27 patients with hepatic involvement went on to develop cirrhosis. The majority of neurologic symptoms are secondary to embolic phenomena, but vascular malformations can occur within the CNS, especially with HHT2 [76].

Endoglin and activin receptor-like kinase I are expressed within endothelium. These proteins are associated with transforming growth factor β (TFGB) receptor complexes. Endoglin is an accessory protein and activin receptor-like kinase is a transmembrane serine/threonine kinase [78, 79]. The many mutations described in HHT ultimately lead to a loss of function of the TGFB signaling pathway. It is suggested that TGFB plays a role in the maintenance of the capillary bed as AVMs in HHT show a progressive disappearance of capillaries.

20.11 Lymphatic Malformations

Lymphatic malformations have the propensity to enlarge more than any other vascular malformation [50]. They occur most commonly in the neck and axilla (55–95%) [50]. These lesions can often become infected, and if located in the head and neck, can compromise the airway. Primary lymphedema, also known as Milroy disease, is an autosomal dominant disorder caused by FL4 missense mutations on 5q35.3. This locale encodes for VEGFR3, and missense mutations here disrupt the kinase domain of the protein, disrupting signaling and ultimately leading to dysregulation of lymphatic endothelium development [50].

20.12 Mixed Lesions

20.12.1 Klippel–Trenaunay Syndrome

Klippel–Trenaunay Syndrome (KTS) has been defined as slow flow, combined capillary, venous and lymphatic malformations involving the limb, or less frequently, the trunk. High-flow arteriovenous fistulas are absent or are a minor component, a key distinction from Parkes-Weber syndrome [50]. The lower limb is involved in the vast majority of cases (95%); however, 15% of patients have combined upper and lower limb involvement [50]. A study of 47 patients exhibited a 53% rate of thrombophlebitis and Kasabach-Merritt syndrome occurred in 45% of patients. Other morbidities of the syndrome in this study included thromboembolism (11%) and high-output heart failure (13%).

The inheritance pattern as well as genes implicated in the pathogenesis of KTS is unclear. Some feel that it is a purely sporadic syndrome, while others have suggested that KTS is a paradominant trait, where the syndrome is linked to a single gene and heterozygotes develop an early somatic mutation, leading to mosaicism [50, 80]. With that in mind, no clear genetic basis for KTS has been found. Whelan et al reported a reciprocal translocation in a patient with KTS at t(5;11) (q13.3;p15.1) and suggested that the culprit gene was on 5q or p11 [81]. Tian et al. identified the VG5Q gene and showed that the translocation found by Whelan et al. results in a threefold increase in gene expression. The VG5Q protein is known to promote angiogenesis, and has been shown to directly bind endothelial cells and promote proliferation. Furthermore, a heterozygous glu133-to-lys substitution (E133K) has been found, which has been shown to increase the activity of VG5Q [82]. Several studies have shown, however, that the E133K substitution can exist in patients without KTS; therefore, the mutation is a polymorphism and does not directly cause KTS [83].

20.12.2 Parkes-Weber Syndrome

Although many feel that Parkes-Weber syndrome is clinically similar to KTS, there are several key differences. In Parkes-Weber, the AVM is the major contributing anomaly, whereas lymphatic malformation, if present, is minor. Lesions are more diffuse in nature and have a rosy color. The upper limb is affected more often than KTS, and patients tend to have a worse prognosis, as their condition can be complicated by heart failure. As mentioned above, the RASA1 gene has been linked to both CM-AVM and Parkes-Weber syndrome. Eerola et al. propose that Ras activity modulators could potentially serve as a targeted therapy for treatment of these patients [84].

20.12.3 Proteus Syndrome

Proteus syndrome is a severe disorder of variable phenotypes involving vascular/lymphatic malformation in addition to asymmetric and disproportionate growth of body parts, connective tissue, epidermal nevi, and adipose tissue [85]. Given the range of phenotypes possible in this disorder, it was aptly named after the Greek god Proteus, also known as "the polymorphous," for his ability to change his shape to avoid capture [86]. Despite the many disparate phenotypes, several studies have sited both lipomatosis as well as hypertrophy of the skin of the soles as a unique feature of the syndrome [87], while it is the connective tissue nevi that are considered pathognomonic for diagnosis [88].

Proteus syndrome is rather uncommon, with an incidence of less than one case per million. And though most cases of Proteus syndrome are considered to be sporadic, reports of cases in monozygotic twins suggest familial transmission and in particular the concept of somatic mosaicism caused by a postzygotic mutation event [89, 90]. This is in support of the hypothesis that Proteus syndrome is caused by a somatic mutation, which is lethal when constitutive [91]. Studies analyzing exon sequencing have also identified an activating missense mutation in the AKT1 gene [92]. The AKT1 gene encodes for the enzyme RAC-α serine/threonine-protein kinase, which is catalytically inactive in fibroblasts and activated by platelet-derived growth factor. Ex vivo studies in cell culture have shown that the prevalence of the mutation is higher in the upper dermis than in the epidermis or lower dermis and that the mutation is absent in glandular tissue, which may explain why certain cell types are more affected than others in this disorder.

20.13 Conclusion

Several types of vascular malformations may have a genetic component, especially if there are various syndromes of vascular malformation.

References

1. Mulliken JB, Fishman SJ, Burrows PE. Mulliken and Young's vascular anomalies: hemangiomas and malformations. Oxford: Oxford University Press; 2013.
2. Nosher JL, Murillo PG, Liszewski M, Gendel V, Gribbin CE. Vascular anomalies: A pictorial review of nomenclature, diagnosis and treatment. World J Radiol. 2014;6:677–92.
3. Mulliken JB, Glowacki J. Hemangiomas and vascular malformations in infants and children: a classification based on endothelial characteristics. Plast Reconstr Surg. 1982;69(3):412–22.
4. Mulliken JB, Glowacki J. Classification of pediatric vascular lesions. Plast Reconstr Surg. 1982;70(1):120–1.
5. International Society for the Study of Vascular Anomalies. ISSVA classification for vascular anomalies (approved at the 20th ISSVA Workshop, Melbourne, April 14, last revision May 2018) 2018.
6. Dasgupta R, Fishman SJ. ISSVA classification. Semin Pediatr Surg. 2014;23:158–61.
7. Paolacci S, Zulian A, Bruson A, Manara E, Michelini S, Mattassi RE, Lee B-B, Amato B, Bertelli M. Vascular anomalies: molecular bases, genetic testing and therapeutic approaches. Int Angiol. 2019;38(2):157–70.
8. Gilbert SF. Developmental biology. 9th ed. Sunderland, MA: Sinauer; 2010.
9. Jain RK. Molecular regulation of vessel maturation. Nat Med. 2003;9(6):685–93.
10. Armulik A, Abramsson A, Betsholtz C. Endothelial/pericyte interactions. Circ Res. 2005;97(6):512–23.
11. Xie C, Ritchie RP, Huang H, Zhang J, Chen YE. Smooth muscle cell differentiation in vitro: models and underlying molecular mechanisms. Arterioscler Thromb Vasc Biol. 2011;31(7):1485–94.
12. Herbert SP, Stainier DY. Molecular control of endothelial cell behaviour during blood vessel morphogenesis. Nat Rev Mol Cell Biol. 2011;12(9):551–64.
13. Millauer B, Wizigmann-Voos S, Schnürch H, Martinez R, Møller NPH, Risau W, Ullrich A. High affinity VEGF binding and developmental expression suggest Flk-1 as a major regulator of vasculogenesis and angiogenesis. Cell. 1993;72(6):835–46.
14. Mustonen T, Alitalo K. Endothelial receptor tyrosine kinases involves in angiogenesis. J Cell Biol. 1995;129(4):895–8.
15. Fischer A, Schumacher N, Maier M, Sendtner M, Gessler M. The Notch target genes Hey1 and Hey2 are required for embryonic vascular development. Genes Dev. 2004;18(8):901–11.
16. You L-R, Lin F-J, Lee CT, DeMayo FJ, Tsai M-J, Tsai SY. Suppression of Notch signalling by the COUP-TFII transcription factor regulates vein identity. Nature. 2005;435(7038):98–104.

17. Carmeliet P, Jain RK. Molecular mechanisms and clinical applications of angiogenesis. Nature. 2011;473(7347):298–307.
18. Gerhardt H, Golding M, Fruttiger M, Ruhrberg C, Lundkvist A, Abramsson A, Jeltsch M, Mitchell C, Alitalo K, Shima D, Betsholtz C. VEGF guides angiogenic sprouting utilizing endothelial tip cell filopodia. J Cell Biol. 2003;161(6):1163–77.
19. Gaengel K, Genové G, Armulik A, Betsholtz C. Endothelialmural cell signaling in vascular development and angiogenesis. Arterioscler Thromb Vasc Biol. 2009;29(5):630–8.
20. Adams RH, Alitalo K. Molecular regulation of angiogenesis and lymphangiogenesis. Nat Rev Mol Cell Biol. 2007;8(6):464–78.
21. Quaegebeur A, Lange C, Carmeliet P. The neurovascular link in health and disease: molecular mechanisms and therapeutic implications. Neuron. 2011;71(3):406–24.
22. Yancopoulos D, Davis S, Gale NW, Rudge JS, Wiegand SJ, Holash J. Vascular-specific growth factors and blood vessel formation. Nature. 2000;407(6801):242–8.
23. Simonavicius N, Ashenden M, Van Weverwijk A, Lax S, Huso DL, Buckley CD, Huijber IJ, Yarwood H, Isacke CM. Pericytes promote selective vessel regression to regulate vascular patterning. Blood. 2012;120(7):1516–27.
24. Potente M, Gerhardt H, Carmeliet P. Basic and therapeutic aspects of angiogenesis. Cell. 2011;146(6):873–87.
25. Suri C, Jones PF, Patan S, Bartunkova S, Maisonpierre PC, Davis S, Sato TN, Yancopoulos GD. Requisite role of angiopoietin-1, a ligand for the TIE2 receptor, during embryonic angiogenesis. Cell. 1996;87(7):1171–80.
26. Maisonpierre PC, Suri C, Jones PF, Bartunkova S, Wiegand SJ, Radziejewski C, Compton D, McClain J, Aldrich TH, Papadopoulos N, Daly TJ, Davis S, Sato TN, Yancopoulos GD. Angiopoietin-2, a natural antagonist for Tie2 that disrupts in vivo angiogenesis. Science. 1997;277(5322):55–60.
27. Herbert SP, Huisken J, Kim TN, Feldman ME, Houseman BT, Wang RA, Shokat KM, Stainier DYR. Arterial-venous segregation by selective cell sprouting: an alternative mode of blood vessel formation. Science. 2009;326(5950):294–8.
28. Brouillard P, Vikkula M. Genetic causes of vascular malformations. Hum Mol Genet. 2007;16(2):140–9.
29. Vikkula M, Boon LM, Carraway KL, Calvert JT, Diamonti AJ, Goumnerov B, Pasyk KA, Marchuk DA, Warman ML, Cantley LC, Mulliken JB, Olsen BR. Vascular dysmorphogenesis caused by an activating mutation in the receptor tyrosine kinase TIE2. Cell. 1996;87(7):1181–90.
30. Morris PN, Dunmore BJ, Tadros A, Marchuk DA, Darland DC, D'Amore PA, Brindle NPJ. Functional analysis of a mutant form of the receptor tyrosine kinase Tie2 causing venous malformations. J Mol Med. 2005;83(1):58–63.
31. Morris PN, Dunmore BJ, Brindle NPJ. Mutant Tie2 causing venous malformation signals through Shc. Biochem Biophys Res Commun. 2006;346(1): 335–8.
32. Sato TN, Tozawa Y, Deutsch U, Wolburg-Buchholz K, Fujiwara Y, Gendron-Maguire M, Gridley T, Wolburg H, Risau W, Qin Y. Distinct roles of the receptor tyrosine kinases Tie-1 and Tie-2 in blood vessel formation. Nature. 1995;376(6535):70–4.
33. Johnson DW, Berg JN, Baldwin MA, Gallione CJ, Marondel I, Yoon SJ, Stenzel TT, Speer M, Pericak-Vance MA, Diamond A, Guttmacher AE, Jackson CE, Attisano L, Kucherlapati R, Porteous ME, Marchuk DA. Mutations in the activin receptor-like kinase 1 gene in hereditary haemorrhagic telangiectasia type 2. Nat Genet. 1996;13(2):189–95.
34. McAllister KA, Grogg KM, Johnson DW, Gallione CJ, Baldwin MA, Jackson CE, Helmbold EA, Markel DS, McKinnon WC, Murrell J. Endoglin, a TGF-beta binding protein of endothelial cells, is the gene for hereditary haemorrhagic telangiectasia type 1. Nat Genet. 1994;8(4):345–51.
35. Bourdeau A, Faughnan ME, Letarte M. Endoglin-deficient mice, a unique model to study hereditary hemorrhagic telangiectasia. Trends Cardiovasc. 2000;10(7):279–85.
36. Dickson MC, Martin JS, Cousins FM, Kulkarni AB, Karlsson S, Akhurst RJ. Defective haematopoiesis and vasculogenesis in transforming growth factor-beta 1 knock out mice. Development. 1995;121(6):1845–54.
37. Abraham S, Kogata N, Fässler R, Adams RH. Integrin beta1 subunit controls mural cell adhesion, spreading, and blood vessel wall stability. Circ Res. 2008;102(5):562–70.
38. Zhang J, Clatterbuck RE, Rigamonti D, Chang DD, Dietz HC. Interaction between krit1 and icap1alpha infers perturbation of integrin beta1-mediated angiogenesis in the pathogenesis of cerebral cavernous malformation. Hum Mol Genet. 2001;10(25):2953–60.
39. Marchuk A, Srinivasan S, Squire TL, Zawistowski JS. Vascular morphogenesis: tales of two syndromes. Hum Mol Genet. 2003;12(Spec No-90001):R97–112.
40. Tille J-C, Pepper MS. Hereditary vascular anomalies: new insights into their pathogenesis. Arterioscler Thromb Vasc Biol. 2004;24(9):1578–90.
41. Hassanein AH, Mulliken JB, Fishman SJ, Greene AK. Evaluation of terminology for vascular anomalies in current literature. Plast Reconstr Surg. 2011;127:347–51.
42. Kollipara R, Dinneen L, Rentas KE, Saettele MR, Patel SA, Rivard DC, Lowe LH. Current classification and terminology of pediatric vascular anomalies. AJR Am J Roentgenol. 2013;201:1124–35.
43. Wassef M, Blei F, Adams D, Alomari A, Baselga E, Berenstein A, Burrows P, Frieden IJ, Garzon MC, Lopez-Gutierrez JC, Lord DJE, Mitchel S, Powell J, Prendiville J, Vikkula M, (2015) On Behalf of the ISSVA Board and Scientific Committee. Vascular anomalies classification: recommendations from

the International Society for the Study of Vascular Anomalies. Pediatrics, 136:e203–e214.

44. Aboutalebi A, Jessup CJ, North PE, Mihm MC. Histopathology of vascular anomalies. Facial Plast Surg. 2012;28:545–53.
45. Nozaki T, Nosaka S, Miyazaki O, Makidono A, Yamamoto A, Niwa T, Tsutsumi Y, Aida N, Masaki H, Saida Y. Syndromes associated with vascular tumors and malformations: a pictorial review. Radiogr Radiol Soc N Am. 2013;33:175–95.
46. Burrows PE. Endovascular treatment of slow-flow vascular malformations. Techniques in vascular and interventional radiology. 2013;16:12–21.
47. Yakes WF. Management of high flow vascular malformations. J Vasc Interv Radiol. 2003;14:P128–33.
48. Castrén E, Salminen P, Vikkula M, Pitkäranta A, Klockars T. Inheritance patterns of infantile hemangioma. Pediatrics. 2016;138:1623.
49. Boull C, Maguiness SM. Congenital hemangiomas. Semin Cutan Med Surg. 2016;35:124–7.
50. Cohen MM Jr. Vascular update: morphogenesis, tumors, malformations, and molecular dimensions. Am J Med Genet A. 2006;140(19):2013–38.
51. Jinnin M, Medici D, Park L, et al. Suppressed NFAT-dependent VEGFR1 expression and constitutive VEGFR2 signaling in infantile hemangioma. Nat Med. 2008;14(11):1236–46.
52. Boye E, Yu Y, Paranya G, Mulliken JB, Olsen BR, Bischoff J. Clonality and altered behavior of endothelial cells from hemangiomas. J Clin Invest. 2001;107(6):745–52.
53. Chou A, Toon C, Pickett J, et al. Endocrine tumor syndromes and their genetics. Front Horm Res. 2013;41:30–49.
54. Chen F, Kishida T, Yao M, et al. Germline mutations in the von Hippel-Lindau disease tumor suppressor gene: correlations with phenotype. Hum Mutat. 1995;5(1):66–75.
55. Crossey PA, Foster K, Richards FM, et al. Molecular genetic investigations of the mechanism of tumourigenesis in von Hippel- Lindau disease: analysis of allele loss in VHL tumours. Hum Genet. 1994;93(1):53–8.
56. Maranchie JK, Afonso A, Albert PS, et al. Solid renal tumor severity in von Hippel Lindau disease is related to germline deletion length and location. Hum Mutat. 2004;23(1):40–6.
57. Kaplan RP, Wang JT, Amron DM, Kaplan L. Maffucci's syndrome: two case reports with a literature review. J Am Acad Dermatol. 1993;29(5 Pt 2):894–9.
58. Lee NH, Choi EH, Choi WK, Lee SH, Ahn SK. Maffucci's syndrome with oral and intestinal haemangioma. Br J Dermatol. 1999;140(5):968–9.
59. Halal F, Azouz EM. Generalized enchondromatosis in a boy with only platyspondyly in the father. Am J Med Genet. 1991;38(4):588–92.
60. Pansuriya TC, van Eijk R, d'Adamo P, et al. Somatic mosaic IDH1 and IDH2 mutations are associated with enchondroma and spindle cell hemangioma in Ollier disease and Maffucci syndrome. Nat Genet. 2011;43(12):1256–61.
61. Duffy K. Genetics and syndromes associated with vascular malformations. Pediatr Clin North Am. 2010;57(5):1111–20.
62. Happle R. Lethal genes surviving by mosaicism: a possible explanation for sporadic birth defects involving the skin. J Am Acad Dermatol. 1987;16(4):899–906.
63. Shirley MD, Tang H, Gallione CJ, et al. Sturge-Weber syndrome and port-wine stains caused by somatic mutation in GNAQ. N Engl J Med. 2013;368(21):1971–9.
64. Kajio F, Nakazawa M. Vascular effects of endothelin-1 in stage 21 chick embryos. Heart Vessels. 1997;12(6):300–5.
65. Van Raamsdonk CD, Fitch KR, Fuchs H, de Angelis MH, Barsh GS. Effects of G-protein mutations on skin color. Nat Genet. 2004;36(9):961–8.
66. Vikkula M, Boon LM, Mulliken JB. Molecular genetics of vascular malformations. Matrix Biol. 2001;20(5-6):327–35.
67. Moodley M, Ramdial P. Blue rubber bleb nevus syndrome: case report and review of the literature. Pediatrics. 1993;92(1):160–2.
68. Bean WB. Blue rubber bleb nevi of the skin and gastrointestinal tract. In: Vascular spiders and related lesions of the skin. Springfield, IL: Charles C. Thomas; 1958. p. 178–85.
69. Kunishige M, Azuma H, Masuda K, et al. Interferon alpha-2a therapy for disseminated intravascular coagulation in a patient with blue rubber bleb nevus syndrome. A case report. Angiology. 1997;48(3):273–7.
70. McDonald J, Bayrak-Toydemir P, Pyeritz RE. Hereditary hemorrhagic telangiectasia: an overview of diagnosis, management, and pathogenesis. Genet Med. 2011;13(7):607–16.
71. Bossler AD, Richards J, George C, Godmilow L, Ganguly A. Novel mutations in ENG and ACVRL1 identified in a series of 200 individuals undergoing clinical genetic testing for hereditary hemorrhagic telangiectasia (HHT): correlation of genotype with phenotype. Hum Mutat. 2006;27(7):667–75.
72. Berg J, Porteous M, Reinhardt D, et al. Hereditary haemorrhagic telangiectasia: a questionnaire based study to delineate the different phenotypes caused by endoglin and ALK1 mutations. J Med Genet. 2003;40(8):585–90.
73. Plauchu H, de Chadarévian JP, Bideau A, Robert JM. Age-related clinical profile of hereditary hemorrhagic telangiectasia in an epidemiologically recruited population. Am J Med Genet. 1989;32(3):291–7.
74. Porteous ME, Burn J, Proctor SJ. Hereditary haemorrhagic telangiectasia: a clinical analysis. J Med Genet. 1992;29(8):527–30.
75. Assar OS, Friedman CM, White RI Jr. The natural history of epistaxis in hereditary hemorrhagic telangiectasia. Laryngoscope. 1991;101(9):977–80.

76. Guttmacher AE, Marchuk DA, White RI Jr. Hereditary hemorrhagic telangiectasia. N Engl J Med. 1995;333(14):918–24.
77. Vase P, Holm M, Arendrup H. Pulmonary arteriovenous fistulas in hereditary hemorrhagic telangiectasia. Acta Med Scand. 1985;218(1):105–9.
78. Attisano L, Cárcamo J, Ventura F, Weis FM, Massagué J, Wrana JL. Identification of human activin and TGF beta type I receptors that form heteromeric kinase complexes with type II receptors. Cell. 1993;75(4):671–80.
79. Barbara NP, Wrana JL, Letarte M. Endoglin is an accessory protein that interacts with the signaling receptor complex of multiple members of the transforming growth factor-beta superfamily. J Biol Chem. 1999;274(2):584–94.
80. Happle R. Klippel-Trenaunay syndrome: is it a paradominant trait? Br J Dermatol. 1993;128(4):465–6.
81. Whelan AJ, Watson MS, Porter FD, Steiner RD. Klippel-Trenaunay-Weber syndrome associated with a 5:11 balanced translocation. Am J Med Genet. 1995;59(4):492–4.
82. Tian XL, Kadaba R, You SA, et al. Identification of an angiogenic factor that when mutated causes susceptibility to Klippel-Trenaunay syndrome. Nature. 2004;427(6975):640–5.
83. Barker KT, Foulkes WD, Schwartz CE, et al. Is the E133K allele of VG5Q associated with Klippel-Trenaunay and other overgrowth syndromes? J Med Genet. 2006;43(7):613–4.
84. Eerola I, Boon LM, Mulliken JB, et al. Capillary malformation–arteriovenous malformation, a new clinical and genetic disorder caused by RASA1 mutations. Am J Hum Genet. 2003;73(6):1240–9.
85. Turner JT, Cohen MM Jr, Biesecker LG. Reassessment of the Proteus syndrome literature: application of diagnostic criteria to published cases. Am J Med Genet A. 2004;130A(2):111–22.
86. Wiedemann HR, Burgio GR, Aldenhoff P, Kunze J, Kaufmann HJ, Schirg E. The proteus syndrome. Partial gigantism of the hands and/or feet, nevi, hemihypertrophy, subcutaneous tumors, macrocephaly or other skull anomalies and possible accelerated growth and visceral affections. Eur J Pediatr. 1983;140(1):5–12.
87. Malamitsi-Puchner A, Dimitriadis D, Bartsocas C, Wiedemann HR. Proteus syndrome: course of a severe case. Am J Med Genet. 1990;35(2):283–5.
88. Biesecker LG, Happle R, Mulliken JB, et al. Proteus syndrome: diagnostic criteria, differential diagnosis, and patient evaluation. Am J Med Genet. 1999;84(5):389–95.
89. Brockmann K, Happle R, Oeffner F, König A. Monozygotic twins discordant for Proteus syndrome. Am J Med Genet A. 2008;146A(16):2122–5.
90. Goodship J, Redfearn A, Milligan D, Gardner-Medwin D, Burn J. Transmission of Proteus syndrome from father to son? JMed Genet. 1991;28(11):781–5.
91. Happle R. Cutaneous manifestation of lethal genes. Hum Genet. 1986;72(3):280.
92. Lindhurst MJ, Sapp JC, Teer JK, et al. A mosaic activating mutation in AKT1 associated with the Proteus syndrome. N Engl J Med. 2011;365(7):611–9.

The Yakes AVM Classification System: Cracking the Code for Curative AVM Endovascular Treatment

21

Alexis M. Yakes, Alexander J. Continenza, and Wayne F. Yakes

Vascular malformations are extremely challenging lesions. The clinical presentations of these congenital abnormalities are protean and range from asymptomatic birthmarks to life-threatening congestive heart failure and exsanguinating hemorrhage. These abnormalities are rare; most clinicians see only a few in a lifetime of practice. Thus, patients afflicted with these disorders often seek help from many different physicians and undergo repetitive examinations, misdiagnosis, and frequent failed attempts at "definitive" therapy that lead to exacerbation of symptoms, lesion recurrences, and disability.

Vascular anomalies were first treated by surgeons. The early surgical solution of proximal arterial ligation of arterial feeders proved futile when the phenomenon of neovascular recruitment rapidly reconstituted arterial inflow to the arteriovenous malformation (AVM) as microfistulous connections became macrofistulous feeders. Complete extirpation of an AVM nidus proved very difficult and very hazardous in that massive hemorrhage often occurred during surgery; necessitation suboptimal partial resections. Partial resections could cause an initial good clinical response, but with time the patient's symptoms usually recurred or worsened.

As stated by D. Emerick Szilagyi, M.D., and coworkers [1], "...with few exceptions, their cure by surgical means is impossible. We had intuitively thought that the only answer of a surgeon to the problem of disfiguring, often noisome and occasionally disabling blemishes and masses, prone to cause bleeding, pain, or other unpleasantness, was to attack them with vigor and with the determination of eradicating them. The results of this attempt at radical treatment were disappointing." In Szilagyi and coworkers' series of 82 patients, only 18 were believed to be operable, and of those, 10 were improved, 2 were the same, and 6 were worse at follow-up [1].

As the discipline of Interventional Radiology developed, embolization of these lesions with particulate matter became widely used in an attempt to completely destroy the lesion, or to "control" the lesion (and hopefully their symptoms), or as a preoperative measure to reduce blood loss and allow a more complete removal [2–4]. With time, however, it was found that complete ablation, or "cure," of an AVM with

A. M. Yakes
University of Kansas Medical Center, The School of Medicine, Kansas City, KS, USA
e-mail: ayakes@kumc.edu

A. J. Continenza
The University of Minnesota Medical Center, Minneapolis, MN, USA

W. F. Yakes (✉)
The Yakes Vascular Malformation Center, Englewood, CO, USA
e-mail: Wayne.yakes@yakesvascularmalformationcenter.com

A. K. Khanna, S. K. Tiwary (eds.), *Vascular Malformations*,
https://doi.org/10.1007/978-981-15-9762-6_21

particulate embolotherapy, proximal coils, and polymerizing agents was truly non-existent [2, 3]. Despite the use of smaller particles and marked improvement in catheter delivery systems, the use of particulate and polymerizing occlusive agents was ultimately also a disappointment for us and so many others. Most AVMs recurred after embolization just as they did after surgery: by neovascular recruitment with reconstitution of arterial inflow into the AVM nidus, as well as by direct recanalization of the embolized vessels themselves.

Liquid agents such as tissue glues, alcohol, sodium morrhuate, and sodium tetradecyl sulfate (Sotradecol) were used sparingly as vascular occlusive agents by Interventional Radiologists for a number of years; these agents were used in the brain, liver, bronchial arteries, muscle tissue, and kidneys [5, 6]. Sodium tetradecyl sulfate was also commonly used to treat superficial venous varicosities with good results. The action of liquid embolic agents appeared to be mediated by a more potent and destructive mechanism than the simple vascular occlusion provided by particles, but intravascular liquids were believed to be far too hazardous for general use. However, in 1986, Yakes et al described curative treatment of an extremity AVM with absolute alcohol. Since then, it has become increasingly apparent that ethanol embolotherapy for vascular malformations can be curative, even for complex AVMs. In this chapter, we discuss the use of alcohol to treat a variety of visceral and truncal high- and low-flow vascular lesions. We believe that alcohol offers significant promise for the patients afflicted with these vascular disorders and now believe it to be the agent of choice for curative vascular malformation therapy [7–9].

21.1 Concepts in the Embryologic Origins of Vascular Malformations

In the embryo, the primitive mesenchyme is nourished by an interlacing system of blood spaces without distinguishable arterial and venous channels. As the embryo matures, the interlacing system of blood spaces becomes differentiated by partial resorption of the primitive vascular spaces and the formation of mature arterial and venous vascular spaces with intervening capillary beds. The classically outlined sequence of events includes (a) the undifferentiated capillary network stage; (b) the retiform developmental stage, characterized by coalescence of the original equipotential capillaries into large, interconnecting, plexiform vascular spaces without an intervening capillary bed; and (c) the final developmental stage, characterized by the resorption of the primitive vascular elements and the formation of mature arterial, capillary, venous, and lymphatic elements [10–13] (Fig. 21.2).

Arrests in development, or the failure of orderly resorption of embryologic primitive vascular elements, results in the persistence of immature vascular structures. Vascular elements retained from the undifferentiated embryonal capillary network stage reveal a strong structural similarity to venous malformations. Failure of orderly resorption of vascular elements from the retiform developmental stage results in the retention of interconnecting channels of immature arteries and veins without an intervening capillary bed. Microfistulous and macrofistulous AVMs correspond to this embryologic stage of vascular development. Other errors in embryologic morphogenesis during the retiform developmental stage could result in other types of vascu-

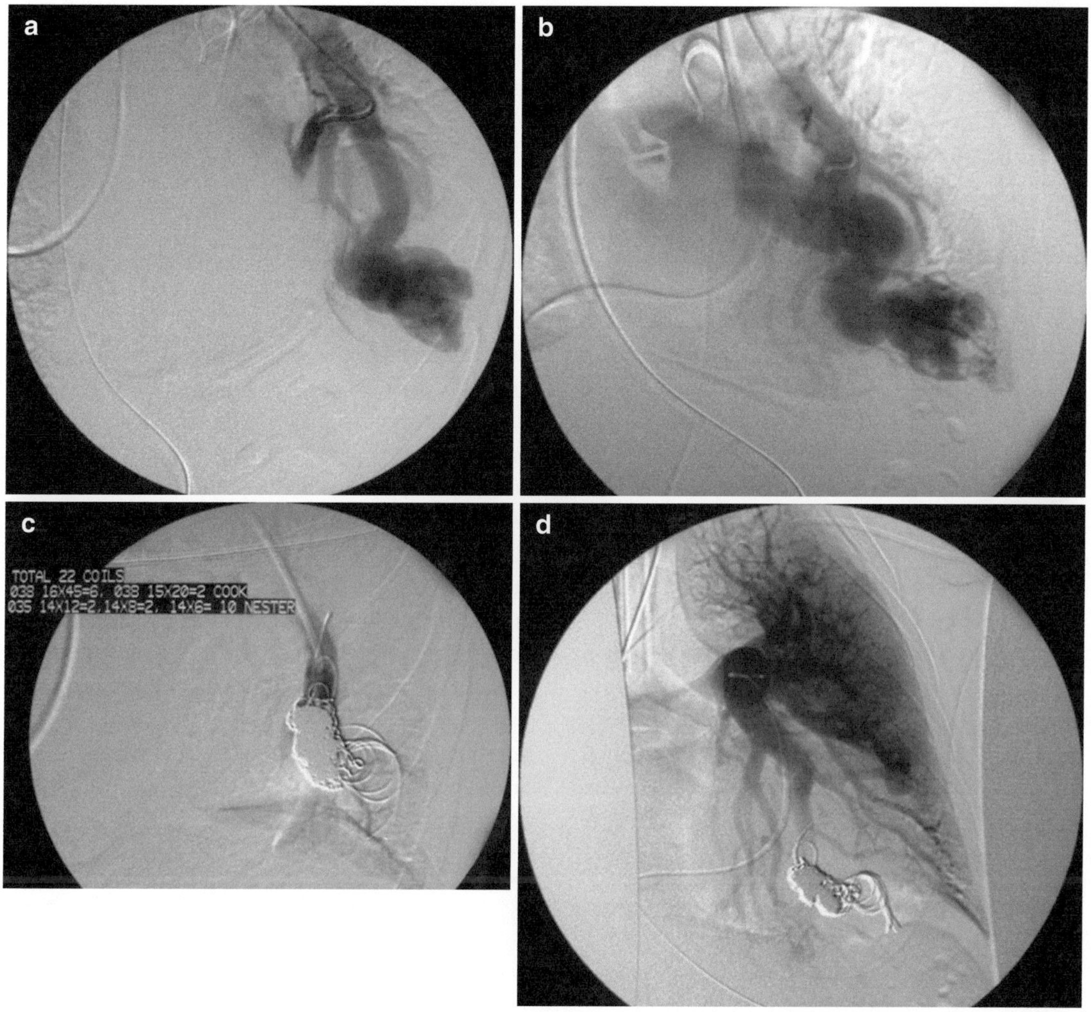

Fig. 21.1 Lt pulmonary AVF in a patient with 40% oxygen saturation on 100% oxygen. (**a**) Lt pulmonary DSA showing Yakes Type I AVM, a massive direct fistula, arterial phase. (**b**) Lt lung pulmonary DSA, venous phase shunt. (**c**) Placement of fibered coils to occlude the AVF with a densely compacted coil pack. (**d**) Lt pulmonary DSA showing total AVF closure. Oxygen saturation immediately rose to 100%

lar malformations. Another example would be retention of primitive capillary elements, which would explain capillary malformations found in port-wine stains. Arteriovenous fistulae (AVF) could result if there was faulty vascular morphogenesis during the later retiform stage. However, due to the constant breakdown and formation of vascular spaces in the embryo, these stages can overlap. This can lead to retained mixed vascular lesions that are complex and contain multiple combinations of these early stages of vascular morphogenesis. As Reid has stated, "In view of the common development on each side of the vascular tree, and in view of the enormous constructive and destructive changes necessary before the final pattern of the vascular tree is reached, it is a marvel not that abnormal congenital communication occasionally, or rarely, occur, but that they do not occur more often" [12] (Fig. 21.3).

Current researchers are now also implicating genetic mechanisms for the development of vascular malformations. Most vascular malformations occur sporadically, but there are syndromes whereby vascular malformations happen (hereditary Hemorrhagic Telangiectasia, Blue Rubber Bleb Nevus Syndrome, Beans Syndrome, Cerebral Cavernous Malformations, etc.) in families as autosomal dominant inheritance. Genetic studies of these families determined mutated genes, directly giving proof of their role in the regulation of angiogenesis [14, 15] (Fig. 21.4).

21.2 Classification of Hemangiomas and Vascular Malformations

Pediatric cutaneous and soft tissue vascular lesions (hemangiomas) and vascular malformations have been classified by Mulliken, Glowacki, and co-workers after research into endothelial cell characteristics, numbers of mast cells present, and endothelial cell in vitro characteristics [16–20]. Most pediatric hemangiomas are not present at birth, clinically manifest within the first month of life, and exhibit a rapid growth phase in the first year. More than 90% of pediatric hemangiomas spontaneously regress to near complete resolution by 5–7 years of age. Hemangiomas occur with a reported incidence of 1–2.6% [16]. Hemangiomas in the proliferative phase are characterized by rapid growth, significant endothelial cell hyperplasia forming syncytial masses, thickened endothelial basement membrane, ready incorporation of tritiated thymidine into the endothelial cells, and the presence of large numbers of mast cells [16–20]. After this period of rapid expansion in the proliferative phase, hemangiomas can stabilize and grow commensurately with the child. Because of the complex nature of hemangiomas, the proliferative phase may continue as the involutive phase slowly begins to progress and dominate. Involuting hemangiomas show diminished endothelial cellularity and replacement with fibrofatty deposits, exhibit

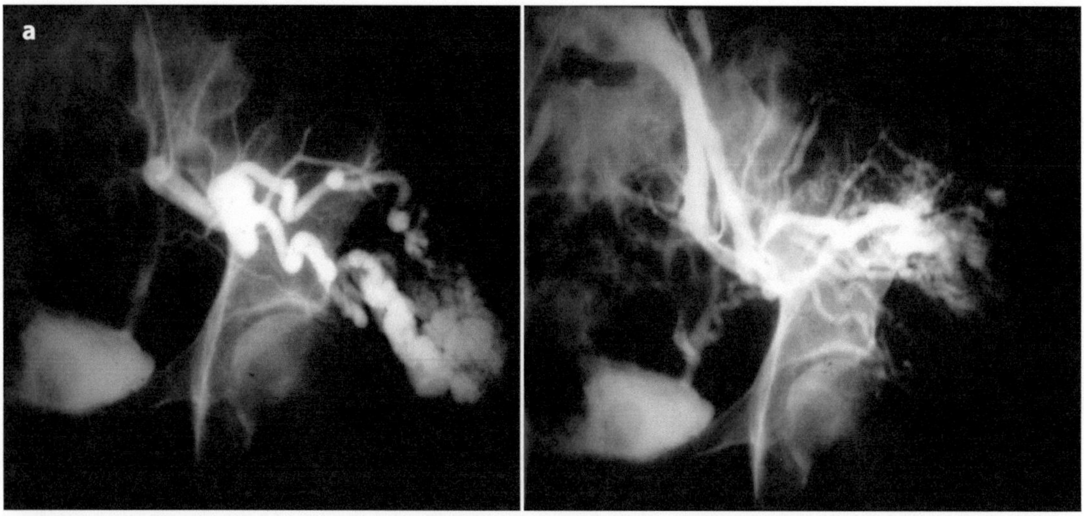

Fig. 21.2 A 42-year-old female with left buttock pain due to Yakes Type IIa AVM with the typical AVM nidus. (**a**) Left superior gluteal artery DSA demonstrating the arterial and venous phase. (**b**) Direct puncture of the AVM nidus in its area of first contrast opacification is performed so that with the ethanol injection, the entire "AVM nidus" would be permeated and sclerosed. (**c**) Direct puncture DSA of the AVM nidus after serial arterial injections through the 18g needle for a total of 31 ml ethanol injected. Thrombosis was achieved. (**d**) Left common Iliac DSA showing total AVM acute occlusion. (**e**) Follow-up Lt pelvis DSA at 2 years demonstrating cure of this AVM

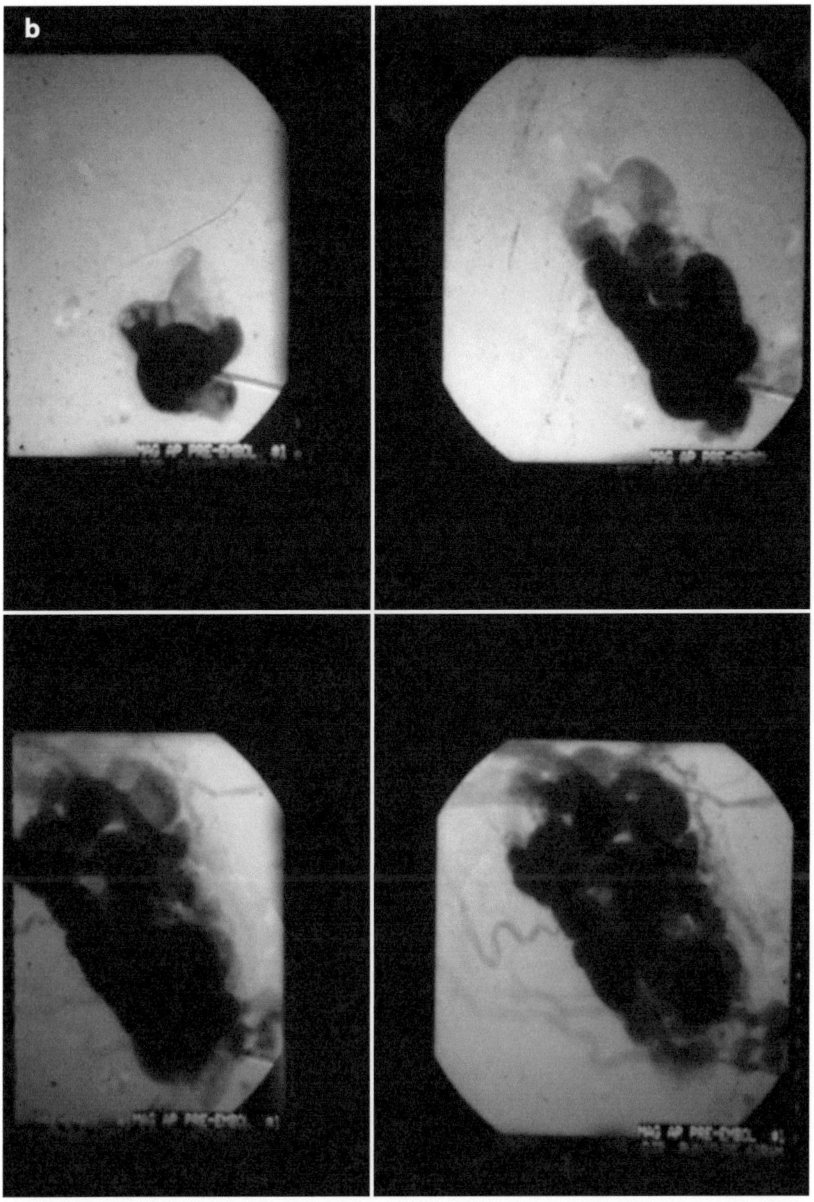

Fig. 21.2 (continued)

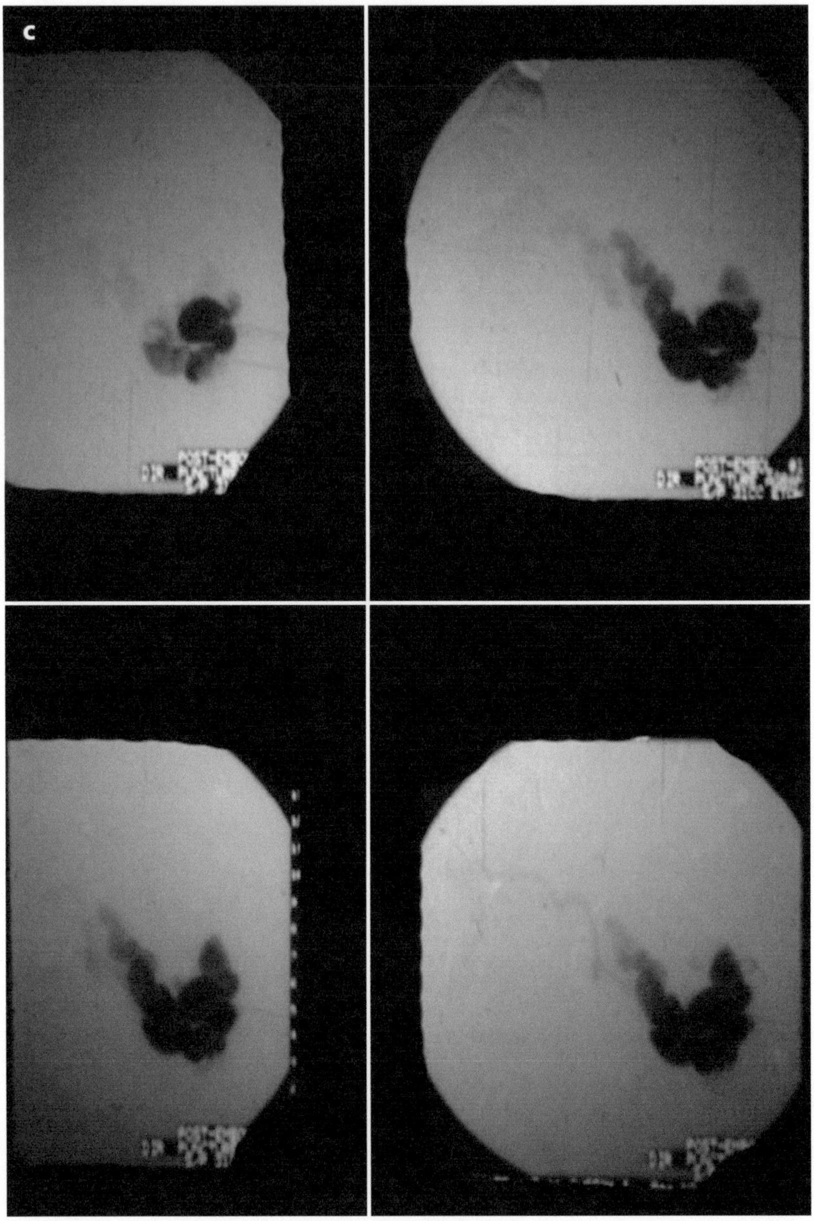

Fig. 21.2 (continued)

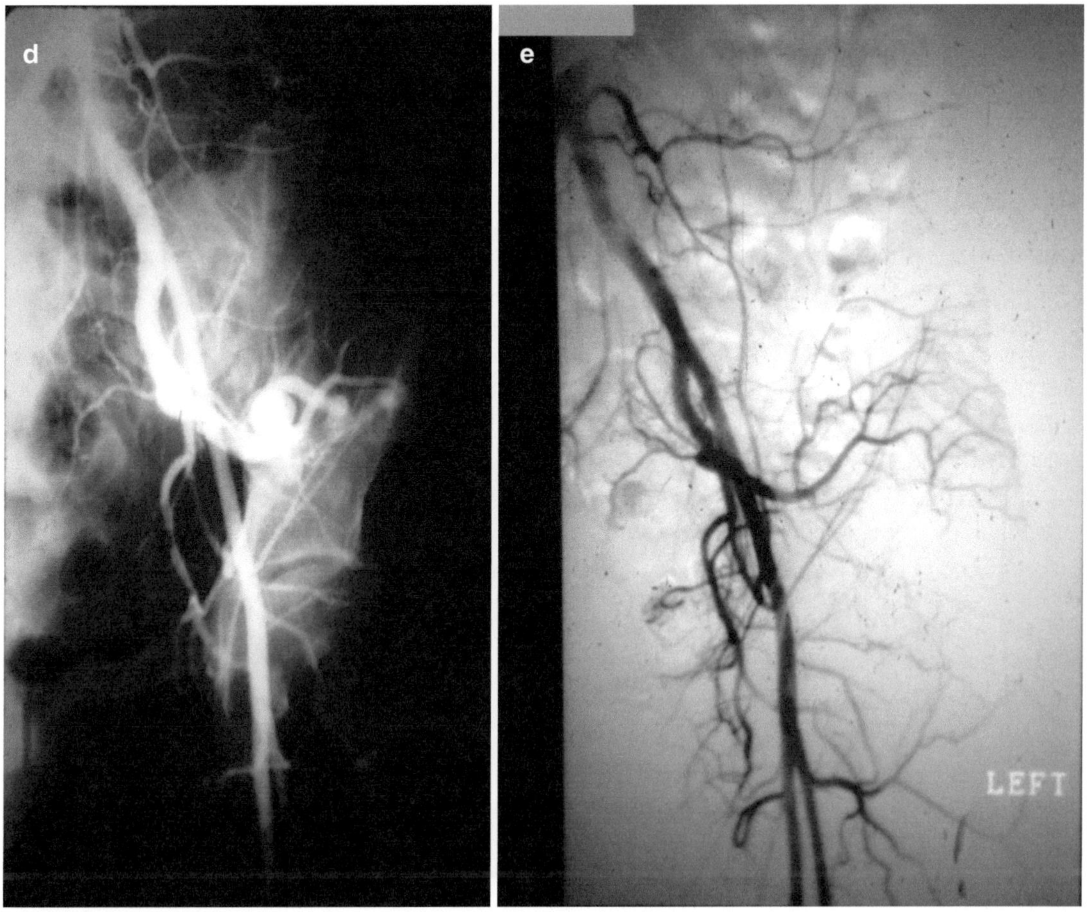

Fig. 21.2 (continued)

a unilamellar basement membrane, demonstrate no uptake of tritiated thymidine into endothelial cells, and have normal mast cell counts [16–20]. Other hemangioma types are congenital pediatric hemangiomas termed "Rapidly Involuting Congenital Hemangiomas" (RICH) and "Non-Involuting Congenital Hemangioma" (NICH). Kaposiform Hemangioendotheliomas (KPH) of the liver can cause heart failure. Kaposiform Hemangioendothelioma of soft tissue causes the Kasabach-Merritt Syndrome of platelet consumption coagulopathy [21, 22]. These two entities have often been confused with vascular malformations. Because of the landmark research of Mulliken and co-workers studying these issues at the cellular level, not at the macro-level, has allowed these diagnoses to be differentiated and defined [16–20] (Fig. 21.5).

Vascular malformations are vascular lesions that are present at birth and grow commensurately with the child. Trauma, surgery, hormonal influences caused by birth control pills, and the hormonal swings during puberty and pregnancy may cause a lesion to expand and grow hemodynamically. Vascular malformations demonstrate no endothelial cell proliferation, contain large vascular channels lined by flat endothelium, have a unilamellar basement membrane, do not incorporate tritiated thymidine into endothelial cells, and have normal mast cell counts. They may be formed from any combination of primitive arterial, capillary, venous, or lymphatic elements with or without direct arteriovenous (AV) shunts. Vascular malformations are true structural anomalies resulting from inborn errors of vascular morphogenesis and the failure of orderly resorption of these primitive vascular elements in the first 4-6 weeks of life of the fetus (Fig. 21.6).

Vascular malformations are categorized into arterial, capillary, and venous malformations (with or without AVF), and lymphatic malformations. The term "hemangioma" should be reserved for the previously described pediatric cutaneous lesions that are not present at birth, except for RICH and NICH, manifest themselves within the first month of life, exhibit a rapid proliferative phase, and then slowly involute to near complete resolution by 5–7 years of age. The old terms describing adult conditions such as "cavernous hemangioma," "hepatic hemangioma," "extremity hemangioma," "vertebral body hemangioma," "cavernous angiomas" and so on, should be replaced with the term "venous malformation." The term "intramuscular hemangioma"

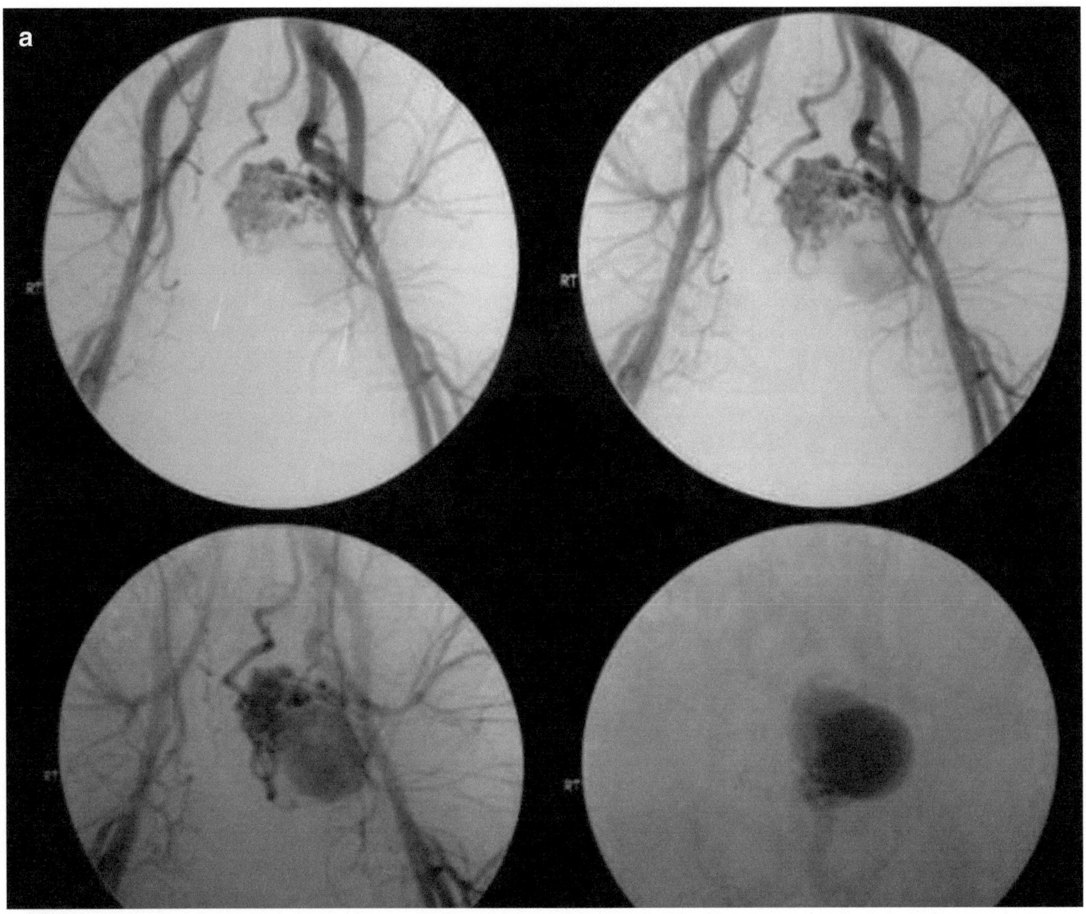

Fig. 21.3 A 37-year-old male with left pelvic pain and arteriograms demonstrating a Yakes Type IIb AVM. (**a**) AP pelvis DSA showing left pelvis AVM. (**b**) Left Internal Iliac artery DSA showing AVM nidus opacified first, and the sole venous drainage is through the outflow aneurysmal vein. (**c**) Selective distal catheter placement into the AVM nidus. Again, the solo outflow aneurysmal vein is present. (**d**) Selective DSA post-total ethanol injection of 25 ml and resultant thrombosis. (**e**) Left Internal Iliac DSA demonstrating cure of the AVM at 4-year arteriographic follow-up

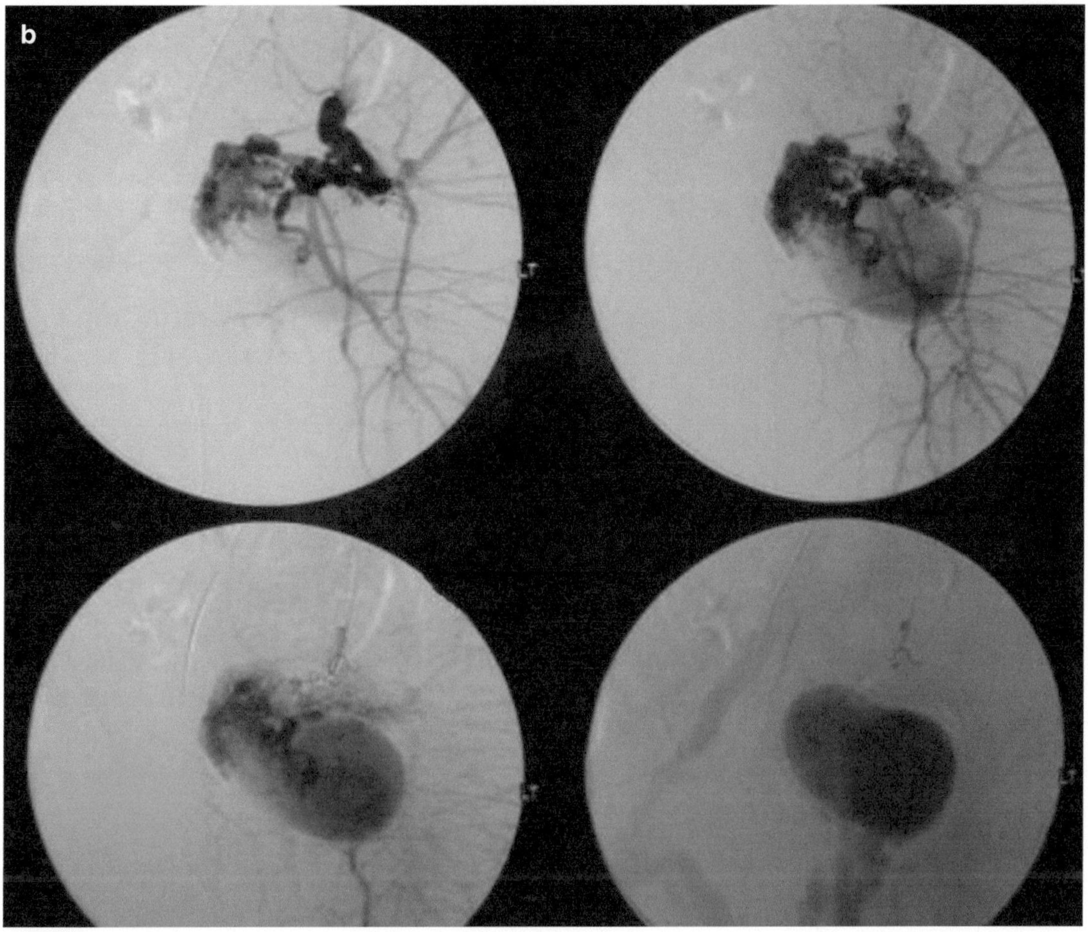

Fig. 21.3 (continued)

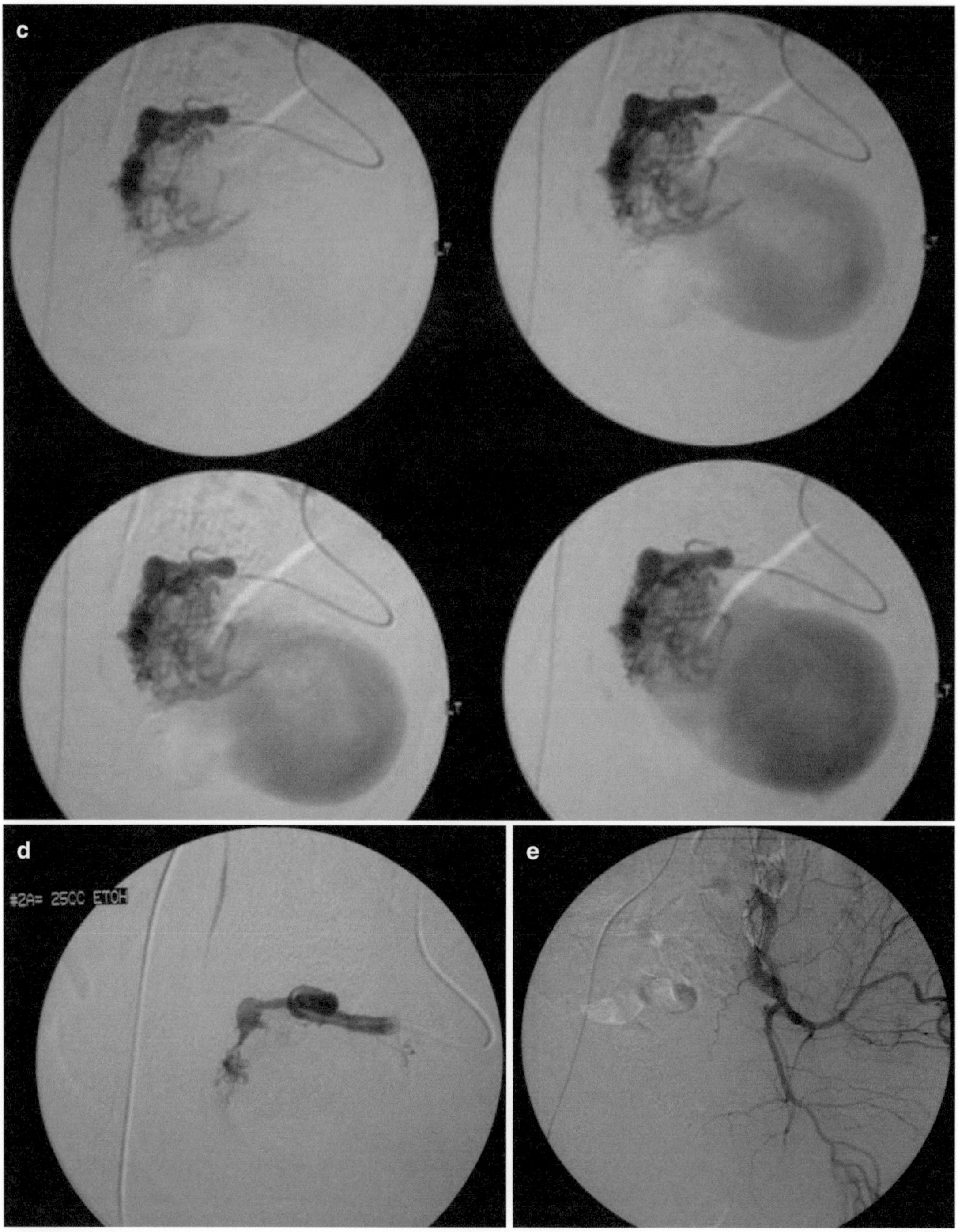

Fig. 21.3 (continued)

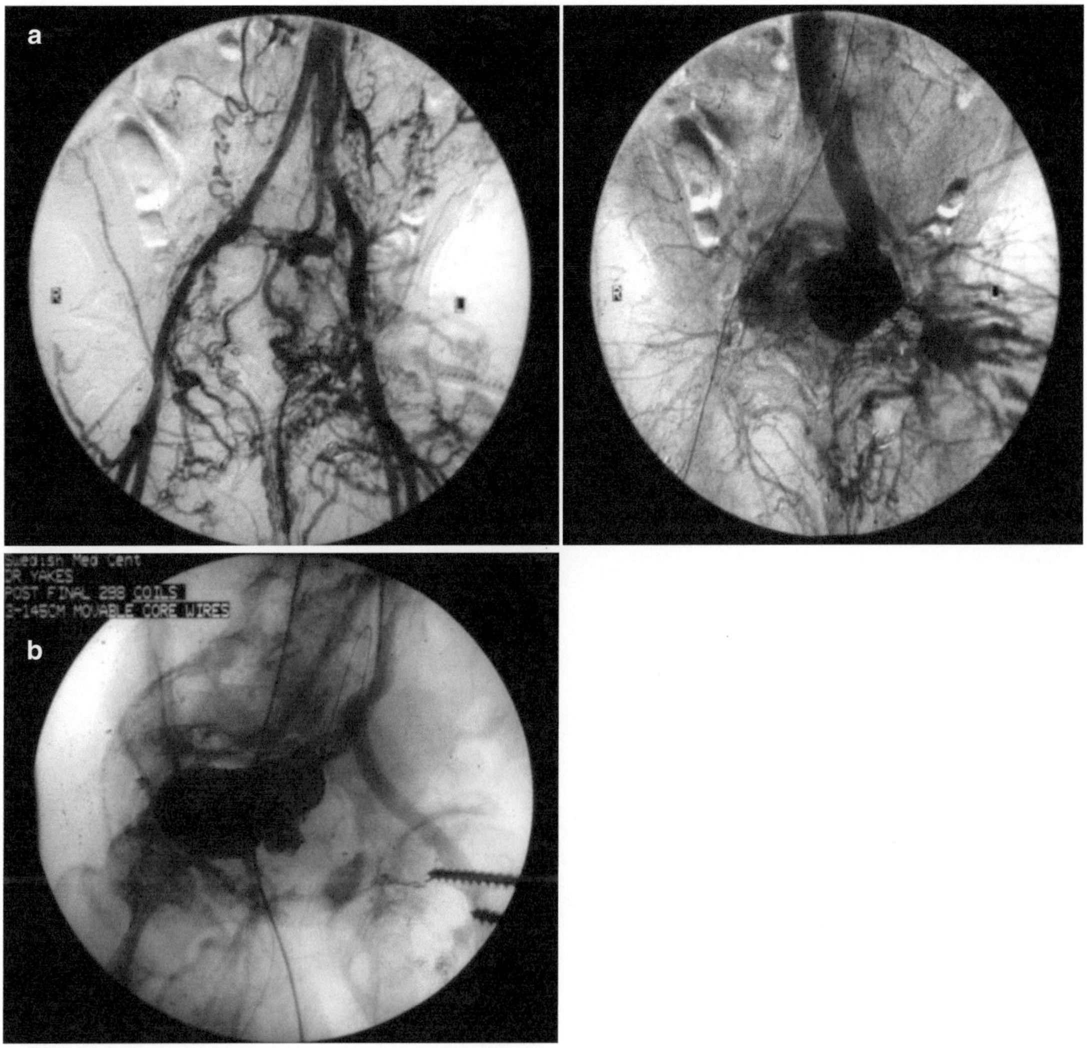

Fig. 21.4 A 32-year-old female developed a nonhealing sacral ulcer after previous coil and glue occlusions of all Lumbar arteries bilaterally and both internal Iliac arteries in the failed attempt to treat the painful left pelvis Yakes IIIa AVM. This created a severely ischemic state for the sacral area and resulted in a nonhealing ulceration. Single outflow vein aneurysm with the AVM niduses in the aneurysmal vein wall. (**a**) Pelvis arteriograms in the arterial and venous phases. Extensive collateral network developed in response to angiogenesis factors released from the endothelial cells lining the AVM vein aneurysm sensing the decreased oxygen tension post-multiple coil embolization. (**b**) Spot film after direct puncture with an 18g needle 15 cm long and placing 298 Cook coils and 3 movable J-core wires of 145 cm length packing into the outflow vein aneurysm. (**c**) Pelvis DSA at 2-year follow-up demonstrating total cure of the Yakes Type IIIa AVM

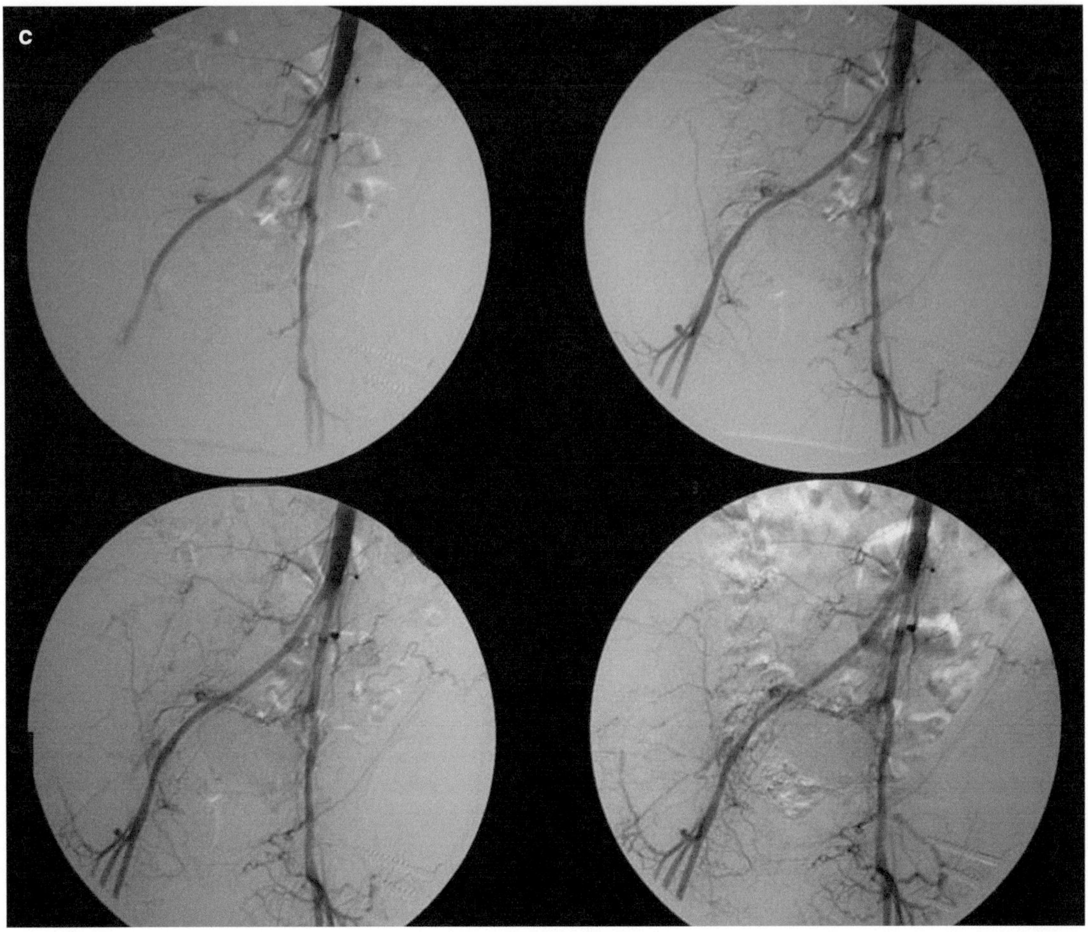

Fig. 21.4 (continued)

should be replaced with "intramuscular venous malformation." The typical port-wine stain, composed of dilated malformed capillary-like vessels, previously incorrectly termed "capillary hemangioma," should instead be termed "capillary malformation." The old terms simple "capillary lymphangioma," "cavernous lymphangioma," and "cystic hygroma" should instead be termed "lymphatic malformations." The old term "hemangio-lymphangioma" should be replaced with "mixed venouslymphatic malformation." The old terms "arteriovenous hemangioma," "arterial angioma," "arteriovenous aneurysm," "cirsoid aneurysm," "red angioma," and "serpentine aneurysm," should be replaced with "arteriovenous malformation" (Table 21.1).

Eponyms have further clouded and confused the nomenclature of hemangiomas and vascular malformations in the world's literature. Maffuci's syndrome (or Kast syndrome) has been defined as a condition whereby the patient has multiple enchondromas and coexistent hemangiomatosis [20]. In the current classification system, hemangiomatosis should be termed venous malformation. The Riley-Smith syndrome has been previously characterized by macrocephaly, pseudopapilladema, and multiple hemangiomas [23]. The term "hemangioma" should be replaced with "venous malformation." Capillary malformations and lymphatic malformations may also be present with the Riley-Smith syndrome. The Riley-Smith syndrome, the Proteus syndrome,

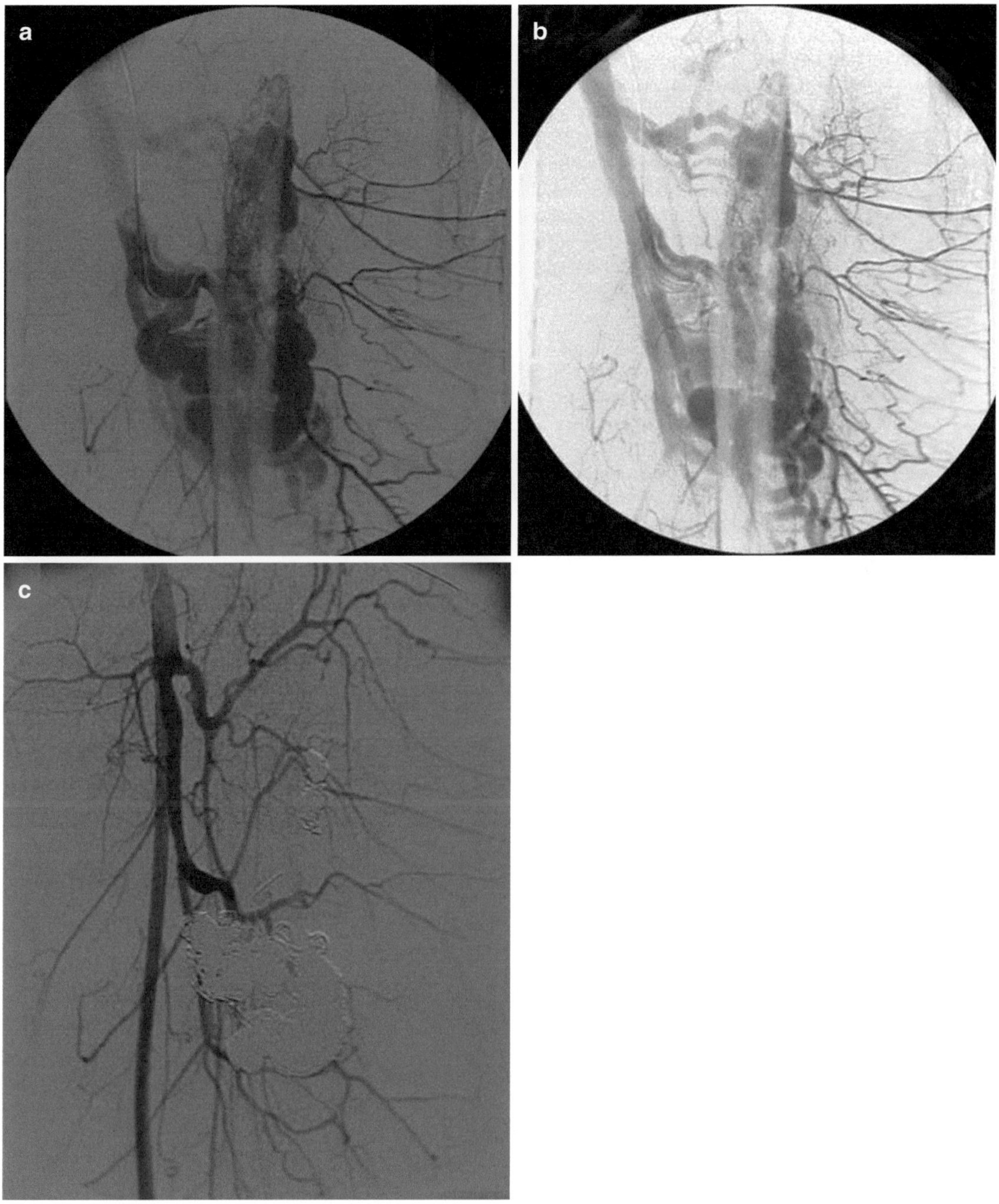

Fig. 21.5 Lt proximal femur intraosseous AVM with multiple vein outflow termed Yakes Type IIb AVM. (**a**) Lt Profunda Femoris DSA showing the arterial phase of the AVM. (**b**) Venous phase showing the multiple vein outflows from this intraosseous AVM. (**c**) Fourteen-month follow-up Left Common Femoral DSA demonstrating persistent cure of the Yakes Type IIIb AVM

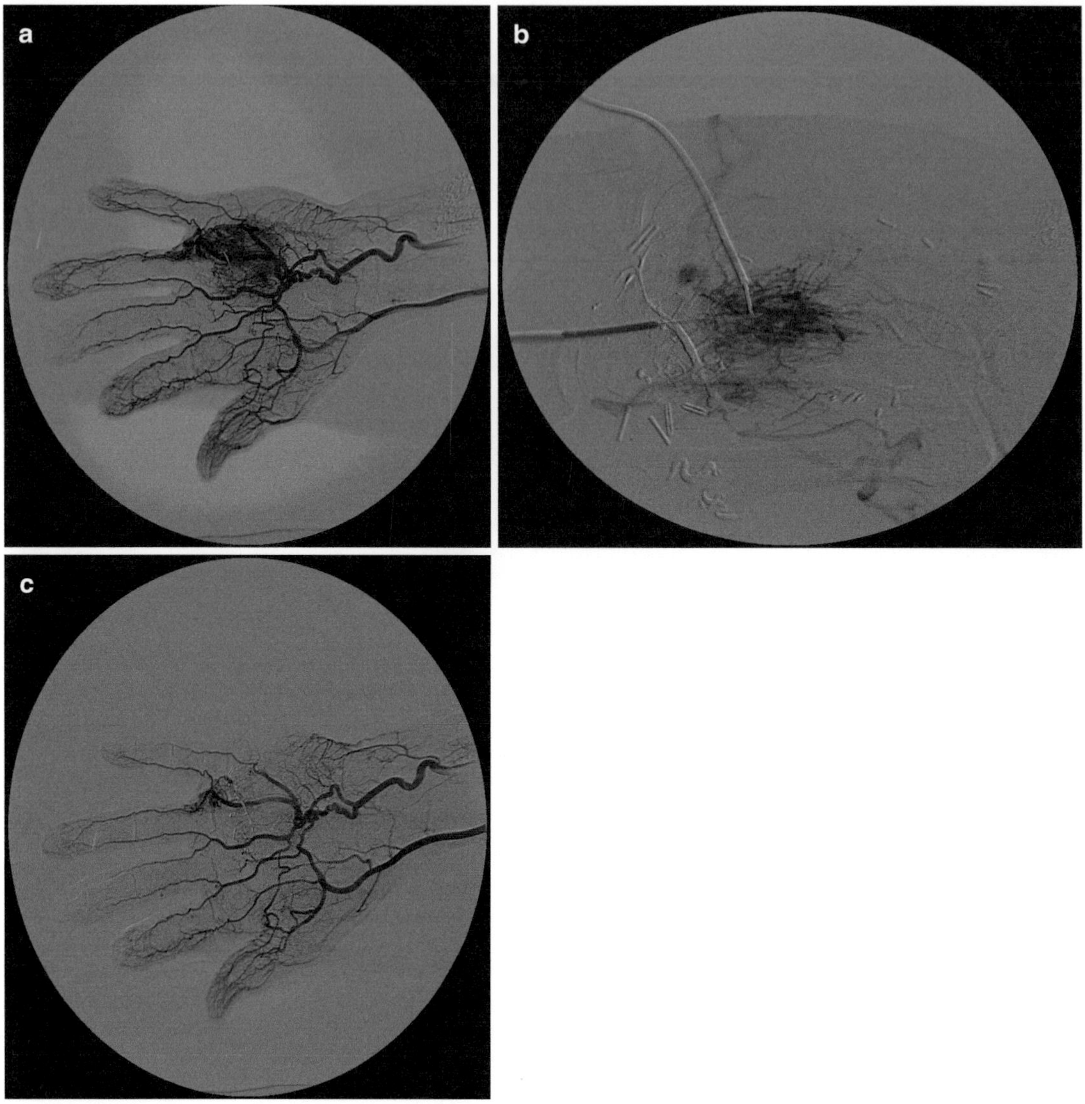

Fig. 21.6 Painful right hand infiltrative Yakes Type IV AVM that failed previous Onyx embolization and with worsening pain symptoms. (**a**) Right Brachial DSA demonstrating an Infiltrative Yakes Type IV AVM at the distal 4th metacarpal area. (**b**) Direct puncture DSA demonstrating the innumerable microfistulae. Note the adjacent Onyx casts. (**c**) One-year follow-up right hand DSA demonstrating persistent cure of the Infiltrating Yakes Type IV AVM

Table 21.1 Schobinger classification of arteriovenous malformation

Stage	Features
I.	Cutaneous blush/warmth
II	Bruit, audible pulsations, expanding lesion
III.	Same as above with pain ulceration, bleeding, infection
IV.	Same as above with cardiac failure

and Bannayan's syndrome are probably a spectrum of similar congenital vascular anomalies [23–26]. Gorham syndrome, Gorham-Stout syndrome, and Trinquoste syndrome are similar entities described as osteolysis (disappearing bone disease) caused by an underlying hemangiomatosis [27]. The term "hemangiomatosis" should be replaced by "venous malformation."

The Blue Rubber Bleb Nevus syndrome (or Bean's syndrome) is another confusing eponym but is unusual in that it is an autosomal dominant heritable condition. It is characterized by subcutaneous (rubbery) venous malformations that spontaneously occur in the extremities and trunk and enlarge. More severe forms can have venous malformations involving the intestines and, in the CNS, that hemorrhage. This can cause neurological deficits or significant GI blood loss. Surgery may be required [28, 29].

Another confusing group of eponyms are Klippel–Trenaunay syndrome, naevus vasculosus osteohypertrophic, naevus verrucous hypertrophycans, osteohypertrophic naevus flammeus, angioosteohypertrophy syndrome, all describe a congenital entity characterized by unilateral lower limb hypertrophy, cutaneous capillary malformations, lymphatic malformations, a normal, hypoplastic, or atretic deep venous system, occasional extension of the vascular malformation into the trunk from the lower extremity, a retained embryonic lateral venous anomaly (Servelle's vein) of the lower extremity, and increased subcutaneous fat in the affected limb. A similar group of eponyms (Parks-Weber syndrome, Giant Limb of Robertson, represents a similar clinical entity that has the same features of the Klippel–Trenaunay syndrome with the coexistence of multiple arteriovenous fistulae. The Klippel–Trenaunay syndrome and Parkes-Weber syndrome usually occur in the lower extremity but can also affect the upper extremity. In the upper extremity, the Parkes-Weber syndrome is more commonly seen, although the Klippel–Trenaunay syndrome is much more common overall [30–32].

These are but a few of the confusing terms used in the literature and in clinical practice. The International Society for the Study of Vascular Anomalies (ISSVA) modern classification system can eliminate the current confusion and all clinicians can finally speak the same language. Accurate terminology will lead to precise identification of clinical entities and to enhanced patient care. The remainder of this chapter will use this modern classification system originated by Mulliken, Glowacki, and coworkers, and adopted by ISSVA, as it is based on the cellular level, not the macro-level [16–20].

21.3 Sclerotherapy of AVMs

Ethanol is a powerful sclerosing agent that denatures blood proteins and destroys vascular endothelial cells by precipitating their protoplasm and denuding them from the vascular wall. These changes occur rapidly and cause thrombosis of the malformation. In malformations, these changes are desirable and account for the curative effects of ethanol endovascular therapy. However, clearly the use of ethanol in a normal vascular structure is to be eschewed, as introduction into vessels supplying structures such as nerves, muscles, or connective tissue will result in necrosis of that tissue end-organ. Ethanol treatment of vascular malformations thus requires significant experience with the agent, as well as extreme caution and a complete understanding of the pathophysiology of the vascular malformation being treated. It should be stressed that some of the most challenging and complex cases seen by vascular specialists involve patients with vascular malformations. These abnormalities should be treated only at medical centers where such patients are seen regularly.

Superselective catheterization and deposition of alcohol directly into the vascular malformation is an essential and vital principle that underlies the safe and effective use of ethanol. As we stated earlier, absolute alcohol destroys tissues, which is the desired effect in vascular malformations but is a toxic and morbid one when normal tissues are involved. Only when alcohol can be accurately placed into the AVM nidus will consistent cures be obtained. Arteriovenous malformations are extremely complex, and their angioarchitecture can be confusing. Even for the experienced Interventionalist, recognition of the nidus of the AVM lesion can be difficult and require all his or her diagnostic skills. Once the nidus is recognized, however, access to the area can be planned and usually achieved by either superselective catheterization or direct puncture so that the appropriate placement and amount of alcohol can be used to destroy the nidus. In our experience, it is common to spend 2–4 h evaluating a lesion with multiple angiographic and/or venographic injections before catheterization or puncture of the vascular malformation can be performed and result in a benefit without complication.

Many tools and techniques can be used to catheterize and treat these lesions, including real-time ultrasound, coaxial microcatheters, and extensive use of digital subtraction arteriography.

Because of the time needed for treatment and the limitations on the total volume of alcohol for use during any one procedure (generally 30–50 mL; maximum 1mL ethanol per kilogram weight), only a segment or a portion of an extensive lesion can be treated in one session. In our experience, the average malformation (arteriovenous or venous) requires four to five sessions, and we have treated some patients with extensive vascular malformations as many as 25 or 30 times to achieve appropriate results. Only a coordinated and dedicated team of specialists consisting of Interventional Radiologists, vascular surgeons, plastic surgeons, anesthesiologists, pediatricians, and pain specialists can handle these patients in an appropriate manner.

21.4 The Cellular Basis for AVM Cure

Without complete surgical extirpation of a vascular malformation, there is a uniform tendency for the malformation (high-flow or low-flow) to recur and for symptoms to worsen. The same can be encountered with embolization techniques if the AVM nidus is not completely obliterated. The reason for this failure to cure partially embolized AVMs is at the cellular level, as all issues in the body are mediated and controlled at the cellular level to affect all things of the macro-level.

Like all blood vessels of the body, AVMs are lined by endothelial cells. When thrombosed with the various embolic agents or when their blood source is interrupted by proximal arterial ligations, endothelial cells sense decreased oxygen tension in their environment. The cell then sends out two factors to rectify the situation and return to its state of normal oxygenation. "Chemotactic cellular factors" are released that cause a cellular macrophage infiltration from the tissues into the thrombosed blood vessel. These macrophages then physically remove the thrombosed embolic elements in the blood vessel. The open channels then become re-endothelialized. This is termed recanalization and is the method by which previously embolized and thrombosed vascular channels are reopened. The other factor secreted by the endothelial cell to rectify its O_2 deprivation is "angiogenesis factor." This factor has not yet been discovered in its chemical form, but we know it exists because of results from various cancer studies as well as peripheral vascular disease models. After sensing decreased oxygen tension because of intravascular thrombosis of the AVM nidus, the endothelial cells release this "angiogenesis factor" and it stimulates a neovascular response. In an attempt to revascularize the thrombosed area and thus increase the oxygen tension level, new blood vessel formation occurs. Microfistulous arteries can become macrofistulous connections to the AVM. This neovascular stimulation phenomenon can be very intense. For example, surgery in the brain must be performed quickly post-embolization before the new blood vessels form and make surgery impossible. These two phenomena of recanalization and neovascular recruitment lead to the routine recurrence of AVMs, all mediated by an intact endothelial cell system.

Neovascular recruitment phenomena and recanalizations do not occur after ethanol embolization of AVMs because the endothelial cell is destroyed. Following ethanol embolization, the endothelial cells are completely denuded from the vascular wall and their protoplasm is precipitated. Blood proteins are also denatured, initiating the clotting cascade. When the vascular wall is denuded of its endothelium and is bare, platelet aggregation occurs with the development of thrombus formation along the vascular wall; the thrombus then propagates until total thrombosis of the lumen is noted. This process can take time; therefore the authors usually waits at least 5–15 min before requesting a follow-up arteriogram to determine if any additional ethanol is required to complete the thrombosis. With the destruction of the endothelial cell, the cells are no longer able to release "chemotactic cellular factor" and "angiogenesis factor," which leads to permanent thrombosis and cure. The amount of ethanol used in each endovascular procedure is tailored to the volume and rate of injection characteristics of the individual compartment of the AVM being injected. No predetermined amount of ethanol is ever considered. Contrast injections must be practiced prior to ethanol embolization. The amount of contrast needed to completely displace blood and not reflux into the proximal normal artery estimates the amount of ethanol required for the embolization. It is unusual to cure an AVM in one session. In the larger lesions, it is preferred to treat individual compartments serially, eventually affecting total treatment over time. We usually wait at least 4 weeks between procedures to allow the patient to return to a new non-edematous baseline prior to further treatment of the AVM lesion.

Endovascular ablation of AVMs with ethanol has ushered in a new era in the therapy of these problematic vascular anomalies. Cures and permanent partial ablations have been well documented in the world's literature [8, 9, 33, 34]. Because neovascular recruitment phenomena and recanalizations have not been observed, partial and complete permanent ablations have led to long-term symptomatic improvement, obviating the need for further treatment.

Various arteriographic AVM classification systems have been proposed to better define endovascular treatment strategies. A cerebrovascular AVM classification system published by Houdart and co-workers in 1993 [35], and a peripheral AVM classification system published by Cho-Do and co-workers in 2006 [36]. Recently, the Yakes AVM classification system further advanced the descriptions of AVM angioarchitectures building on these two previously published classification systems. Furthermore, refinement has led to more specific endovascular treatment strategies related to Yakes Types I, II, IIIa, IIIb, and IV [33, 34].

21.5 Arteriovenous Malformations: The Yakes Classification and Its Therapeutic Implications

The Houdart Classification of Intracranial Arteriovenous Fistulae and Malformations of high-flow lesions and the Cho-Do Classification of AVMs of the peripheral arterial circulation are strikingly similar despite their anatomic locational differences (CNS vs. peripheral vasculatures). Both authors also suggest similar therapeutic approaches based on their arteriographic classification. Houdart Classification states: Type A (AVF multiply into a large aneurysmal vein with single outflow drainage), Type B (multiple microfistulae into an aneurysmal vein with single outflow vein), and Type C (multiple shunts between arterioles and venules connected to each other). The Cho-Do et al. Classification based on "nidus morphology" states: Type I (arteriovenous fistulae with no more than three separate arteries shunt to the initial single venous component), Type II (arteriovenous fistulae (with) multiple arterioles shunt to the initial part of a plexiform appearance into a single venous component), Type IIIa (arteriovenous fistulae with non-dilated fistulae with fine multiple shunts are present between arterioles and venules), and Type IIIb (arteriovenulous fistulae with dilated fistulae with multiple shunts are present between arterioles and venules).

Houdart Type A is the same as the Cho-Do Type I, Houdart Type B is the same as the combination of the Cho-Do types IIIa and IIIb. Therapeutic implications are also similar as well. The Houdart Type A and Type B and Cho-Do Types I and II, proffer retrograde approaches to occlude the vein aneurysm outflow as being a potential for curative treatment of these AVM types. The first publication illustrating the retrograde vein occlusion techniques for high flow was malformations first published in 1990. Later, Jackson et al published the retrograde vein approach in 1996. The Do Group in Seoul, Korea published their successful experience with the retrograde vein approach in 2008 [36].

The Yakes AVM Classification has some similarities to both classification systems, and some stark differences. The Yakes AVM Classification system are: Yakes Type I AVM (is a direct arteriovenous fistula, a direct artery to vein connection (typified by pulmonary AVF and renal AVF, for example), Yakes Type II AVM (AVM characterized by usually multiple in-flow arteries into a "nidus" pattern with direct artery–arteriolar to vein–venular structures that may, or may not, be aneurysmal), Yakes Type IIIa AVM (multiple arteries–arterioles to an enlarged aneurysmal vein sac with the niduses that are within the vein wall, with an enlarged single outflow vein), Yakes Type IIIb AVM (multiple arteries–arterioles into an enlarged aneurysmal vein sac with the niduses that are within the vein wall extending into the multiple aneursymal out-flow veins), and Yakes Type IV AVM (microfistulous innumerable arteriolar structures to innumerable venular connections that diffusely infiltrate a tissue such as ear AVMs that infiltrate the entire cartilage of the pinna). What is different in this Yakes Type IV AVM is that there are admixed among the innumerable fistulae are capillary beds in the tissue. If it only had AVFs, the tissue would not be viable. No other AVM angioarchitecture has this duality of AVFs (without intervening capillary beds) and adjacent nutrient capillaries in the affected tissue.

As an aside, the term "nidus" is rampant in the medical literature ("AVM nidus", "nidus of infection", etc.). Unfortunately, the initial unknown author was only partially familiar with the Latin language. "Nidus" is thought to mean "nest" in Latin, and indeed it does. However, "nidus" with the ending "us" denotes the male gender. In the Latin language, the true term meaning "nest" is, in fact, "nidum.". The ending "um" denotes a neuter gender which a "nest" truly is. Thus, the original author accurately describing "nest-like" conglomeration of vascular structure was woefully inaccurate penning the word as "nidus" (masculine) instead of the true word "nidum" (neuter). Being rife in the literature for decades, it is not foreseeable for any correction of this term.

21.6 Summary

- **Yakes Type I:** Can be permanently occluded, with mechanical devices such as coils, fibered coils, Amplatzer Plugs, and other occluding devices.
- **Yakes Type II:** Can be permanently occluded with undiluted absolute ethanol.
- **Yakes Type IIIa:** Can be permanently occluded by dense coil packing of the vein aneurysm with or without ethanol embolization into the vein aneursym. This can be accomplished via direct puncture of the vein aneurysm, or by retrograde vein catheterization of the vein aneurysm.
- **Yakes Type IIIb:** Can be permanently occluded by dense coil packing of the vein aneurysm and the multiple aneurysmal outflow veins with or without ethanol injection into the vein aneurysm. This can be accomplished via direct puncture of the vein aneurysm, or by retrograde vein catheterization of the multiple aneurysmal out-flow veins and the main vein aneurysm itself.
- **Yakes Type IV:** Can be permanently occluded via transarterial superselective embolization with 50% mixture of non-ionic contrast and ethanol that treats the micro-AVFs and spares the higher resistance normal capillaries. Or by direct puncture of the AV fistulas themselves can be performed and to use pure ethanol on the direct injections.

References

1. Szilagyi DE, Smith RF, Elliott JP, et al. Congenital arteriovenous anomalies of the limbs. Arch Surg. 1976;111:423–29. 1976/04/01.
2. Gomes AS, Mali WP, Oppenheim WL. Embolization therapy in the management of congenital arteriovenous malformations. Radiology. 1982;144:41–9. 1982/07/01. https://doi.org/10.1148/radiology.144.1.7089264
3. Kaufman SL, Kumar AA, Roland JM, et al. Transcatheter embolization in the management of congenital arteriovenous malformations. Radiology. 1980;137:21–9. 1980/10/01. https://doi.org/10.1148/radiology.137.1.7422847.

4. Doppman JL, Pevsner P. Embolization of arteriovenous malformations by direct percutaneous puncture. AJR Am J Roentgenol. 1983;140:773–8. 1983/04/01. https://doi.org/10.2214/ajr.140.4.773.
5. Klimberg I, Hunter P, Hawkins IF, et al. Preoperative angioinfarction of localized renal cell carcinoma using absolute ethanol. J Urol. 1985;133:21–4. 1985/01/01.
6. Sarin SK, Sethi KK, Nanda R. Pulmonary hemodynamic changes after intravariceal sclerotherapy with absolute alcohol. Gastrointest Endosc. 1988;34:403–6. 1988/09/01.
7. Yakes WF, Parker SH. Diagnosis and management of vascular anomalies. Interv Radiol. 1992;1:152–89.
8. Yakes WF, Pevsner P, Reed M, et al. Serial embolizations of an extremity arteriovenous malformation with alcohol via direct percutaneous puncture. AJR Am J Roentgenol. 1986;146:1038–40. 1986/05/01. https://doi.org/10.2214/ajr.146.5.1038.
9. Yakes WF, Parker SH, Gibson MD, Haas DK, Pevsner PH, Carter TE. Alcohol embolotherapy of vascular malformations. Semin Interv Radiol. 1989;6:146–61.
10. Woollard HH. The development of the principal arterial stems in the forelimb of the pig. Contrib Embryol. 1922;14:139–54.
11. Rienhoff WF. Congenital arteriovenous fistula: an embryological study with the report of a case. Johns Hopkins Hosp Bull. 1924;35:271–84.
12. Reid MR. Studies on abnormal arteriovenous complications acquired and congenital. I. Report of a series of cases. Arch Surg. 1925;10:601–38.
13. DeTakats G. Vascular anomalies of the extremities. Surg Gynecol Obstet. 1932;55:227–37.
14. Vikkula M, Boon LM, Mulliken JB. Molecular genetics of vascular malformations. Matrix Biol. 2001;20:327–35. 2001/09/22.
15. Zabramski JM, Wascher TM, Spetzler RF, et al. The natural history of familial cavernous malformations: results of an ongoing study. J Neurosurg. 1994;80:422–32. 1994/03/01. https://doi.org/10.3171/jns.1994.80.3.0422.
16. Mulliken JB, Glowacki J. Hemangiomas and vascular malformations in infants and children: a classification based on endothelial characteristics. Plast Reconstr Surg. 1982;69:412–22. 1982/03/01.
17. Mulliken JB, Zetter BR, Folkman J. In vitro characteristics of endothelium from hemangiomas and vascular malformations. Surgery. 1982;92:348–53. 1982/08/01.
18. Glowacki J, Mulliken JB. Mast cells in hemangiomas and vascular malformations. Pediatrics. 1982;70:48–51. 1982/07/01.
19. Finn MC, Glowacki J, Mulliken JB. Congenital vascular lesions: clinical application of a new classification. J Pediatr Surg. 1983;18:894–900. 1983/12/01.
20. Young AE. Pathogenesis of vascular malformations. In: Vascular birthmarks: hemangiomas and malformations. 1988; p. 107–13.
21. Warrell RP, Jr, Kempin SJ. Treatment of severe coagulopathy in the Kasabach-Merritt syndrome with aminocaproic acid and cryoprecipitate. N Engl J Med. 1985;313:309–12. 1985/08/01. https://doi.org/10.1056/NEJM198508013130507.
22. Bowles LJ, Kostopoulos-Farri E, Papageorgiou AN. Perinatal hemorrhage associated with the Kassabach-Merritt syndrome. Clin Pediatr (Phila). 1981;20:428–9. 1981/06/01. https://doi.org/10.1177/000992288102000611.
23. Riley HD Jr, Smith WR. Macrocephaly, pseudopapilladema, and multiple hemangiomata: a previously undescribed heredofamilial syndrome. Pediatrics. 1960;26:293–300.
24. Wiedemann HR, Burgio GR, Aldenhoff P, et al. The Proteus syndrome. Partial gigantism of the hands and/or feet, nevi, hemihypertrophy, subcutaneous tumors, macrocephaly or other skull anomalies and possible accelerated growth and visceral affections. Eur J Pediatr. 1983;140:5–12. 1983/03/01.
25. Bannayan GA. Lipomatosis, angiomatosis, and macrencephalia. A previously undescribed congenital syndrome. Arch Pathol. 1971;92:1–5. 1971/07/01.
26. Higginbottom MC, Schultz P. The Bannayan syndrome: an autosomal dominant disorder consisting of macrocephaly, lipomas, hemangiomas, and risk for intracranial tumors. Pediatrics. 1982;69:632–4. 1982/05/01.
27. Gorham LW, Stout AP. Massive osteolysis (acute spontaneous absorption of bone, phantom bone, disappearing bone); its relation to hemangiomatosis. J Bone Joint Surg Am. 1955;37-A:985–1004. 1955/10/01.
28. Fishman SJ, Smithers CJ, Folkman J, et al. Blue rubber bleb nevus syndrome: surgical eradication of gastrointestinal bleeding. Ann Surg. 2005;241:523–8. 2005/02/25. https://doi.org/10.1097/01.sla.0000154689.85629.93.
29. Bean WB. Blue Rubber-Bleb nevi of the skin and gastrointestinal tract. In: Vascular spidders and related lesions of the skin; 1958. p. 178–85.
30. Baskerville PA, Ackroyd JS, Browse NL. The etiology of the Klippel-Trenaunay syndrome. Ann Surg. 1985;202:624–7. 1985/11/01. https://doi.org/10.1097/00000658-198511000-00015.
31. Gloviczki P, Hollier LH, Telander RL, et al. Surgical implications of Klippel-Trenaunay syndrome. Ann Surg. 1983;197:353–62. 1983/03/01. https://doi.org/10.1097/00000658-198303000-00017.
32. Phillips GN, Gordon DH, Martin EC, et al. The Klippel-Trenaunay syndrome: clinical and radiological aspects. Radiology. 1978; 128:429–34. 1978/08/01. https://doi.org/10.1148/128.2.429.
33. Yakes W, Baumgartner I. Interventional treatment of arterio-venous malformations. Gefasschirurgie. 2014;19:325–30.

34. Yakes WF, Yakes AM. Arteriovenous malformations: The Yakes classification system and its therapeutic implications. Egyptian J Vasc Endovasc Surg. 2014;10:9–23.
35. Houdart E, Gobin YP, Casasco A, et al. A proposed angiographic classification of intracranial arteriovenous fistulae and malformations. Neuroradiology. 1993;35:381–5. 1993/01/01.
36. Cho SK, Do YS, Shin SW, et al. Arteriovenous malformations of the body and extremities: analysis of therapeutic outcomes and approaches according to a modified angiographic classification. J Endovasc Ther. 2006;13:527–38. 2006/08/25. https://doi.org/10.1583/05-1769.1.

22 Obstructive Malformations of the Internal Jugular Vein

Marian Simka

The internal jugular veins (IJV) constitute the primary outflow route from the head and neck in humans. However, blood flows out from the cranial cavity differently, depending on body posture [1–5]. In the supine body position, a majority of blood flows through the IJVs (Fig. 22.1) while in the sitting or standing humans a substantial part of venous outflow is shifted toward vertebral veins (Fig. 22.2). These different outflow patterns are possible because in the area of the foramen magnum of the skull there are several connections between the bulb of the internal jugular vein (the anatomical structure joining the sigmoid sinus and the internal jugular vein, which is located at the posterolateral aspects of the jugular foramen and collects most of the blood flowing out of the brain) and the vertebral veins. These connections are primarily executed through the suboccipital cavernous sinus, which is a huge venous plexus surrounding the vertebral artery at the level of the first cervical vertebra, just below the foramen magnum [6–8]. Still, even in the upright body position, the IJVs remain an important outflow route from the brain.

Each of the IJV is a direct continuation of the sigmoid sinus, then it passes through the jugular foramen and descends in the carotid sheath of the neck downwards, finally draining into ipsilateral brachiocephalic vein. Although the IJV is a paired vein, it is typically asymmetric. Usually, a wider IJV can be found on the right side. This asymmetry of the IJVs is associated with their embryological development. These veins develop from the precardinal veins found in the embryo. During normal embryological development the precardinal veins connect to the common cardinal veins, while a part of the left common cardinal vein involutes. In addition, the left brachiocephalic vein, which is not present during early phase of venous embryogenesis, develops during its late stage in order to provide venous drainage from the left subclavian and jugular veins to the superior vena cava [9]. This asymmetric involution and development of veins found in the embryo, together with typical asymmetry of the confluence of cerebral sinuses (a majority of humans present with asymmetric *torcular*, which means that most of the cerebral venous outflow is directed toward only one of the transverse sinuses, usually the right one), is probably responsible for the typically dominant right IJV. Still, in some individuals, this is the left IJV that has a larger diameter, while there are some people with similarly sized IJVs [10]. The aforementioned asymmetry of the IJVs in most humans is without clinical relevance; still it should be taken into consideration during cannulation of these veins.

Since an adult pattern of jugular veins emerges relatively late during embryogenesis,

M. Simka (✉)
Department of Anatomy, University of Opole, Opole, Poland

A. K. Khanna, S. K. Tiwary (eds.), *Vascular Malformations*,
https://doi.org/10.1007/978-981-15-9762-6_22

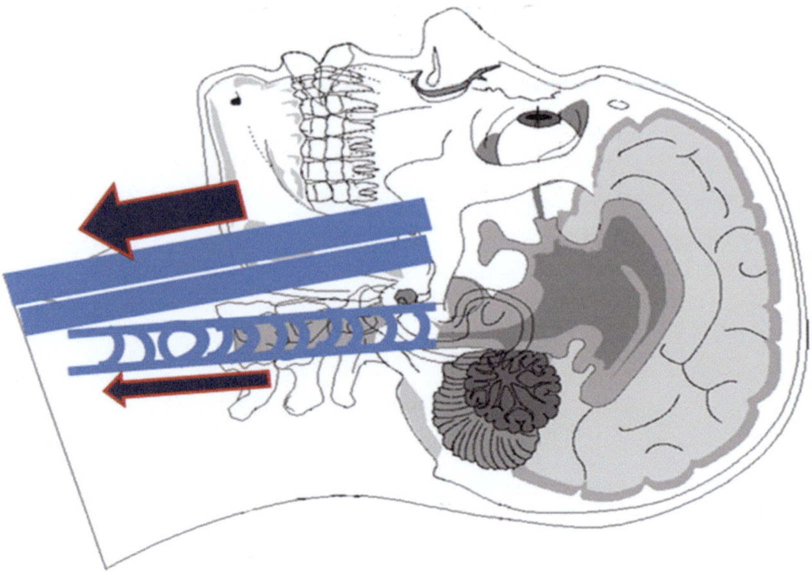

Fig. 22.1 In the supine body position, blood flow out of the brain primarily through the internal jugular veins

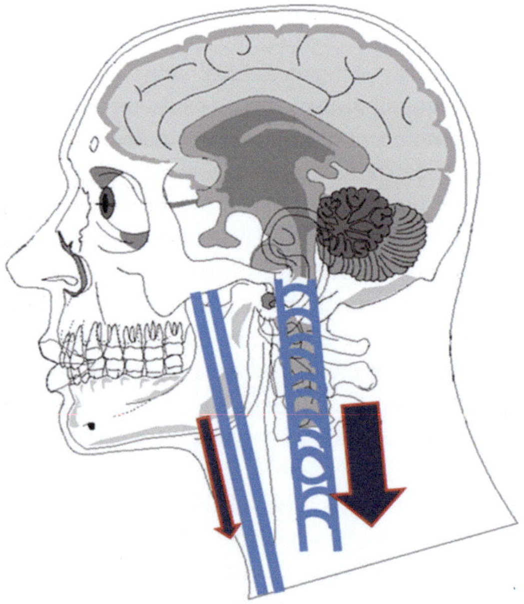

Fig. 22.2 In the upright body position, a majority of cerebral venous outflow is shifted toward vertebral veins and spinal epidural plexus

the so-called extratruncular—according to the Hamburg classification [11]—malformations do not affect these veins. On the contrary, truncular malformations of the IJVs, which result from abnormal development during formation of veins in the fetus, are quite prevalent. Similar to other venous truncular malformations, there can be obstructive, as well as aneurysmatic malformations of the IJV. Aneurysmatic dilatations of the IJV, which are usually found in its proximal and middle portions, represent a well-known clinical problem [12], and therefore will not be thoroughly discussed in this chapter. These lesions are usually diagnosed in children, most cases are asymptomatic and, except for cosmetic indications, do not require medical intervention. It remains unclear if these dilatations are actually associated with an increased risk of thrombosis (unless they are symptomatic, very large, or saccular) and whether a prophylactic surgery, typically comprising partial excision and plasty, is really justified, especially considering the risk associated with such an invasive treatment.

Obstructive malformations of the IJVs represent a relatively new clinical problem that—of as yet—has not been fully understood. Stenotic lesions of the IJV were described for the first time in 2009 by the team led by an Italian vascular surgeon, *Paolo Zamboni*. Using catheter venography they have demonstrated abnormalities of the IJVs in a group of multiple sclerosis patients [13, 14].

Since these vascular lesions compromised venous outflow from the central nervous system, they coined the term "chronic cerebrospinal venous insufficiency" that depicted this anomaly [15]. Chronic cerebrospinal venous insufficiency has been recognized by *the Consensus Document of the International Union of Phlebology on the diagnosis and treatment of venous malformations*, as venous truncular lesions obstructing main outflow routes from the central nervous system [11].

The most frequent abnormality of the IJV found in multiple sclerosis patients is a stenotic "over-competent" jugular valve [16–20]. Further research on this issue has also revealed other stenotic lesions, not related to the valves, for example, external compression by an aberrant omohyoid muscle [21], or hypoplasia of this vein, usually localized just below the jugular foramen (Fig. 22.3).

Nonetheless, these abnormalities are much less prevalent than stenotic valves. Furthermore, abnormal jugular valves, although prevalent in multiple sclerosis patients [22–24], are not unique to this neurological disease [25, 26]. Obstructive abnormalities of jugular valves can also be found in healthy subjects, still less frequently than in patients with cerebral disease. Other neurological pathologies associated with stenotic jugular valves and other obstructive malformations of the IJVs comprise Parkinson disease, lateral amyotrophic sclerosis, and Ménière disease [27, 28].

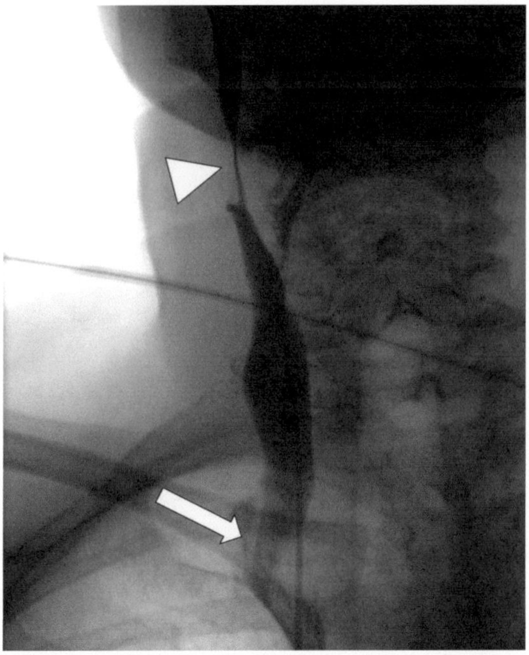

Fig. 22.3 A tandem malformation of the left internal jugular vein: hypoplastic segment of this vein below the jugular foramen (upper arrow) and stenotic jugular valve (lower arrow)

In normal subjects, the IJV is a valveless vein, except for a single valve that is located just above its junction with the brachiocephalic vein. Normal jugular valves are equipped with leaflets that allow blood flow toward the heart and prevent a backward flow. Competent jugular valves play an important role in establishing physiological venous outflow from the brain during increased intrathoracic pressure, which occurs during coughing, sneezing, or defecation [29]. These valves make also impossible a backward flow in such clinical situations as cardiopulmonary resuscitation or blunt chest injury. Normal jugular valves are bicuspid, their leaflets are mobile, and the length of the leaflets is adequate to the diameter of the IJV. Mono- and tricuspid valves have also been described; such valves, as long as they do not impair the flow, should be regarded normal [31–34]. On the contrary, some jugular valves, irrespective of the number of leaflets, significantly compromise the flow (Figs. 22.4 and 22.5). This flow impairment that develops at the proximity of jugular valve, either result from an abnormal macroscopic structure of the venous wall, or from an impaired mobility of leaflets, even if these leaflets macroscopically seem normally structured [34–36]. In some individuals, an increased stiffness of valve leaflets is related to their abnormal biochemical and histological structure [37, 38]. In these cases, an atypical collagen composition in the area of jugular valve, as well as lack of endothelium on malformed valve leaflets has been described.

Classification of abnormal jugular valves has been suggested by *Al-Omari* and *Al-Bashir*. They have categorized [39] abnormal valves into four groups:

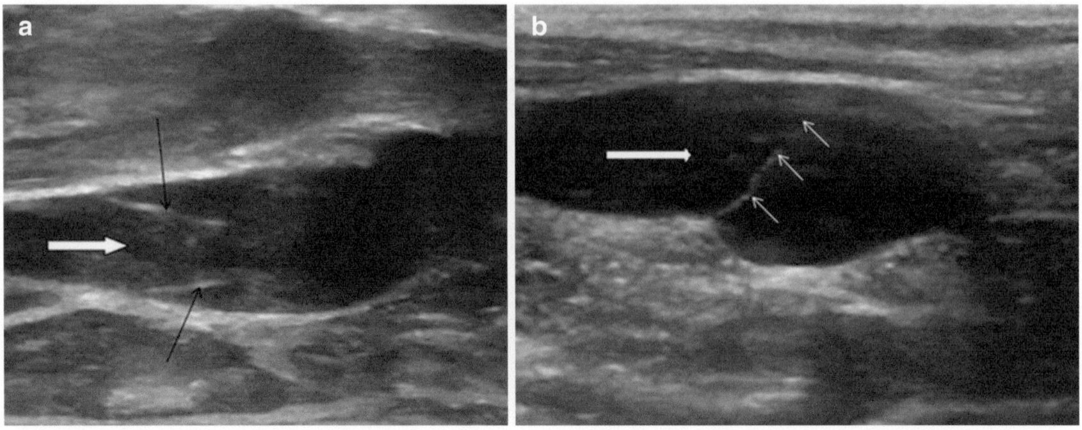

Fig. 22.4 Sonography of the jugular valve: (**a**) normally structured valve and (**b**) membranous malformation of the jugular valve severely disturbing the flow

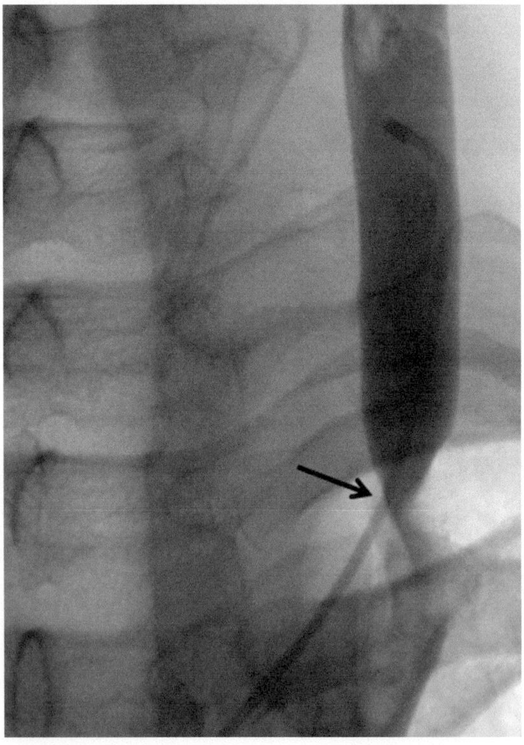

Fig. 22.5 Typical venographic appearance of stenotic jugular valve

- Stenotic jugular valves without severe structural abnormalities.
- Jugular valves with abnormal valve leaflets (accessory, ectopic, or abnormally long leaflets).

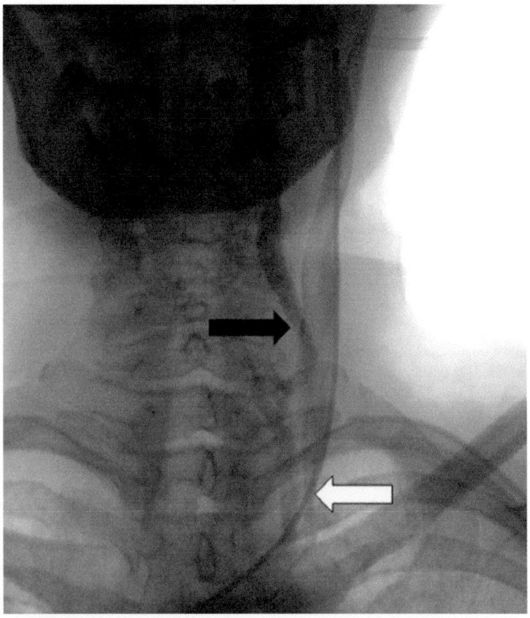

Fig. 22.6 Significant stenosis of the left internal jugular vein caused by malformed jugular valve (white arrow). Huge outflow through collateral network (black arrow), primarily constituted by the anterior jugular vein

- Septum-like or membranous obstructions at the level of jugular valve.
- Severely malformed jugular valves (such as inverted, double, or sigmoid valves).

There is a whole spectrum of the flow abnormalities associated with malformed jugular veins. They can be rather minor or very severe (Fig. 22.6).

Ludyga et al. have categorized venographic findings [34, 40] associated with an impaired venous outflow through the IJVs into four grades:

- *Grade 1:* Venous outflow slowed down, but no reflux detected
- *Grade 2:* Venous outflow slowed down, mild reflux and/or pre-stenotic dilatation of the vein
- *Grade 3:* Venous outflow slowed down, with reflux and outflow through collaterals
- *Grade 4:* No outflow through the vein, huge outflow through collaterals

Similarly to other venous malformations, a malformed IJV may have a different hemodynamic impact on their relevant vascular system, namely the brain, depending upon location of the malformation, its extent and severity, and natural compensation through collaterals. Since physical effects play an important role in regulating venous outflow, and these effects are of paramount importance in the upper part of the human body (above the heart), it seems indispensable to presents some basic physical principles governing the flow in the tubes [41]. Flow in human veins is basically a flow at a low velocity through collapsible tube. In this context, it significantly differs from arterial flow, which—from a physical point of view—is less complex and primarily depends on the pressure gradient. Flow in the veins is significantly affected by two factors that are negligible in the arteries: a collapse of venous wall resulting from negative transmural pressure, and increased viscosity of blood at low-velocity flow.

A majority of veins, from physical point of view, can be considered collapsible tubes [42, 43]. Venous walls, if not supported by adjacent tissues (which is not the case of the IJV) can spontaneously collapse. A degree of such a collapse depends on the value of transmural pressure. Transmural pressure is defined as the difference between the pressure inside and outside the vascular wall.

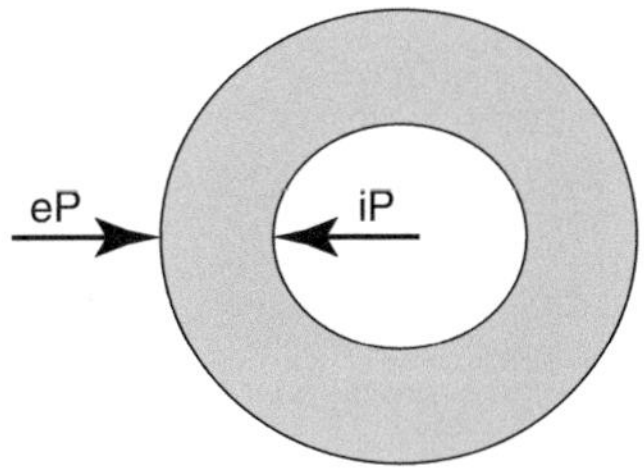

$$\text{tmP} = \text{iP} - \text{eP}$$

where

tmP—transmural pressure
iP—pressure inside the vessel
eP—pressure outside the vessel

At negative transmural pressure, which occurs when a particular vein is higher than the right atrium of the heart, such a vein can collapse. Partial collapse is usually associated with decreased volumetric flow rate, because flow resistance in such a collapsed vein is much higher than in fully opened blood vessel. According to *the Hagen-Poiseuille's Law*, the resistance of the tube is inversely proportional to the fourth power of its radius. Therefore, even a partial collapse results in significant increase in the resistance.

The Hagen-Poiseuille's equation:

$$Q = \frac{\Delta P \cdot \pi \cdot r^4}{8\eta L}$$

where

Q—volumetric flow rate
ΔP—pressure gradient
r—radius of the vessel
η—dynamic viscosity of the fluid
L—length of the vessel

and its transformation presenting the relationship between flow resistance and radius of the vessel:

$$R = \frac{8\eta L}{\pi r^4}$$

where

R—flow resistance
η—dynamic viscosity of the fluid
L—length of the vessel
r—radius of the vessel

Furthermore, flow resistance in the veins is also affected by flow velocity. Blood is a non-Newtonian, shear-thinning fluid, and its viscosity increases at a low flow velocity. At low shear blood viscosity increases by a factor of 4–5. Consequently, according to *the Hagen-Poiseuille's Law*, flow resistance increases by the same factor. In addition, the area of a malformed jugular valve exhibits regions with stagnant flow. In these regions there may develop physical barriers, the so-called *Lagrangian coherent structures* [44] that dynamically divide regions in the fluid flows (Fig. 22.5). Most likely, these regions are associated with a much higher flow resistance than it could be assumed based solely on the degree of the stenosis.

An increased flow resistance in the IJVs results in shifting blood flow from these veins toward alternative pathways: the vertebral veins and the epidural venous plexus of the spinal canal, and also toward deep cervical veins and other veins of the neck (Fig. 22.7). These collateral routes, however, are not likely to sufficiently substitute the jugular pathway. Consequently, an impaired cerebral venous drainage may emerge.

It is well known that multiple sclerosis patients, in comparison with healthy individuals, exhibit a decreased cerebral blood flow. This diminished flow is particularly seen in the periventricular regions of the brain, the area that is routinely affected by multiple sclerosis plaques [45]. MR investigations have demonstrated that decreased cerebral perfusion in multiple sclerosis patients presenting with chronic cerebrospinal venous insufficiency is proportional to the severity of extracranial venous pathology [46–49]. Other studies have revealed that patients with chronic cerebrospinal venous insufficiency also exhibit an abnormal pattern of the flow of the cerebrospinal fluid [50].

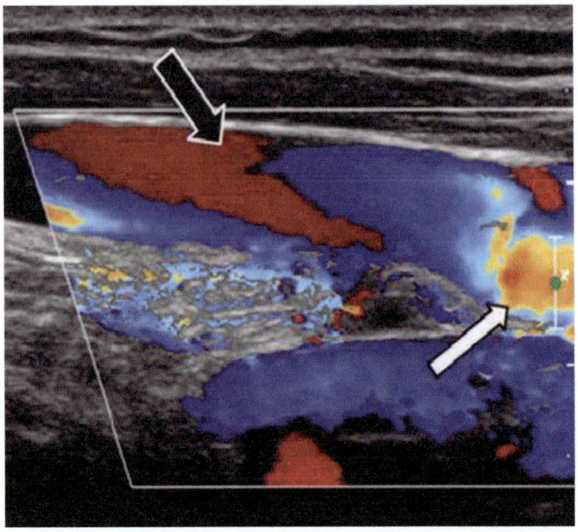

Fig. 22.7 Separated regions in the fluid flows (arrows) in the area of stenotic jugular valve revealed by color Doppler sonography

For the time being an actual clinical relevance of pathological jugular valves and other malformations of the IJVs remains elusive. Although these malformations are very prevalent in multiple sclerosis patients, it is rather unlikely that these lesions are directly evoking this neurological disease. But it is possible that they represent a permissive lesion, which may modify the clinical course of multiple sclerosis. Similarly, regarding Parkinson disease, lateral amyotrophic sclerosis and Ménière disease, a direct causative role of obstructive malformations of the IJVs in these neurological entities remains unclear. Still some authors suggested that obstructive extracranial venous abnormalities may promote neurodegeneration [50–54]. Ten years ago, when a seminal *Zambonis*'s work was published, this hypothetical link between venous abnormality and neurodegeneration was elusive. But some years later, the so-called glymphatic system of the brain has been discovered. The glymphatic system, utilizing the aquaporin-4 water channels, enables the convective flow of the interstitial fluid from the periarterial to the perivenous space. In this way, this system clears the brain from waste products, including also substances that are suspected to play a role in the pathogenesis of neurodegenerative diseases, e.g., β-amyloid [55]. Since the glymphatic system is closely related to small cerebral veins, it is possible that an abnormal venous drainage affects functioning of this system. Therefore, malformed jugular valves and other obstructive malformations of these veins may play a role in the pathogenesis of multiple sclerosis. One of the possible pathomechanisms includes an accumulation of β-synuclein within cerebral parenchyma, a protein that is thought to be responsible for neurodegeneration in multiple sclerosis [56]. This may occur in patients with the impairment of the glymphatic system due to extracranial venous pathology. However, more studies in this field are required to find out whether such a link between glymphatic system, chronic cerebrospinal venous insufficiency, and cerebral disease actually exists [57].

References

1. Andeweg J. Consequences of the anatomy of deep venous outflows from the brain. Neuroradiology. 1999;41:233–41.
2. Cirovic S, Walsh C, Fraser WD, et al. The effect of posture and positive pressure breathing on the hemodynamics of the internal jugular vein. Aviat Space Environ Med. 2003;74:125–31.
3. Doepp F, Schreiber SJ, von Műnster T, et al. How does the blood leave the brain? A systematic ultrasound analysis of cerebral venous drainage patterns. Neuroradiology. 2004;46:565–70.
4. Gisolf J, van Lieshout JJ, van Heusden K, et al. Human cerebral venous outflow pathway depends on posture and central venous pressure. J Physiol. 2004;560:317–27.
5. Schreiber SJ, Lürtzing F, Götze R, et al. Extrajugular pathways of human cerebral venous blood drainage assessed by duplex ultrasound. J Appl Physiol. 2003;94:1802–5.
6. Arnautović KI, Al-Mefty O, Pait TG, et al. The suboccipital cavernous sinus. J Neurosurg. 1997;86:252–62.
7. Caruso RD, Rosenbaum AE, Chang JK, et al. Craniocervical junction venous anatomy on enhanced MR images: the suboccipital cavernous sinus. AJNR Am J Neuroradiol. 1999;20:1127–31.
8. Takahashi S, Sakuma I, Omachi K, et al. Craniocervical junction venous anatomy around the suboccipital cavernous sinus: evaluation by MR imaging. Eur Radiol. 2005;15:1694–700.
9. Lee BB, Laredo J, Neville R. Embryological background of truncular venous malformation in the extracranial venous pathways as the cause of chronic cerebrospinal venous insufficiency. Int Angiol. 2010;29:95–108.
10. Beards SC, Yule S, Kassner A, et al. Anatomical variation of cerebral venous drainage: the theoretical effect on jugular bulb blood samples. Anaesthesia. 1998;53:627–33.
11. Lee BB, Bergan J, Gloviczki P et al. Diagnosis and treatment of venous malformations. Consensus Document of the International Union of Phlebology (IUP)-2009. Int Angiol. 2009;28:434–51.
12. Paleri V, Gopalakrishnan S. Jugular phlebectasia: theory of pathogenesis and review of literature. Int J Pediatr Otorhinolaryngol. 2001;57:155–9.
13. Zamboni P, Consorti G, Galeotti R, et al. Venous collateral circulation of the extracranial cerebrospinal outflow routes. Curr Neurovasc Res. 2009;6:204–12.
14. Zamboni P, Galeotti R, Menegatti E, et al. Chronic cerebrospinal venous insufficiency in patients with multiple sclerosis. J Neurol Neurosurg Psychiatry. 2009;80:392–9.
15. Zamboni P, Galeotti R. The chronic cerebrospinal venous insufficiency syndrome. Phlebology. 2010;25:269–79.
16. Al-Omari MH, Rousan LA. Jugular vein morphology and hemodynamics in patients with multiple sclerosis. Int Angiol. 2010;29:115–20.
17. Bavera PM, Agus GB, Alpini D, et al. Results from 823 consecutive duplex exams for CCSVI in a vascular centre. Acta Phlebol. 2012;13:141–8.
18. Dolic K, Marr K, Valnarov V, et al. Intra- and extraluminal structural and functional venous anomalies in multiple sclerosis as evidenced by 2 noninvasive imaging techniques. AJNR Am J Neuroradiol. 2012;33:16–23.
19. Giaquinta A, Beggs CB, Veroux M, et al. Catheter venous angiography for the evaluation of cerebral venous outflow. Ital J Vasc Endovasc Surg. 2018;25:273–6.
20. Krsmanović Ž, Živković M, Lepić T, et al. Small internal jugular veins with restricted outflow are associated with severe multiple sclerosis: a sonographer-blinded, case-control ultrasound study. BMC Neurol. 2013;13:90.
21. Simka M, Majewski E, Fortuna M, et al. Internal jugular vein entrapment in a multiple sclerosis patient. Case Rep Surg. 2012;2012:293568.
22. Bastianello S, Romani A, Viselner G, et al. Chronic cerebrospinal venous insufficiency in multiple sclerosis: clinical correlates from a multicentre study. BMC Neurol. 2011;11:132.
23. Simka M, Latacz P, Ludyga T, et al. Prevalence of extracranial venous abnormalities: results from a sample of 586 multiple sclerosis patients. Funct Neurol. 2011;26:197–203.
24. Veroux P, Giaquinta A, Perricone D, et al. Internal jugular veins outflow in patients with multiple sclerosis: a catheter venography study. J Vasc Intervent Radiol. 2013;24:1790–7.
25. Dolic K, Weinstock-Guttman B, Marr K, et al. Risk factors for chronic cerebrospinal venous insufficiency

(CCSVI) in a large cohort of volunteers. PLoS One. 2011;6:e28062.
26. Zivadinov R, Marr K, Cutter G, et al. Prevalence, sensitivity, and specificity of chronic cerebrospinal venous insufficiency in MS. Neurology. 2011;77:138–44.
27. Alpini DC, Bavera PM, Hahn A, et al. Chronic cerebrospinal venous insufficiency (CCSVI) in Meniere disease: case or cause? ScienceMED. 2013;4:9–15.
28. Menegatti E, Tessari M, Vannini ME, et al. High resolution m-mode evaluation of jugular vein valves in patients with neurological and neurosensory disorders. Curr Neurovasc Res. 2017;14:316–22.
29. Fisher J, Vaghaiwalla F, Tsitlik J, et al. Determinants and clinical significance of jugular venous valve competence. Circulation. 1982;65:188–96.
30. Harmon JV Jr, Edwards WD. Venous valves in subclavian and internal jugular veins. Frequency, position and structure in 100 autopsy cases. Am J Cardiovasc Pathol. 1987;1:51–4.
31. Lepori D, Capasso P, Fournier D, et al. High-resolution ultrasound evaluation of internal jugular valves. Eur Radiol. 1999;9:1222–6.
32. Lin BS, Kong CW, Tarng DC, et al. Anatomical variation of the internal jugular vein and its impact on temporary haemodialysis vascular access: an ultrasonographic survey in uraemic patients. Nephrol Dial Transplant. 1998;13:134–8.
33. Valecchi D, Bacchi D, Gulisano M, et al. Internal jugular valves: an assessment of prevalence, morphology and competence by color Doppler echography in 240 healthy subjects. Ital J Anat Embryol. 2010;115:185–9.
34. Simka M, Hubbard D, Siddiqui AH, et al. Catheter venography for the assessment of internal jugular veins and azygos vein: position statement by expert panel of the International Society for Neurovascular Disease. Vasa. 2013;42:168–76.
35. Zamboni P, Morovic P, Menegatti E, et al. Screening for chronic cerebrospinal venous insufficiency (CCSVI) using ultrasound - recommendations for a protocol. Int Angiol. 2011;30:571–97.
36. Zivadinov R, Bastianello S, Dake MD, et al. Recommendations for multimodal noninvasive and invasive screening for detection of extracranial venous abnormalities indicative of chronic cerebrospinal venous insufficiency: a position statement of the International Society for Neurovascular Disease. J Vasc Interv Radiol. 2014;25:1785–94.e17.
37. Coen M, Menegatti E, Salvi F, et al. Altered collagen expression in jugular veins in multiple sclerosis. Cardiovasc Pathol. 2013;22:33–8.
38. Zamboni P, Tisato V, Menegatti E, et al. Ultrastructure of internal jugular vein defective valves. Phlebology. 2015;30:644–7.
39. Al-Omari MH, Al-Bashir A. Internal jugular vein valve morphology in the patients with chronic cerebrospinal venous insufficiency (CCSVI); angiographic findings and schematic demonstrations. Rev Recent Clin Trials. 2012;7:83–7.
40. Ludyga T, Kazibudzki M, Simka M, et al. Endovascular treatment for chronic cerebrospinal venous insufficiency: is the procedure safe? Phlebology. 2010;25:286–95.
41. Zaniewski M, Simka M. Biophysics of venous return from the brain from the perspective of the pathophysiology of chronic cerebrospinal venous insufficiency. Rev Recent Clin Trials. 2012;7:88–92.
42. Chow KW, Mak CC. A simple model for the two dimensional blood flow in the collapse of veins. J Math Biol. 2006;52:733–44.
43. Katz AI, Chen Y, Moreno AH. Flow through a collapsible tube. Experimental analysis and mathematical model. Biophys J. 1969;9:1261–79.
44. Shadden SC, Taylor CA. Characterization of coherent structures in the cardiovascular system. Ann Biomed Eng. 2008;36:1152–62.
45. Simka M, Zaniewski M. Reinterpreting the magnetic resonance signs of hemodynamic impairment in the brains of multiple sclerosis patients from the perspective of a recent discovery of outflow block in the extracranial veins. J Neurosci Res. 2010;88:1841–5.
46. Feng W, Utriainen D, Trifan G, et al. Characteristics of flow through the internal jugular veins and cervical C2/C3 and C5/C6 levels for multiple sclerosis patients using MR phase contrast imaging. Neurol Res. 2012;34:802–9.
47. Feng W, Utriainen D, Trifan G, et al. Quantitative flow measurements in the internal jugular veins of multiple sclerosis patients using magnetic resonance imaging. Rev Rec Clin Trials. 2012;7:117–26.
48. Haacke EM, Feng W, Utriainen D, et al. Patients with multiple sclerosis with structural venous abnormalities on MR imaging exhibit an abnormal flow distribution of the internal jugular veins. J Vasc Interv Radiol. 2012;23:60–8.
49. Hartel M, Kluczewska E, Simka M, et al. Magnetic resonance venography of chronic cerebrospinal venous insufficiency in patients with associated multiple sclerosis. Pol J Radiol. 2011;76:59–62.
50. Beggs CB. Venous hemodynamics in neurological disorders: an analytical review with hydrodynamic analysis. BMC Med. 2013;11:142.
51. Chung CP, Beggs C, Wang PN, et al. Jugular venous reflux and white matter abnormalities in Alzheimer's disease: a pilot study. J Alzheimer Dis. 2014;39:601–9.
52. Simka M. What is the relationship between chronic cerebrospinal venous insufficiency and multiple sclerosis? Rev Vasc Med. 2013;1:66–70.
53. Zhou D, Ding JY, Ya JY, et al. Understanding jugular venous outflow disturbance. CNS Neurosci Ther. 2018;24:473–82.

54. Zivadinov R, Chung CP. Potential involvement of the extracranial venous system in central nervous system disorders and aging. BMC Med. 2013;11:260.
55. Plog BA, Nedergaard M. The glymphatic system in the CNS health and disease: past, present and future. Annu Rev Pathol. 2018;13:379–94.
56. Lodygin D, Hermann M, Schweingruber N, et al. β-Synuclein-reactive T cells induce autoimmune CNS grey matter degeneration. Nature. 2019;566:503–8.
57. Simka M, Skuła M. Potential involvement of impaired venous outflow from the brain in neurodegeneration: Lessons learned from the research on chronic cerebrospinal venous insufficiency. Rev Recent Clin Trials. 2019;14(4):235–6.

MIX
Papier aus verantwortungsvollen Quellen
Paper from responsible sources
FSC® C105338

If you have any concerns about our products,
you can contact us on
ProductSafety@springernature.com

In case Publisher is established outside the EU,
the EU authorized representative is:
Springer Nature Customer Service Center GmbH
Europaplatz 3, 69115 Heidelberg, Germany

Printed by Libri Plureos GmbH
in Hamburg, Germany